The Advance of American Nursing

The Advance of

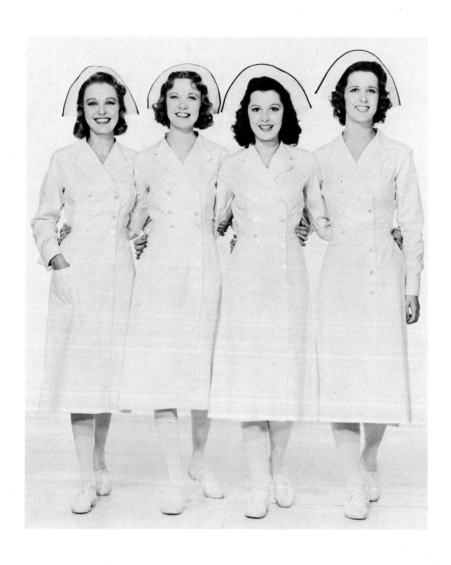

American Nursing

Philip A. Kalisch, Ph.D.

Associate Professor of History and Politics of Nursing,
School of Nursing, University of Michigan, Ann Arbor, and
Adjunct Associate Professor of Nursing,
College of Nursing, Wayne State University, Detroit

Beatrice J. Kalisch, Ed.D.

Shirley C. Titus Professor of Nursing,
Chairperson, Department of Parent-Child Nursing, and
Project Director, Pediatric Nurse Practitioner Program,
School of Nursing, University of Michigan, Ann Arbor

Little, Brown and Company   Boston

Preface

Change characterizes today's nursing in America, and the modern nurse constantly faces decisions involving new technology, new ideas, new values, and new problems. Since on-the-spot solutions to contemporary problems are usually inadequate, nurses need a new orientation, derived from a study of the past, to help them cope successfully with change and develop a keener sensitivity about their roles as health care providers. The history of American nursing includes many clinical, social, cultural, psychological, and educational aspects with critical implications for all modern decision making in the field. Hence, knowledge of past experience can create a better understanding of the present and can cast some light on the pathway to planning the future. We cannot see ahead without looking back.

This textbook was written to provide a modern historic approach to understanding nursing in the United States without assuming the reader's prior knowledge of nursing, medical, or social history. Consequently, it can be used effectively in a wide variety of professional nursing courses in baccalaureate degree, associate degree, and diploma programs. It should also prove helpful to practicing nurses; knowledge of their professional history may increase their effectiveness. When nurses view their work against a multidimensional backdrop, they are better able to define, classify, and confront the problems they face. This book endeavors to present just such a backdrop.

Grateful acknowledgment is made to the American Journal of Nursing Company for permission to reprint material in Chapter 7 that we previously published in *Nursing Research*, and to Alice Clarke for permission to reprint material in Chapter 2 that we previously published in *Nursing Forum*.

We wish to express our appreciation to the following individuals for their helpful insights and support in carrying out the research and writing of this book: Esther Lucille Brown, former Director of Studies, Russell Sage Foundation; Christopher Campbell, Editor, Nursing Department, Little, Brown and Company; M. Elizabeth Carnegie, Editor, *Nursing Research*; Alice Clarke, Editor, *Nursing Forum*; Virginia Cleland, Professor of Nursing, Wayne State University; Carolyne Davis, Associate Vice President for Academic Affairs, University of Michigan; Rheba De Tornyay, Dean, College of Nursing, University of Washington; Katharine Densford Dreves, former Dean, School of

Nursing, University of Minnesota; Edna Fagan, Assistant Administrator for Nursing, Nebraska Methodist Hospital; M. Louise Fitzpatrick, Dean, School of Nursing, Villanova University; Susan Gortner, Chief, Nursing Research and Practice Branches, Division of Nursing, U.S. Public Health Service; Constance Holleran, Director, Government Relations, American Nurses' Association; Virginia Jarrat, Dean, Harris College of Nursing, Texas Christian University; Anne Kibrick, Chairman, Department of Nursing, Boston State College; Madeleine M. Leininger, Dean, College of Nursing, University of Utah; Lucile Petry Leone, former Chief Nurse Officer, U.S. Public Health Service; and Edith Lewis, Editor, *Nursing Outlook.*

We would also like to acknowledge the support of Ingeborg Mauksch, Professor of Nursing, Vanderbilt University; Mary Kelly Mullane, Executive Secretary, American Association of Colleges of Nursing; Helen Nahm, former Dean, School of Nursing, University of California, San Francisco; Marie O'Koren, Dean, School of Nursing, University of Alabama at Birmingham; Gretchen Osgood, Associate Director, Division of Nursing, U.S. Public Health Service; Isabelle Payne, Dean, School of Nursing, Michigan State University; Edith Rathbun, Special Assistant to the Director, Division of Nursing, U.S. Public Health Service; Congressman Paul G. Rogers of Florida, Chairman, Subcommittee on Health, House Interstate and Foreign Commerce Committee; Jessie Scott, Assistant Surgeon General and Director, Division of Nursing, U.S. Public Health Service; Ruth Sleeper, former Director of Nursing, Massachusetts General Hospital; and Margretta Styles, Dean, School of Nursing, University of California, San Francisco. Lastly, the firm support of Dean Mary Lohr, University of Michigan School of Nursing, was invaluable in facilitating our work.

P. A. K.

B. J. K.

Ann Arbor, Michigan

Contents

*To our students
in the hope that their generation
will be better equipped than ours
to realize nursing's full potential*

1
From Hippocrates to Florence Nightingale: The Birth of Modern Nursing

*N*ursing is as old as mankind, although the origins of the profession as we know it today go back less than a century and a half. The word *nurse* is a reduced form of the Middle English *nurice*, which was derived, through the Old French *norrice*, from the Latin *nutricius* (nourishing). In Roman mythology, the goddess Fortuna, in addition to her usual function as goddess of fate, was also worshipped as Jupiter's nurse (Fortuna Praeneste) and prayed to for hygiene in the public baths (Fortuna Balnearis). From the dawn of civilization mankind has sought to acquire a knowledge of pain-relieving remedies and to discover additional means of preventing disease. To alleviate human suffering, man has also developed nursing roles.

Dawn of Civilization
Primitive peoples looked upon natural phenomena as the work of the gods. The sun was carried across the heavens in the chariot of Apollo. Wind was the breath of a god. Storms and earthquakes were the works of angry gods or demons. Sicknesses with intense suffering were thought to be caused by some evil spirit in possession of the sufferer. In an effort to scare away this evil spirit, friends of the sufferer, wearing hideous masks and making terrifying noises, danced about him. Evil spirits might be kept away by wearing an amulet, by setting up horrible images about the camp, or by making offerings and sacrifices. Usually, among primitive peoples, there were medicine men who were believed to possess the "magic" necessary to drive away the evil spirits or to appease the offended demons. These medicine men were held in reverence, for they were thought to be able to intercede with the gods on behalf of those afflicted with illness.

It is not surprising, therefore, that in the earliest civilizations the priests served as physicians. This was true in Babylon, Egypt, Israel, and Greece. Among the ancient Greeks, Apollo was the god of health. When angered, he visited plagues and epidemics on mankind, and his favor insured health.

Apollo's son Aesculapius was a skillful healer—so skillful, according to legend, that he was killed by Zeus out of fear that men would cease to die. Later he was worshiped as god of medicine, and temples were erected in his honor beside health-giving mineral springs, on wooded mountains where the invigorating air

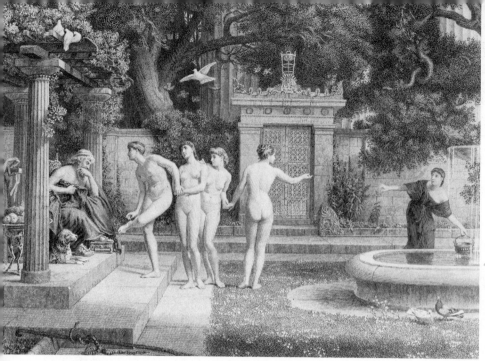

A Visit to Aesculapius.

Hippocrates of Cos.

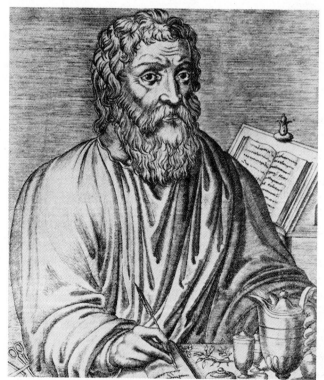

restored the sick, and in other healthful locations. These temples became sanitariums where the priests of Aesculapius acquired skill in treating disease. Hygeia and Panacea, daughters of Aesculapius, were among the earliest of these temple attendants. The sanitariums were known as Asclepieia. A famous one was located at Cos.

A typical incident from ancient mythology was quaintly and succinctly related by the Elizabethan poet Thomas Watson:

In time long past, when in Diana's chase,
  A bramble bush prickt Venus in the foot,
Olde Aesculapius healpt her heavie case,
  Before the hurte had taken any roote [1].

Centuries later, a Victorian English painter, Thomas Poynter, vividly depicted this scene in a large painting. In that work, Aesculapius sits on the honeysuckle-covered porch of his house, which faces a garden in which a fountain plays softly and soothingly. The gate in the garden wall leads to his temple, seen partly through a grove of large ilex trees. Venus, attended by the Three Graces, leans upon one of them for support as she shows Aesculapius her wounded foot. Behind Aesculapius stands Hygeia, holding a small box of medicines. One of the Graces holds out her hand, hastening an attendant who fetches water from the fountain. Doves and sparrows, sacred to Venus, flit about; a serpent, the physician's special attendant, twines round Aesculapius's staff.

Four thousand years ago Egyptian physicians and nurses possessed an abundant pharmacopoeia with which to cure the ill. The Ebers Papyrus lists more than 700 remedies for ailments from snakebite to puerperal fever. The Kahun Papyrus (circa 1850 B.C.) prescribed suppositories apparently used for contraception. The tomb of an Eleventh Dynasty queen yielded a medicine chest containing vases, spoons, dried drug compounds, and medicinal roots. Because the composition of prescriptions reflected a curious mixture of medicine and magic, the most repulsive concoctions were thought to provide the most efficacious remedies. Lizard's blood, swine's ears and teeth, putrid meat and fat, tortoise brains, old books boiled in oil, milk of a lying-in woman, water of a chaste woman, lice, and excreta of men, donkeys, dogs, lions, and cats are examples of some of the ingredients that were used.

Greek and Roman Era (460 B.C.–A.D. 476)

In ancient Greece nearly 2000 years thereafter, Hippocrates of Cos (460–370 B.C.), "the father of medicine," emphasized the rational treatment of sickness as a natural rather than god-inflicted phenomenon. Hippocrates systematically arranged the oral and written teachings on remedies and diseases, which had once been the secrets of priests, into a textbook of medicine that was used for centuries thereafter. He recognized the fundamental truth that making accurate observations of and drawing general conclusions from actual phenomena form the basis of sound medical reasoning.

The notion most persistent and most damaging to the practice and theory of medicine was the doctrine of the four humors, first elaborated by Empedocles of Acragas (493–433 B.C.). Because Empedocles was a philosopher as well as a physician, he readily incorporated his cosmologic ideas into his medical theory. He believed that the same four elements, or "roots of things," of which the universe was supposedly made had to be found in man and in all animate beings. Empedocles, following ancient, mythical teachings, considered man to be a microcosm, a small world within the macrocosm, or great world. The four humors of the body—blood, bile, phlegm, and black bile—corresponded to the four elements of the world—fire, air, water, and earth. Depending on the predominating humor, a person was either sanguine, choleric, phlegmatic, or melancholic.

This doctrine gave rise to a fallacious though seemingly rational system of medicine that was for centuries to supersede the practical art of medicine of the Hippocratic school. Treatment was aimed at restoring the appropriate balance of humors, through the control of their corresponding elements, by the manipulation of two sets of opposite qualities: hot and cold, wet and dry. Fire was hot and dry, air was hot and wet, water was cold and wet, and earth was cold and dry. If a man had a fever he needed more cold; if he had a chill he needed more heat. Because these theories bore practically no relation to actual physiology, medical practice based on them was rarely, if ever, effective.

Another outstanding figure in the development of Greek science was Aristotle (384–322 B.C.), who demonstrated that the hearts of animals were the source of the blood vessels. Because religious bans forbade the touching of the dead human body, however, this new knowledge was not utilized. Theophrastus of Lesbos (372–288 B.C.), a pupil of Aristotle, rather than delving into the human body, followed the example of his master in the study of natural history by arranging and systematizing plants. Ignorance, rooted in the doctrines of Empedocles, continued for several centuries until it was attacked by Galen of Pergamum (A.D. 129–199).

Aristotle had distinguished the arteries from the veins, but he had considered the arteries to be air vessels. Galen refuted this theory by demonstrating that the arteries, when opened, always gushed blood. He profited from this knowledge by tying the arteries for the purpose of stopping hemorrhage. He also displayed insight through his accurate assessment of the human skeleton and the organs of motion, and he identified the muscular filaments, blood vessels, and nerves. Through experiments on animals he detected the spinal marrow, the nerves of the brain, and the nerves of sensation and motion. Galen enumerated and classified the nerves into pairs and groups and even discovered several of the ganglia. He recognized the natural division of the human body into cavities and was familiar with the locality and appearances of the chief organs. Indeed, his knowledge of particular body structures was generally so correct that it formed the basis for most subsequent anatomic classification.

There was little advance in nursing or medicine during the rise and fall of the Roman Empire. Nursing practice remained in the hands of well-meaning relatives and friends, for the most part, although with the spread of Christianity there was an increased association of nursing with religion. Roman physicians such as Celsus (53 B.C.–A.D. 7) relied heavily on Greek medicine. After A.D. 300, the advance of medical knowledge was abruptly halted by the gradual collapse of the Empire. Some three centuries later, medical knowledge had practically disappeared in the western world. Although copies of the works of Hippocrates and Galen were extant, few could read and understand them. Thus, the embryo of medical and nursing theory died in western Europe, a victim of invading barbarian hordes.

Byzantine and Islamic Influences (476–1096)

In the Eastern Roman or Byzantine Empire, the knowledge of medicine and nursing did not sink so low as it did in the West. Constantinople survived successive attacks by the Turks and preserved its libraries, and its Greek-speaking inhabitants had a high regard for learning, which they zealously pursued when conditions permitted. Elsewhere, the Arabs, an able people whose ancestors had lived at the edge of all the great Mediterranean civilizations, fostered a respect for erudition. Once firmly in control of a vast empire, the Moslems supported learning. The great caliphs had camel caravans laden with Greek and Latin books brought to Baghdad, where they engaged Nestorians, Jews, and Persians to translate these works into Arabic. Among these translators were brilliant scholars such as Janus Damascenus (circa 850), Avicenna (980–1037), Moses Maimonides (1135–1204), Avenzoar (circa 1150), and Averroes (1131–1216). This knowledge was disseminated through the new schools that arose in Baghdad, Cairo, and ultimately in Cordova, in Spain.

In western Europe, scientific medicine survived the Dark Ages chiefly through the efforts of Jewish physicians who translated Greek and Arabic medical treatises into Latin and who circulated Greco-Arabic medical knowledge throughout Christendom. About 1060, Constantinus Africanus (1030–1087) brought a cargo of Islamic medical treatises to Salerno and, with the aid of his translations of Greek and Arabic medical works, spurred the revival of medicine in Italy. Ideally situated to take advantage of such external influences, the famous school of Salerno remained the leading medical institution in western Europe until the twelfth century. There women studied nursing and obstetrics; *Mulieres Salernitanae* were probably midwives trained at the school. One of the most famous Salernitan products is an early-twelfth-century obstetrical treatise by a midwife named Trotula, entitled *Trotulae curandarum aegritudinum muliebrum* (*Trotula on the Cure of Diseases of Women*).

Fighting Male Nurses of the Crusades

During the eleventh century the attention of western Europe turned to the Holy Land. About 1050, European merchants secured permission from the Moslem ruler of Egypt to build a hospital in Jerusalem for receiving and sheltering Christian pilgrims who had fallen ill during visits to the Holy Land. This hospital was dedicated to St. John, and the nursing duties were performed by Benedictine monks under the leadership of a man called Gerard. After the capture of Jerusalem

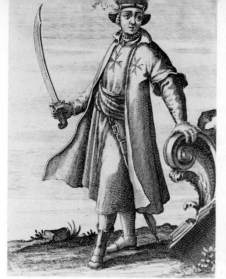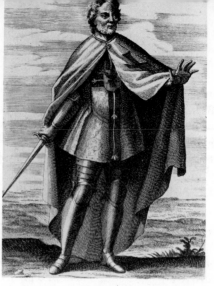

Religious and military nursing orders fought in the Holy Land during the twelfth century.

by the Crusaders in 1099, a number of wealthy nobles, having witnessed the excellent nursing care given to wounded Christians, endowed the hospital with land both in Europe and in the Holy Land.

When some of the crusaders observed the outstanding patient care provided by the Hospital of St. John, they decided to join its nursing force. As the battle for the Holy Land raged back and forth in later years, the hospital workers organized into a separate military-nursing order: The Knights Hospitalers of St. John of Jerusalem. Gerard became Grand Master of the Order, drew up a code of rules, and introduced as a uniform for the brethren the well-known black robe with a white maltese cross which later became a familiar sight on the battlefields of the Holy Land. Organized into a hierarchy of knights, priests, and serving brothers, the Knights took oaths of poverty, humility, and chastity and followed a democratic constitution under which the major decisions were determined by vote.

The Hospitalers soon became famous and highly esteemed, providing thousands of pilgrims and crusaders in the Holy City with hospitality and care. Each year they increased their possessions, wealth, and network of hospitals and commanderies, and they attracted large numbers of recruits. In time, besides performing works of nursing and charity, the Hospitalers, many of whom were monks and priests, undertook to defend the Holy Land by becoming soldiers as well. Gradually the Order developed into a full-fledged fighting force, although its paramount activity continued to be that of caring for the pilgrims, the sick, and the poor.

The next religious military order founded was that of the Knights Templars, in 1118, followed in 1190 by the third and most famous, the Knights of the Teutonic Order. After they had been summoned to help fight the pagan Prussians in 1225, the Teutonic Knights concentrated more and more upon military pursuits. The Knights Hospitalers, on the other hand, never lost sight of their nursing duties. A less important and ill-fated order was founded especially for knights who had contracted the dreaded disease of leprosy endemic in the Near East: the Knights Hospitalers of St. Lazarus, whose Grand Master was always a leper.

For nearly two centuries, from 1096 to 1291, successive waves of Europeans swept down upon the Levant, first in order to retake the Holy Land from the Moslems and later to protect it from reconquest. They came in the tens of thousands: pilgrims, mercenaries, children, small companies of men-at-arms following their feudal lords, and even whole armies. As an instrument of papal foreign policy, the Crusades were designed to secure the Holy Land and to protect the pilgrim routes. They were also useful in channeling the aggressive energy of warring and often lawless nobles into a constructive war outside the confines of Europe.

Throughout the Crusades the Templars and the Hospitalers played the dominant role in military and religious activites. They were the finest fighting force in the Holy Land. In battle after battle they were deployed in positions of honor: Templars on the right, Hospitalers on the left. Large numbers of women were allowed to form a separate chapter of the Hospitalers, and they soon helped found scores of additional hospitals under the auspices of the Hospitaler Dames of the Order of St. John of Jerusalem.

The thirteenth century in the Holy Land was characterized by the ever-growing wealth and pretentions of the Templars and Hospitalers, their ferocious rivalry, and a series of military disasters for the Knights. Gradually, control of the conquered territories slipped from their hands. While important hospitals, almshouses, preceptories, and commanderies were built and soon flourishing in

Hospitaler Dame of the Order of St. John of Jerusalem.

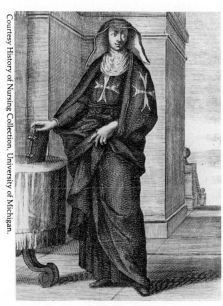

France, Germany, Spain, and England, and while the Knights in high offices of the great Orders appeared at the courts of leading princes and churchmen, the unity of Christendom overseas, already riddled by internal dissension, began to crumble under Islamic counteroffensives. The Hospitalers remained in the Mediterranean as Christendom's front-line defense against the Moslem threat; the Knights of the Teutonic Order withdrew to found a state of their own in northern Europe; knights of other religious military orders continued to fight the Moslems outside the Holy Land.

After the Hospitalers had been expelled from the Holy Land by the Turks, they annexed the island of Rhodes in 1309. When Rhodes fell to the Turks in 1530, the Hospitalers obtained Malta from the Holy Roman Emperor. One of the best descriptions of the nursing activities of the Knights in the Malta Hospital is recorded in the diary of British naval chaplain Henry Teonge, who visited Malta aboard H.M.S. *Assistance* in 1674: "The Hospital is a vast structure, wherein the sick and wounded lye. This so broade that twelve men may with ease walke abreast up the midst of it; and the bedds are on each syde, standing on four yron pillars with white curtens and vallands, and covering, extremely neate, and kept cleane and sweete . . ." Almost everyone who visited the Hospital commented on its cleanliness and that the Knights themselves attended the patients. Throughout these centuries, the Knights Hospitalers were known primarily for their incessant warfare against the Moslems. Nevertheless, these Knights continued to perform their original and foremost function: nursing.

Medieval Medicine and Nursing (1096–1438)

Early in the fourteenth century, the medical school of Salerno was surpassed by that of Bologna, due to the latter's revival of human dissection. In 1315 Mondino de Luzzi (1270–1326), a professor at Bologna, wrote an illustrated account of dissections he had performed on the bodies of two women. This work became the bible of anatomy students for the next 250 years. To de Luzzi belongs the credit for having been the first to add pictorial illustrations to anatomic descriptions. His dissection, however, was scarcely less crude than that practiced by the ancients. "Beneath the veins of the forearm," he remarked, "we see many muscles and many large and strong cords to which it is not necessary to attend in the anatomy of such a corpse."

The corpse was used only as a teaching aid and not as a source of anatomic knowledge. Anatomic dissections were established as a regular part of the curriculum in most medical schools, however, and a standard procedure was developed. The cadaver was laid on a table, around which the students clustered. The actual dissection was performed by a demonstrator (often a surgeon) while the professor on his high lecture platform read from Galen. Students abruptly disregarded any anatomic evidence that conflicted with Galen's statements, despite the mental gymnastics necessary in making the facts of anatomy conform with that revered authority. Certain corpses were thus considered "defective" when they failed to uphold Galen's speculations. De Luzzi insisted that the best

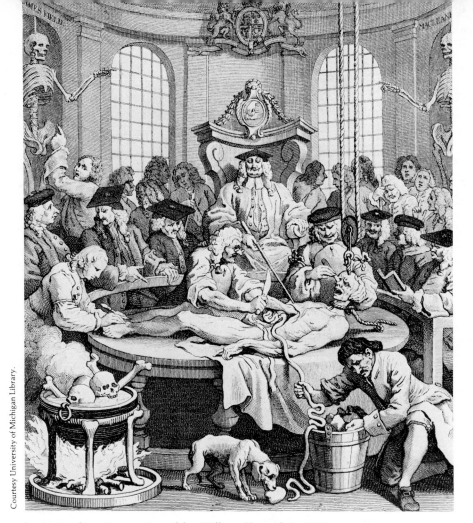

Anatomic dissection portrayed by William Hogarth in 1751.

corpse for the purposes of dissection was one that had been dried in the sun for three years.

It was the religious orders that revived the embryo of nursing during the Middle Ages. St. Benedict's Rule decreed that every monastery have a hospital, and although care for the ailing was at first directed mainly toward members of the Order, workers on church-owned estates were eventually included. The masses, however, still had to depend on their womenfolk for treatment and care during illness.

The increase in the tempo of hospital founding during the twelfth and thirteenth centuries can be attributed to monastic and papal reform movements then taking place and to an accompanying upsurge of intense religious feeling. The oldest actual hospital in Europe seems to have been the *Hôtel Dieu* in Lyons, founded about 542 by Childbert I, King of France. The famous *Hôtel Dieu* in Paris was founded about 652 by St. Landry, Bishop of Paris. The oldest hospital in Italy

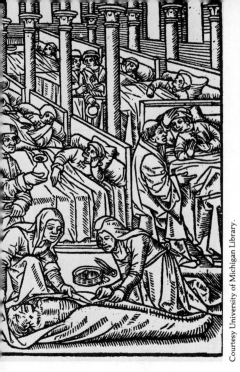

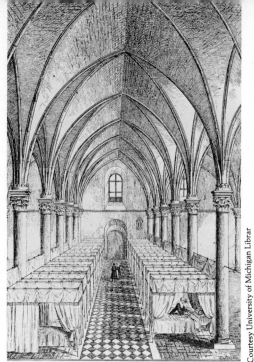

Medieval hospital interior.

Interior of Hôtel Dieu *in Angers.*

is believed to be Santa Maria della Scala in Sienna, established in 890. During the Middle Ages, charitable institutions, hospitals, and medical schools multiplied, and Popes, princes, and priests exemplified their devotion to the religious sentiment of the age by personally nursing the sick and the wounded.

Hôtels Dieu for the sick and aged were developed as a result of the institution of religious nursing orders. These orders commonly followed the Rule of St. Augustine; as the most lenient of the monastic rules, it was peculiarly suited to men and women who had a hard nursing task to perform in addition to their prescribed religious ritual. In France, *chanoinesses hospitalières* were assigned to serve the *Hôtel Dieu* in Abbeville (1158), in Beauvais (1158), for the *Hôtel Dieu* Saint Gervais (1177), and for the *Hôtel Dieu* Saint Oppostune in Paris (1188). The Ordre Hôspitalier du Saint-Esprit was founded in Montpellier about 1195 to tend for the sick, the poor, foundlings, pilgrims, and strangers; by 1198 it had established six or seven daughter houses. Funds were solicited by traveling brethren who displayed relics to the faithful in churches.

Other orders were created to provide hospital service to those suffering from certain diseases: the Lazarites looked after lepers, and the Antonites cared for those afflicted with skin diseases. In France alone, by the end of the reign of St. Louis (1226–1270), there were an estimated 800 Lazarite houses in which lepers could be segregated and tended to. By the middle of the fourteenth century there were 59 houses in the diocese of Paris alone. They comprised small, separate dwellings for the lepers and a modest house for the nurses who looked after them.

Like the infirmaries of monasteries, the monastic *Hôtels Dieu* were built on a churchlike plan of nave and transept with an altar at the head of the building. The great hospital hall at Angers, nearly 200 feet long and more than 70 feet wide, was remarkable for its tall columns and high-pitched vaults, for its 16 windows, and for its light and elegant proportions. The men patients occupied the right aisle, the women patients occupied the left, and the middle aisle was kept empty. The tombs of the founders were located near the door, where there was a great statue of the bound Christ. A cloister opened off the great hall and led to a small frescoed chapel. Nearby were the large barns for the hospital and quarters for the staff. Some 40 nursing sisters provided nursing care here, with 25 men to help them and two canons to serve the chapel.

By the mid-fifteenth century a new type of hospital began to develop in Italy. Its first example was Santa Maria Nuova in Florence, founded in 1286 by Folco Portinari. In 1334 a new men's department was built, in which the four wards radiated in the cruciform manner from a central altar—the east-west wards were much shorter than the north-south wards. Later, an east-west ward for women was added. The men were looked after by lay brothers, and the women were attended by lay sisters.

Hospital Work in the Fifteenth Century

In the fifteenth century, Florence had 35 hospitals, each generously supported by public and private donations. Some hospitals were notable examples of architecture, and some of their halls were adorned with inspiring works of art. Martin Luther later described several of these hospitals:

Ward scene Hôtel Dieu *in Paris.*

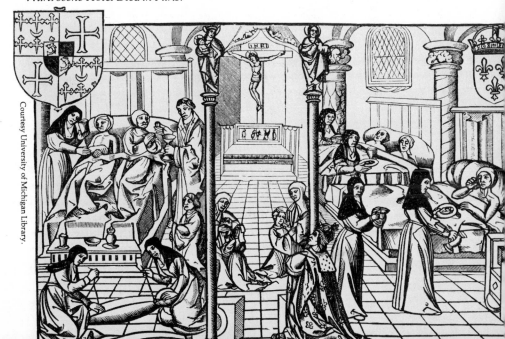

In Italy the hospitals are handsomely built, and admirably provided with excellent food and drink, careful attendants, and learned physicians. The beds and bedding are clean, and the walls are covered with paintings. When a patient is brought in, his clothes are removed in the presence of a notary who makes a faithful inventory of them, and they are kept safely. A white smock is put on him, and he is laid on a comfortable bed, with clean linen. Presently two doctors come to him and servants bring him food and drink in clean vessels . . . . Many ladies take turns to visit the hospitals and tend the sick, keeping their faces veiled, so that no one knows who they are; each remains a few days and then returns home, another taking her place . . . . Equally excellent are the foundling asylums of Florence, where the children are well fed and taught, suitably clothed in a uniform, and altogether admirably cared for [2].

Early European hospitals were more like hospices or homes for the aged. The sick were part of a group of helpless individuals including paupers, pilgrims, travelers, orphans, and the aged, for whom Christian charity provided food and shelter. Usually the sick were received for the purpose of ministering to their physical and spiritual needs until they were well enough to return to work. Nursing was handled by various religious orders.

In a typical hospital of the 1400s, the daily work of the nurses began at 5:00 A.M., when, after rising and washing, they went downstairs to church service. Then the sister nurses went about their work in areas such as the laundry, the wards, and the hall for admittance. When the patients were awake, each sister would make the rounds with a basin in one hand and a towel in the other. Later, while beds were being made, the healthier patients were allowed to get up while the more seriously ill were moved to vacant beds. Each bed, a straw-filled mattress suspended on cords stretched from four corner posts, held at least two and in many cases three patients. The patient lay with his head encircled by a piece of rolled linen. The bed was covered by a counterpane of heavy gray cloth draped over both sides.

Sister nurses were forbidden to witness childbirths, to help with gynecologic examinations, or even to diaper boy babies. Close contact with male patients, such as administering enemas, was also prohibited, as was the care of patients suffering from venereal diseases. Servants were employed to carry out these tasks. Most medicines were derived from herbs, although these were often combined with offensive substances such as urine, animal excreta, powdered earthworms, and the like.

Plague and Pestilence

During the Middle Ages a series of horrible epidemics, including St. Anthony's Fire (erysipelas), leprosy, typhus, and bubonic plague, ravaged the civilized world. The Black Death was one of the names given to the bubonic plague, which devastated Europe, Asia, and Africa in the fourteenth century. It was characterized by acute inflammation of the lungs, burning sensations, unquenchable thirst, and inflammations of various parts of the body. The Black Death derived its name from the black spots symptomatic of the circulatory arrest and putrefactive decomposition evident in one of its stages upon the skin and in the inflamed parts.

The first plague epidemic, which flared up in A.D. 540 during the reign of the Byzantine emperor Justinian, was called the Plague of Justinian. This outbreak lasted 60 years and was a catastrophe equivalent to any nuclear holocaust. The English historian Edward Gibbon states in *The History of the Decline and Fall of the Roman Empire* that the estimated death toll of 100 million is a figure "not wholly inadmissible." The plague leaped, writes a contemporary chronicler, "to the ends of the hospitable world" beginning at the seaports and spreading inland.

The most fatal and widespread plague epidemic, believed to have originated in China about 1340 to 1345, spread to nearly all parts of the known world. Advancing westward, it invaded Persia, Arabia, North Africa, and Palestine; carried over caravan routes, it proceeded along the coasts of the Mediterranean and Black Seas, arrived in Constantinople about 1347, and by means of sailing vessels eventually reached the seaports of Italy. From so many foci of contagion it soon established itself in Europe by sweeping in one great wave over Italy, Austria, Germany, France, and finally England in 1348.

In China, 13 million people were said to have perished from the plague, while in the rest of Asia it claimed nearly 24 million lives. A moderate estimate places the number who perished in Europe at 25 million, contributing to an overall total of more than 60 million deaths. In many parts of Europe, only one-fourth of the population survived, and in some places there were not enough left to bury the dead. Hardly anyone afflicted by the plague survived the third day of the attack. The black spots and tumors sealed a doom that even the best of physicians and nurses were powerless to avert. So great was the fear of contagion that parents even deserted their plague-stricken children; family ties were dissolved and the sick were left to die alone. Ships overtaken by the epidemic, their decks strewn with dead, putrefying bodies, drifted unmanned through the North, Black, and Mediterranean seas.

Professors at the University of Paris attributed the outbreak of the plague to the astrologic conjunction of Saturn, Jupiter, and Mars in the house of Aquarius on March 20, 1345, at 1:00 P.M. The conjunction of Saturn and Jupiter dictated death and disaster; that of Mars and Jupiter brought forth pestilence. The cataclysmic epidemic was thus believed to have been duly ordained by the heavens, and mankind was helpless against it.

Mostly, the atmosphere was blamed for the spread of disease, especially between seasons, when it was warm and moist and when sudden, radical changes in temperature were most common. Once contagion broke out, nothing could stop it. Epidemics that started at the end of winter usually lasted until the heat of summer, at which point they gave way to other diseases, such as malaria. Plague and puerperal fever dispatched victims quickly, especially in the towns, with their narrow streets and closely packed houses. There, epidemics took the greatest toll.

14

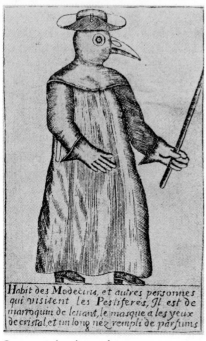

Habit des Medecins, et autres personnes
qui visitent les Pestiferes, Jl est de
marroquin de levant, le masque a les yeux
de cristal, et un long nez rempli de parfums

Costume of a plague doctor.

Courtesy National Library of Medicine.

Changing Concepts of Disease and Medicine

Traditionally, illness was regarded as a foreign element that lodged in the bodies of the sick and had to be expelled—a concept partly based on the belief in magic. It was considered effective treatment to exorcise an affliction in cases of unjustified bodily invasion of the pious. Diseases were ascribed not to external agents invading the body but rather to internal imbalances of the four humors. Thus, diseases did not exist as separate entities: there were only diseased states of the body. Few medicines were derived from mineral sources, for the ancient Greek philosophers and the medieval scholars were not greatly interested in chemical substances or properties, even though some chemical problems had been studied by alchemists during late antiquity and in the Middle Ages. A few of these alchemists became interested in the application of alchemy to medicine. This interest culminated in the work of Paracelsus (1493–1540), a Swiss physician who attempted to develop a new medical science by combining medicine with alchemy. Throughout the ages alchemy had involved the practice of chemical crafts and mysticism.

Paracelsus rejected the belief that physical health was determined by the four constitutional humors. He devised the theory that the human body was essentially a chemical system composed of the two principal elements, mercury and sulphur, plus a third—salt—his own addition. Salt had been recognized earlier as a fundamental substance, but it was not generally regarded as a basic chem-

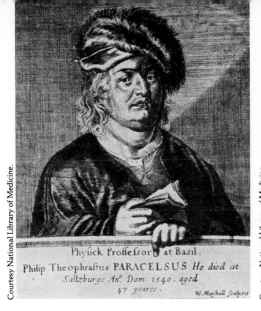

Phyſick Proffeſſorʃ at Basil.
Philip Theophraſtus PARACELSUS *He died at
Saltzburge An. Dom: 1540. aged
47 yeares.* W.Marſhall ſculpſit

Paracelsus (1493–1540).

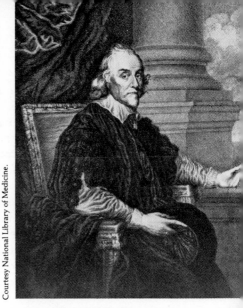

William Harvey (1578–1657).

ical until the time of Paracelsus. In his opinion, disease was caused by an imbalance of the principal elements, just as the physician-followers of Empedocles believed that diseases arose from a lack of harmony among the humors. According to Paracelsus' theory, however, the balance could be restored not by organic remedies but by mineral medicines. The followers of Paracelsus were distinguished from the Galenic school by their use of chemical compounds in medical practice. No doubt they killed many patients, but in so doing they learned through experimentation. Largely by accident, they soon discovered a number of useful drugs that added to their chemical knowledge.

The Renaissance (1438–1600)

The revival of learning during the Renaissance spurred the advance of medicine. Ambroise Paré (1510–1590), a barber surgeon of Paris, began his successful career as surgeon to Marshal de Monte in 1536. Freed from the confines of ancient dogma that had for centuries enveloped medicine in superstitious blindness, Paré determined to observe things for himself and to accept only the evidence derived from personal experience. In his opinion, medical practice based on accurate observation would surpass the fallacious doctrines of the ancients. Paré revived Galen's method, long in disuse, of tying the blood vessels for the purpose of stopping hemorrhage. He was probably the first to employ ligatures instead of cauterization after amputations. Hitherto, gunshot wounds, which had been considered poisonous, had been treated by the application of boiling oil, hot pitch, or red-hot iron. After observing that wounds not treated in such a severe fashion were more likely to heal, Paré rejected these drastic methods.

In 1543 a Flemish doctor, Andreas Vesalius (1514–1564), published an elaborate treatise on surgery and anatomy. Since this work, based on his experience in numerous dissections, dared to refute Galen, it was violently attacked and

Vesalius' findings were hotly disputed. Not until six decades later, in the time of the English physician William Harvey (1578–1657), who discovered the process by which the heart keeps the blood circulating throughout the body, was the scientific spirit of Vesalius reaffirmed. The methodology of Harvey's researches was based on the new, analytical principle of induction, a process in which data were carefully collected and considered.

Before Harvey, it had been the practice of centuries to place at the head of all medical treatises certain axioms, improperly called "principles," which were to be taken as medical canon. By the beginning of the seventeenth century, however, scientific discoveries had finally refuted the fallacies of the ancients. By using the inductive process, Francis Bacon (1561–1626) soon devised what would come to be known as the scientific method.

Seventeenth- and Eighteenth-Century Hospitals

Throughout Europe the average life span was still wretchedly short. People married at very early ages, and widows of 15 and younger were found in every town. The high mortality rate accounted for the prestige of the "graybeards" to whom places of honor were accorded for having passed the age of 40 in a society where

Paris Foundling Hospital.

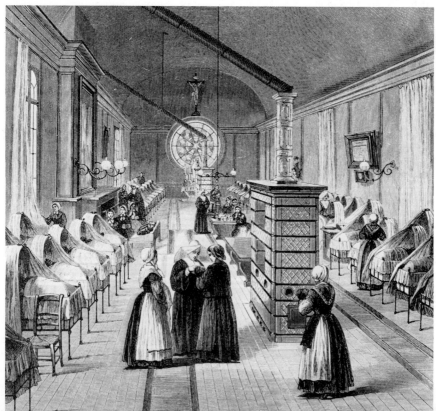

it was common to die young. The birth rate was high, but not high enough to compensate for the brevity of life—about 20 years.

The slums of the growing cities contributed to a rate of infant mortality sometimes as high as 50 percent. In London, 58 percent of all children died before their fifth birthday and abandonment of infants was common. Between 1771 and 1777, nearly 32,000 infants were admitted to the Paris Foundling Hospital at the rate of 89 per day; 80 percent died before the age of one. The spread of dry nursing—replacement of the breast by the bottle—contributed greatly to infant mortality in the eighteenth century. Sir Hans Sloane estimated the death rate of bottlefed infants to be three times that of breastfed infants. Unsterilized dry feeding became especially popular among the French upper class until the publication of Rousseau's *Emile* in 1762 made breastfeeding fashionable. Some progress was evident, however. In Geneva, the average life span increased from 21.21 years in the sixteenth century, to 25.67 years in the seventeenth century, and to 33.62 years in the eighteenth century.

Hospitals could not satisfy the need for institutional care. They grew in number, but quality declined and mortality was still high between 1737 and 1748. The *Hôtel Dieu* in Paris received 251,178 patients, of whom 24 percent died. The demands made on this "Mansion of God" led to its putting three, four, five, or even six persons in each bed. The year 1788 saw the publication of a valuable study on hospitals, *Mémoires sur les hôspitaux de Paris*, by French surgeon J. R. Tenon. Informative and well-organized, the book contained ample statistical tables and a colorful narrative, including unsavory passages on hospital latrines. The description of the operating room, in which those who were to be operated upon next day lay beside those who had been operated upon that morning, was especially terrifying.

Although thousands were admitted into hospitals, thousands more in times of pestilence were turned away and died in the streets. Milton's description of a contemporary hospital serves as an appropriate commentary:

Hôtel Dieu *in Paris, early 1700s.*

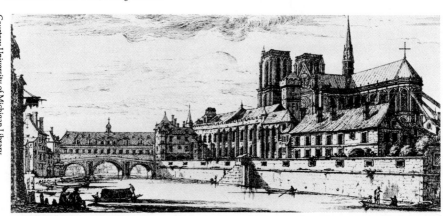

Immediately a place
Before his eyes appeared, sad, noisome, dark;
A lazar-house it seemed, wherein were laid
Numbers of all diseased—all maladies
Of ghastly spasm, or racking torture, qualms
Of heart-sick agony, all feverous kinds,
Convulsions, epilepsies, fierce catarrhs,
Intestine stone and ulcer, colic pangs,
Demoniac phrensy, moping melancholy,
And moon-struck madness, pining atrophy,
Marasmus, and wide-wasting pestilence,
Dropsies and asthmas, and joint-racking rheums.
Dire was the tossing, deep the groans; Despair
Tended the sick, busiest from couch to couch;
And over them triumphant Death his dart
Shook, but delayed to strike, though oft invoked
With vows, as their chief good and final hope [3].

In England, John Howard's *An Account of the Principal Lazarettos in Europe* appeared in 1789 and contained plans of and remarks about lazarettos in Marseilles, Genoa, Leghorn, and Spezia, as well as a lengthy commentary on hospital conditions in London and in some of the provinces. Howard's remarks mixed praise with criticism. He noted that in London Hospital "there are no cisterns for water; the vaults are often offensive . . . . Medical and chirurgical are together. . . . In a dirty room in the cellar there is a cold and a hot bath which seemed to be seldom used." Of St. Bartholomew's Hospital, Howard commented: "The wards . . . were clean . . . the windows were open." Of St. Thomas's Hospital: "The wards are fresh and clean . . . there were not water closets." Of St. George's: "The kitchens . . . are underground and were neither neat nor clean. A good old coal bath, but not used." Of Bethlehem (Bedlam): "There is no separation of the calm and quiet from the noisy and turbulent, except those who are changing theirselves. To each side of the house there is only one vault: very offensive." Of St. Luke's: "This noble hospital was neat and clean" [4].

Care of the Sick in Colonial America

Meanwhile, across the Atlantic in the British colonies of America, hospital care was no better. During the seventeenth and eighteenth centuries colonial hospitals were either almshouses or pesthouses, and hospitals proper did not yet exist. Hospitals for contagious diseases, called pesthouses, were erected in most of the major cities, not so much out of humane motives but rather to protect the public from the spread of infectious diseases, which often broke out among immigrants during the long voyage from Europe.

The medical profession could offer little help against rampant disease and sickness. Patients were often subjected to such crude forms of treatment as bleeding and purgatives, which actually aggravated illnesses. Medicine was not as developed in America as it was in Europe, and colonial physicians were in general

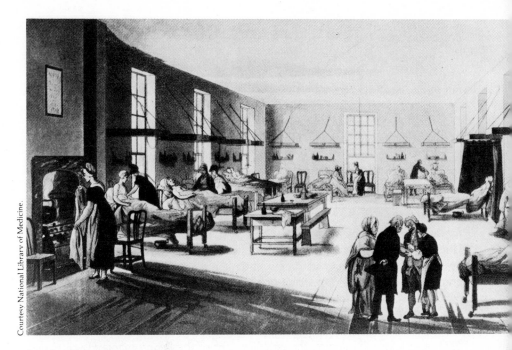

Courtesy National Library of Medicine.

London Hospital scene, 1780s.

poorly educated. As a rule, they acquired their skills not in colleges and hospitals but as apprentices to those already engaged in practice. After taking a short course of readings in medical books, a young man might then ride out with an older physician to gather herbs and run other errands for him. In this way, he would be initiated into the mysteries of healing. At the end of his term of apprenticeship, with this inadequate training, he was turned loose on the public. Fees were small, and frequently he had to engage in some other occupation on the side, most commonly the barber's trade.

A few colonial physicians received a regular medical education in Great Britain, mainly at the University of Edinburgh, and by the end of the eighteenth century, 117 Americans had been graduated from this university. Two medical schools had been established in America by the end of the colonial period: the Medical College of Philadelphia in 1765 (later affiliated with the University of Pennsylvania) and the medical department of King's College in 1767. Consequently, by 1770 a few first-class physicians and surgeons were practicing in America. Except for a few religious orders, however, nursing remained in the hands of the uneducated.

Average life expectancy at birth was estimated to be only 35 years. Plagues were a constant nightmare. Smallpox, which afflicted about one person in five—including the heavily pockmarked George Washington—was especially dreaded. A crude form of inoculation was introduced in 1721 despite the objections of many physicians and a few clergymen who opposed "tampering with the will of

God." Powdered toad was a favorite prescription for smallpox, and sanitation was primitive.

During the eighteenth century, yellow fever was reported to have caused 41,000 deaths in New Orleans, 10,000 in Philadelphia, and 3400 in New York. "Bring out your dead!" was the daily cry of the drivers of the death wagons. Dr. Benjamin Rush, the foremost physician of the time, believed that the Philadelphia epidemic of 1793 arose from the fumes of a coffee shipment that had spoiled on the docks, and although he noted that mosquitoes were numerous that summer, he failed to realize their significance. In 1797 he observed that one patient had developed the fever after smoking a cigar and that wind direction seemed to have had some influence upon the number of persons infected.

First Hospitals in America

Hospitals developed slowly in the thirteen colonies. In 1751 the first hospital deserving the name was founded in Philadelphia at the suggestion of Benjamin Franklin. To justify its construction, he maintained that it was the duty of the public to provide the same quality of care for the poor, friendless, sick, and insane inhabitants native to Philadelphia as was afforded to newly arrived immigrants. A petition written by Franklin was presented to the Pennsylvania Assembly in 1751, and a bill authorizing the establishment of the Pennsylvania Hospital was passed in the same year. Nearly $14,000 was raised by popular subscription to erect the building, and the colony appropriated an additional $10,000. The second colonial hospital was New York Hospital, founded in 1770 under a charter granted by George III at the request of several New York physicians seeking to prevent the spread of infectious diseases by sailors and immigrants. Due to the outbreak of the Revolutionary War, however, the hospital was not opened until 1791.

These early general hospitals were organized along French and English lines. Patients too poor to afford a private physician could pay only very small sums for their hospital care. Part-time staffs of physicians served without remuneration in order to increase their experiences and reputations through hospital affiliations. Each of the early colonial hospitals had an agreement with a nearby medical school whereby teaching was permitted in the hospital wards. In most instances, the important teaching positions in the school were held by members of the hospital staff. The original hospitals were privately managed and funded by public subscription and by generous gifts and bequests from wealthy families. Additional financial support was provided by contributions from the colonial governments.

The first hospital in the colonies for treatment of the insane was established in Philadelphia as a department of the Pennsylvania Hospital in 1752. A second such institution was founded at Williamsburg, Virginia in 1773. A third, the Friends' Hospital at Frankfort, near Philadelphia, was established in 1817. There followed the McLean Hospital at Charlestown, Massachusetts (1818), the Bloomingdale Hospital near the city of New York (1821), and the South Carolina Hospital at Columbia (1822). Forms of treatment for mental patients ranged from the cruel to the absurd, such as the frequent use of the rotating swing. By 1840 there were

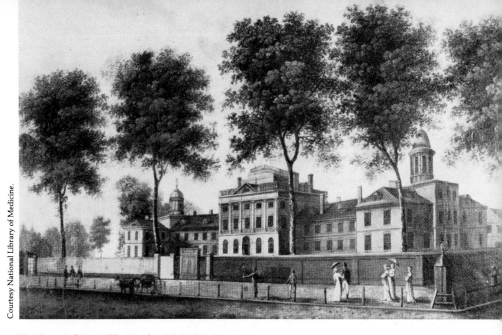

The Pennsylvania Hospital in Philadelphia.

Rotating swing used in hospitals for the insane, about 1820.

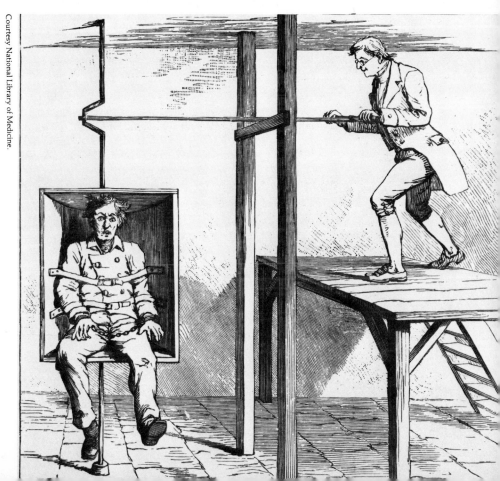

22

only eight hospitals for the insane in the United States. The overflow were confined to poorhouses and prisons.

The admission list of the Pennsylvania Hospital for the Insane for the year 1842 reveals the nebulous state of mid-nineteenth-century psychiatric diagnosis [5]:

Admissions	Men	Women	Total
Ill health of various kinds	22	24	46
Intemperance	20	0	20
Loss of property	17	6	23
Dread of poverty	2	0	2
Disappointed affections	2	4	6
Intense study	5	0	5
Domestic difficulties	1	5	6
Fright at fires	2	3	5
Grief—loss of friends	4	16	20
Intense application to business	2	0	2
Religious excitement	8	7	15
Want of employment	9	0	9
Use of opium	0	2	2
Use of tobacco	2	0	2
Mental anxiety	4	1	5
Unascertained	73	50	123
Total	173	118	291

Dorothea Lynde Dix, pioneer worker for the better care of mental patients in the United States.

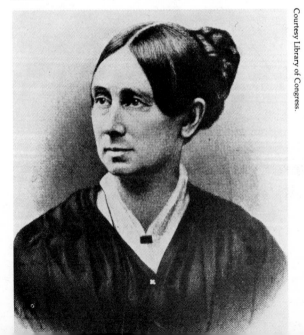

Courtesy Library of Congress.

Dorothea Dix, a frail, soft-spoken, middle-aged schoolteacher from New England, almost single-handedly wrought a revolution in the field of mental health care. Infinitely compassionate, she journeyed thousands of wearisome miles to investigate existing conditions in mental institutions and to appeal to state legislatures for improved treatment of the insane. Despite the powerful public prejudice against women in medicine, she succeeded in obtaining improved facilities and better-trained attendants.

Miss Dix's petition to Congress on June 27, 1848, which requested a grant of land to be used for the relief and support of care for the mentally disturbed, reveals the results of her travels and research on the subject:

At A_____, in the cell first opened, was a madman. The fierce command of his keeper brought him to the door, a hideous object: matted locks, an unshorn beard, a wild, wan countenance, disfigured by vilest uncleanness; in a state of nudity, save the irritating incrustations derived from that dungeon, reeking with loathsome filth. There, without light, without pure air, without warmth, without cleansing, absolutely destitute of everything securing comfort or decency, was a human being—forlorn, abject, and disgusting, it is true, but not the less a human being—nay more, an immortal being, though the mind was fallen in ruins, and the soul was clothed in darkness . . . .

At R_____, and M_____, and L_____, and B_____, were repetitions of the like dismal cells, heavy chains and balls, and hopeless sufferings. After my visit to L_____, I found one of the former inmates at the hospital in the charge of Dr. Brigham. He bore upon his ankles the deep scars of fetters and chains, and upon his feet evidence of exposure to frost and cold.

At E_____, the insane were confined in cells crammed with coarse, dirty straw, in the basement, dark and damp. "They are," said the keeper, "taken out and washed (buckets of water thrown over them) and have clean straw, once every week."

In H_____, were many furiously crazy. Several of the women were said to be the mothers of infants, who were in an adjoining room pining with neglect, and unacknowledged by their frantic mothers. . . .

Do you turn with inexpressible disgust from these details? It is worse to witness the reality. Is your refinement shocked by these statements? There is but one remedy; the multiplication of well-organized hospitals; and to this end, creating increased means for their support [6].

Although Congress did eventually enact legislation based on Miss Dix's plea for aid to the insane, the bill was vetoed by President Franklin Pierce as an unwarranted intrusion by the federal government into purely State matters.

The Pennsylvania Hospital of Philadelphia, the New York Hospital, and the Massachusetts General Hospital in Boston, situated in the three largest cities of the country, furnish the best examples of hospital construction in the United States in the early nineteenth century. Designs followed the block plan and buildings resembled large barns. Although hospitals appeared in most of the important coastal cities and in inland locations such as Cincinnati (1821), Pittsburgh (1847), Buffalo (1845), and Rochester (1847), most facilities were housed in large buildings converted into temporary quarters. Later, as a result of the increase in population and wealth of the communities which they served, many of these institutions built more suitable buildings.

During the 1850s, the Massachusetts General Hospital began construction of three pavilion wards. Each was a separate building accommodating about 30 patients. They were high-ceilinged, well-ventilated, and generally well-planned for that time. In the belief that in 20 years they would become so contaminated that it would be unsafe to continue to house patients in them, these buildings were built of wood so that they could be easily torn down and replaced.

The pavilion-type hospital developed from the idea that it was necessary to segregate patients and to replace buildings frequently. It represented a great improvement over the old block plan by providing fresh air, sunlight, and ample space for each patient. It was also expected to prevent gangrene and infectious diseases, which were believed to be airborne and the result of poor ventilation, but this reasoning was soon disproved. The pavilion-type hospital occupied very large areas and was costly to construct, heat, and maintain, but its use persisted because it represented an excellent means of providing the patients with light, air, and space.

Slow Medical Advances

By 1850, although nearly 100 years had passed since the first general hospital had been established in the United States, hospitals were still regarded as institutions for the accommodation of strangers and the sick poor—in other words, as places for the care rather than the cure of patients. No self-respecting woman ever thought of having her baby in a public hospital. Conditions in some of these institutions, notably in the surgical wards, defied description. A mid-nineteenth-century student might think his teacher to be excessively fussy if he prohibited spitting in the wards. Infection and cross-infection were frequent. Several diseases became so common in hospitals that they were known as "hospital diseases": erysipelas, pyemia, septicemia, and gangrene. Before the discovery of antisepsis, a surgeon often prided himself on the condition of his blood-encrusted apron, the degree of filth indicating to some extent his experience. Nurses in these pioneer hospitals were normally drawn from the tough, charwoman class that regarded nursing as distasteful drudgery rather than as a humanitarian calling.

Surgery, although improved by an increased knowledge of anatomy, dealt chiefly with physiologic emergencies such as fractures, amputations, and superficial growths. Patients in surgical operations were ordinarily tied down and sometimes braced with a stiff shot of whiskey. The surgeon then sawed or cut with breakneck speed, undeterred by the shrieks of his patient. Even if the operation was a success, there was little hope that the patient would survive the inevitable postsurgical "hospitalism," the term applied to a variety of septic infections virtually endemic in hospital wards. "Hospitalism" was fatal in about one of every three surgical patients. Committing surgical patients to hospitals came almost to be regarded as tantamount to signing their death certificates in advance.

By the 1850s the physical environment of the rapidly growing urban areas was beginning to constitute a worsening health hazard. The cities were not properly drained, and in none of them was there proper disposal of refuse.

Rubbish was thrown into the gutters, and garbage was allowed to accumulate in alleys and backyards. In some places the air was polluted by vile odors emanating from slaughterhouses and manufactories. Packs of dogs were allowed to run loose on the streets and numerous rats lived under the wooden sidewalks. The hogs that roamed at will served as scavengers and often were a nuisance when they impeded traffic and dug unsightly wallows in the streets. The public was not protected against the sale of milk from diseased cows, and it was charged that 8000 children lost their lives annually in New York as a result of infection from milk.

In the period before the Civil War, medical standards declined, unable to keep pace with the demands of a fast-growing population for more trained physicians. Medical schools, as a rule, conferred full degrees upon completion of annual courses of four-months' duration over a two year period. Both first and second year students attended the same lectures each year. Regular attendance was not required and the examinations were generally cursory. A common saying was that "a boy who is unfit for anything else must become a doctor." It was hoped that medical students would spend the months between the two lecture courses in practical observation of patients with their preceptors and in some study and review of what they had listened to during the first term. The University of Virginia Medical School, considered to be one of the best in the country, was actually giving *two* courses of lectures in the same calendar year, with little time in between.

Physicians were so inadequately trained that they often aggravated rather than alleviated disease. Emetics, purgatives, and bleeding remained the three mainstays among the therapeutic treatments of the typical mid-century practitioner. Bloodletting, the prevailing cure for most ailments, contributed to the death of Zachary Taylor in 1850. After consuming iced milk and chilled cucumbers on a hot Fourth of July, the President came down with gastroenteritis, which his physicians diagnosed as *cholera morbus*. They drugged, bled, and blistered the President for five days until he finally succumbed to the standard practices of mid-nineteenth-century medicine.

Normally a physician was required only to treat a limited variety of diseases, and his chief bedside problem was in administering the proper portion of medicine. In addition to the favored use of calomel, medicines most frequently given were quinine, jalap, and occasionally opium (laudanum).

Until the late nineteenth century, brandy and whiskey were favorite remedies for many of the severe febrile illnesses. In the treatment of such prevalent diseases as typhus, puerperal fever, and septic conditions, large quantities of alcohol were used: a patient might be dosed with a whole quart of whiskey within 24 hours. Whiskey was considered to be so valuable in the treatment of pneumonia that one distinguished New York physician famous for his diagnostic ability in pulmonary diseases declared that if he were given a choice between using all the drugs of the pharmacopeia *without* whiskey, or using whiskey *without* all the drugs of the pharmacopeia for the treatment of pneumonia, he would choose the latter alternative, confident that whiskey alone would save far more of his patients. Medical textbooks of the 1860s recommended brandy and whiskey for the treatment of many diseases and medical lectures extolled the virtues of their use.

Quack Doctors and Self-Medication

One hindrance to good health was the use of patent medicines and fake remedies. Americans placed much faith in folk medicines. For example, some believed that whooping cough should be treated by hanging a bag of live groundbugs around the patient's neck, or if this was inconvenient, the patient might be advised to eat the shed skin of a snake or eggs obtained from a person whose name had not been changed by marriage. According to popular belief, a vegetable-free diet protected against cholera, a horse chestnut in one's pocket healed piles (hemorrhoids), and mercury chloride served as a universal balm.

In 1854 S. S. Fitch boasted that 100,000 copies of his *Health Almanac* had been sold in six years: Fitch, who claimed to be an M.D., sold a wide variety of patent medicines through the mail. Offering to diagnose any ailments that were described in letters written to him, he would, upon receipt of the money requested, forward his secret-formula medicines. Directions for the use of all 20 were the same:

Begin with one-quarter of the smallest dose printed on each box or bottle.

If using two or more medicines, mix the doses together, if to be taken at or near the same time of day.

Increase one or two drops of each daily, until you arrive at the full doses, if no inconvenience is previously felt.

Shake each bottle before using.

For each distinct disease you have, use the medicine directed for it. The medicines do not injure each other, and used as directed will not injure any one. For their effects see the letters in this Guide.

Consult me as soon as possible, either by letter or personally, and I will give you all needful advice [7].

Two of the more popular concoctions sold by Fitch were advertised as follows:

HEART CORRECTOR

Persons subject to palpitation, spasms about the chest and left side, stoppage of the action of the heart, beating of the heart, trembling all over and about the heart, water about the heart, and all ossifications of the heart, rheumatism about the heart, and in angina pectoris, and debility of the heart, will find this a most valuable remedy; it is above all price, and will perfectly cure a great many cases of heart trouble; it will never injure but always do good, and has been used many years by a great many persons, with lasting benefit. For sleepless, restless patients, this is valuable; and where the person experiences great sinking and debility, it helps greatly, and takes away the allgone feeling of many persons. No person having any trouble of the heart should be without this medicine. Keep it in your bedroom, take it with you on journeys, and everywhere, especially if liable to sudden attacks. It is a noble and useful remedy. See remarks on Heart Diseases, in my Lectures.

NERVINE

In almost every case of chronic disease the nerves become weak, and something is required to sooth and strengthen them, and to prevent sinking and debility, and wasting of the nervous system. In all of these cases the Nervine is an invaluable medicine, and should be faithfully used. Begin with three drops, and increase one drop a day until you get up to fifteen drops, which is as much as is generally useful. You may then suspend its use for four days, that it may not lose its effect. It is highly useful, and assists the effects of other medicines. I feel as if I could not cure consumption without it. It is most useful in consumption, heart disease, liver complaint, dyspepsia, costiveness, diarrhea, bronchitis, neuralgia, rush of blood to the head, confusion in the head, restlessness, rheumatism, and all humors, kidney disease, female complaints, piles, scrofula, skin disease, all varieties of head-ache, catarrh, white swellings, tic doloreux, etc.; in all affections of the throat, loss of voice, etc. Toothache it promptly cures. Put a little in the tooth, on cotton, and rub a little over that affected tooth, on the cheek, and on the gum, etc. It is valuable in all spinal diseases, disposition to apoplexy, and nervousness. In neuralgia, rub it freely on the part, etc. It acts on all these by its control over the nervous system [8].

So backward was medical science that Dr. Oliver Wendell Holmes felt justified in making this severe indictment of his fellow practitioners in 1860: ". . . if the whole materia medica, as now used, could be sunk to the bottom of the sea, it would be all the better for mankind—and all the worse for the fishes" [9].

Oliver Wendell Holmes.

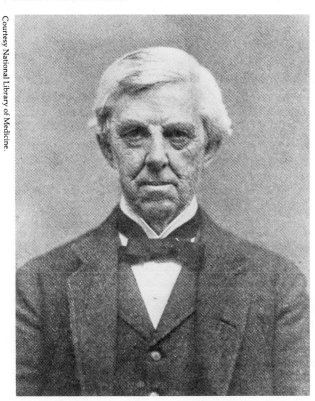

The Sairy Gamps

By today's standards, most of the hospitals in the United States in the early nineteenth century were disgraceful. Dirty, unventilated, and contaminated by infections, they actually facilitated the spread of disease. Hospital wards were filled with patients with discharging wounds, which made the atmosphere so offensive that the use of perfume was required. Nurses of the period adopted the use of snuff in order to make working conditions more tolerable. The same bed linen served several patients. Pain, hemorrhage, infection, and gangrene were rife in the wards.

Nursing was considered an inferior, undesirable occupation. During the previous century religious attendants had been largely replaced by lay people who were employed without any attention given to their selection. Often drawn from the criminal class and lacking a spirit of self-sacrifice, they exploited and abused the patients. Often the only lay nurses available were aged inmates or women who could obtain no other employment and who were willing to perform menial tasks along with their nursing duties. Work was not subject to inspection or discipline. There was practically no nursing service at night except in cases of childbirth and impending death, at which times a "watcher" would be hired. Many of these nurses were widows with large families. Some drowned their grievances in alcohol. Others stooped to accepting bribes from patients and their relatives. Vice was rampant among these women, who sometimes "aided" the dying by removing pillows and bedclothes and by performing other morbid activities designed to hasten the end.

In 1844, in England, Charles Dickens accurately portrayed this class of nurses in *Martin Chuzzlewit* through the characters of Sairy Gamp and Betsy Prig. In a later preface to the novel, dated November, 1849, he noted:

Mrs. Sarah Gamp is a representation of the hired attendant on the poor in sickness. The Hospitals of London are, in many respects, noble institutions; in others, very defective. I think it not the least among the instances of their mismanagement, that Mrs. Betsy Prig is a fair specimen of Hospital Nurse; and that the Hospitals, with their means and funds, should have left it to private humanity and enterprise, in the year Eighteen Hundred and Forty-nine, to enter on an attempt to improve that class of persons [10].

Mrs. Gamp first appears in Chapter 19, when she is summoned by Mr. Pecksniff to prepare the body of Anthony Chuzzlewit for burial. After first awakening all the neighbors, Mr. Pecksniff finally rouses Mrs. Gamp, who consents to accompany him:

Mrs. Gamp had a large bundle with her, a pair of patterns and a species of gig umbrella; the latter article in colour like a faded leaf, except where a circular patch of a lively hue had been dexterously let in at the top . . . . She was a fat old woman, this Mrs. Gamp, with a husky voice, and a moist eye, which she had a remarkable power of turning up and showing the white of it. Having very little neck, it cost her some trouble to look over herself, if one may say so, to those to whom she talked. She wore a very rusty black gown, rather the worse for snuff, and a shawl and bonnet to correspond. In these dilapidated articles of dress she had, on principle, arrayed herself, time out of mind, on such occasions

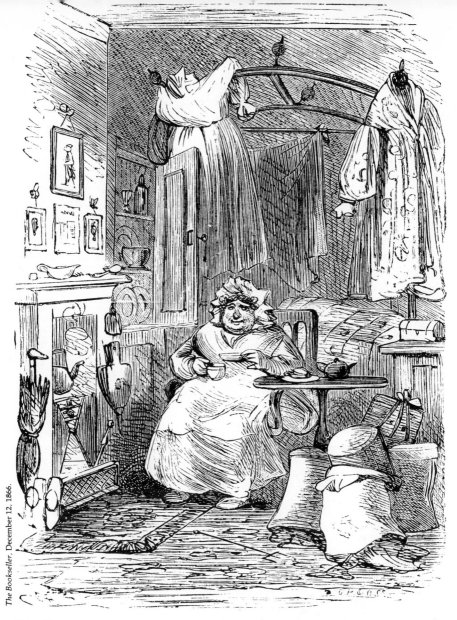

Sairy Gamp.

as the present; for this at once expressed a decent amount of veneration for the deceased, and invited the next of kin to present her with a fresher suit of weeds: an appeal so frequently successful, that the very fetch and ghost of Mrs. Gamp, bonnet and all, might be seen hanging up, any hour in the day, in at least a dozen of the second-hand clothes shops about Holborn. The face of Mrs. Gamp—the nose in particular—was somewhat red and swollen, and it was difficult to enjoy her society without becoming conscious of a smell of spirits. Like most persons who have attained to great eminence in their profession, she took to hers very kindly; insomuch, that setting aside her natural predilections as a woman, she went to a lying-in or a laying-out with equal zest and relish [11].

An idea of the irresponsibility of the hospital nurses may be derived from the following extract describing an epidemic of cholera that occurred in the Philadelphia General Hospital during the spring of 1833:

In the house the cases increased daily until a general panic took place. Nurses became clamorous for an increase in wages, which was granted. Those between terror and want of moral sense were seized with a kind of mad infatuation. They drank the stimulants provided for the sick, and in one ward where the pestilence raged in its most fearful forms, and where between the dead and the dying the sight was most appalling, these furies were seen lying drunk upon or fighting over the dead victims of the disease. In this state of disorder, application was made to Bishop Kendrick for Sisters of Charity. The request was granted, and these devoted ministers of mercy at once entered upon their mission of danger, restoring order and diffusing hope by the calm and self-possessed manner with which they moved among the diseased. These Sisters remained at their post until the 20th of May 1833 [12].

Nursing in Modern Religious Orders

The Sisters of Charity had been founded in Paris in 1633 by Saint Vincent de Paul, assisted by Mlle Louise Le Gras (Ste. Louise de Marillac). Instead of taking perpetual vows, the Sisters took simple vows, which were renewed annually.

Elizabeth Bayley Seton.

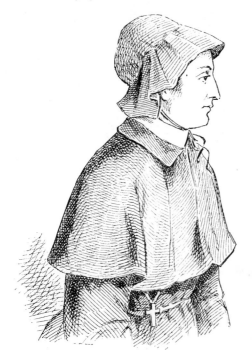

Courtesy Library of Congress.

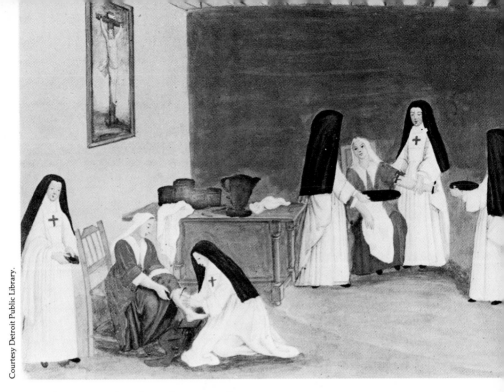

Sister nurses at work in the early nineteenth century.

They also took a fourth vow binding themselves to the care of the sick. In the United States the Sisters of Charity began their charitable works under the direction of Elizabeth Bayley Seton. Mother Seton's first community, known as The Sisters of Charity of Saint Joseph, was established at Emmitsburg, Maryland, in July, 1809. Soon many orders and branches of orders in the Roman Catholic Church bore the name of Sisters of Charity. Some of them were also called "Gray Sisters" or "Gray Nuns," "Daughters of Charity," and "Sisters of Saint Vincent de Paul."

Also deeply involved in nursing were the Sisters of Mercy, an order founded in Dublin in 1827 by Catherine McAuley, who later served as its mother superior. Besides their three primary vows, the Sisters took a fourth by promising to devote their lives to the service of the poor, the sick, and the ignorant—an obligation that was zealously observed. The order was introduced into the United States in December, 1843, when seven Sisters came from Carlow, Ireland, to establish a convent in Pittsburgh.

Several other Catholic orders were closely associated with nursing at this time. In 1822 the Sisters of Bon Secours were organized by the archbishop of Paris to care for the sick in their homes and for orphans in asylums. During the early 1840s this order began its nursing activities in the United States. The Sisters of the Holy Cross were founded at Le Mans, France in 1839. Their goals included the care of the sick in hospitals and orphanages. Their first American novitiate was opened at Bertrand, Michigan in 1844.

The Birth of Modern Nursing

During the nineteenth century deaconess orders, which had previously existed back near the time of Christ, were revived by Protestant churches that felt the need for the assistance of women in conducting religious work.

The first modern order of deaconesses was established in 1836 by the German Pastor Theodor Fliedner of Kaiserswerth, who needed an organized corps of nurses for his new infirmary. This experiment proved so successful that it was immediately copied by Lutheran organizations in other parts of Europe. As instituted by Pastor Fliedner, the Order of Deaconesses of the Rhenish Province of Westphalia comprised three classes of members: the first class devoted itself to the care of the sick poor and to the rescue of fallen women by the means of Magdalen homes; the second class served as teachers; the third class, known as visitation deaconesses, assumed the responsibilities of regular parochial work.

It was in the little German town of Kaiserswerth that the modern movement for nursing education began. Here Pastor Fliedner and his devoted wife Friederike established a refuge for discharged prisoners. Aroused by the lack of facilities for the care of the sick and by physicians' bitter complaints "of the hireling service by day and night, of the drunkenness and immorality of the attendants" then available, they opened a small hospital with a training school for deaconesses in 1836. The first candidate, Gertrude Reichardt, was so disheartened when she saw the sparse facilities and poor equipment—"a shabby table, some brokenbacked chairs, worn-out knives, two-pronged forks, worm-eaten beds and appliances to match"—that she was about to return home in despair. But soon a large bundle arrived containing a quantity of new bed linen, clothing, and ward fittings. She regarded this windfall as a providential sign and remained to become the first of the deaconesses dedicated to a new ideal of nursing. Thus, the efforts of the Fliedners resulted in the birth of modern nursing and prepared the way for Florence Nightingale [13].

Eighteen years later, soon after the outbreak of the Crimean War—in which Britain, France, and Turkey fought against Russia for control of access to the Mediterranean from the Black Sea—ugly rumors of the neglect and mismanagement of casualties began to reach England. Reports dispatched by William Howard Russell, special correspondent to the *London Times*, and printed on October 9 and 12, 1854, revealed that the hospitals contained "neither surgeons, dressers, nurses, nor the commonest appliance of a workhouse sick ward." Later, after observing that the French were receiving nursing care from the Sisters of Charity, Russell demanded, "Why have we no Sisters of Charity?"

In regard to conditions in British hospitals, correspondent Russell wrote that "the commonest accessories of a hospital are wanting; there is not the least attention paid to decency or cleanliness; the stench is appalling; the fetid air can barely struggle out to taint the atmosphere, save through the chinks in the walls and roofs; and, for all I can observe, these men die without the slightest effort being made to save them." He added that "the sick appear to be tended by the sick, the dying by the dying" [14].

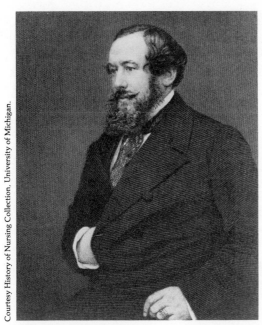

William Howard Russell.

The corridors and wards of the Barrack Hospital at Scutari were paved with dirty broken stones. The damp, filthy building was in a bad state of repair and infested with rats and vermin. Sanitary arrangements were appalling. No steps had been taken to clean the rooms, beds, and bedding, and all necessary equipment was lacking. Russell noted that "the manner in which the sick and wounded are treated is worthy only of the savage . . . . The hospitals have not the commonest appliances of a workhouse sick ward" [15].

The Duke of Newcastle, as Secretary for War, was responsible for the administration of the Army, and Sir Sidney Herbert, as Secretary at War, was placed in charge of its finances. Even though Newcastle was grossly overworked, he quickly decided to send a commission to investigate Russell's allegations. Meanwhile Herbert, who for years had been interested in the care of the sick, took control of the situation. Russell had contrasted the deplorable medical and sanitary conditions of the British with those of the French, for whom 50 Sisters of Charity were providing admirable nursing care. Herbert saw no reason why Britain too should not send a group of women nurses. He knew that there would be some opposition in Parliament, but he was determined to make the attempt.

Florence Nightingale: Pioneer

Herbert's thoughts turned at once to Miss Florence Nightingale. On Sunday, October 15, 1854, he wrote to Miss Nightingale explaining the situation and the need for women nurses in the Crimea. He claimed that she was the only person

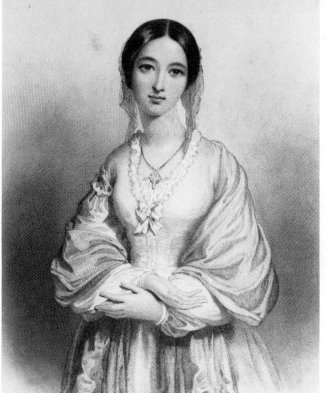

Florence Nightingale.

in England capable of organizing and supervising such a plan. "Would you listen to the request to go and superintend the whole thing," he stated, "deriving your authority from the Government, your position would secure the respect and consideration of everyone" [16]. With Miss Nightingale's acceptance of this challenge, nursing took one of its longest steps forward.

Florence Nightingale had been born in Florence 34 years before, on May 13, 1820, and had been named after the city of her birth. Born of wealthy, influential English parents, she was raised in England and, unlike the average English girl of the time, received a thorough education. She and the only other child of the family, Parthenope, were tutored by governesses, and as the girls grew older, their father took an active part in their education. Early in her teenage years Florence mastered the fundamentals of Greek and Latin, read Plato, studied history, mathematics, and philosophy, and wrote essays on subjects designated by her father. She was a shy, sensitive child, inclined to be pensive and somewhat morbid.

Soon after her seventeenth birthday Florence returned to Italy. Later she took other trips with her parents or in the company of family friends. During these travels, in addition to the usual itinerary of art, architecture, and nature study, she invariably took notes on the laws and social conditions of the lands which she visited. Her sister, on the other hand, as an average girl of a prominent family, preferred social activities. Upon returning from their first continental trip, the girls were presented at Court.

At an early age, Florence expressed to her parents a desire to enter the nursing field, but they were convinced that nursing was a profession suited only for women like Sairy Gamp. While Florence fully appreciated her parents' viewpoint, she determined that it would not be necessary for her to degrade herself in order to become a nurse. Moreover, she considered it unfair to condemn an occupation because of its existing poor reputation. Rather, she thought it better to correct the evils in nursing.

Her decision to train in an English hospital at the age of 25, nine years prior to Herbert's summons, was met by the determined objections of her mother, who naturally expected Florence to marry wisely and to assume her inherited place in society. Florence rejected matrimony, however, and took advantage of every opportunity to acquaint herself with nursing conditions.

In the autumn of 1849, Miss Nightingale departed on a tour with family friends. They wintered in Egypt, and Florence spent time in Alexandria with the Sisters of Charity of Saint Vincent de Paul. Spring, 1850, found her in Athens, from where she set out, unaccompanied, for Kaiserswerth. Arriving in July, 1850, she remained there for two weeks and came away firmly resolved to return there to train as a nurse, despite the objections of her family.

The following year, when her ailing sister Parthenope was about to journey to the mineral springs of Carlsbad, Florence insisted on going to Kaiserswerth for nurses' training while Mrs. Nightingale and Parthenope stayed at the resort. Permission was granted on condition that no one outside the family was to know where she went. Florence reached the deaconess institution early in July, 1851, and stayed three months.

Finally, after Florence returned from Germany and the Nightingales were setteled back home in England, provisions were made for her to enter her chosen profession. After arrangements had been made for Florence to go to France to work with several Catholic nursing sisters, her mother induced her to postpone the trip. It was 1853 before she reached Paris, where, granted an official permit, she inspected hospitals and religious institutions and observed surgeons at their work. While in France she negotiated for a position in England as superintendent of the Establishment for Gentlewomen During Illness, a charity hospital for governesses run by titled ladies. She assumed this position upon her return to London, but friends soon persuaded her to leave the institution, for she was handicapped by an intolerant board of directors with little knowledge of good hospital management. Negotiations were under way for her appointment as the superintendent of nurses at King's College Hospital when the outbreak of the Crimean War presented her with a brilliant and unexpected opportunity for achievement.

At Herbert's insistence, the British government conferred on Miss Nightingale the inspiring title "Superintendent of the Female Nursing Establishment of the English General Hospitals in Turkey." This lofty title was a misnomer, for there was not yet any female nursing establishment to superintend, but this deficiency was soon remedied by a frantic recruiting drive in London. Two days after receipt of her orders, on October 21, 1854, the newly appointed superintendent set out for the Dardanelles with 38 self-proclaimed nurses of varied experience, of

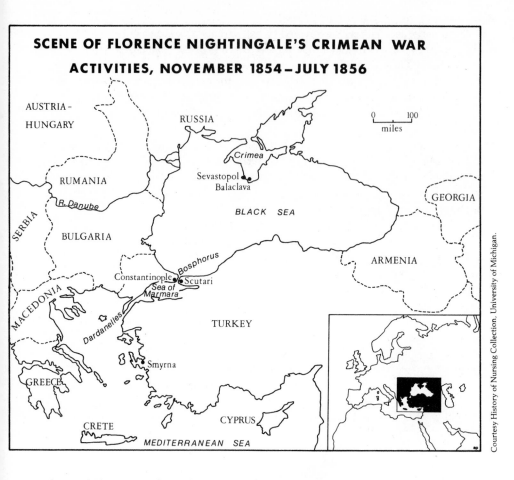

Scene of Florence Nightingale's Crimean War activities.

whom 24 were nuns. The other 14 also claimed some nursing experience—which generally meant very little.

Florence Nightingale and her nursing force arrived at Scutari, a suburb of Constantinople on the Asiatic side of the Bosphorus, on November 4, 1854. It was here that the British military hospital had been established in a huge building called Selimah Kishler. Previously housing Turkish artillery, it had been requisitioned because it had appeared to offer suitable accommodations. Renamed the "Barrack," this building had acquired an ignominious reputation. There were no beds, no furniture, no eating utensils, no medical supplies, and no blankets. The latrines were clogged and the tubs standing in the passage were never emptied. Men lay naked on the floor in their own excrement. It was later estimated that three-quarters of all the casualties suffered by the British Army in the Crimean War resulted from such diseases as dysentery, typhoid, and cholera, which were contracted in the hospital. The Barrack Hospital had proved to be a death trap rather than a sanatorium. Moreover, it had been the subject of extremely unfavorable journalistic reports, much to the consternation of Dr. John Hall, Chief of Medical Staff for the British Expeditionary Force.

Even though some medical officers complained to each other about the ineptitude of the Medical Department and privately acknowledged both the verity of William Howard Russell's exposés in the *Times* and the value of sending Miss Nightingale and her nurses, the majority resented this outside interference and drew together into "a defensive phalanx" to justify and protect themselves. Most medical officers, like Dr. Hall, regarded Miss Nightingale as an intruder who would undermine military authority. A powerful, mutual hatred soon developed between the two. When Dr. Hall was awarded the K.C.B. (Knight Commander of the Order of the Bath), Miss Nightingale sarcastically referred to him as the "Knight of the Crimean Burial Grounds."

Because no accommodations had been arranged for Miss Nightingale's group of 39 women, they crowded into six small rooms in one of the hospital's towers. Each room could hold only two with comfort. Meanwhile the corresponding accommodations in the other tower were fully occupied by one major. There was no furniture in the dirty rooms, which were swarming with vermin, and one of them even contained a long-neglected corpse. The Nightingale nurses wore gray tweed dresses, gray worsted jackets, plain white caps, short woolen cloaks, and brown scarves embroidered in red with the words "Scutari Hospital."

The Barrack Hospital at Scutari was designed to accommodate 1700 patients, but between 3000 and 4000 were tightly packed into it when Miss Nightingale arrived. There were four miles of beds situated 18 inches apart. The mattresses on the beds, the tiles of the unglazed, unwashed floor, and even the plaster on the walls were soaked with liquid excrement. The building was standing in "a sea of sewage." Lice, maggots, rats, and countless other forms of vermin were crawling around everywhere. Describing the conditions to Sidney Herbert, Florence wrote graphically that "the vermin might, if they had but unity of purpose, carry off the four miles of beds on their backs and march them into the War Office" [17].

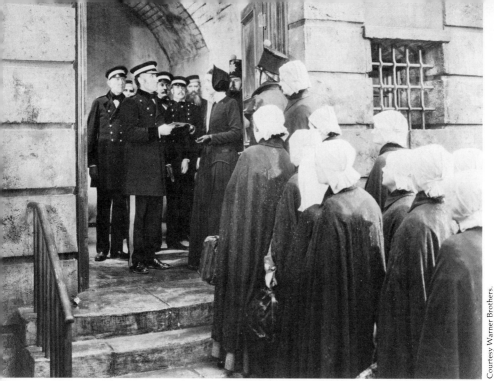

Florence Nightingale and her nurses are met by unappreciative surgeons at the Barrack Hospital at Scutari in the motion picture biography White Angel, *starring Kay Francis. (From the Warner Brothers release* White Angel © *1936 Warner Bros. Pictures, Inc. Copyright renewed 1963.)*

Within 10 days of her arrival, Miss Nightingale had set up a kitchen for special diets and had rented a house which she converted into a laundry. After she had hired soldiers' wives to do the washing, clean linen finally began to appear on the hospital wards. Unable to obtain any money from the authorities, Miss Nightingale utilized the *Times* Relief Fund and even her own personal resources to purchase medical supplies, food, and hospital equipment for virtually an army. Once satisfied with the improvement in hospital conditions, she initiated social service work among the soldiers. This program of social welfare, however, earned her the criticism of the surgeons, who reproached her for "spoiling the brutes" [18].

In the small room where Florence sat at a plain wooden table and wrote requests, orders, letters, and reports, there was a narrow bed, in which she seldom slept. In addition to her heavy administrative burden, she spent long hours in the wards nursing. Robert Robinson, a disabled 11-year-old drummer boy from the Sixty-eighth Light Infantry, served as her personal attendant, delivering messages and carrying her lamp at night while she went among the crowds of wounded to help during an operation or sit by a dying man.

It was not uncommon for Miss Nightingale to spend eight hours at a time, sometimes on her knees, dressing wounds and comforting the soldiers. At other times she stood for as long as 20 consecutive hours distributing stores, directing her staff, and assisting in operations. On one occasion, when she saw five soldiers laid aside as hopeless cases, she asked permission to care for them. Next morning they were ready to be operated on. "Before she came," one soldier wrote home, "there was cussin' and swearin', but after that it was holy as a church." Another wrote, "What a comfort it was to see her pass even. She would speak to one and nod and smile to as many more, but she could not do it all, you know. We lay there by hundreds, but we could kiss her shadow as it fell, and lay our heads on the pillow again content." "She was all full of life and fun when she talked to us," said another, "especially if a man was a bit downhearted" [19].

Correspondent M. W. Macdonald of the *Times* filed a memorable report on Miss Nightingale's work:

Wherever there is disease in its most dangerous form, and the hand of the despoiler distressingly nigh, there is this incomparable woman [Florence Nightingale] sure to be seen; her benignant presence is an influence for good comfort, even amid the struggles of expiring nature. She is a "ministering angel," without any exaggeration, in these hospitals; and as her slender form glides quietly along each corridor, every poor fellow's face softens with gratitude at the sight of her. When all the medical officers have retired for the night, and silence and darkness have settled down upon those miles of prostrate sick, she may be observed alone, with a little lamp in her hand, making her solitary rounds [20].

The compassion and success of Florence Nightingale and her nurses captured world-wide attention. (From the Warner Brothers release White Angel *© 1936 Warner Bros. Pictures, Inc. Copyright renewed 1963.)*

Courtesy Warner Brothers.

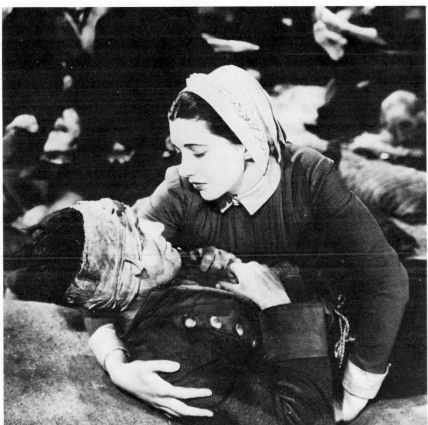

Victorian poet R. N. Cust immortalized Miss Nightingale for the British public in his poem *Scutari Hospital*.

Moaning in agony,
  Writhing in pain,
Fighting the dreadful flight
  Over again;
Hearts yearning for home,
  Yearning in vain,
Tears over manly cheeks
  Pouring like rain.
Thus through the dreary day
  And dreary night
Lie England's soldiers
  After the fight!

Flitting like angels
  From bed to bed,
Cooling the parched lips
  And aching head,
Of the poor mangled limb
  Loosening the bands,
Wiping the clammy brows
  With tender hands.
Thus through the dreary night
  And dreary day
To England's nurses
  Hours pass away!

Many a blessing,
  Many a prayer,
Burst from rough lips for
  Those angels there.
England sends gladly
  Her mighty sons,
With implements of war
  And battering guns.
And England's daughters
  Proudly repair,
In Liberty's battle,
  Perils to share [21]!

The difficulties that Miss Nightingale encountered and the prejudices that she had to overcome were enormous. The revolutionary aspect of her work, which did more than just reorganize military hospitals and procure comfort for thousands of wounded soldiers, cannot be fully measured. As a result of the unprecedented introduction of women nurses into the British Army, she succeeded in overcoming age-old prejudices and in elevating the status of all nurses. Probably for the first time in history, the overwhelming support of public opinion forced an antagonistic military hierarchy to accept a lady administrator with extensive authority.

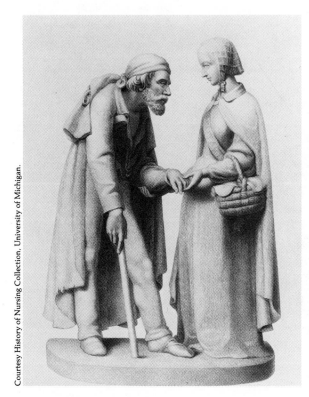

Courtesy History of Nursing Collection, University of Michigan.

"The Wounded at Scutari."

Six months later, in early May, 1855, when conditions at the Barrack Hospital were reasonably satisfactory, Miss Nightingale journeyed across the Black Sea to the Crimea. Two British hospitals were located there, both near the seaport of Balaclava. One, the General Hospital, had been established near the harbor upon the arrival of the British in September, 1854. The enormous numbers of sick from cholera, from wounds received at the battles of Balaclava (October 25, 1854) and Inkerman (November 5, 1854), and from the undernourishment and exposure during the winter of 1854–55 had necessitated further accommodations, and a cluster of huts had been erected on the heights near the old Genoese Castle above Balaclava. This complex, which constituted the second hospital, was accordingly called the Castle Hospital.

Accompanying Miss Nightingale to the Crimea was Alexis Soyer, chef at the Reform Club in London, whose task it was to supervise the army's diet. Because he had studied how to cook large quantities of food economically and at the same time serve delicious dishes, he rapidly trained the cooks in the hospital kitchens to prepare excellent meals made strictly with army rations. He invented a special cooking oven, the Soyer boiler, which was used long afterward, and the "Scutari teapot," which could brew tea for half a company of men.

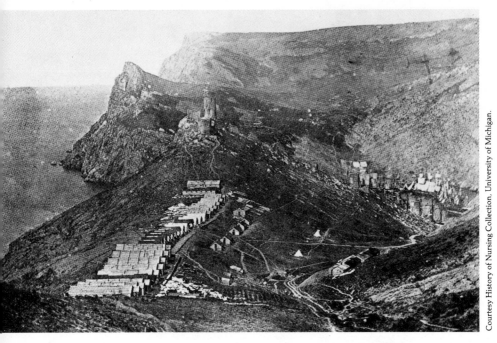

Hospitals at Balaclava.

After visiting the front and the hospitals, Florence contracted "Crimean fever" and was taken to the Castle Hospital, where she nearly died. She was evacuated to Scutari, where she narrowly avoided an underhanded effort by Dr. John Hall to ship her directly to England in order to eliminate her "interference" with Medical Staff affairs. Soldiers wept when news of her illness reached them, and all England awaited the outcome in anxious suspense. Within a few weeks she had recovered and resumed her duties at Scutari, but the strain and responsibility of providing nursing care had undermined her health to such an extent that she would never again be able to work with her previous physical vigor.

By the end of the Crimean War, Florence had supervised 125 nurses—a small number by later standards, but large when one considers the opposition of the Army physicians. When she first arrived at the Barrack Hospital, its mortality rate stood at 60 percent; she left it at a fraction over 1 percent. The general improvement in all British military hospitals is perhaps best indicated by the overall drop in the mortality rate from 42 percent to 2.2 percent. Miss Nightingale's immense courage and indomitable perseverance forced the military authorities to acknowledge that there was a place for women nurses in Army hospitals. In recognition of her services, Queen Victoria presented her with a distinctive brooch bearing the inscription "Blessed are the merciful."

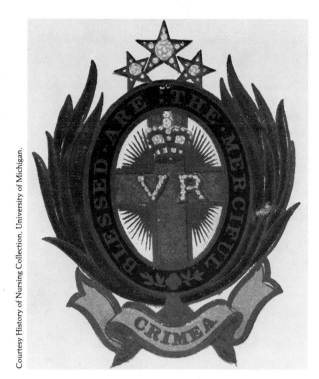

Courtesy History of Nursing Collection, University of Michigan.

Illustration of Miss Nightingale's decoration, obverse. The engraving on the back reads: "To Miss Florence Nightingale, As a Mark of Esteem and Gratitude for Her Devotion Towards the Queen's Brave Soldiers. From Victoria R., 1855."

After the Crimean War ended early in 1856, the hospitals were closed one by one, and the nurses returned to England. Miss Nightingale was among the last to leave in July, 1856. Upon her return from the Crimea, she immediately began pursuing the two goals most vital to her: reform of Army sanitary practices and the establishment of a school for nurses. The latter task was aided by the donation of more than $220,000 by the British public.

When the nurse training school was begun as an experiment at St. Thomas' Hospital in London, the overwhelming majority of London physicians opposed the project. Of the 100 physicians asked, only four favored the school. Most replied that because nurses occupied much the same position as housemaids, they needed little instruction beyond poultice-making, the enforcement of cleanliness, and attention to the patient's personal needs. Miss Nightingale's ill health prevented her from taking charge of the program, but for years she acted as its chief adviser.

In addition to establishing the training school, Miss Nightingale worked to improve the health standards of the British Army. She was determined that the lessons taught by the Crimean War be used to prepare for the future. In order to influence Parliament and the general staff of the British Army, she wrote a study entitled *Notes on Matters Affecting the Health, Efficiency, and Hospital*

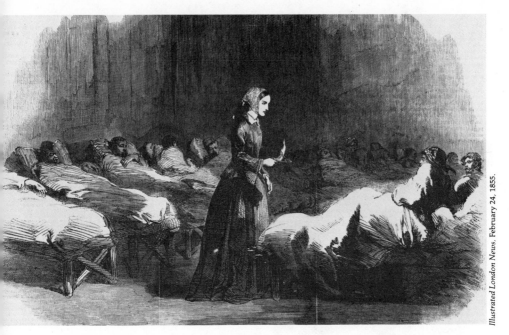

"The Lady with a Lamp"—Florence Nightingale in the Barrack Hospital at Scutari.

Administration of the British Army (1858), which was respectfully received by Her Majesty's government. Her *Notes on Hospitals* (1858) was a seminal work, and her *Notes on Nursing* (1859) served for decades as the standard text on nursing. Upon completion of these studies, she undertook the enormous project of investigating sanitary conditions in India.

While the Crimean War caused untold suffering, it also led to one of the greatest humanitarian advances of history: modern military nursing, from which developed professional nursing in general. If it had not been for the horrible conditions in the British hospitals and camps at the beginning of this war, there would have been no nursing reform by Florence Nightingale. Possibly her indomitable spirit would have achieved its goal in some other way, but the frightful things that the "Lady with a Lamp" saw and the heroic things that she did reached the newspapers and gave her the backing of public opinion.

Across the Atlantic, Henry Wadsworth Longfellow paid popular tribute to the "Saint of the Crimea" with his poem *Santa Filomena:*

Whene'er a noble deed is wrought,
Whene'er is spoken a noble thought,
   Our hearts, in glad surprise,
   To higher levels rise.

The tidal wave of deeper souls
Into our inmost being rolls,
   And lifts us unawares
   Out of all meaner cares.

Honour to those whose words or deeds
Thus help us in our daily needs,
   And by their overflow
   Raise us from what is low!

Thus thought I, as by night I read
Of the great army of the dead,
   The trenches cold and damp,
   The starved and frozen camp—

The wounded from the battle plain,
In dreary hospitals of pain—
   The cheerless corridors,
   The cold and stony floors.

Lo! in that house of misery,
A lady with a lamp I see
   Pass through the glimmering gloom,
   And flit from room to room.

And slow, as in a dream of bliss,
The speechless sufferer turns to kiss
   Her shadow, as it falls
   Upon the darkening walls.

As if a door in heaven should be,
Opened, and then closed suddenly,
   The vision came and went—
   The light shone and was spent.

On England's annals, through the long
Hereafter of her speech and song,
   That light its rays shall cast
   From portals of the past.

A lady with a lamp shall stand
In the great history of the land,
   A noble type of good,
   Heroic womanhood.

Nor even shall be wanting here
The palm, the lily, and the spear,
   The symbols that of yore
   Saint Filomena bore [22].

Summary

The ancient Greeks prepared the way for modern medical science by emphasizing the rational treatment of disease as a natural rather than god-inflicted phenomenon.

During the Middle Ages the medical knowledge of the classical world practically vanished in Western Europe but was preserved in the East, through the efforts of Byzantine and Arab scholars.

During the Crusades several religious and military nursing orders, the most famous of which was the Knights Hospitalers, were established to care for the sick and wounded.

Numerous hospitals were founded throughout Western Europe during the twelfth and thirteenth centuries, largely as a result of monastic and papal reform movements and an accompanying upsurge of intense religious feeling. Hôtels Dieu for the sick and the aged were established by religious orders dedicated to nursing.

The slums of European cities, which grew rapidly in the seventeenth and eighteenth centuries, served as breeding grounds for disease. The mortality rate was high and the average life expectancy extremely short. Hospitals could not satisfy the increasing need for institutional care.

The first hospitals in the United States were founded in the late eighteenth and early nineteenth centuries. During the 1840s, Dorothea Dix dedicated herself to improving the miserable conditions in mental institutions.

By 1850, the few hospitals that existed in America were still regarded as places for the accommodation of indigents and the homeless and not as institutions for care of the general public or as the proper setting for the delivery of babies. The quality of nursing care was notoriously poor, and one of every three surgical patients succumbed to a variety of septic infections called "hospital diseases."

In the 1850s, poor sanitary conditions in the fast-growing cities constituted major health hazards. Bleeding, purging, and the administration of emetics and large quantities of alcohol were standard medical practices of the mid-nineteenth century. Quack medicine proliferated in the period following the Civil War.

In the mid-nineteenth century nurses were often recruited from the most depraved elements of society. Charles Dickens' character Sairy Gamp is an effective caricature of the crude nurse-midwife of that era.

In 1836, Pastor Theodor Fliedner instituted a nurse training course for his Order of Deaconesses in Kaiserswerth, Germany. This innovation marked the dawn of the modern era of nursing and served as a model for future developments.

In 1854, Sidney Herbert, British Secretary at War, appointed Florence Nightingale to organize a corps of nurses for the Crimean War. Miss Nightingale and her staff journeyed to Scutari in order to alleviate the miserable conditions in the Barrack Hospital. By the end of the war, the mortality rate in this hospital had dropped from 60 percent to just over 1 percent.

Florence Nightingale's efforts during the Crimean War helped to eliminate many prejudices against better class women entering nursing. After the war, she returned to England to help found a nurse training school at St. Thomas' Hospital in London, despite strong opposition from the physicians. Her achievements generated the impetus for the development of professional nursing in the modern era.

References

1. Edward Arber, ed., *Thomas Watson Poems* (Westminister: A. Constable & Co., 1895), p. 56.
2. Theodore G. Tappert, Helmut T. Lehmann, ed., trans. *Luther's Works* (Philadelphia: Fortress Press, 1967), vol. 54, p. 296.
3. David Masson, ed., *The Poetical Works of John Milton* (New York: Macmillan Co., 1903), p. 255.
4. John Howard, *An Account of the Principal Lazarettos in Europe; with Various Papers Relative to the Plague; Together with Further Observations on Some Foreign Prisons and Hospitals; and Additional Remarks on the Present State of Those in Great Britain and Ireland* (Warrington: T. Cadell, 1789), pp. 1–259.
5. Pennsylvania Hospital for the Insane, *Annual Report of the Physician-in-Chief and Superintendent to the Board of Managers for 1842* (Philadelphia: The Hospital, 1843), p. 6.
6. Dorothea Dix, *Memorial of D. L. Dix, Praying for a Grant of Land for the Relief and Support of the Indigent Curable and Incurable Insane in the United States* (Washington, D.C.:   Tippin and Streeper, 1848), pp. 1–21.
7. Samuel Sheldon Fitch, *Dr. S. S. Fitch's Health Almanac for 1854* (New York: S. S. Fitch & Co., 1854), p. 19.
8. *Ibid.*, p. 20.
9. Oliver Wendell Holmes, *Currents and Counter-Currents in Medical Science* (Boston: Ticknor and Fields, 1860), pp. 39–40.
10. Charles Dickens, *Martin Chuzzlewit* (New York: Macmillan Co., 1910), p. xxviii.
11. *Ibid.*, pp. 312–313.
12. L. P. Bush, "Reminiscences of the Philadelphia Hospital and Remarks on Old-Time Doctors and Medicine," *Philadelphia General Hospital Reports*, vol. 1 (January, 1890):68–78.
13. M. Adelaide Nutting and Lavinia L. Dock, *A History of Nursing* (New York: G. P. Putnam's Sons, 1907), vol. 2, p. 15.
14. *Times* (London), October 9 and 12, 1854.
15. *Times* (London), November 18, 1854.
16. Eliza F. Pollard, *Florence Nightingale* (London: S. W. Partridge Co., 1902), pp. 74–78.
17. Arthur Hamilton-Gordon Stanmore, *Sidney Herbert of Lea: A Memoir* (New York: E. P. Dutton & Co., 1906), vol. 1, pp. 393–394.
18. Alexis Soyer, *Soyer's Culinary Campaign* (London: G. Routledge and Co., 1857), p. 154.
19. Henry Tyrrell, *History of the War with Russia 1854–1856* (London: W and R. Chambers, 1856), p. 310.
20. *Times* (London), November 20, 1854.
21. R. N. Cust, "Scutari Hospital," *Notes and Queries*, vol. 9 (August 25, 1908):337.
22. Henry Wadsworth Longfellow, "Santa Filomena," *Atlantic Monthly*, vol. 1 (November, 1857): 22–23.

2
Untrained but Undaunted:
The Women Nurses of the Blue and the Gray

*W*hen the United States entered the Civil War in 1861, the concept of the trained nurse was still only being talked about. "It seems strange that what the aristocratic women of Great Britain have done with honor is a disgrace for their sisters on this side of the Atlantic to do," fretted a young Southern girl just after the war's outbreak [1].

The alleged "disgrace" was the nursing of sick and wounded soldiers by women. For decades foreign visitors had remarked that American wives and mothers seemed to have been placed upon a higher pedestal than had their European sisters. All agreed that American women excelled in modesty, humility, piety, and chastity, and American men generally concurred. Woman's place in society was dictated by her physical delicacy: smaller and weaker than man, she was obviously mentally and physically inferior as well. American men did acknowledge, however, that women were morally superior, but that superiority would unquestionably be endangered if they were permitted to engage in activities such as nursing strange men on the battlefield. Yet unless someone did this tremendous job, thousands of sick and wounded would die of neglect.

The American Civil War lasted from April, 1861, to April, 1865, and was fought under conditions guaranteed to swell the casualty lists. Huge armies faced each other, firing as they advanced until one or the other gave ground. Combat, waged with rifled muskets and cannon, was often more dangerous than it would come to be in World Wars I and II. By the time it was over, of a total of 14 million free males nearly two million were under arms—over one million in the blue of the North and over 900,000 in the gray of the South—a higher proportion than in any other American War. Either as battle casualties or as victims of disease, 618,000 men died in service—360,000 Union troops and 258,000 Confederates. Many died on the battlefield; the less seriously wounded faced the hazards of primitive sanitary conditions and a comparatively inept medical corps.

A Lesson from England
Florence Nightingale had been internationally celebrated for her tremendous contributions to the health of the British Army in the Crimean War, and her methods had been called to the attention of America through the publication

of her *Notes on Nursing: What It Is, and What It Is Not;* but the ambition of a few American women to engage in professional nursing service had been more than counterbalanced by opposition from the medical profession.

According to Miss Nightingale, nurse training was necessary in order to:

> ... teach not only what is to be done, but how to do it. The physician or surgeon orders what is to be done. Training has to teach the nurse how to do it to his order; and to teach, not only how to do it, but *why* such and such a thing is done, and not such and such another; as also to teach symptoms, and what symptoms indicate what of disease or change, and the "reason why" of such symptoms.
> Nearly all physicians' orders are conditional. Telling the nurse what to do is not enough and cannot be enough to perfect her—whatever her surroundings. The trained power of attending to one's own impressions made by one's own senses, so that these should *tell* the nurse how the patient is, is the *sine qua non* of being a nurse at all. The nurse's eye and ear must be trained—smell and touch are her two right hands—and her taste is sometimes as necessary to the nurse as her head .... Merely looking at the sick is not observing. To look is not always to see. It needs a high degree of training to look, so that looking shall tell the nurse aright, so that she may tell the medical officer aright what has happened in his absence ... [2].

Of significance to well-meaning amateur nurses was Miss Nightingale's warning that:

> ... life or death may lie with the good observer. Without a trained power of observation, no nurse can be of any use in reporting to the medical attendant. The best one can hope for is that he will be clever enough not to mind her, as is so often the case. ... It is most important to observe the symptoms of illness; it is, if possible, more important still to observe the symptoms of nursing; of what is the fault not of the illness but of the nursing. Observation tells *how* the patient is; reflection tells *what* is to be done; training tells *how* it is to be done. ... Reflection needs training, as much as observation. The nurse is told by the medical attendant, "If such or such a change occurs, or if such or such symptoms appear, you are to do so and so, or to vary my treatment in such or such a manner." In no case is the physician or surgeon always there. The woman must have trained powers of observation and reflection, or she cannot obey. The patient's life is lost by her blunder ... and people say, "The doctor is to blame"; or, worse still, they talk of it as if God were to blame—as if it were God's will. God's will is *not* that we should leave our nurses, in whose hands we must leave issues of life or death, without training to fulfill the responsibilities of such momentous issues [3].

American Women Answer the Call

Almost before the echo of the first gun fired on Fort Sumter had died away, scores of Northern women were offering their services to the government. The President's call for 75,000 militia volunteers on April 14, 1861 was also answered by wives, sisters, and mothers. Within three weeks, 100 women had been selected, out of many hundreds of applicants, to take a special short course of training under physicians and surgeons in New York City. On June 10, 1861, Dorothea Lynde Dix, already well-known as a humanitarian on behalf of the mentally ill, was appointed by Secretary of War Simon Cameron to superintend the women nurses.

*Prevalence of Major Diseases in the Union Army during the Civil War**

Cases		Deaths	
Disease	Number	Disease	Number
Diarrhea and dysentery	1,700,000	Diarrhea and dysentery	44,500
Malaria	1,300,000	Typhoid fever	34,800
Rheumatism	286,000	Pneumonia	20,000
Respiratory	283,000	Malaria	10,000
Typhoid fever	148,000	Smallpox	7,000
Syphilis and gonorrhea	80,000	Tuberculosis	7,000
Pneumonia	77,000	Measles	5,000
Measles	76,000	Meningitis	2,600
Jaundice	70,000	Scurvy	770
Scurvy	47,000	Rheumatism	710
Tuberculosis	29,000	Respiratory	500
Smallpox	19,000	Jaundice	400
Liver abscess	12,000	Yellow fever	400
Sun stroke	6,600	Liver abscess	300
Meningitis	4,000	Sun stroke	261
Insanity	2,600	Syphilis and gonorrhea	150
Yellow fever	1,300	Insanity	90

*United States War Department, Surgeon General's Office, *The Medical and Surgical History of the War of the Rebellion (1861–1865)* prepared in accordance with acts of Congress under the direction of the Surgeon General, Joseph K. Barnes, United States Army (Washington, D.C.: Government Printing Office, 1870–1888), three parts in six volumes.

Her wide-ranging commission, dated April 23, 1861, theoretically gave her the power to organize hospitals for the care of all sick and wounded soldiers, to appoint nurses, and to "receive, control and disburse" special supplies donated by individuals or associations for distribution among the troops [4]. These were sweeping powers far in excess of those enjoyed by Florence Nightingale or, indeed, desired by Miss Dix. Working as an individual, Miss Dix had never had occasion to run an office force or to organize groups of workers for any sort of complicated program.

Even before Miss Dix's appointment was made public, other agencies and individuals had already begun relief work. The Medical Department of the United States Army had begun organizing the hospitals, and the United States Sanitary Commission had been authorized to channel supplies and comforts contributed by the home folks for the boys in the hospitals. Miss Dix was left with the duty of organizing a corps of female nurses.

The eagerly awaited circular issued by Miss Dix in 1862 stated that no woman under 30 need apply. All nurses were required to be plain-looking women, to wear simple brown or black dresses, and to eschew all bows, curls, jewelry, and especially hoop skirts. Good morals and common sense were the only other nec- . essary qualifications. But plain-looking women over 30 were not the only ones who burned with impatience to take an active part in the conflict in which their

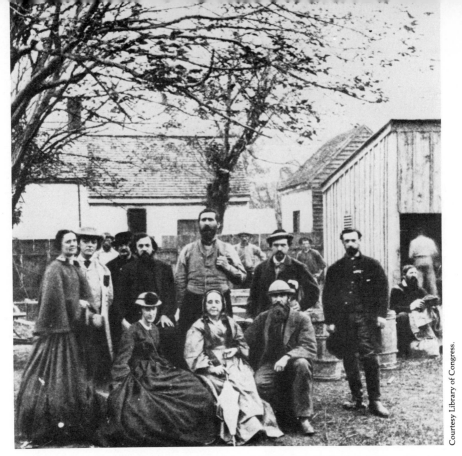

Nurses and officers of the United States Sanitary Commission at Fredericksburg, Virginia, in 1864.

husbands and brothers were engaged. Many who were unable to meet Miss Dix's requirements ignored them completely and nursed all through the war without official recognition or financial compensation: those who had been regularly appointed received $12 a month from the government.

In the North, the war quickly inspired a call for greater numbers of female nurses. On May 11, 1861, *American Medical Times* warned: "We must not wait to learn by bitter experience what the Crimean War taught England and France; and we must now resolve that our intelligence shall anticipate and provide against all dangers not essentially fortuitous." An editorial pointed out that during the Crimean War female nursing in military hospitals had been put to a practical test and that the opinions of those who had witnessed its efficiency were worthy of consideration. Dr. E. A. Parkes, who had been in charge of the Renkioi Civil Military Hospital on the Dardanelles during the Crimean War, was cited as having testified: "I have a very high opinion of female nurses, if they have been trained and are proper nurses." The Medical Director of the British Civil Military Hospital at Smyrna, Turkey, was quoted as having said that "they worked uncommonly well; out of 22 female nurses only one was removed for any misconduct. . . . Several of the ladies that we had did the work uncommonly well, and it would have been very difficult to have got a larger class of severe cases of fever attended to so well by night and day except by the agency of those ladies, who were thoroughly to be relied on, not only from their superior intelligence but also from their devotion to the work" [5].

Mary Livermore (1820–1905), a nurse in the United States Sanitary Commission and later a temperance and suffrage leader, asserted (rather naively) that the pain of men in battle was nothing next to the agony that women felt in sending their loved ones off to war "knowing full well the risks they run—this involves exquisite suffering, and calls for another kind of heroism." Miss Livermore reasoned that the more highly cultivated and refined a volunteering lady was, the better a nurse she would make; such women were sure to submit to inconvenience and privation with much better grace than could those of the lower classes [6].

Walt Whitman Writes of Hospital Nursing

But it was a male nurse, Walt Whitman (1819–1892), who most poignantly captured the mood of nursing amid the carnage of battle. Journeying to Washington in December, 1862, in search of his brother who had been wounded while serving with the Army of the Potomac in Virgina, Whitman found him to be safely recovered but also saw enough of the misery of war to come to the decision to devote himself to nursing wounded soldiers in the various hospitals of the city. He worked entirely on his own, going about the wards to talk with the soldiers or to read to them, bringing gifts of fruit, jelly, and candy, and on occasion writing letters that they dictated for their families.

He also assisted at wound-dressing and eloquently described his work in verse;

Bearing the bandages, water and sponge,
Straight and swift to my wounded I go,
Where they lie on the ground after the battle brought in,
Where their priceless blood reddens the grass, the ground,
Or to the rows of the hospital tent, or under the roof'd hospital,
To the long rows of cots up and down each side I return,
To each and all one after another I draw near, not one do I miss,
An attendant follows holding a tray, he carries a refuse pail,
Soon to be fill'd with clotted rags and blood, emptied, and fill'd again.

I onward go, I stop,
With hinged knees and steady hand to dress wounds,
I am firm with each, the pangs are sharp yet unavoidable,
One turns to me his appealing eyes—poor boy! I never knew you,
Yet I think I could not refuse this moment to die for you, if that
  would save you [7].

Although a few people approved and promoted the idea of women nursing in military hospitals, many others held that it was not the proper thing for a respectable woman to do. Even the liberal Whitman concluded "It remains to be distinctly said that a few or no young ladies, under the irresistible conventions of society, answer the practical requirements of nurse for soldiers" [8]. Physicians

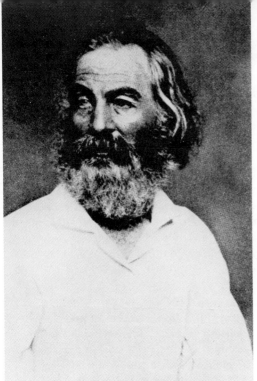

Courtesy Corcoran Gallery of Art.

Walt Whitman. Photograph by Mathew Brady.

disliked the idea of women in the hospitals for other reasons. They charged that many of the women were opinionated, unreliable, and gossipy, and that they showed favoritism. Military hospitals had traditional rules and regulations, and untrained, undisciplined women nurses did not fit in. Thus from the very beginning some of the medical directors refused to accept the nurses Dorothea Dix had assigned to them or, when forced to allow them in, treated the nurses so badly that they soon took ill or quit in disgust.

The duties of a Civil War nurse when she did win admittance to the wards were extremely diverse. Many of the surgeons resented the presence of the women nurses, and because they often came in without instruction in their proper duties, they were frequently assigned to any housekeeping job that needed to be done, such as scrubbing the wards or supervising the laundry. Generally they would be called upon for direct patient care only in moments of crisis, such as when a trainload of wounded troops arrived and hundreds had to be washed, fed, and put quickly to bed. Miss Dix, on the other hand, expected the same women nurses to supervise the wards (including the male nurses), to dress wounds, and to administer medications.

Hospitals and Hospital Routine

Large military hospitals were an obvious necessity throughout the war. Prior to this time, the largest in existence had been the 41-bed facility at Fort Leavenworth, Kansas. Base hospitals, both Union and Confederate, were at first located

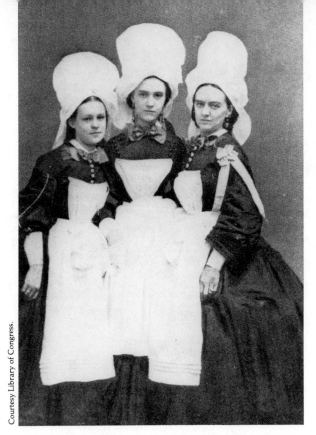

United States Sanitary Commission nurses dressed for work.

in nearby hotels, churches, factories, warehouses, schools, academies, and private dwellings such as the National Hotel, Georgetown College, Odd Fellows Hall in Washington, and the Tishomingo Hotel in Corinth, Mississippi. Unlikely places such as the Georgetown Prison in the District of Columbia, the Capitol Rotunda, church pews, farmhouses, pigsties, and the Lee Mansion were also used to house Federal casualties.

As casualties poured in from the great battles, additional wards were constructed around many of these buildings. Finally, separate groups of roof-ventilated, one-story wooden pavilions were constructed, arranged radially around a central administration building, and connected by covered passageways. The first of these facilities was a barn-like wooden structure erected in 1862 at Parkersburg, West Virginia. Others, such as the Satterlee Hospital in Philadelphia and the Mower Hospital in nearby Chestnut Hill, had over 3000 beds and covered acres of ground. The North eventually had over 200 military hospitals situated in most of the major cities, with 16 located in the Washington area alone.

Rigid rules concerning the work and behavior of both nurses and patients were instituted by the administrative surgeons. At Jarvis Army General Hospital in Baltimore the edicts read as follows:

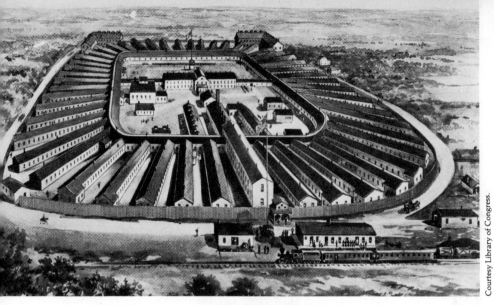

Mower United States General Hospital at Chestnut Hill, Pennsylvania, 1863.

The Nurses will be under the direct supervision of the Stewards and Chief Wardmaster. They will be held responsible for the proper administration of their wards, and they will take particular pains to carry out all orders emanating from the proper authority and pertaining to the welfare of the sick.

The Patients will obey all lawful orders and instructions given them by the Nurses. They will be careful to be cleanly, and their conduct must be exemplary. All swearing, vulgar language, and indecent exposure strictly prohibited, under penalty of severe punishment.

The Wards must be thoroughly ventilated and cleaned once each day, and the beds must be arranged as often as they may require—care being taken to have things in proper condition at all times for inspection.

The Nurses will guard against fires, and not use lights in their wards when not required, and they must report to the Surgeon in attendance on their Wards anything unusual occurring therein.

If a patient needs medical or surgical attendance, the Nurse must at once see the Medical Officer of the Day, and request him to visit the person who is complaining. The interests of the afflicted require that the Nurses be mild and humane in waiting on their more unfortunate companions, and the Surgeon in Charge expects this of them.

Should a patient not in sound mind be troublesome, the Nurses must bear with him: but if a patient, in his rational senses, conducts himself improperly, the Nurse will report the facts in the case to the Medical Officer of the Day.

No lounging on beds or smoking in wards will be tolerated, and each bed, when not occupied, must be covered with clean bedding, which should be thoroughly changed at least once a week.

The Female Nurses must be treated with the utmost respect and it must be remembered, a true soldier is always known by his good conduct.

Convalescents must render every assistance to their companions who are disabled and assist in keeping their wards in proper police.

Patients must take baths at regular intervals, and, when indicated by nature they must have their hair and beard cut, as there is no excuse for vermin in a well-regulated Hospital.

The Female Nurse will not be allowed in the wards after tattoo: and while all lady friends and relatives of Patients will be treated with proper courtesy and respect when visiting the Hospital, they will not be allowed in any of the wards after dark, except by special permission from the Surgeon in Charge [9].

Louisa May Alcott's Experiences

A little book entitled *Hospital Sketches*, written by Louisa May Alcott (1832–1888), gives an idea of some of the work done in Civil War hospitals by volunteer nurses. The time span covered in Miss Alcott's narrative was the month following the Battle of Fredericksburg, fought in December, 1862, and the story amply portrays the character and value of Civil War nursing. The improvised hospital, in what had formerly been a Georgetown tavern and hotel, accommodated about 300 patients, most of whom had been brought in shortly after the battle in all stages of injury and disease.

Having had no preliminary instructions, Louisa Alcott was placed in charge of a ward of 40 beds, where she spent her shining hours washing faces, serving rations, and giving medicine. Her assigned station was a very hard chair, "with pneumonia on one side, diphtheria on the other, two typhoids opposite, and a dozen dilapidated patriots hopping, lying, and lounging about." Miss Alcott concluded that the surgeons were fairly capable; some had seen service in the Crimean War. She did not think that it was necessary, however, for nurses to observe the numerous amputations and other operations, for the "patient needs no care but such as the surgeons can best give." She thought that the nurse's

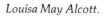

Louisa May Alcott.

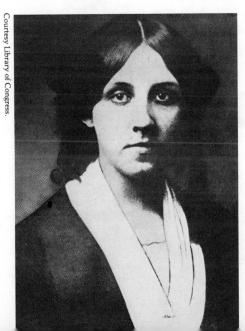

Courtesy Library of Congress.

work should begin afterward. It was then that she should "soothe and sustain, tend and watch" [10].

Apparently, the nurses soon became efficient in their work—at least those of them who remained. Some, as Miss Alcott pointed out, soon learned that nursing was not their vocation. Her experiences revealed that the sick and wounded longed for the care and support of women, and she told many touching stories of the soldiers' gratitude for the help that had been given them by the women nurses.

Louisa walked the rounds at night on her assigned ward, carrying out duties such as dressing Patrick Murray's wounded knee, reading Dickens to Sergeant Bane, and soothing John Suhre—who was meeting his approaching death with great serenity as the hours passed. Sometimes, too, she had time to write letters to the folks back in Concord, signing them "Tribulation Periwinkle" and describing the watchman's long, thin legs and green cloth shoes; Sergeant Bane's attempts to write to Dearest Jane with his unwounded left hand; and the chaplain's gloomy preaching of resignation to men who had breathed death in the air at Fredericksburg. As a budding young writer, she found that there was no longer any need for her to invent situations or search out exotic backgrounds to amuse the neighbors at home. Here, between two rows of iron beds within the papered walls of a hotel room converted to meet the exigencies of war, was material enough for a lifetime of letters and stories.

In her journal for Monday, January 4, 1863, she wrote:

A Union Army hospital ward, Christmas, 1864.

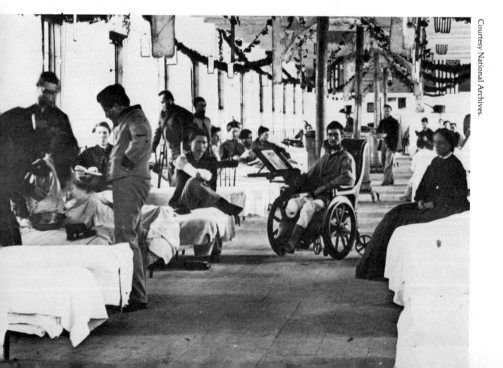

Up at six, dress by gaslight, run through my ward and throw up the windows, though the men grumble and shiver. But the air is bad enough to breed a pestilence, and as no notice is taken of our frequent appeals for better ventilation, I must do what I can. Poke up the fire, add blankets, joke, coax and command—but continue to open doors and windows as if life depended on it. Mine does, and doubtless many another, for a more perfect pestilence box than this house I never saw—cold, damp, dirty, full of vile odors from wounds, kitchens, washrooms, stables. Till noon I trot, trot, trot, giving out rations, cutting up food for helpless "boys," washing faces, teaching my attendants how beds are made or floors are swept, dressing wounds, dusting tables, sewing bandages, keeping my tray tidy, rushing up and down after pillows, bed linens, sponges, and directions until it seems as if I would joyfully pay down all I possess for fifteen minutes' rest. At twelve comes dinner for the patients and afterward there is letter writing for them or reading aloud. Supper at five sets everyone running that can run . . . evening amusements . . . then, for such as need them, the final doses for the night [11].

Mother Bickerdyke's Adventures

Another of the more famous untrained Civil War nurses was a little-educated but superbly shrewd Illinois woman in her 40s named Mary Ann Bickerdyke (1817–1901). She was soon called "Mother" Bickerdyke by the troops. When, in 1861, she agreed to accompany medical supplies to Cairo, Illinois, she promised: "I'll go to Cairo, and I'll clean things up there. You don't have to worry about that, neither. Them generals and all ain't going to stop me. This is the Lord's work you're calling me to do" [12]. Numerous stories were soon being told about "Mother's" exploits:

Looking from his tent at midnight, an officer observed a faint light flitting hither and thither on the abandoned battlefield, and, after puzzling over it for some time, sent his servant to ascertain the cause. It was Mother Bickerdyke, with a lantern. Stooping down [among the dead] and turning their cold faces towards her, she scrutinized them searchingly, uneasy lest some might be left to die uncared for. She could not rest while she thought any were overlooked who were yet living.

Observers recalled a hospital boat:

Incessant cries of "Mother, Mother, Mother" rang through the boat, in every note of beseeching anguish. And to every man she turned with a heavenly tenderness, as if he were indeed her son. She moved about with a decisive air, and gave directions in such decided, clarion tones as to ensure prompt obedience [13].

On one occasion a disrespectful Union officer snapped at Mrs. Bickerdyke: "Madam, you seem to combine in yourself a sick-diet kitchen and a medical staff. May I inquire under whose authority you are working?" Without pausing in her work, Mother answered: "I have received my authority from the Lord God Almighty. Have you anything that ranks higher than that?" This bold nurse was especially outraged when she saw lazy or corrupt medical officers, and the great efforts she made to secure their dismissals were often successful—although such action created much ill will among the physicians. Mrs. Bickerdyke wielded considerable power, largely because of her firm friendship with General Ulysses S. Grant and General William T. Sherman [14].

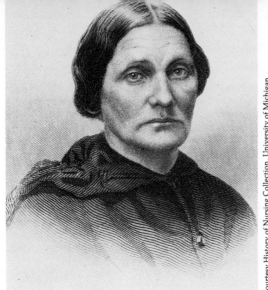

Mary Ann Bickerdyke.

Jane Stuart Woolsey.

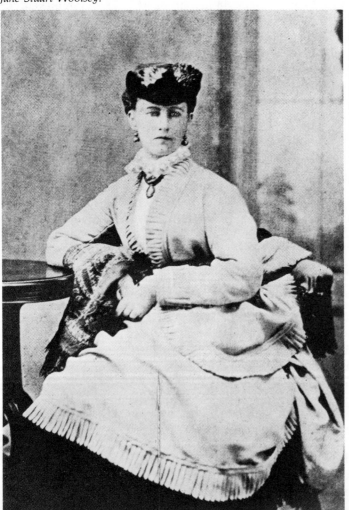

Not all the women nurses of the North were as successful as Miss Alcott and Mrs. Bickerdyke. Surgeons generally condemned them, although seldom citing any specific shortcomings. From their own accounts, the nurses did not always obey orders and sometimes substituted their own prescriptions for those of the physicians. Others fed men the food they wanted but were not supposed to have, while some lavished attention on favorite patients and were jealous of other nurses who had proved themselves more popular. A few took advantage of the weaknesses of the patients in order to reform them or to push upon them a particular brand of religion.

Jane Stuart Woolsey's Observations

According to the astute observations of Jane Stuart Woolsey (1830–1891), a wide range of women were employed as nurses by the government:

Mrs. A_____ had "come out," she told me, "to crush the rebellion," which she conceived she could best do by distributing inordinate quantities of what she called "sanitary jel." She had a difference with Mrs. C_____ who considered pickled cucumbers the proper weapons to use against the enemies of the country.

Mrs. M_____ announced with dignity, at our first interview, "I am a daughter of Pennsylvania. You must have heard of Curtin's daughters? I have been in the field with the [such and such] brigade, in [such and such] battles, and [such and such] skirmishes. All this may be found in my journal." Then, after a little conversation, she revealed that she had given us the "sign" or password of two or three orders, and as none had been "taken up," she inferred we "was all right." She had registered a vow not to serve with any "Sisters," or with members of any secret society . . . . Whether the new administration was disappointing or fresh fields of laurels unfolded elsewhere, I do not know, but in a few weeks "letters requiring her presence at home" arrived and the daughter of Pennsylvania was seen no more [15].

On the other hand, more sensitive but still inadequate "nurses" were much in evidence:

Miss D_____ was an excellent little creature, gently-mannered, delicate, tremulous, full of intense and indignant patriotism. Night and day found her unflagging in her place. Watch had to be kept over her lest she should never get proper food or rest. She could not work by rule or method. She lost the law in the exceptions. She took what she thought "shortcuts," and hand-to-mouth ways of doing what systematic effort would have accomplished in half the time. She was full of goodness and devotion. When she was not at a patient's pillow she was hurrying eagerly to the storeroom to collect comforts and tell the abuses and atrocities she had seen. She thought all military restriction atrocious. She wanted "to go and see Mr. Lincoln about it." Her health gave way before the end of the war and she went home. We were very sorry to part with her. I am afraid the generous heart that beat so fast is scarcely beating now.

Mrs. H_____, wife of the commissary sergeant, one of the most capable and faithful of our men, had a placid, sweet face, that might do a sick man good to look on. Her dress was simple and fresh, her voice, even her manner, quiet and soothing. She had a fever while she was at the Hospital, and was too delicate to do much service in nursing; but it was comfortable to know that she was moving about the ward, restraining roughness by her gentle presence, and overlooking the distribution of the food and stimulants [16].

Nursing on the Mississippi

Another scene of nursing service took place on the muddy waters of the Mississippi, where the war saw the first use of a Navy hospital ship. The steamer *Red Rover*, captured from the Confederates, was converted into a floating hospital to serve with the Federal flotilla. The Western Sanitary Commission contributed $3500 to be used in her conversion, and she was ready for service on June 10, 1862. The medical officer aboard made use of the services of some Catholic nuns who had volunteered to nurse the wounded after the aborted first siege of Vicksburg in 1862. In effect, these Sisters of Mercy were among the first Navy nurses.

The description of the *Red Rover*, given by George D. Wise in the following excerpt from a letter to Flag Officer A. H. Foote, shows that no effort had been spared to provide excellent facilities for the care of the sick.

I wish that you could see our hospital boat, the *Red Rover*, with all her comforts for the sick and disabled seamen. She is decided to be the most complete thing of her kind that ever floated, and is in every way a decided success. The Western Sanitary Commission gave us, in cost of articles, $3,500. The icebox of the steamer holds 300 tons. She has bathrooms, laundry, elevator for the sick from the lower to the upper deck, operating room, nine different water closets, gauze blinds to the windows to keep the cinders and smoke from annoying the sick, two separate kitchens for sick and well, a regular corps of nurses, and two water closets on every deck . . . [17].

Nursing in the South

In the Confederate states the bulk of nursing duty fell into the rough hands of infantrymen who were detailed against their wishes to this type of duty. Many of these men were convalescent soldiers, selected more often because they were not strong enough for field duty than for any degree of aptitude or experience in caring for the sick. Moreover, as they grew well enough to be of any real help they were usually whisked off to their line regiments. This gap in medical care was due to the South's slow recognition of the desirability of women as regular members of the Medical Department of the Army. For the first year and a half of the war, women had worked in the hospitals only as volunteers, and few of them had undergone any sort of training. Not until September, 1862, did the Confederate Congress grant them official status.

In the Confederate states especially there was widespread public prejudice against women serving in hospitals. It was generally held that an occupation involving such intimate contact with strange men was unfit for self-respecting women to pursue. There was no tolerance whatever of young, unmarried women in these positions. "The simple truth is," wrote one Southern lady in withdrawing her application for a nursing position, "that my family is much opposed to my doing so, especially my brothers . . . . The boys have heard so much about ladies being in the hospitals that they cannot bear for me to go" [18].

Valor was exhibited by others not so easily discouraged, however. "I had never been inside of a hospital, and was wholly ignorant of what I should be called

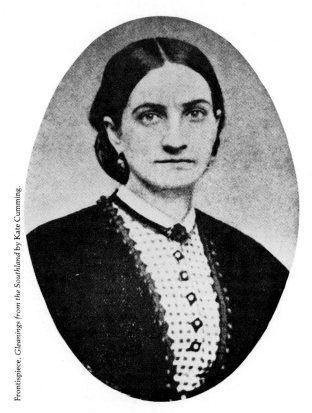

Kate Cumming.

upon to do, but I knew that what one woman [Florence Nightingale] had done another could" wrote Kate Cumming (1828–1909) of Mobile, of her decision to volunteer as a nurse. She later recorded:

There is a good deal of trouble about the ladies in some of the hospitals of this department. Our friends here have advised us to go home, as they say it is not considered respectable to go into one. I must confess, from all I had heard and seen, for awhile I wavered about the propriety of it; but when I remembered the suffering I had witnessed, and the relief I had given, my mind was made up to go into one if allowed to do so [19].

Miss Cumming stayed with the hospital service of the Army of Tennessee after the Battle of Shiloh and served with distinguished ability.

Nursing in the Confederate Army, often under primitive conditions, was exhausting and frustrating work. On November 13, 1864, Miss Cumming, then serving at a hospital in Atlanta, noted in her diary:

Our wounded are doing badly; gangrene in its worst form has broken out among them. Those whom we thought were almost well are now suffering severely. A wound which a few days ago was not the size of a silver dime is now eight or ten inches in diameter.

The surgeons are doing all in their power to stop its progress. Nearly every man in the room where they were so full of jokes has taken it; there is very little laughing among them now. It is a most painful disease, and plays sad havoc with the men in every way. We cannot tempt them to eat, and we have very little sweet milk, and that is the cry with them all. Many a day I have felt as if I could walk any distance to get it for them [20].

Of the work of such female nurses, Dr. S. H. Stout, Medical Director of Hospitals of the Army and Department of Tennessee, wrote:

The gratitude of the soldiers was always manifest whenever these female nurses came into the wards. For they served them as amanuenses by writing letters to the families and friends of the disabled. They prayed for and with them when requested. They cooked appropriate and delicate food for them when needed. They wiped the sweat from the brows of the dying and closed the eyes of the dead. Often entrusted to send the last messages of the dying to their families and friends at home, these faithful matrons never failed to perform their promises [21].

On the other hand, Mary Boykin Chesnut (1823–1886), in *A Diary from Dixie*, reveals the reactions of a more typical woman of the Southern aristocracy, whose sentiments were later effectively mirrored in the experiences of Scarlett O'Hara in *Gone With the Wind*:

August 19th, 1864. Began my regular attendance in the Wayside Hospital. Today we gave wounded men, as they stopped for an hour at the station, their breakfast. Those who are able to come to the table do so; the badly wounded remain in wards prepared for them where their wounds are dressed by nurses and surgeons, and we take bread and butter, beef, ham, hot coffee to them there . . . . They were awfully smashed-up objects of misery, wounded, maimed, diseased. I was really quite upset and came home ill. This kind of thing unnerves me quite. As I came into my room I stood there on the bare floor and made Ellen undress me and take every thread I had on and throw them all into a washtub out of doors. She had a bath ready for me, and a dressing-gown [22].

Evaluation of Civil War Nursing

Close to 10,000 women served as nurses during the war. In the North, the 3214 nurses appointed by Miss Dix and other officials held legal status as employees of the Army and received salaries of 40 cents and one ration in kind each day. A second group of nurses were the several hundred Sisters of Charity or nuns of various orders. A third group consisted of those employed out of necessity over short periods to do the menial hospital chores. A fourth group consisted of black women employed under the General Orders of the War Department at a salary of $10 a month. An estimation of the number of women serving in the third and fourth groups was set by the Federal Pension Office at 4500. A fifth group was made up of an unknown number of uncompensated volunteers. A sixth group consisted of women camp followers. The seventh and last group consisted of women employed by various relief organizations. Very few of these women had actual hospital experience or qualifications other than physical strength and willingness to serve. Probably at least 9000 women performed nursing duties of one kind or another in the North; less than 1000 did so in the South.

Jane Stuart Woolsey in *Hospital Days*, a rare monograph printed for private circulation in 1870, summarized her views of the women war nurses. These views, the result of observation and experience of a woman superintendent of nurses in military hospitals during the war, are probably a fair analysis of the true status and character of the Civil War nurses. "Was the system of women nurses in hospitals a failure?" she asked. Indeed, there had never been any system, she concluded. So far as she knew, the experiment of a compact, general organization was never even tried. Hospital nurses were of "all sorts, and came from various sources of supply; volunteers, paid or unpaid; soldiers' wives and sisters who had come to see their friends, and remained without any clear commission or duties; women assigned by the General Superintendent of Nurses; sometimes, as in a case I knew of, the wife or daughter of a medical officer drawing the rations, but certainly not doing the work, of a 'laundress' " [23].

These women were set adrift in a hospital—8 to 20 of them, slightly educated, for the most part, without training or discipline, without company organization or officers. They did their own "reporting" to the surgeons or to the General Superintendent, which was very much "as if Private Robinson should 'report' to General Grant" [24].

Similarly, a first-hand investigation of the nursing system of the United States Sanitary Commission concluded:

It is to be regretted that a more favorable account of the way in which the nurses have been received and treated in the hospitals cannot be given. They have not been placed, as they expected and were fitted to be, in the position of head nurses. On the contrary, with a very efficient force of male nurses, they have been called on to do every form of service, have been overtasked and worn down with menial and purely mechanical duties, additional to the more responsible offices and duties of nursing. They have encountered a certain amount of suspicion, jealousy and ill-treatment, which has rendered their situation very trying . . . . women nurses in military hospitals . . . are objects of continual evil speaking among coarse subordinates, are looked at with a doubtful eye by all but the most enlightened surgeons, and have a very uncertain, semi-legal position, with poor wages and little sympathy, except from the sick and wounded men they comfort and bless. Nothing but the most patriotic and humane motives could sustain women in this position [25].

Although the nursing system was defective and the doctors did not approve of the women, there were certain parties to the experiment who deemed it an unqualified success: the patients. The basis of the men's approval was not too well reasoned and was rather sentimental and undiscriminating. As one of them replied when asked what he would have: "Anything just so it has a woman's finger on it" [26]. Another recalled:

Connected with our hospital was a lady who acted as matron. She frequently passed through the wards with some delicacy for the sick in her hands; this she gave to such as could take it; often the poor fellow had no stomach for anything, but the pleasure of receiving anything from the fair hands of a woman was too tempting to resist, and down it went, stomach or no stomach. Again she would pass from cot to cot, saying a kind word to each occupant, adjusting the blanket for this one, wiping the sweat from another's brow, and maybe writing to mother or wife for one too feeble to use a pen [27].

In contrast, far too many women flooded Civil War hospitals as merely curious visitors and not in order to render any useful service. According to the account of one Indiana volunteer:

The females . . . go gawking through the wards, peeping into every curtained couch, seldom exchanging a word with the occupant, but as they invariably "hunt" in couples giving vent to their pent up "pheelinks" in heart-rending outbursts of "Oh, my Savior," "Phoebe, do look here," "Only see what a horrid wound," "Goodness, gracious. how terrible war is," "My, my, my. Oh, let's go—I can't stand it any longer." And as they near the door, perhaps these dear creatures will wind up with an audible—"Heavens, what a smell. Worse than fried onions" [28].

A second class of women visitors who frequented the hospitals were generally in the company of "flashy youths got up in the latest style." These women were:

. . . wasp-waisted, almond-eyed, cherry-lipped, finely-powdered damsels, carrying tiny baskets, containing an exquisitely embroidered handkerchief, highly perfumed, and a vial or two of restoratives (to be used in case of sudden indisposition). This batch of "sight seers," do-nothings, idlers, time-killers, fops, and butterflies skip through the hospital and like summer shadows, leave no trace behind [29].

Although lacking a rigorous training for nursing, the more successful Civil War nurses had been driven by sentiment to enter hospital work. They saw nursing in a manner reminiscent of Longfellow, who had immortalized the work of Florence Nightingale in verse.

Postwar Developments

After the war, several of the women who had been nurses helped lead the movement for the establishment of nurse training schools. Prominent among them were the Woolsey sisters—Abby, Jane, and Georgeanna. Abby (1828–1893) wrote one of the first books on the subject, *A Century of Nursing with Hints Toward the Organization of a Training School*, published in 1876. As directress of the Presbyterian Hospital in New York, Jane reorganized the nursing force, while Georgeanna (1833–1906) helped found the Connecticut Training School for Nurses in New Haven in June, 1873.

About this time in England, Florence Nightingale was elaborating on what made a good training school for nurses:

A year's practical and technical training in hospital wards, under trained head-nurses who themselves have been trained to train.

The training of probationers should be as much a part of the duty of the head nurse ("sister") as directing the under-nurses or seeing to the patients.

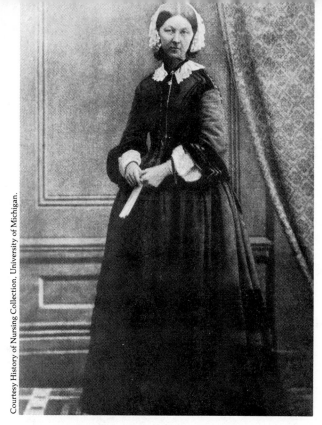

After the Civil War. Florence Nightingale's ideas about the organization of nurse training schools began to receive increasing attention in the United States.

To tell the training, you require weekly records . . . kept by the head-nurses of the progress of each probationer (pupil) in her ward-work, and in the moral qualities necessary in her ward-work; a monthly record by the matron of the results of the weekly records; and a quarterly statement by her as to how each head-nurse has performed her duty to each probationer. The whole to be examined periodically by the governing body.

Clinical lectures from the hospital professors . . . elementary instruction in chemistry . . . physiology . . . and general instruction on medical and surgical topics; examinations, written and oral, at least four of each in the year, all adapted to nurses; as also lectures and demonstrations with anatomical, chemical and other illustrations, adapted especially to nurses—all in the presence and under the care of the matron (Lady Superintendent) and mistress of probationers (Class-mistress and "Home"-sister); together with instruction from a medical instructor, one of the hospital professors and hospital medical staff, specially selected to teach the nurses.

A good nurses' library of professional books, not for the probationers to skip and dip in at random, but to be made careful use of, under the medical instructor and class-mistress.

Classes for a competent mistress to drill the professorial teaching into the probationers' minds; the mistress of probationers to be above all a "home"-sister, capable of making the "home" a real home, and of training and disciplining the probationers there in all good—in moral qualities, customs, and habits, and manners, without which no woman can be a nurse, and in their duty and feeling to God as well as to their neighbor.

The authority and discipline over all the women of a trained lady-superintendent . . . who is herself the best nurse in the hospital, the example and leader of her nurses in all that she wishes her nurses to be . . .

An organization not only to give this training systematically, and to test it by current tests and examinations, but also to give the probationers, by proper help in the wards, time to do their work as pupils as well as assistant-nurses, and above all to make it a real moral as well as nursing probation—for nursing is a probation as well as a mission.

Accommodation for sleeping, classes, and meals; arrangements for time and teaching and work; surroundings of a moral and religious, and hard-working and sober, yet cheerful tone and atmosphere, such as to make the training-school and hospital a "home" which no good young woman of any class need fear by entering to lose anything of health of body or mind; with moral and spiritual helps, and an elevating and motherly influence over all, such as to make the whole a place which will train really good women, who can withstand temptation and do real work, and neither be "romantic" nor "menial." For, make a hospital as good as you will, hospital-nurses require more such helps, and get less, than women either in their own homes or in domestic service.

Every hospital should have and be such a school for training nurses for itself and other institutions . . . [30].

Almost three decades later Mary Livermore, one of the last of the famous untrained nurses of the Civil War, addressed the sixth annual convention of the Nurses' Associated Alumnae (later the American Nurses' Association) on June 10, 1903, and declared "I find all that is within me rising up in this presence in a semi-reverential attitude. A congregation of trained women nurses. Something that in my earlier days I never expected to see." Here was evidence of a new profession that had grown in part from the seeds of the collective Civil War nursing experience [31].

While Mary Livermore and her associates had fought for "the right to tread so softly beside the couch of pain" and "to watch beside the dying in the still small hours of the night," the new generation of nurses was being trained in scientific principles of patient care and was finding that nursing demanded an abundance of strength, both of mind and body [32]. The romantic concept of the nurse as a guardian angel watching through the night and ceaselessly concerned with the patients ignored the reality of the woman with the scrub brush, the lady of soap and water, and the tireless cook of gruel and custard. But, no matter how beholders saw the wartime nurses and their work, the untrained Civil War nurses conferred upon the women of the United States a great practical gift. Although most were amateurs, their humble efforts and the positive effects of their femininity upon the sick and wounded troops made it legitimate for respectable women to enter the field of nursing and helped to create a new profession.

Summary

Prior to the Civil War, nursing was not commonly practiced by respectable American women. At the outbreak of the war, a stigma was attached to the nursing of strange men on the battlefield.

The publication of Florence Nightingale's Notes on Nursing acquainted American women with the concept of professional nursing and stimulated many of them to offer their services to the Union Army after the outbreak of the Civil War in 1861.

Dorothea Dix was appointed by the Secretary of War to superintend the women nurses. She was empowered to organize hospitals, to provide equipment and supplies, and to train nurses.

Miss Dix required female nurses to be at least 30 years old and plain in appearance and dress.

Nearly 10,000 women served as nurses during the Civil War: about 9000 in the North and fewer than 1000 in the South. Several recounted their Civil War nursing experiences in journals.

Military hospitals were small and crowded and consisted of improvised structures. They were usually located in converted buildings such as hotels, churches, factories, and schools.

Nursing services on the first American hospital ship, the Federal steamer Red Rover, *were provided by the Sisters of Mercy.*

The activities of women nurses included household duties such as scrubbing and laundering as well as washing, feeding, putting the patients to bed, dressing wounds, and administering medications.

In the Confederate States there was widespread public prejudice against women serving in hospitals; unmarried women nurses were particularly harassed. Nursing care was furnished primarily by convalescent infantry men.

The lack of formal training programs throughout the war produced a defective system of nursing service. The negative social attitudes toward women nurses was influential in limiting the number of women who served as nurses.

The collective nursing experiences of the Civil War were to be instrumental in the establishment of the first training schools for nurses.

References

1. Kate Cumming, *Journal of Hospital Life in the Confederate Army of Tennessee from the Battle of Shiloh to the End of the War; with Sketches of Life and Character and Brief Notices of Current Events During That Period* (Louisville: John P. Morton, 1866), p. 28.
2. Florence Nightingale, "Nurses, Training of," in Richard Quain, ed., *A Dictionary of Medicine* (New York: Appleton & Co., 1883), pp. 1038–1039.
3. *Ibid.*, p. 1039.
4. L. P. Brockett and Mary C. Vaughan, *Woman's Work in the Civil War: A Record of Heroism, Patriotism and Patience* (Philadelphia: Seigler, McCurdy, 1867), pp. 102–103.
5. *American Medical Times*, vol. 3 (July 13, 1861):25.
6. Mary A. Livermore, *My Story of the War; a Woman's Narrative of Four Years' Personal Experience as Nurse in the Union Army, and in Relief Work at Home, in Hospitals, Camps and at the Front, During the War of the Rebellion. With Anecdotes, Pathetic Incidents, and Thrilling Reminiscences Portraying the Lights and Shadows of Hospital Life and the Sanitary Service of the War* (Hartford: A. D. Worthington, 1889), p. 110.

7. Walt Whitman, *The Works of Walt Whitman* (New York: Funk and Wagnalls, 1968), vol. 1, p. 285.
8. Mark Van Doren, *Walt Whitman* (New York: Viking Press, 1945), p. 557.
9. Rules for Nurses and Patients, Jarvis U.S.A. General Hospital, July 21, 1864 (Placard). Copy in Library of Congress, Washington, D.C.
10. Louisa M. Alcott, *Hospital Sketches* (Boston: Roberts Brothers, 1885), pp. 29–30.
11. Ednah D. Cheney, ed., *Louisa May Alcott: Her Life, Letters, and Journals* (Boston: Little, Brown and Company, 1889), pp. 143–144.
12. Nina Brown Baker, *Cyclone in Calico: The Story of Mary Ann Bickerdyke* (Boston: Little, Brown and Company, 1952), p. 11.
13. Florence Shaw Kellogg, *Mother Bickerdyke as I Knew Her* (Chicago: Unity Publishing Co., 1907), p. 30.
14. Margaret B. Davis, *The Woman Who Battled for the Boys in Blue—Mother Bickerdyke* (San Francisco: Pacific Press Publishing House, 1886), pp. 23–51.
15. Jane Stuart Woolsey, *Hospital Days* (New York: D. Van Nostrand, 1870), p. 45.
16. *Ibid.*, pp. 45–49.
17. Louis H. Roddis, "The U.S. Hospital Ship *Red Rover* (1862–1865)," *Military Surgeon*, vol. 77 (August, 1935): 92.
18. Kate Cumming, *Gleanings from the Southland* (Birmingham: Roberts & Son, 1895), pp. 37–38.
19. Richard B. Harwell, ed., *Kate: The Journal of a Confederate Nurse* (Baton Rouge: Louisiana State University Press, 1959), p. 169.
20. *Ibid.*, p. 169.
21. S. H. Stout, "Reminiscences of Medical Officers of the Confederate Army and Department of Tennessee," *St. Louis Medical and Surgical Journal*, vol. 64 (April, 1893): 228.
22. Mary Boykin Chesnut, *A Diary from Dixie*, ed. by Ben Ames Williams (Boston: Houghton Mifflin Co., 1949), pp. 430–431.
23. Woolsey, *op. cit.*, pp. 41–42.
24. *Ibid.*, p. 42.
25. U.S. Sanitary Commission, *Report Concerning the Woman's Central Association of Relief at New York, to the United States Sanitary Commission at Washington, October 12, 1861* (New York: The Commission, 1861), pp. 18–19.
26. Elvira J. Powers, *Hospital Pencilings* (Boston: Edward L. Mitchell, 1866), p. 172.
27. Charles B. Johnson, *Muskets and Medicine* (Philadelphia: F. A. Davis, 1917), p. 60.
28. "Prock's Letters from Camp, Battlefield and Hospital," *Indiana Magazine of History*, vol. 34 (January, 1938):96.
29. *Ibid.*, pp. 96–97.
30. Nightingale, "Nurses, Training of," *op. cit.*, pp. 1039–1041.
31. Mary A. Livermore, "Nurses in the Civil War," *Proceedings of the Sixth Annual Convention of the Nurses' Associated Alumnae of the United States, June 10, 11, and 12, 1903* (Philadelphia: J. B. Lippincott Co., 1903), pp. 1–6.
32. "Night Duty," *Trained Nurse and Hospital Review*, vol. 41 (October, 1908):239.

3
The Founding of Early Schools of Nursing in America

During the nineteenth century common law and biblical tradition bound women to an inferior status. William Blackstone, the great British legal authority, had disposed of the independent rights of women by the simple common law rule: "The husband and wife are one, and that one is the husband." In this state of wardship, the wife had no control over her property or her person. As a ward, she could not initiate a lawsuit by herself. If she ran away, her husband could forcibly reclaim and beat her as if she were a slave. If she resorted to divorce—where religious factors or complicated legal procedures permitted it —she might lose her home, her children, and her property. A drunken husband might sell his wife's clothing or require her employer—if she were employed— to turn over her earnings to him. It was even possible to circumvent the complaints of a wife overly conscious of her human rights by committing her to an insane asylum.

The American Woman's Place in Nineteenth-Century Society

The sentimentality of the age produced an exaggerated chivalry and etiquette that was as confining to intellectually vigorous or sensitive women as the whalebone corsets and steel hoops that encased their bodies. Popular Victorian literature in America idealized the fragile "lady" subject to self-induced faints, indifferent to exercise after marriage, languidly playing with her ringlets, idly moving her delicate fingers over the piano keys, and faithful to the minute ritual of etiquette books. Corseted tightly in gowns, these women decorated themselves with an assortment of laces, silks, trinkets, and rings, sat in parlors receiving visitors, changed ensembles several times a day, and patiently awaited their fathers' or husbands' return from the hectic business world.

Much of this routine was decidedly unhealthy. Dr. Robert L. Dickinson, a lecturer on obstetrics at the Long Island College Hospital, published a paper in the 1870s in *The New York Medical Journal* entitled "The Corset: Questions of Pressure and Displacement." The results of his experiments and observations of corset pressure indicated that:

The maximum pressure of the corset was 1.625 pounds to the square inch during inhalation, making the total estimated pressure 30 to 80 pounds.

The capacity of expansion of the chest was restricted by one-fifth when the corset was on the body.

The thoracic character of women's breathing was largely caused by wearing corsets.

The abdominal wall was thinned and weakened by the pressure of stays; the liver suffered great direct pressure and was more frequently displaced than any other organ.

The pelvic floor was bulged downwards, by tight-lacing, one-third of an inch [1].

Women were educated for marriage in a patriarchal society that revolved about their fathers and brothers and stressed property relationships rather than marital companionship. Despite women's reproductive functions, they were expected to know as little as possible about sex and to accept without complaint the double standard of morality.

The young lady of gentle background who wanted to step out of a strict family relationship in order to relieve the economic burden on her father or to seek an opportunity for self-development faced a real problem. Aside from teaching as a private governess or in the schoolroom and various types of handiwork such as dressmaking, millinery, and embroidery, few occupations were considered proper for a young woman to undertake.

Mary Wollstonecraft had passionately argued in the name of human dignity for justice to women. In her influential *Vindication of the Rights of Women* (1792), she had urged that the trades and professions be opened to women according to their abilities, that women be educated in coeducational schools, and that society abolish the existing double standard of morality. Some of her ideas were popularized in the 1840s by novelist Charles Brockden Brown and by transcendentalist Margaret Fuller, whose *Women in the Nineteenth Century* (1845) made a plea for the economic and intellectual emancipation of women.

First Instruction of Nurses and Midwives

Intermittently throughout the first 70 years of the nineteenth century, physicians gave lectures to nurses and midwives at state hospitals in several large Eastern cities of the United States, but these activities could in no way be construed as formal courses of instruction. Just before the turn of the century, Dr. Valentine Seaman, an attending physician at New York Hospital, had conceived and initiated the first comprehensive course of instruction for nurses on the North American continent. This achievement was commemorated in an inscription placed below his portrait in the original hospital building: "In 1798 he organized in the New York Hospital the first regular training school for nurses, from which other schools have since been established and extended their blessings throughout the Community"[2]. In connection with the maternity department of New York Hospital, Dr. Seaman, far ahead of his time, had organized a course of 24 nursing lectures, including outlines of anatomy, physiology, and the care of children. The three concluding lectures were published in 1800 as *The Midwives Monitor, and Mothers Mirror, Being Three Concluding Lectures of a Course of Instruction of Midwifery; Containing Direc-*

tions for Pregnant Women; Roles for the Management of Natural Births, and for Early Discovering When the Aid of a Physician is Necessary and Cautions for Nurses, Respecting Both the Mother and Child. To Which is Prefixed, a Syllabus of Lectures on that Subject.

The practice of obstetrics by male physicians had been practically unknown in the British colonies of North America. Early public disapproval of this practice was indicated in 1646 when a man was arrested and heavily fined for practicing as a midwife in Massachusetts. But in 1752, when Dr. James Lloyd returned to Boston after having studied in London and announced himself as a physician and man midwife, he introduced a new vogue. Twenty years later, a female midwife moving from Boston to Salem felt compelled to announce in an advertisement that her reason for relocating was that men midwives were too numerous in Boston. The practice of obstetrics by male physicians became so common that the male designation of "man midwife" had disappeared by 1800.

Another training course for nurses was organized by liberal Quaker physician, Joseph Warrington, who in 1828 established the Philadelphia Lying-in Charity. Dr. Warrington, a graduate of the University of Pennsylvania, was obstetric physician to the Philadelphia Dispensary for the Medical Relief of the Poor, founded in 1786. While working in this capacity he became aware of the urgent need for trained midwives who would deliver, without fee, the babies of poor women in their homes. On May 7, 1832 he formed an additional institution, incorporated as The Philadelphia Lying-in Charity for Attending Indigent Females in Their Own Homes.

Warrington began to train nurses in midwifery during classes with his medical students. Later, he expanded the training program to include experience in medical and surgical nursing. In 1839 Dr. Warrington wrote *The Nurses' Guide, Containing a Series of Instructions to Females Who Wish to Engage in the Important Business of Nursing Mother and Child in the Lying-in Chamber.* Faced with a shortage of applicants, Dr. Warrington in 1854 wrote a six-page pamphlet entitled *An Appeal for the Supply of a Greater Number of Intelligent Women to Become Trained as Nurses for the Sick.*

In Boston Dr. Samuel Gregory helped found a second school for nurse-midwives in 1846. Dr. Gregory published a number of pamphlets urging more courses and better instruction in this field. One of his addresses was entitled *Man Midwifery Exposed and Corrected; or the Employment of Men to Attend Women in Childbirth, shown to be a Modern Innovation, Unnecessary, Unnatural and Injurious to the Physical Welfare of the Community and Pernicious in its Influences on Professional and Public Morality.* Dr. Gregory wanted to make it possible for aspiring women midwives to acquire some scientific knowledge as a basis for their practice. In that era the skill of midwives was acquired primarily through trial and error.

Dr. Gregory also wrote a pamphlet that was published in February, 1846, under the title *Licentiousness, Its Cause and Effects.* It stated that "There is demanded now, as formerly, a supply of female accoucheurs [midwives]; also a class of female physicians, qualified at least to attend to the peculiar complaints of their own sex" [3]. Dr. Gregory cited the success of Mme Lachapelle and Mme Boivin of Paris, who were so skilled in saving the lives of mothers and babies that the mortality among patients confined in Paris was much less than that in Boston. It was obvious that midwives in the United States needed instruction in anatomy and physiology, especially in the physiology of pregnancy and parturition.

Elizabeth Blackwell Opens Medicine to Women

Before the Civil War, females were generally admitted on an equal basis to elementary and secondary schools, but the doors of most colleges were closed to them. A few private colleges for women had been founded, but very few schools (three, to be exact) admitted women to study with men. An application for admission to attend medical lectures at Harvard was made as early as 1847 by Harriet K. Hunt. It was refused, but, without benefit of a medical degree, she gained some success both as a practitioner of hydropathy and as a lecturer on temperance, phrenology, the evils of tobacco, and sex hygiene.

The first woman to study medicine in America—and in modern times the first anywhere—was Elizabeth Blackwell. Born in England in 1821, she immigrated to the United States with her parents, who eventually settled in Cincinnati, in 1832. Upon completion of her education, Elizabeth and her younger sister Emily engaged in school teaching. Elizabeth was first inspired to seek a medical education by the remarks of a friend, dying slowly of cancer, whom she was nursing. "Why don't you study medicine?" the patient asked. "It would have been so much less harassing for me to have been taken care of by a woman than by a man." Elizabeth found it impossible, however, to secure the opportunity to pursue a regular medical education [4].

In 1845 Elizabeth met Dr. Joseph Warrington, the liberal Quaker physician. He believed that there was no obstacle, either mental or physical, to prevent a woman from studying medicine. He suggested to Elizabeth that she wear men's clothing, as Dr. Mary Edwards Walker later did, because he felt that a woman would be less conspicuous in trousers, but Elizabeth refused to disguise herself. Dr. Warrington tried to help her gain admission to one of the Philadelphia medical schools. She followed up her applications with personal appeals to faculty members, but although many of them were impressed by her poise, attractive personality, and obvious preparation, she was turned down by every medical school in Philadelphia and New York and also by Harvard, Yale, and Bowdoin. Disheartened but still determined, she began studying anatomy in the private school of Dr. Joseph M. Allen and applied to several rural medical schools.

All told, Elizabeth Blackwell applied for admission to 12 different medical colleges and was rejected by all of them. Finally, in October, 1847, the faculty of the Geneva Medical School of Western New York decided to refer the decision on her pending application to the all-male student body. The circumstances

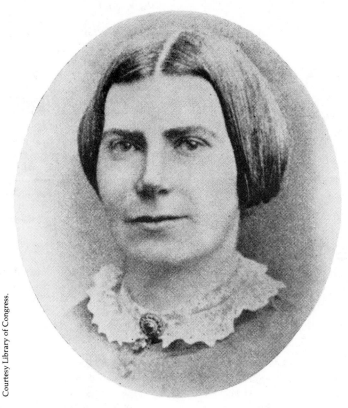

Dr. Elizabeth Blackwell.

surrounding this incident were later recalled by Dr. Stephen Smith, an eyewitness to the proceedings:

> Being located in the country, the class of students was largely made up of the sons of farmers, tradesmen, and mechanics. A common saying among the people of that vicinity was that a boy who proved to be unfit for anything else must become a doctor. And the "royal road" to a medical degree was made remarkably easy at that time. The full term of study was three years and the fee was reduced to a minimum.
>
> Under these circumstances the class contained a large element of rude and uncouth country youths whose love of "fun" far exceeded their love of learning. During the interval of lectures every form of athletic sport might be witnessed with occasional "fisticuff" exercises which elicited ear-splitting shouts of the spectators. Nor did the excitement cease with the commencement of the lecture, but often continued through it to the great annoyance of those students who were attentive and studious. The rowdyism of the class may be realized when it is stated that the residents in the vicinity endeavored to have the college declared and treated as a public nuisance.
>
> One morning early in the session, the Dean of the Faculty, an elderly, courtly, nervous gentleman, entered the classroom with a letter in his hand. He stated, with trembling voice, that the Faculty had received a very important communication from an eminent physician of Philadelphia and he had been requested to lay the letter before the

class and ask its serious and thoughtful consideration of the request which the writer made.

A profound silence fell upon the class-room as he proceeded. The writer stated that he had a lady medical student who had attended a course of lectures in a college in Cincinnati; that he wished to have her attend one of the Eastern city colleges and graduate, but that everyone had refused her admittance; that he thought that a country college like Geneva might not object to her entrance; that if refused admission, she would be compelled to go to Edinburgh, Scotland to graduate. The Dean remarked that the request was so unusual, and so vitally interested the members of the class, that the Faculty decided to submit the question of admission of a woman student to its judgment, and had determined that, if there was one negative vote, the faculty would deny the request.

It was subsequently learned that the Faculty was unanimously opposed to the admission of a woman to the class, but did not care to take the responsibility of opposing the request of the eminent Philadelphia physician. Believing that the class would quite unanimously reject the proposal, the Faculty determined to place their denial upon the action of the students. To make the action of the class certainly negative they decided that a single vote against the request would enable the Faculty to refuse admission.

But the Faculty did not understand the tone and temper of the class. For a minute or two, after the departure of the Dean, there was a pause, then the ludicrousness of the situation seemed to seize the entire class, and a perfect babble of talk, laughter, and catcalls followed. Congratulations upon the new source of excitement were everywhere heard, and a demand was made for a class meeting to take action on the Faculty's communication.

A meeting was accordingly called for the evening, and a more uproarious scene can scarcely be imagined. Fulsome speeches were made in favor of admitting women to all the rights and privileges of the profession, which were cheered to the echo. At length the question was put to vote, and the whole class arose and voted "Aye" with waving of handkerchiefs, throwing up hats, and all manner of vocal demonstrations.

When the tumult had subsided, the chairman called for the negative votes, in a perfectly perfunctory way, when a faint "Nay" was heard in a remote corner of the room. At that instant, the class arose as one man and rushed to the corner from which the voice proceeded. Amid screams of "cuff him," "crack his skull," "throw him down stairs," a young man was dragged to the platform screaming, "Aye, aye! I vote 'aye.' " A unanimous vote in favor of the woman student had thus been obtained by the class, and the Faculty was notified of the result [5].

Initially ostracized by the townspeople of Geneva and by the faculty, both of which groups regarded her as immoral or "queer," Elizabeth gradually won acceptance through her diligence and enthusiasm for her studies. During her 1848 summer vacation she gained admittance to the wards of Philadelphia General Hospital, where she pursued clinical study and helped combat an epidemic of typhus that had broken out among the patients. This experience inspired her to write her M.D. thesis on the subject of typhus and the importance of sanitary measures in combating disease. On January 23, 1849, Elizabeth Blackwell graduated at the head of her class.

Immediately after graduation she went to Europe and spent two years in several hospitals of London and Paris to which she had been able to gain admittance. Perplexed male authorities first suggested, as Dr. Warrington had done, that she dress as a man, but they finally admitted her in her usual attire. She studied at La Maternité, the famous school of midwifery in Paris, where life was "infernal." It seemed that the female midwifery students were "pretty generally the mistresses of the students." While passing through England in April, 1851, she visited Florence Nightingale. One afternoon during the visit, Dr. Blackwell openly admired the facade of Embley Estate, where she was staying. "Do you know what I always think when I look at that row of windows?" said Miss Nightingale. "I think how I should turn it into a hospital and just where I should place the beds" [6].

After studying privately with the demonstrator of anatomy at Cincinnati Medical College, Elizabeth's sister Emily applied for admission to the medical college at Geneva in 1851 but was refused. The faculty agreed that the presence of Elizabeth had resulted in a positive effect upon the conduct and attainments of the other students, but they would not consider Elizabeth's admission as a precedent and feared that if they opened their doors to women in general, they would become unpopular, thereby decreasing their enrollment. After Emily's applications had been rejected by several other medical schools, Rush Medical College in Chicago admitted her as a student for the first year of the program but, after censure by the State Medical Society of Illinois, refused to allow her to proceed with the second year. Finally, her application was accepted by the Medical Department of Western Reserve University in Cleveland, where she was graduated in 1854.

In the meantime, concern over the Blackwells' difficulties had induced a group of Quakers to aid in establishing a full medical course for women in Philadelphia. The Quakers' initiative laid the foundation for the Woman's Medical College of Pennsylvania, which opened in March, 1850, and graduated its first eight female physicians on December 31, 1851. They possessed only a theoretical knowledge of medicine, however, because the College could not gain access to clinical facilities. Although male physicians could not prevent women from studying medicine, they felt unwilling to introduce them, as they did their male students, into the houses of even their poorest patients for fear that they might lose their clientele by making themselves odious as reformers.

The Need for Trained Nurses Recognized

In 1849 the Massachusetts Legislature appointed a state sanitary commission to propose plans for promoting public health. The commission recommended in its report early in 1850 "that institutions be formed to educate and qualify females to be nurses of the sick." To this end, the education of nurses was one of the purposes included in the 1850 charter of the New England Female Medical College. The College's annual catalogues urged aspiring nurses to attend the medical college lectures. A few women were given bedside training in nursing during the three years in which the medical college operated a hospital. A desire to establish a more complete course of instruction for nurses was mentioned in the manuscript records of the trustees, who at one time contemplated applying to the state legislature for funds with which to found a school for nurses [7].

Founding of First Hospitals for Women

After her return from Europe, Dr. Elizabeth Blackwell settled in New York in 1851. The few patients who availed themselves of her counsel did not nearly constitute a "practice." In fact, there was not yet a woman physician in any city who could support herself entirely from the results of her medical studies. No respectable family in a good neighborhood would rent rooms to a "female physician"—a term then used by the notorious New York City abortionist Ann Trow Lohman. Even friends refused to help. Dr. Blackwell was forced to buy a house in order to obtain the privilege of publicly offering her services as a regularly educated physician.

The editor of the *Buffalo Medical Journal* later speculated: "If I were to plan with malicious hate the greatest curse I could conceive for women, if I would estrange them from the protection of women and make them as far as possible loathsome and disgusting to men, I would favor the so-called reform which proposes to make doctors of them" [8]. The *Medical and Surgical Reporter* declared: "The opposition of medical men arises because this movement outrages all their enlightened estimate of what a woman should be. It shocks their refined appreciation of woman to see her assume to follow a profession with repulsive details at every step, after the disgusting preliminaries have been passed" [9]. It was asserted that much of a man's more delicate feeling and refined sensibility had to be subdued before he could study medicine. In females, therefore, such delicate feeling and sensibility would be entirely destroyed. Nowhere were women who sought entrance to medical schools met by legitimate objections. Their requests were simply refused as obnoxious and inspired by an obsession to intrude into affairs outside their proper sphere.

By the mid-1850s, although there were medical schools for women in Philadelphia and Boston, the level of instruction offered was inadequate and in no way comparable to the training given to men. Dr. Blackwell decided that there was a definite need for a medical school to give women proper training and for a hospital to provide women physicians with clinical experience. By speaking frequently before various civic organizations, she eventually obtained financial support from an influential group of New York women. In 1853 Elizabeth Blackwell established a small dispensary in a New York tenement district. Four years later she expanded this facility into the New York Infirmary for Women and Children, with herself and Drs. Emily Blackwell and Marie E. Zakrzewska as administrative physicians. This institution was the first of its kind in the world. It offered care to the poor as a dispensary and soon opened a lying-in ward with 12 beds.

After the opening of The New York Infirmary for Women and Childen on May 12, 1857, Dr. Zakrzewska wrote: "We kept true to our promise to begin at once a system for training nurses although the time specified for that purpose was only six months" [10]. The school began with two nurses, one of whom remained for several years to become invaluable as a head nurse. Dr. Zakrzewska was evidently not satisfied with the success of this first system, however, for eight months later she said:

We . . . began to make more positive plans for the education and training of nurses. The first women who presented themselves . . . were unwilling to give a longer time than four months. During this time they received no compensation except their keeping and one weekly lesson from me on the different branches of nursing [11].

At that time the New York Infirmary was the only place in New York, other than the debauched and dissolute wards of Bellevue and Blackwell's Island, where an unwed pregnant girl could find refuge. When the Civil War broke out, Dr. Blackwell tried to obtain a post with the Union Army, but she was refused. In May, 1861, she converted Bellevue Hospital into a training center for nurses in which an intensive, four-week course prepared about 100 women for service in military hospitals.

Meanwhile, in March, 1861, the Woman's Hospital of Philadelphia was founded as an adjunct to the Woman's Medical College of Pennsylvania. Dr. Ann Preston, a member of the first graduating class of the College, was the leading force behind the establishment of this Hospital, the purpose of which was to treat women's and children's diseases and to provide obstetric care, clinical instruction, and "practical training of nurses." About one year later Dr. Preston instituted a six-month training course for nurses and wrote a pamphlet entitled *Nursing the Sick and the Training of Nurses* in which she described the ideal nurse as having "maternal tenderness, common sense, and a training in 'the greatness of little things.' " She noted that the nurse had to have "the patience of hope [and] the faith of love. The good nurse is an artist!" Nurse training accordingly became part of hospital routine, and although initially the hospital awarded no formal diploma, it was soon able "to send out capable nurses into private families" [12]. The first known graduate was Harriet Neuton Phillips, who completed her training in 1869 and immediately assumed the position of head nurse at the hospital at a salary of $4 per week.

Nursing Service Personnel Woefully Inadequate

During the 1860s the nursing service at most hospitals was haphazard and disorganized. While some women developed an aptitude for nursing and achieved positive results in caring for the sick, the majority of nurses at that time were uneducated and often morally unfit to assume responsibility for patient care. This was especially true in large city hospitals, where nurses were often recruited from among the poor who had sought shelter in almshouses.

At Bellevue Hospital in New York the wards were staffed by former inmates of the workhouse on Blackwell's Island called "ten-day women." Arrested for public drunkenness or disorderly conduct and sentenced to 10 days in the workhouse, they were paroled as soon as they had recovered sufficiently to be of service, provided that they agreed to undertake nursing in the Bellevue wards. One of these so-called nurses was enlisted for every 20 patients, a proportion that was increased in times of severe epidemic.

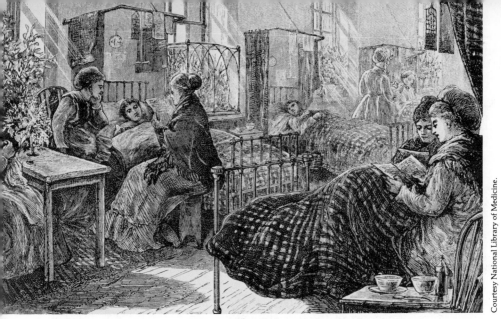

Convalescents attending the sick, about 1870.

In American hospitals of the 1850s, religious orders provided exemplary nursing service.

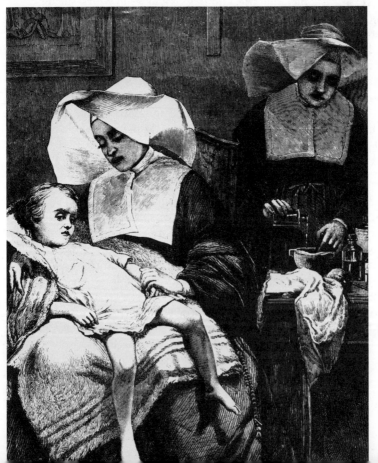

The Philadelphia General Hospital employed so few nurses that it could not adequately care for the patients. Sometimes the nurses' inability to read directions on medicine bottles resulted in unexpected disasters and even in loss of life. Little more could be expected of these nurses, however, when one examined the conditions under which they were forced to live. In 1866 the Hospital's warden, Dr. T. N. McLaughlin, wrote:

While we have some excellent nurses, some that cannot be improved upon, the majority are not what we desire. With a few exceptions we have been obliged to utilize the convalescent patients, who have had no training, and from their previous habits and vocations do not possess the requirements to make good nurses. They are illiterate and have never been accustomed to any refinement, and that feeling of sympathy which is so essential is entirely wanting. They are . . . compelled to sleep in small, overcrowded and ill-ventilated rooms adjoining the wards, and in some instances in the wards. Four or five persons are often crowded into one room that is only of sufficient size to accommodate one, where they inhale the impure atmosphere of the hospital and are annoyed by the cries and moans of the suffering . . . [13].

Most of the better American hospitals utilized the services of Catholic sisters and Protestant deaconesses. Saint Luke's Hospital in New York, for example, had been staffed, since its foundation in 1853, by a Protestant order of nurses, and a similar order provided care in the Syracuse Hospital. Even though these nursing sisters were far superior to the women otherwise hired, they were still untrained, and their best intentions were no substitute for adequate knowledge of medical procedures.

Physicians Express Need for Trained Nurses

At the 1868 meeting of the American Medical Association, the AMA President, Dr. Samuel D. Gross, advocated the training of nurses:

I am not aware that the education of nurses has received any attention from this body; a circumstance the more surprising when we consider the great importance of the subject. It seems to me to be just as necessary to have well trained, well instructed nurses as to have intelligent and skillful physicians. I have long been of the opinion that there ought to be in all the principal towns and cities of the Union institutions for the education of men and women whose duty it is to take care of the sick and to carry out the injunctions of the medical attendant. There is hardly one nurse, of either sex, in twenty who has a perfect appreciation of the requirements of the sick room, or who is capable of affording the aid and comfort so necessary to a patient when oppressed by disease or injury. It does not matter what may be the skill of the medical practitioner, how assiduous or faithful he may be in the discharge of his functions as guardian of health and life, his efforts can be of comparatively little avail unless they are seconded by an intelligent and devoted nurse. Myriads of human beings perish annually in the so called civilized world for the want of good nursing [14].

The following year Dr. Gross presented a committee report that called attention to the absence of organized efforts to upgrade nursing care. This report

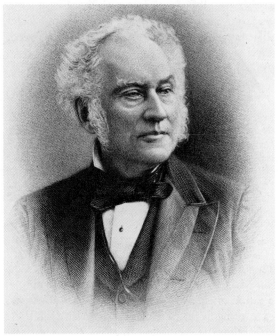

Courtesy National Library of Medicine.

Samuel D. Gross, M.D.

emphasized the importance of nursing care and concluded that nursing should be of universal interest because of its impact on every class of society and its importance as a complement to the services of physicians everywhere. Dr. Gross also recounted the history of nurse training efforts in other countries and referred to the large number of women in the United States who were potential candidates for such training. In conclusion he suggested that schools of nursing be attached to hospitals, that instruction be provided by the medical staff and by the resident physician of each hospital, and that nursing schools be formed under the aegis of county medical societies throughout the nation.

Popular Agitation for Nurse Training

For years Sarah Josepha Hale of Philadelphia edited the popular women's magazine *Godey's Lady Book,* which had a monthly circulation of more than 150,000. Although this magazine was devoted mainly to fashion plates and sentimental tales, Mrs. Hale encouraged middle-class women to learn to enjoy their leisure time without inhibition by discarding their tight corsets and engaging in activities such as swimming, horseback riding, sponsoring and patronizing public playgrounds, and enjoying the family "picnic"—a term which she popularized. More importantly, she influenced the generations before and after the Civil War to create greater social and educational opportunities for women. In the spring of 1871 Mrs. Hale made a plea for "lady nurses":

Much has been lately said of the benefits that would follow if the calling of [the] sick nurse were elevated to a profession which an educated lady might adopt without a sense of derogation . . . . There can be no doubt that the duties of a sick nurse, to be properly performed, require an education and training little, if at all, inferior to those possessed by members of the medical profession. To leave these duties to untaught and ill-trained persons is as great a mistake as it was to allow the office of surgeon to be held by one whose proper calling was that of a mechanic of the humblest class . . . Every medical college should have a course of study and training especially adapted for ladies who desire to qualify themselves for the profession of nurse; and those who had gone through the course, and passed the requisite examination, should receive a degree and diploma, which would at once establish their position in society. The "graduate nurse" would in general estimation be as much above the ordinary nurse of the present day as the professional surgeon of our times is above the barber-surgeon of the last century.

When once the value of the "graduate nurses" became known, there is no doubt that the demand for them would be very great. Every village of a thousand inhabitants would, with the country about it, give occupation for two or three, at least. In any case of severe and protracted illness, their services would be called for as a matter of course, when the circumstances of the family allowed it . . . .

There would be the further advantage that the nurse would not be an ignorant and unrefined person, with whom association would be unpleasant, but an educated lady, who would form an acceptable addition to the family circle during a period of anxiety and trouble—one who could give useful counsel on many subjects besides those of the sick chamber, and who would know how to economize not only her own health and strength, but the health and strength of the household . . . . In short, whenever such a profession is once established, it will soon be deemed as useful and respectable as any other [15].

The following year Dr. J. P. Chesney of New Market, Missouri declared:

As a nurse a woman's physical capacities are incomparably superior to those of man . . . . Who ever heard of a woman succumbing to the toils and exhausting vigils incident to nursing those in whom she was interested? Her eye is never closed, her ear is never deaf, her feet are never weary while the necessities of the sick have a claim upon her. The morning's dews or the gloom of midnight deter her not from her humane ministrations; no one like her can smooth the painful couch, make sweet the bitter draught, or calm the aching heart; no one so ready to gratify the childish caprices or soothe the distempered imagination when "thick coming fancies" oppress the troubled brain. In fact, it would appear that there is a strange compatibility between women and the chamber of the sick; their benevolence relieving it of many of its terrors, while in its solemn precincts they learn, and teach, those lessons of humility and self-sacrifice [16].

At about the same time, Dr. Horatio Storer in his pamphlet *Nurses and Nursing* clearly described the organization of nursing schools as they would exist in the following decade: "There must, sooner or later, be established, in connection with all large hospitals, scholarships, as it were, for nurses, corresponding somewhat to those already provided for ambitious medical students, who, for six months or a year, receive the appointment of resident or house physician" [17]. Dr. Storer believed that many capable women would gladly offer their services for room and board only, in exchange for the privilege of caring for patients and for a certificate indicating the faithful completion of hospital training.

Birth of the First Training School for Nurses

The associate of the Blackwells, Dr. Marie Zakrzewska (or "Dr. Zak," as she was called), also exerted a profound influence upon nursing. Born in Berlin in 1829, she demonstrated at an early age a keen interest in medicine. In 1851 she graduated from the school for midwives at the Charité Hospital in Berlin, where she obtained the appointment of chief midwife and professor in the following year. The knowledge and experience that she gained from this position increased her desire to practice medicine. Since German medical schools refused to accept her, however, she decided to immigrate to the United States, where she expected to find a more tolerant attitude toward women wishing to study medicine. In May, 1854, she was introduced to Dr. Elizabeth Blackwell, who advised her to learn English and secured her admission to the Medical Department of Western Reserve University. Two years later, in March 1856, she received her M.D. degree.

Marie Zakrzewska, M.D.

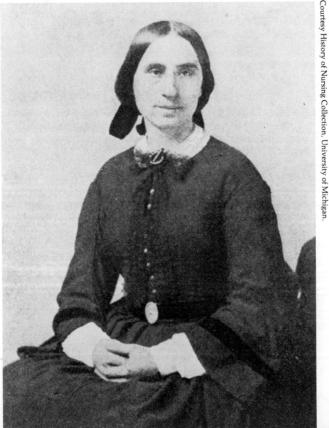

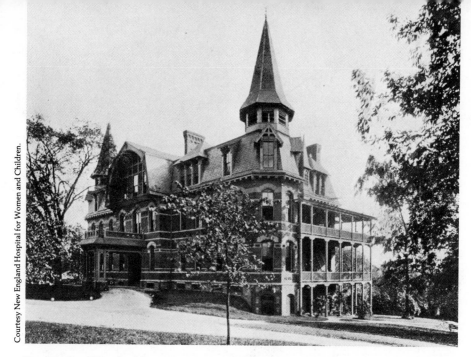

New England Hospital for Women and Children, about 1873.

After working with the Drs. Blackwell for two years at the New York Infirmary, Dr. Zakrzewska in 1859 accepted an appointment from the New England Female Medical College of Boston as professor of obstetrics and resident physician of a proposed woman's hospital. After a dispute with the College's administrators, she succeeded in founding her own institution, the New England Hospital for Women and Children, which opened July 1, 1862. Its act of incorporation expressly stated that the training of nurses was to be one of its fundamental purposes. In connection with the nurse training course, the board of directors proudly announced: "We offer peculiar advantages for training nurses for their important duties, under the superintendence of a physician" [18]. Students were required to attend the course for six months. After a probationary period of one month, they were granted a small wage, board, and laundry service. Despite these incentives, few women were willing to invest the required six months' time.

Because Dr. Zakrzewska experienced difficulty in attracting qualified female physicians for the new hospital, she began the practice of employing one female premedical student in the wards each year in order to give her practical experience and to induce her to return to the hospital upon completion of her medical studies. In 1867 Susan Dimock, a young Southern girl of 18, came to the hospital for such preparation. Acting on the advice of Dr. Zakrzewska and Dr. Lucy Sewall, both of whom recognized her outstanding potential, she applied successfully to the medical school of the University of Zurich.

Four years later, in 1871, Miss Dimock graduated with high honors—the the sixth woman to obtain a medical degree from Zurich between 1867 and

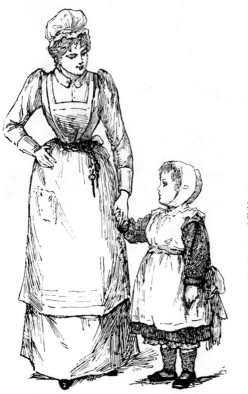

Courtesy New England Hospital for Women and Children.

Student nurses at the New England Hospital for Women and Children aided the head nurse in all aspects of nursing care.

1872. The topic of her dissertation, written in German, was "The Different Forms of Puerperal Fever." After graduation she spent six months in Vienna and three in Paris for further study and observation in hospitals. In July, 1872, she returned to the United States to assume the post of resident physician at the New England Hospital for Women and Children. Dr. Dimock's three-year appointment provided her with an annual salary of $300, board, an office in the hospital, and the privilege of a private practice. As a result of her superb training in Europe, she brought with her the most recent diagnostic methods, the correct procedure for taking medical history, and the latest surgical techniques.

Immediately after completion of a new hospital building in July, 1872, the New England Hospital nursing course was expanded into the "first general training school for nurses in America." Organized and equipped to give full general training along modern, practical lines, it employed a staff of physician-instructors in all medical branches and offered a hospital service program that included medicine, surgery, and obstetrics. The school's administration announced in its 1872 report:

In order more fully to carry out our purpose of fitting women thoroughly for the profession of nursing, we have made the following arrangements. Young women of suitable acquirements and character will be admitted to the hopsital as school nurses for one year. This year will be divided into four periods: three months will be given respectively to the practical study of nursing in the medical, surgical, and maternity wards, and [of] night nursing. Here the pupil will aid the head nurse in all the care and work of the ward under the direction of the attending and resident physicians and medical students. In order to enable women entirely dependent upon their work for support to obtain a thorough training, the nurses will be paid for their work from one to four dollars per week after the first fortnight, according to the actual value of their services to the hospital. A course of lectures will be given to nurses at the hospital by physicians connected with the institution, beginning January 21st. Other nurses desirous of attending these lectures may obtain permits from our physicians. Certificates will be given to such nurses as have satisfactorily passed a year in practical training in the hospital.

The report continued:

As long as we were in the old hospital, with space so inadequate to our needs, we were able to carry out only partially our plans for training nurses, but finding the demand so constant for those we have already trained, and the need of good nurses so great in the community, we have now determined to use our increased facilities to the utmost, and each year to send out a small band of trained nurses [19].

While in Europe Dr. Dimock had visited Florence Nightingale, from whom she had learned something about the essentials of a legitimate training school. Miss Nightingale had stressed the organization of the nursing staff along authoritarian lines. Just as the superintendent regarded the probationers as her children, the head nurses, who were responsible for training both the probationers and student nurses, were supposed to consider their charges as students rather than servants. In addition, physicians were to lecture once a week on pertinent medical and surgical topics.

Based on these guidelines the first American nurse training school to offer a graded course in scientific nursing began, with five probabtioners, on September 1, 1872. The students worked from 5:30 A.M. to 9:00 P.M. and slept in rooms placed near the ward so that they could be quickly awakened for emergencies during the night. In return for their one year of service, they received 12 lectures, given by several women physicians on medical, surgical, and obstetric nursing, which were organized as follows: Dr. Marie Zakrzewska, one lecture on "Positions and Manners of Nurses in Families"; Drs. Emily and Augusta Pope, four lectures on "Physiological Subjects"; Dr. Lucy Sewall, one lecture on "Food for the Sick"; Dr. Susan Dimock, two lectures on "Surgical Nursing"; Dr. Helen Morton, two lectures on "Childbed Nursing"; Dr. Emma Call, one lecture on "The Use of Disinfectants to Prevent Contagion"; and Dr. Marie Zakrzewska, one lecture outlining "General Nursing."

The nursing students received a small allowance upon completion of a quarter of the 12-month course. On October 1, 1873, the first diploma was awarded to 32-year-old Linda Richards—America's first professionally trained nurse. It must be remembered, however, that the New England Training School was

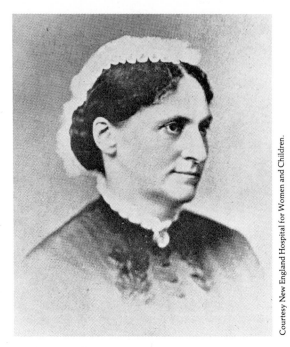

Courtesy New England Hospital for Women and Children.

Linda Richards.

not located in a general hospital, that the training course was short, and that the lectures were comparatively meager. Dr. Dimock's untimely death in 1875 aboard the steamship *Schiller*, which sank en route to England, cut short a promising career, but not before she had organized a definite curriculum and working plan for the School. As a memorial, a street adjacent to the hospital was renamed in her honor.

Establishment of the First Nightingale School

Even as Linda Richards was graduating, three more nurse training schools were opening in New York, New Haven, and Boston. The New York Training School, which was attached to the Bellevue Hospital, was the first in the United States to be modeled after Florence Nightingale's school at the famous St. Thomas' Hospital in London.

In 1872 the prominent New York socialite Louisa Schuyler, a descendant of both Alexander Hamilton and Revolutionary War major-general Philip Schuyler, convened a group of society ladies in her home. Organized as the State Charities Aid Association of New York, these citizens regularly visited the various charitable institutions of the city and took note of needed reforms. One committee of the Association was assigned to visit Bellevue Hospital. Including such prominent women as Mrs. Joseph Hobson, Mrs. William H. Osborn, Miss Julia Gould, and the Misses E. and B. Van Rensselaer, the com-

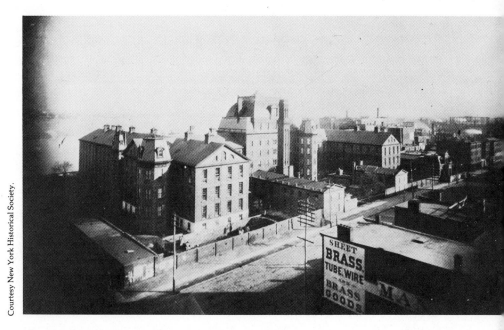

Courtesy New York Historical Society.

Bellevue Hospital, about 1880.

mittee followed a route from the Schuyler home to Bellevue Hospital that was described as "the fashionable promenade of the city."

At Bellevue the visitors found 900 patients, most of them in terrible distress and in need of a great deal more nursing care. Many were forced to sleep on the floor, without blankets or pillows, because there was no extra bedding except for the unwashed blankets of recently deceased patients. There were no night nurses and only three night watchmen for hundreds of patients. These watchmen sometimes drugged patients with morphine to keep them quiet and to counteract the stimulants that they had taken during the day. In the kitchen, tea and soup were frequently made in the same boiler. Moreover, the coffee was nauseating and the beef dry and hard. "Special diets" generally existed in name only. In the event that they were cooked they stood little chance of reaching the patients, for much of the food was confiscated on its way up from the kitchen by the "ten-day" women who had been committed to the workhouse on Blackwell's Island for drunkenness and disorderly conduct and had subsequently been transferred to Bellevue Hospital as "nurses."

The official statistics were dismal. In 1871, about 15 of every 100 patients had died on the premises. Of 1102 hospital deaths, 69 were attributed to infections acquired from within the wards. The risk of delivering a baby at Bellevue was high: 33 of 376 mothers (or 9 percent) died of puerperal fever. Surgery was even more dangerous. During the 18 months beginning in January, 1872, there were 58 amputations, 28 of which ended in deaths because of shock, hospital gangrene, exhaustion, and tetanus. Amazingly, although many of these operations were relatively simple, three of five hand amputations proved fatal, as did five of seven arm removals, and four of eight foot amputations. The committee recalled the words of Florence Nightingale, who had insisted, "The most delicate test of sanitary conditions in hospitals is afforded by the progress and termination of surgical cases after operation, together with the complications which they present"[20].

In view of these gloomy statistics the committee concluded that to delay a massive reform of Bellevue Hospital would be "simply criminal." The members were convinced that the Hospital could not function effectively until the nursing service had been completely reorganized. Inspired by the success of similar projects begun in England by Florence Nightingale, they boldly attacked the problem but received little encouragement from the medical profession. One distinguished physician stated: "I do not believe in the success of a training-school for nurses at Bellevue. The patients are of a class so difficult to deal with, and the service is so laborious, that the conscientious, intelligent woman you are looking for will lose heart and hope long before the two years of training are over." A clergyman who was well acquainted with the Hospital echoed this opinion and thought it "not a proper place for ladies to visit" [21].

In order to organize a nurse training school in the most effective manner, the committee dispatched Gill Wylie, a young resident physician, to London, where he observed the methods of the training school which Florence Nightingale had established at St. Thomas' Hospital. Returning with a favorable impression of this school, Dr. Wylie strongly recommended that the one at Bellevue Hospital be similarly organized, even though he realized that some features of the British system would be unsuitable for it. He even suggested that the governing board of Bellevue invite the school at St. Thomas' Hospital to send some of its nurses to New York to assist in the establishment of an American counterpart.

This recommendation was referred to a committee consisting of Drs. James R. Wood, Alonzo Clark, and Stephen Smith. Only Dr. Smith favored the complete implementation of Dr. Wylie's proposals. By contrast, Drs. Wood and Clark maintained that women who had received medical training would automatically consider themselves capable of practicing medicine and would immediately go out into the country to do so. Since state laws regulating medical practice were rather lax at that time, it was theoretically possible for a trained nurse to practice as a physician without legal interference. In order to alleviate fears of local physicians, the exact limits of the nurses' duties were defined with particular care.

Fully aware of the controversial nature of this plan, Miss Schuyler's group raised more than $23,000 to establish the nurse training school and rented a house near the Hospital for the nurses to live in. Finding a person capable of taking charge of the new school, however, proved to be an arduous task. "Sister Helen" Bowden of the Sisterhood of All Saints was finally selected to fill this position.

Recruiting enough qualified students for the school, which opened on May

24, 1873, was difficult because strict admission requirements deterred many who might otherwise have come. These requirements included a solid previous education, strong constitution and freedom from physical defects (including those of eyesight and hearing), and excellent references. The recruiting effort for the first class was far from satisfactory because, of 73 applicants from states as far away as California, only 29 were considered worthy of acceptance. Of these, 10 were dismissed for various reasons before the first nine months had expired.

The story of the gradual replacement of the old order was later recounted by Dr. Stephen Smith: "The school soon proved so efficient that it was not long before the old nurses were entirely supplanted"[22]. These displaced women left in a foul disposition, however, venting their wrath on Bellevue authorities with coarse expletives and throwing stones at the new student nurses.

Until this experiment proved to be a success or failure, the students were given charge of only the women's wards at Bellevue. Even though conditions in the men's wards were far worse than in the women's, there had been no serious thought of asking "lady nurses" to care for male patients. When Dr. Smith, who had found the student nurses so successful with his female patients, proposed sending them into his male wards, he encountered tremendous opposition from the medical board. It was argued that the male patients of Bellevue were "nothing but a raft of bums from Five Points and the Bowery, and to send women nurses among them would be an outrage"[23]. Undaunted, Dr. Smith sent one of the students to work on the male wards. She proved to be quite successful, and within a week additional students improved conditions to a level comparable with those in the female wards. This improvement was so remarkable that Dr. James Wood, who at first had been particularly opposed to the new idea, soon asked that nurses be assigned to his male wards.

The course of training consisted of dressing wounds, applying fomentations, making beds, positioning, bathing, and caring for helpless patients. Moreover, the nursing students were taught to prepare and apply bandages, make rollers, and line splints. They also learned how to cook and serve food for patients. Instruction in the best methods of securing fresh air and of warming and ventilating the sickroom were stressed. Exemplary deportment, patience, perseverance, and obedience were expected as a matter of course throughout the training program.

Although the program lasted two years, the trainees received instruction for the first year only. During this time they attended lectures by experienced physicians and were considered to be under the supervision of the superintendent of the school. These first-year students received $10 per month after a probationary period of one month. During the second year, the salary of the students, who now simply provided service without receiving additional instruction, was slightly increased. Not until each student had satisfactorily completed the entire two-year program did she receive her coveted, ornate diploma.

The Connecticut Training School For Nurses
at New Haven State Hospital

Meanwhile, the New Haven State Hospital was also starting a nurse training school based on the Nightingale plan. On May 21, 1873, the founding committee for what was to become the Connecticut Training School for Nurses held its first formal meeting to appoint a superintendent of nursing. This was not an easy task, inasmuch as the pool of experienced nurses from hospitals that had conducted nursing courses was very small. After many inquiries and visits the committee selected Miss Bayard, superintendent of the recently upgraded Training School for Nurses of the Woman's Hospital of Philadelphia. Of 21 student applicants, six were finally selected, but two of these failed to appear because of illness when the course of instruction began on October 6, 1873.

The four student nurses and their superintendent immediately found themselves faced with demanding duties. The north ward of the hospital was filled with 10 typhoid fever patients. The founding committee's journal relates:

Our nurses for the first five weeks did very hard work. The fever cases were severe, some of the patients entirely delirious, throwing themselves out of bed, or getting up and dragging their sheets and blankets out into the entry. . . . The four nurses in turn sat up night after night and did duty during the day in the other wards or diet kitchen, where the special diet for thirty [patients] was cooked and distributed to all parts of the hospital by the nurse who cooked it [24].

One of the first problems that had to be resolved was the elimination of the students' trailing skirts and superfluous jewelry, which did not constitute proper nursing attire. Dr. Francis Bacon later recalled: "I remember one morning I was met by the head nurse with the despairing question, 'What *shall* I do with Miss_____? She appeared at breakfast with all her long hair curled down her back' ". Dr. Bacon suggested the use of large caps and soon no one needed to be told that elaborate hairstyles were out of place in a sickroom. He further related that when the hospital surgeons were assured of the provision of good nursing care to combat the danger of "hospital disease," they began to undertake surgery never before attempted in the hospital [25].

On March 26, 1874, six months after the school opened, the hospital committee, which had ordered an evaluation of the performance of the student nurses, concluded: "In regard to the work undertaken by the school in the care of the sick and disabled, we find for it many general commendations. The physicians and surgeons report a decided improvement in the nursing, and speak strongly of the good already accomplished." By the end of the first year, nearly 100 applications for admission to the school were on file, but the majority of the young women withdrew their names after learning of the large amount of work required [26].

By the end of the second year of operation the Connecticut Training School for Nurses was able to supply trained graduates for the field of private duty nursing; by the fourth year it began to graduate candidates for jobs as superintendents of nursing in other hospitals; and by the sixth year the school faculty had published their own handbook of nursing.

The Boston Training School for Nurses

In November, 1873, the third American school of nursing modeled after the Nightingale system began operation in Boston as the Boston Training School for Nurses at Massachusetts General Hospital. The *Report of the United States Commissioner of Education for 1873* contains the following description of this school, which was

giving a systematic training to women who wish to become nurses. With a small and manageable number for a beginning, an influential body of ladies and gentlemen has made arrangements with the trustees of the Massachusetts General Hospital for exercise of the pupils in their wards. Lodging and boarding at a house near the hospital, these pupils are to receive instruction there in the theoretic part of their profession and in the preparation of diet for the sick, and for a year will practice in the wards under the direction of the hospital-physicians. During that year they will receive $10 a month for clothing and personal expenses. At the expiration of the year they will become full nurses and receive as such a salary sufficient for their support, but must remain another year for further practice and instruction. This full term of two years completed, they will, if approved, receive diplomas certifying their knowledge of nursing, their physical ability, and good character [27].

The first superintendent, Mrs. Billings, was a former nurse with the Union army during the Civil War. She was succeeded three months later, in January, 1874, by Mary Phinney von Olnhausen, a German baroness who had also served as a volunteer nurse with the Union army and later with the German army during the Franco-Prussian War. Only one of the staff physicians at Massachusetts General supported the establishment of the nurse training school. Because the others refused to cooperate in providing instruction for the student nurses, women physicians from the New England Hospital for Women and Children came over to help give the weekly lectures. In November, 1874, Linda Richards became superintendent of nurses at an annual salary of $600 and continued in this capacity for the next two and one-half years.

Throughout the next decade Linda Richards enjoyed phenomenal success in organizing training schools for nurses. Linda, who had served as night superintendent at Bellevue Hospital during its first year (1873), not only supervised the early development of the Boston Training School for Nurses at Massachusetts General Hospital but also organized or reorganized five other important schools in subsequent years, including the new school at Boston City Hospital in 1878. It is significant that these early "Nightingale" training schools for nurses, each of which was affiliated with a general hospital, enjoyed semi-autonomous status. Very soon, however, this trend toward autonomy was reversed as nursing "schools" tended to become the nursing service departments of their respective hospitals. Because these early schools lacked substantial endowments and permanent independent budgets, they were totally

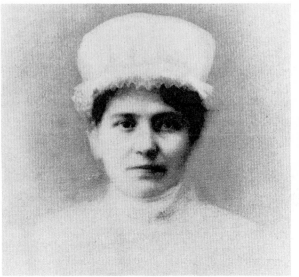

Annual Report, 1886. McLean Hospital, Waverly, Massachusetts.

Photographic composite of pictures of all 15 members of the Class of 1886 of the McLean Asylum Training School for Nurses, Waverly, Massachusetts. (Negatives of 15 individual portraits were overlaid to make this composite.)

dependent upon private donations and the good will of hospital authorities for their funding.

The Nurse Training School Experience in the Late 1870s

If you had been one of the student pioneers in one of the early nurse training schools over a century ago, your experience as a probationer would have conformed to the following general pattern. At the time of your entrance to the school you would have been between the ages of 25 and 35. Prior to your admission you would have completed an application form in which you would have stated your marital status (single or widowed, for married women were not accepted), present occupation, height, weight, education, and state of health (in particular whether or not your sight and hearing were perfect). Any physical defect, especially pulmonary, would have disqualified you. Two persons would already have submitted character references.

Once admission was granted, you immediately entered the hospital. You did not arrive as part of a group of students, for students were not usually received in classes but were admitted as needed. The initial experience was quite unlike any other that you had previously had. One of the older trainees showed you to your room, which was actually a six- to eight-foot high stall containing three separate beds. These stalls were erected under the dome of what had once been the operating theater of the hospital and had later been converted into the servants' quarters. There was no heat and no light except for that which filtered

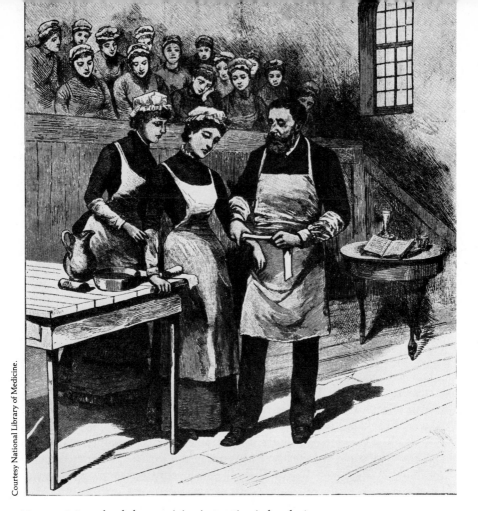

Nurse training school class receiving instruction in bandaging.

through the painted white glass of the dome, which seemed to be at least a hundred feet above the room. There was no privacy because the servants who came up to their rooms at all hours of the day and night chatted, scolded each other, and told stories. Except for the beds, which were in fairly good condition, the rooms were sparsely furnished. Your roommates might not be at all congenial, for they too were undergoing much emotional strain.

Later, at dinner time, you were taken to another part of the hospital for your first of many institutional meals. You found that the food was of poor quality, for the cook, despite all her years of service, seemed to hate nurses in training and regarded you as an intruder with no rights. You soon discovered that many of the student nurses spent nearly all their monthly wages on additional food. Later, when you had mustered up enough courage to complain about the fare, you found that your complaints were to no avail and actually jeopardized your future in the school.

After dinner you were given a notebook and pencil and told to proceed to an operating theater to hear your first lecture. Since you had just arrived at the school, you were not too tired that first evening, but you found the lecturing physician to be exhausted from his long day at work. The next week, however, when you attended the second lecture, you too were tired and unable to get much out of his presentation.

After class that first night you noticed that there was no place where you could really socialize with the other students. Soon you sensed a cliquishness: as a new student occupying one of the stalls in the oldest part of the hospital, you were looked down upon as inferior by the more advanced students, who enjoyed the privilege of occupying the rooms adjacent to the superintendent's quarters. You also encountered favoritism and ingratiating types who curried favor with the superintendent by offering her dainties, making her a cup of tea, or sewing a seam for her.

Early the next morning you put on one of the wash dresses that you had brought from home and at 6:30 A.M. began your probationer's duties on the hospital wards. As you entered the ward you were introduced to the head nurse. At first you were asked to do only simple work, like arranging the linen closet and folding clothes. Later you were given more arduous tasks, such as sweeping and cleaning, polishing the floors and furniture, and washing and ironing. You were surprised that you even had to beg for the materials with which to do this drudgery. In folding the linen you were told to do the sheets, the towels, the pillowslips, and then the washcloths, in that order. You also learned that all the sheets had to be folded to exactly the same size and that the folded items were to be placed in neat, separate piles in the linen cupboard. The appearance of this closet was a major source of pride for the nurses.

Before coming to the school you had considered yourself particularly well suited for nursing, and, having read Florence Nightingale's *Notes on Nursing*, you had become somewhat informed about nursing duties. As the first clinical day progressed, however, you discovered that you were not required to know *anything*. In fact, the head nurse preferred to work with raw material, so to speak, who had no preconceptions about nursing. What *was* required was receptiveness, intelligence, and, above all, an energetic nature. If you did have any prior knowledge or opinions of nursing, it was wise to keep them to yourself! On the wards you adhered to principles of order and decorum that absolutely subordinated the nurses to the physicians.

As the afternoon wore on you found yourself looking at the clock and waiting for 8:00 P.M. to come so that you could go off duty. The hospital atmosphere, a combination of strange sights and sounds and the smell of drugs and other unavoidable odors most perceptible to the uninitiated, had managed to produce in you a mild case of first-day shock. You were unable to sleep that night, and by the end of the week you found yourself crying in bed with pain in your feet and legs. You kept these little ailments to yourself, however, because you were anxious to satisfy your superiors and perform your duties as directed. By the end of the first week you were grateful for the half-day off. Although you worked only

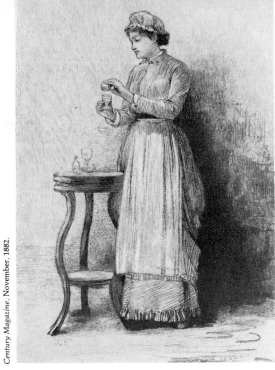

Century Magazine, November, 1882.

A student nurse, about 1882.

Taking a patient's pulse, about 1888.

Scribner's Magazine, June, 1888.

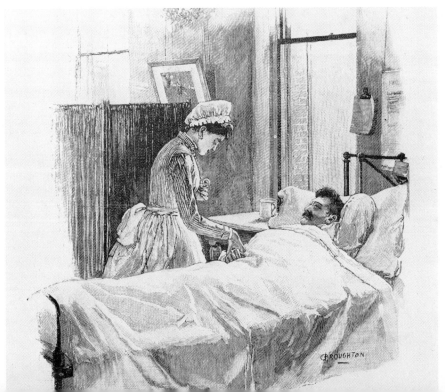

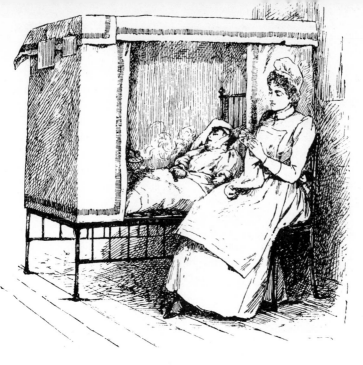

Night duty was an exciting but anxious experience.

Giving medicines, about 1888.

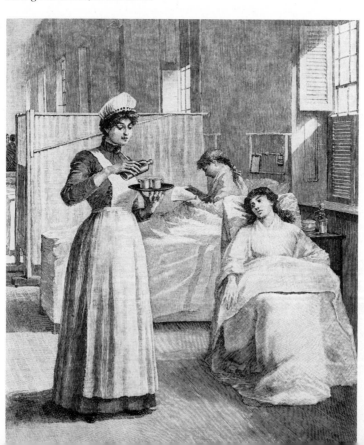

six hours that day, you were so exhausted that you spent your free time resting indoors instead of leaving the hospital for recreation.

With the second week came greater responsibility. You were given charge of 10 to 15 patients. The head or senior nurse went around the ward with you for the first time and demonstrated how to make beds, change soiled linen, move an invalid from one bed to another, cover a patient and avoid fatiguing her while sitting her up to have her bed made, and get a patient in and out of bed. You also learned the importance of having patients make their own beds when they were able. The latter part of the day was spent in waiting on your patients and keeping your side of the ward in order at all times. The first month was a probationary period, during which you had to master a host of difficult techniques and procedures. Instruction was given by visiting and resident physicians, by surgeons, and by the superintendent, assistant superintendent, and head nurses (who were themselves students). Demonstrations took place from time to time, and examinations were administered at regular intervals.

To your great satisfaction you finally passed through the probationary period and became a junior nurse. Having shown yourself qualified, you were required to sign the following agreement: "I hereby agree to remain for two years in the Training-School for Nurses as a pupil nurse and to obey the rules of the school and hospital." Board, lodging, and laundry were furnished, and a monthly stipend of $7 was provided for clothes, textbooks, and incidental expenses. This stipend, you were told, represented an allowance rather than wages.

For three more months you engaged in the same work that you had done as a probationer, and then you went on night duty. You were beginning to feel somewhat independent by this time, although you had not yet acted completely alone because there was always an experienced nurse on the top floor from whom you could seek help in case of emergency. Since you had probably never before remained awake the entire night, your first night duty was rather exciting and anxious. You were alert and wide awake until about two o'clock in the morning when the effort to keep awake began to grow painful. With the aid of an antiquated lantern that cast large shadows and a tiny ray of light, you peered about the large ward. Sometimes the miserable little lamp went out while the wick spit and sputtered. To your dismay, you found that patients had a way of dying during the night despite your utmost efforts to keep them alive until dawn. It required considerable nerve on your part to "lay out" a dead patient in the small hours of the morning. There was something uncanny in the air that first night in the silent, gloomy wards, but you got used to it after a time. Since your night duty lasted 14 hours, you began to feel completely exhausted about 5:00 A.M. You braced yourself, however, and summoned up a last spurt of energy to get through the early day's work until 8 A.M., when you collapsed, without breakfast, into bed.

Your nurse's training was divided into several "services." You spent so many months in each of the different branches—medical, surgical, maternity, gynecologic, eye, skin, and throat, and pediatric—unless you were needed by another service. Then you found that the training school's rotation plan was quickly overlooked. About six months of your training period was devoted to night duty, which was spread out over two years. During the day, each of the 30-bed wards of the hospital had four nurses: two juniors, one senior, and a head nurse, who were also responsible for the "special cases" in adjacent private rooms.

When you became a senior nurse at the beginning of the second year, your duties changed somewhat and you now felt more important. You were no longer required to attend evening lectures or take bothersome quizzes, and your monthly allowance was increased to $12. You were given charge of the linen closets, you assisted in serving food and dispensing medicine, and you carried out orders for various patients' treatments. The prescription list for patients carried 30 names, and some patients received as many as five or six different medicines. After sufficient practice and with the assistance of another nurse, you were able to dispense all medications within 30 to 40 minutes.

When you were elevated to the position of head nurse, you were given charge of an entire ward. You were responsible for the condition of this ward, for the care of its patients, and for the instruction of less experienced student nurses—in fact, for whatever was done or not done on the ward. Dealing with the various personalities of the physicians who relied upon you to carry out their orders faithfully required mature judgment and tact. After receiving the notes of the night nurse and seeing that all the work was proceeding smoothly, you went around with a notebook in hand and examined the condition of each patient. You questioned him, listened to what he had to say, and made your own observations. In this way you became acquainted with all your patients and were able to report every important detail to the attending physicians.

Each week, as you proceeded with your training, you gained confidence in yourself while others gained confidence in you. There was no time for dreaming, and amidst sickness and death you invariably acquired a matter-of-fact disposition. Except for an annual two-week vacation and the one-half day off every other week, you devoted seven days a week to nursing. After you had made up any sick days that you had been granted during your two years of training, a board of physicians gave you a final examination, and, after passing it, you received a fancy diploma signed by the examining board and by a committee of the training school board of directors. Since your name was now listed on the school rolls, a patient or physician needing a nurse could summon you. At last you were ready to begin a career in private duty nursing in the homes of patients.

Uniforms and Caps

The new graduate was always proud to wear her school cap and uniform on her private duty nursing assignments. The practice of wearing uniform and cap, important symbols of nursing, seems to have grown out of its military and religious heritage, which had always placed high value on the wearing of uniforms. Until the 1850s, the religious orders had been the dominant factor in the evolution of nursing service. After this time, Florence Nightingale's military nursing experi-

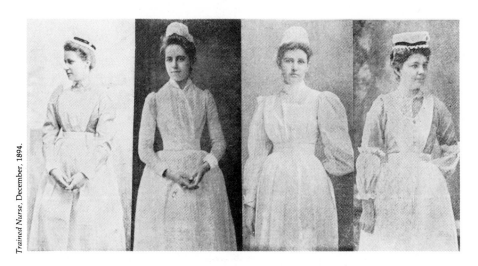

Trained Nurse, December, 1894.

Uniforms and caps of nurses at four New York hospitals, 1894.

ence during the Crimean War exerted a powerful influence on the subsequent development of professional symbols.

The New York Training School for Nurses at Bellevue Hospital was the first school to adopt a standard uniform for student nurses. After the school had been operating for about a year, the board of directors decided that the students should wear a gingham apron in the morning and a white one in the afternoon, in addition to the required dark woolen dresses and variously shaped white caps. For reasons of economy as well as neatness, the Training School committee concluded in 1876 that the adoption of a standard uniform, which would have the same psychological effect on nurses as on a company of military recruits, was both necessary and advantageous.

The most well-bred woman of the first Bellevue class was Euphemia Van Rensselaer of New York, whose aristocratic relatives held high positions in business and government. After her father, Union Army Brigadier General Henry B. Van Rensselaer, died of typhoid fever during the Civil War, she resolved to become a trained nurse. In describing Euphemia's return from the New York Training School, a relative, Mrs. John King Van Rensselaer, wrote: "When she returned to her family's home, she entered the basement, took off her verminous clothes, and then stood on a sheet while her old nurse cleansed her body and combed her hair. Only after this purification would she permit the rest of the household to greet her."

It was Euphemia who introduced the uniform, apron, and cap of the Bellevue Training School for Nurses. At first the students had opposed the wearing of uniforms, which were commonly worn by servants at that time. After certain members of the Training School committee decided to grant Euphemia two days' leave of absence to have a uniform made for herself, she returned to the hospital

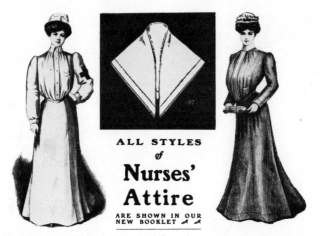

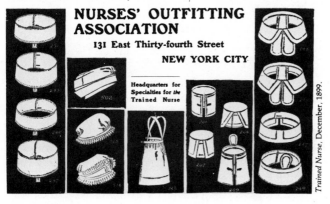

Trained Nurse, December, 1899.

The latest styles in nurses' attire at the turn of the century.

in her new attire. When the other students saw how attractive she looked in her tailored uniform, they were eager to adopt it as standard dress. The new outfit consisted of a long gray dress for winter and a calico version for summer, both with white apron and cap and brown linen cuffs covering the sleeves from the wrist to the elbow. In 1880 the gray dress for winter was replaced by an easily laundered dress that could be worn throughout the year.

Not until the 1890s was a regulation uniform generally established as a distinguishing mark of each nurse training school. The use of stripes and checks on student nursing uniforms was derived from the old calico summer attire. The bib and apron, which were also worn in early European nurse training schools, were similar to those worn by gentlewomen while performing their household duties.

Many early uniforms seem to have been designed as concessions to modesty and contemporary fashions rather than to comfort, convenience, or hygiene. Charming frills and laces, layers of starched petticoats, long, full skirts, tight bodices, and long, stiff cuffs and high collars were characteristic features of these uniforms. Since it was considered immodest for nurses to show their ankles, long dresses were required, and high stiff collars and shirtfronts were worn to conceal the upper part of the body. A nurse working on an infectious case could not be on duty half an hour without getting her sleeves contaminated. Although these sleeves were carriers of infection, nurses who rolled up their cuffs or sleeves were soundly rebuked, for such an appearance suggested the usual demeanor of laundresses or scrubwomen. Students who had been caught with their sleeves rolled up and cuffs removed invariably alleged that they "had just taken them off" or "were just putting them on."

Despite the disadvantages of these confining uniforms, however, their effect on the public was pronounced. In a popular account of the nursing students at Saint Luke's Hospital in New York, a reporter for *Munsey's Magazine* raved that their appearance was "all that the most inveterate reader of sentimental war stories could desire." The nurses of Saint Luke's wore a neat uniform of blue and white striped gingham. Their bibbed white aprons, neckbands of stiff linen, and crisply erect and airily poised little caps of sheer white mull conjured up an image of exquisite orderliness that was believed capable of inspiring hope in the hearts of their patients. The reporter thought that "it would be impossible to conceive of anything so manifestly out of place as disease daring to persist near them" [28]. In every ward there was a head nurse who could easily be recognized by the black velvet band upon her cap.

The original purpose of the nurses' cap was to cover the long hair that was fashionable during the late nineteenth century. The first ones resembled dust caps and were quite large. Each school developed its own distinctive cap, and the black bands on some caps indicated a student's rank. The mandatory use of a standard cap style was first introduced at Massachusetts General Hospital in 1878, along with a regulation uniform.

Nurses continued to wear their school caps, uniforms, and school pins after graduation, whether as private duty nurses or superintendents. Physicians and patients therefore began to recognize the various caps and uniforms and to associate them with the reputations of the various training schools. The distinctive uniform and pin began to symbolize the nurse's pride in the high standards of the training school from which she had graduated.

The origins of professional nursing in the United States can be attributed to the desire of respectable women for a broader occupational role, to the pioneering efforts of the first female physicians, to humanitarian sentiments among certain liberal physicians and magazine editors, and to the financial support of various civic and philanthropic groups in New York, New Haven, and Boston. In the beginning, the training schools were involved in a desperate struggle to prove their worth to society in the face of constant criticism from the medical profession. Their success in convincing the public of their usefulness enabled them to impart a higher degree of professionalism to their graduates.

Summary

In nineteenth-century America, severe societal restrictions confined most women to domestic roles that did not permit their involvement in the professions.

On-the-job instruction given to nurses and midwives was haphazard and incomplete. In 1798 Dr. Valentine Seaman developed an organized course for nurses at New York Hospital that consisted of lectures on anatomy, physiology, and the care of children.

Until it was initiated in the 1750s, the practice of obstetrics by male physicians was practically unknown in the British colonies of North America but subsequently became fashionable throughout New England. This practice evoked criticism for causing "licentiousness."

Another nursing course was initiated by Dr. Joseph Warrington, a Philadelphia Quaker, as part of the Philadelphia Lying-in Charity, in 1828. He was particularly interested in preparing nurses and midwives for work among the poor.

Elizabeth Blackwell was the first woman to study medicine. After refusal by 12 medical schools, she was admitted in 1847 to the Geneva Medical College of Western New York, where she graduated at the head of her class. As a reaction to the prejudice against Dr. Blackwell and other early female physicians, the Women's Medical College of Pennsylvania was founded in 1850. Seven years later, Dr. Blackwell opened the New York Infirmary for Women and Children.

During the 1860s, hospital nursing service was generally disorganized and often supplied by paroled women convicts, convalescent patients, and illiterate persons of low morals. Hospitals served by religious nursing orders received a much higher level of nursing care.

Marie Zakrzewska, an associate of Drs. Elizabeth and Emily Blackwell, founded the New England Hospital for Women and Children in 1862. One of her major aims was to offer a six-month nurse training course in connection with the hospital, but it attracted few interested applicants.

Dr. Susan Dimock, trained in Switzerland, introduced European diagnostic and surgical techniques during her tenure at the New England Hospital. In 1872 a nurse training school, the first in America to offer a graded course in scientific nursing, was opened in affiliation with the hospital.

Meanwhile, a committee of the New York State Charities Aid Association began to inspect conditions at Bellevue Hospital. The members were determined to improve the quality of nursing service by organizing a training school along the lines of the Nightingale system. Despite opposition from local physicians, the New York Training School for Nurses was opened in 1873.

Similar schools based on the Nightingale system were founded that same year at the New Haven State Hospital in Connecticut and at the Massachusetts General Hospital in Boston. Although the first training schools were fairly autonomous within the hospitals to which they were attached, this trend was soon reversed.

The experience of being a student nurse in a training school of the 1870s was arduous. Living conditions, working hours, and responsibilities required tremendous physical and emotional endurance. Students worked long hours and were required to sign contracts in return for a course of lectures, on-the-job training, and small allowances. In general, graduates of these early schools engaged in private duty nursing.

Although students initially resisted the idea of uniforms, which to them signified servant status, standardized uniforms for each school were widely used by the 1890s. As concessions to modesty and fashion, early uniforms were confining, inconvenient, and often nonhygienic.

References

1. Robert L. Dickinson, "The Corset: Questions of Pressure and Displacement," *New York Medical Journal*, vol. 46 (November 5, 1887), 507–516.
2. M. Adelaide Nutting and Lavinia L. Dock, *A History of Nursing* (New York: G. P. Putnam's Sons, 1907), vol. 2, p. 339.
3. Samuel Gregory, *Licentiousness, Its Causes and Effects* (Boston: G. Gregory, 1857), p. 6.
4. Elizabeth Blackwell, *Pioneer Work in Opening the Medical Profession to Women: Autobiographical Sketches* (New York: Longmans, Green & Co., 1895), p. 23.
5. Stephen Smith, "In Memory of Dr. Elizabeth Blackwell and Dr. Emily Blackwell," *Bulletin of the New York Academy of Medicine*, vol. 25 (January, 1911): 3–7.
6. Rachel Baker, *The First Woman Doctor: The Story of Elizabeth Blackwell, M.D.* (New York: Julian Messner, 1944), pp. 161–175.
7. Commonwealth of Massachusetts, *Report of a General Plan for the Promotion of Public and Personal Health, Devised, Prepared, and Recommended by the Commissioners Appointed under a Resolve of the Legislature of Massachusetts Relating to a Sanitary Survey of the State* (Boston: Dutton and Wentworth, 1850), 544 pp., passim.
8. Editorial, *Buffalo Medical Journal*, vol. 24 (July, 1869): 191.
9. "Women as Physicians," *Medical and Surgical Reporter*, vol. 44 (May, 1881): 354–356.
10. Agnes C. Vietor, *A Woman's Quest: The Life of Marie E. Zakrzewska, M.D.* (New York: Appleton & Co., 1924), p. 360.
11. *Ibid.*, p. 361.
12. Ann Preston, *Nursing the Sick and the Training of Nurses* (Philadelphia: King and Baird, 1863), pp. 1–14.
13. Philadelphia General Hospital, *Annual Report of the Philadelphia General Hospital for 1866* (Philadelphia: The Hospital, 1866), p. 7.
14. "Report of the Committee on the Training of Nurses," *Transactions of the American Medical Association*, vol. 20 (1869): 161.
15. Sarah J. Hale, "Lady Nurses," *Godey's Lady's Book*, vol. 92 (March, 1871): 188–189.
16. J. P. Chesney, "Woman as a Physician," *Richmond and Louisville Medical Journal*, vol. 11 (January, 1871): 1–15.
17. Horatio Storer, *Nurses and Nursing* (Boston: Lee and Shepard, 1868), p. 10.
18. New England Hospital for Women and Children, *Annual Report of the Officers to the Society and Friends, 1862–1863* (Boston: The Hospital, 1863), p. 3.
19. _____. *Annual Report of the Officers to the Society and Friends, 1871–1872* (Boston: The Hospital, 1872), p. 5.
20. New York State Charities Aid Association, *Report of the Committee on Hospitals, Dec. 23, 1872 on the Training School for Nurses to be Attached to Bellevue Hospital* (New York: The Association, 1873), pp. 11–16.

21. *Ibid.*, pp. 16–17.
22. *New York Evening Sun*, March 11, 1911.
23. *Ibid.*
24. Francis Bacon, "Founding of the Connecticut Training School for Nurses," *Trained Nurse*, vol. 15 (October, 1895), p. 187.
25. *Ibid.*, pp. 188–189.
26. *Ibid.*, p. 189.
27. U.S. Commissioner of Education, *Annual Report of the U.S. Commissioner of Education for 1873* (Washington, D.C.: Government Printing Office, 1874), p. 60.
28. K. Hoffman, "St. Luke's, N.Y.: Model Hospital," *Munsey's Magazine*, vol. 22 (January, 1900): 487–496.

4
The Rise of Scientific Medicine and Its Impact on Nursing

Physicians of the centennial year 1876 did their best to control the prevailing diseases, but the profession was still hampered by ignorance and superstition inherited from the past. Much of its thinking was still clouded by the erroneous Hippocratic concept of the "epidemic constitution of the atmosphere." Even as late as 1882 the superintendent of health of Providence, Rhode Island, reported that he had known of one situation in his city where nearly all the residents of a large house had developed typhoid fever due to the decomposition of a large quantity of potatoes stored in the basement. Medical literature still contained references to the "zymotic" (fermentative) diseases—a term applied to specific infections such as Asiatic cholera, smallpox, typhus, diphtheria, dysentery, typhoid, whooping cough, and syphilis.

Yellow Fever Epidemics
In the summer of 1878 one of these scourges—yellow fever—reappeared in New Orleans. The outbreak was noted in the *New York Times* of July 24, 1878, which told of four deaths occurring in 48 hours. Before the end of the month the newspaper announced that other cities along the Mississippi had become alarmed and were establishing a rigid quarantine on vessels and travelers from New Orleans. In spite of this precaution the disease spread rapidly up river, causing serious outbreaks in eight states. Hysteria permeated the entire South.

Memphis was hit hardest. Over half its population fled. Of the 20,000 who remained, over 17,000 developed yellow fever within three months, and 5000 of those people died. Many who ran away carried the seeds of yellow fever with them and set off new outbreaks in other parts of the country. Even physicians and nurses who stayed to care for the sick fell ill: in one group of 39 volunteer helpers, 32 developed yellow fever and 12 of them died. The cost of this great epidemic in money, suffering, and lives was enormous. New Orleans, Vicksburg, and Memphis bore the brunt of the outbreak, but hundreds of other communities were attacked. Commerce was practically stopped in the Lower Mississippi Valley, and the economic loss was estimated in the millions of dollars. No one knew what caused yellow fever or how it was spread, and therefore no one knew how to cure or prevent it.

The medical journals were filled with speculation about the cause of the disease and with heated controversy about its prevention and treatment. Because Americans had been so thoroughly frightened by the epidemic, Congress appointed a special commission to investigate the causes and existing remedies of yellow fever. The commission failed. Americans of the 1870s would remain exposed to yellow fever—and a host of other diseases of unknown cause.

Lag in Medical Knowledge

Because of the comparatively primitive state of medical knowledge and practice in the 1880s, it is doubtful that the medical profession exerted any significant net influence on the morbidity or mortality of infants and young children of the time. Records of vital statistics for the large cities of America show similar patterns of astonishingly high mortality rates among the very young.

Reliable official lists of live births and of burials indicate that the infant mortality rate (number of deaths occurring during the first year of life per 1000 live births) varied between 250 and 500. The highest rates were among artificially fed babies confined to foundling homes, with between 75 and 90 percent of such babies dying within their first year. Some metropolitan records show that more than half the total deaths from all causes in the average community occurred among children under five years of age. Three-fourths of the total occurred among children under 12. These high mortality rates of the late nineteenth century accounted in large measure for the average life-span's remaining at 35 to 38 years. Although adequate records are not available, it can be assumed that the morbidity rates of the time were also extremely high. Enteric disorders, malnutrition, and the common respiratory and contagious diseases constituted the major causes of death.

In the pharmaceutic field the latest drugs in use during the 1870s were coal tar products that were displacing calomel and whiskey as the panacea for febrile illnesses. There were very serious abuses. Antipyrin, which came first, was used to such an extent during earlier epidemics of influenza in this country that it often produced serious, if not fatal, results. Acetanilid, which followed, became a favorite popular remedy for headaches and probably did more harm than antipyrin. The salicylates, introduced for rheumatism and supposed for a long time to be a specific for that affliction, came to be used for all possible aches and pains. A series of coal tar hypnotics, each introduced with the definite assurance that it had all the advantages and none of the disadvantages of opium, proved in succession to have serious, lasting side effects that rendered them unsafe when used over long periods. By the 1890s the ten most important drugs in medical practice were: (1) ether, (2) morphine, (3) digitalis, (4) diphtheria antitoxin, (5) smallpox vaccine, (6) iron, (7) quinine, (8) iodine, (9) alcohol, and (10) mercury.

A few physicians intelligent enough to realize the inadequacy of their American training went to Europe to complete their educations. There they found a different world—a world of laboratories and carefully controlled experiments. They learned to use the microscope to distinguish between normal and abnormal

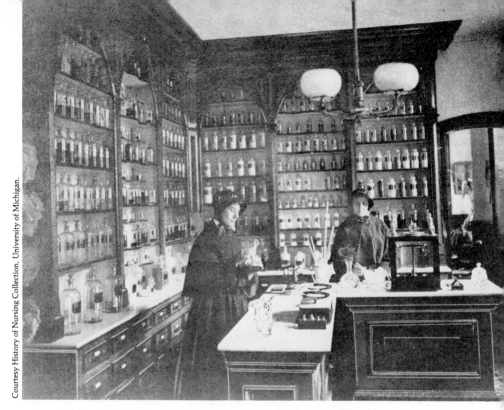

Nurses in the pharmacy of the New York Foundling Hospital, about 1892.

tissue and to identify the conditions that accompanied certain diseases. Pathology and physiology, barely recognized in American medical schools, were well advanced abroad. Bacteriology—the science, more than any other, destined to revolutionize medicine—was in a stage of vigorous youth. European scientists turned to projects relating to the cause and prevention of disease, and American graduate students crossed the Atlantic to learn the new techniques and to bring "modern medicine" back to their schools and hospitals.

Founders of Bacteriology and Antisepsis

During the last quarter of the nineteenth century there was an almost unbelievable advance in medicine brought on by an unusual number of medical discoveries characterized by the development of scientific methods in the approach to problems of medicine. The growth of work in the basic sciences and the use of the experimental process in seeking answers greatly accelerated understanding in bacteriology and pathology and laid the groundwork for developments in biochemistry, physiology, and pharmacology.

In the 1840s a Hungarian obstetrician, Ignaz Semmelweiss, had made a study of postmortem tissues of women who had died of puerperal infection in Vienna hospitals. He believed that medical students working on dissections prior to attending obstetric cases were responsible for the high mortality rate. He con-

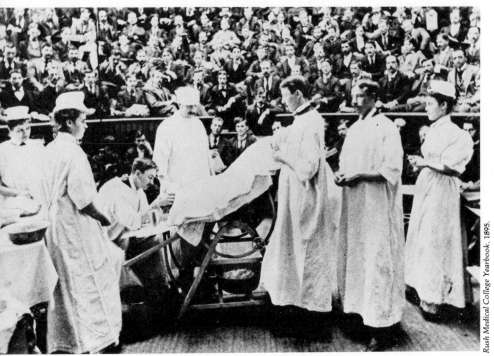

American doctors educated in Germany returned to demonstrate the elements of scientific medicine. Surgical Clinic at Rush Medical College, Chicago, about 1894.

Pasteur's battle against deadly microbes was brought to life in The Story of Louis Pasteur, *which won three 1936 Academy Awards. (From the Warner Brothers release* The Story of Louis Pasteur © *1936 Warner Bros. Pictures, Inc. Copyright renewed 1963.)*

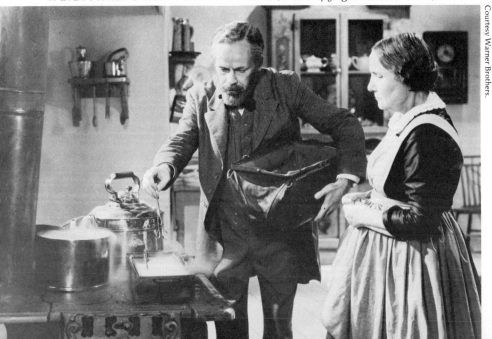

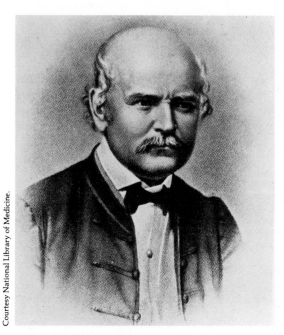

Courtesy National Library of Medicine.

Ignaz Semmelweiss, about 1861.

cluded that unclean hands, dirty clothes, and the unsanitary conditions in hospitals were transmitting puerperal fever, which was causing a death rate of 12 to 15 percent on the maternity wards. His book, *The Aetiology, Concept and Prophylaxis of Childbirth Fever*, gave the world theories and methods of treatment that had been validated when he reduced the death rate in the maternity wards by over 90 percent between 1846 and 1848—through the simple expedient of cleanliness. Semmelweiss, in advocating antisepsis, pointed the way to elimination of maternal mortality, but professional approval was withheld, and his ideas were ridiculed both in America and in Europe for a long time afterward.

Later, the French chemist Louis Pasteur demonstrated the scientific basis for Semmelweiss' theory when he proved that bacteria were living microorganisms. These bacteria increased through reproduction, not by spontaneous generation, but they could be destroyed by heat and chemical action. In 1864 Pasteur officially introduced the germ theory to science. A year later, medicine received its first dividend from Pasteur's work: Joseph Lister, a surgeon of Glasgow, Scotland, applied Pasteur's findings by using carbolic acid to disinfect the wound of a compound fracture in a patient at the Glasgow Infirmary, thus beginning the era of antisepsis in surgery. Lister's success with carbolic acid sprays as antiseptics in surgical operations after 1865 not only hastened wound healings but reduced the mortality rate in his hospital from 45 to 12 percent. Antisepsis, the forerunner of aseptic surgery, could be deliberately planned, thus greatly increasing the number and extent of operative procedures and the treatment of conditions amenable to surgery.

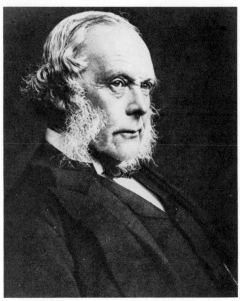

Courtesy National Library of Medicine.

Joseph Lister.

Under antisepsis, infected wounds were opened widely and antiseptics used freely in them in the hope of killing the infectious agents. Unfortunately, the earlier antiseptics were extremely toxic and often killed tissue cells to a greater extent than the bacteria present. The better surgeons used drainage tubes to flush the wound surfaces thoroughly with antiseptic solution at regular intervals. Gradually, fewer and fewer badly infected wounds were seen. Skepticism persisted, however, in Pasteur's own country and elsewhere. As late as 1886, Dr. Morris Longstreth of Philadelphia published a serious, 16-page dissertation "Against the Germ Theory of Disease" in *The Therapeutic Gazette*.

As a result of antiseptic techniques, puerperal sepsis was no longer "childbed fever," but streptococcal septicemia. To understand the effect of the antiseptic principle in extending the scope of surgery, one has but to remember that in the days before listerism the mortality for amputation ran around 40 to 60 percent due to infection and secondary hemorrhage. Lawson Tait, a famous British surgeon, had enjoyed remarkably good results in ovariotomy by applying the principle of scrupulous cleanliness, although he steadfastly opposed Lister and denied the existence of bacteria. From Lister's antisepsis and Lawson Tait's cleanliness came the acceptance of asepsis, which is the cornerstone of surgical technique today. In 1891 William Halsted of Baltimore introduced the use of rubber gloves—initially, it must be admitted, to protect the skin of the hands of his scrub nurse. It was later that the face mask was generally adopted. These developments were of great significance in the continued development of hospitals, since the ability to limit infections soon became a necessary preliminary to gaining the public's confidence.

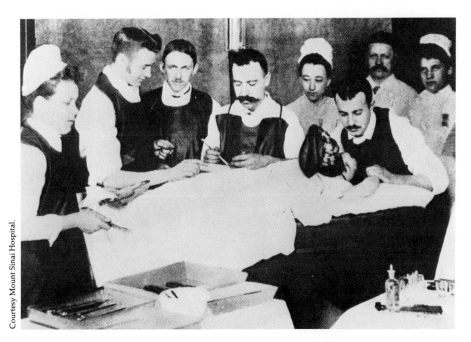

Courtesy Mount Sinai Hospital.

Operating room at Mount Sinai Hospital in New York City, about 1880.

Surgical Risks Reduced by New Advances

Related to antiseptic surgery was the development of anesthesia: with anesthesia the degree of surgery that could be undertaken with safety and with promise of success was tremendously increased and the danger to patients correspondingly lessened. The use of ether as an anesthetic agent had been demonstrated by Crawford Long of Georgia in 1842 and by William Morton of Boston in 1846. In 1847 James Y. Simpson of England introduced chloroform. These events proved to be a boon to patient and surgeon alike. To the patient it meant relief of pain; to the surgeon it meant that he could dispense with the practice of extremely rapid but inaccurate operating and adopt instead the slow, painstaking anatomic technique.

The first nurse anesthetists were chosen by the surgeons with whom they were to work. They were women who seemed especially qualified for this type of duty, and it was believed that the nurse would devote her entire attention to the conduct of the anesthesia—as opposed to the intern, whose interest would naturally be divided between the anesthesia and the surgical procedure. By the time the intern had become proficient in administering anesthesia, his term of service usually ended; in contrast, the nurse would stay on indefinitely and become increasingly valuable.

In the late 1890s the administration of ether was not easy for the nurse. Patients commonly came to the operating room expressing greater repugnance and fear

ETHER INHALERS.

Various devices for the administration of ether in the 1880s.

toward the anesthesia than toward the actual operation. Little innovation had been made in the administration of ether since its inception. An ether-cone, so-called, was fashioned from a folded newspaper or butcher's straw cuff, covered snugly with a folded towel, and fastened tight at the top by safety pins; its inside was stuffed with fluffed gauze. An indefinite amount of ether, ranging from a dram or two to an ounce or two according to the judgment of the nurse anesthetist, was poured into the gauze, and the cone was applied near to or in contact with the patient's face. Then, as now, followed the constant admonition to "take a deep breath."

Too often the ether vapor was so strong that one or two deep breaths would nearly choke the patient, but according to the prevailing practice this was to be expected, and it was assumed that the only thing to do was to rush the patient through the agony as quickly as possible. So, the more the patient choked and struggled for air, the more the ether was pushed and force applied to keep him sufficiently still. Inhalation of ether vapor at first stimulated the mucuous glands: the stronger the vapor, the greater the stimulation. If the patient was lucky, the anesthetist might accidentally allow him to return to a lighter ether-tension stage, and coughing and vomiting might clear out the frothy mucus; thus the anesthesia maintenance stage would be much improved. But all too often the anesthesia was kept at too deep a level; the mucus remained in the air passages (more or less obstructing them and causing a subcyanosis due to poor respiratory exchange); and irritation of the bronchial epithelium was followed by prolonged postoperative nausea and vomiting, which were aggravated by swallowing ether-laden mucus. Under these conditions—although anesthesia had been accomplished, the operation had been performed, and the patient was usually still alive—the horror of "taking ether" could not easily be forgotten.

The advent of antiseptic surgery necessitated a rearrangement of operating rooms in all hospitals. In the early hospitals operations were done in connection with the surgical wards, but the necessities of medical teaching soon rendered it essential that amphitheaters be built to permit medical and nursing students to view clinics and surgical operations. No special effort was made in these amphitheaters to guard against the possibility of infection from the surroundings of the patient or from those who came in contact with him. The patient was usually brought in under the influence of an anesthetic, the operation was done before the students, and subsequent dressings were made on the ward or in some adjoining room. The advent of antiseptic surgery, however, rendered it essential to meet the altered conditions of surgical work with the provision of new operating rooms.

Antiseptic surgery and anesthesia both increased the demand for hospitals. Anesthesia could be more conveniently administered in a hospital than in a home, and the operating room equipment for antiseptic surgery and administration of anesthesia demanded a highly specialized department, furnished with technical equipment, that could seldom be found outside a hospital. Thus the developing complexities of the operating room began to make the hospital more and more a necessity.

The development of blood transfusion also had great effect on the craft of surgery. It appears that transfusion was first practiced as early as 1867, but the modern period began in 1901 when it became possible to describe the four blood groups, thus making compatible blood transfusions possible and opening the way for the development of blood banks and for a method of supportive therapy that has become basic to much of the success of modern surgical treatment.

Improved Diagnostic Instruments
One of the most striking developments in the medical practice of the era came with the introduction of the thermometer. It seems almost impossible now to understand why physicians were so slow to accept this indispensable diagnostic

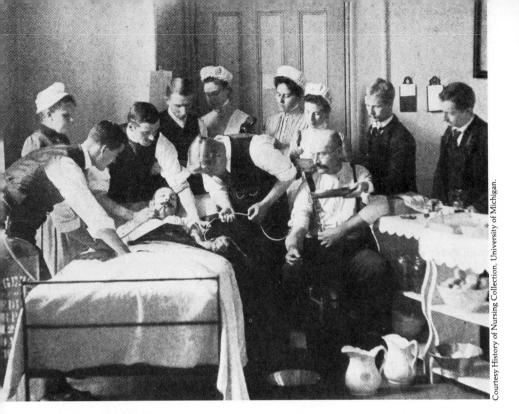

Blood transfusion, circa *1890.*

aid. Not until the 1880s was the thermometer generally used by city physicians in the United States, and it was nearly 1890 before it was generally employed in country practice. Older physicians made all sorts of objections to its use, asked why a physician should bother to carry such a toy around with him, and some fretted over the possibility of delirious patients injuring themselves with broken thermometers. The introduction of the thermometer quite literally revolutionized the study and treatment of various illnesses.

Other instruments were equally important. A new stimulus was given to therapeutics when Dr. George Elliott of New York brought with him from Edinburgh, in 1860, the hypodermic syringe. Because of professional conservatism and the fear that, since the hypodermic was used for injection of opium and other narcotic drugs, it might readily lead to drug abuse, it took over 20 years for this to become a common instrument in the hands of physicians. The double stethoscope (an American modification of the basic instrument that had been around since 1816) added to the knowledge of diseases of the chest as well as of the condition of the fetus at any given time. Also, that long-used instrument, the microscope, soon came into much greater use.

More precision instruments were invented during this period, all of them contributing to more accurate diagnoses. Among these w re the ophthalmoscope and laryngoscope, developed before 1860; the gastroscope, the sphygmomanometer, and the cystoscope (before 1883); and the bronchoscope, in 1898. Thomas Edison's invention of the incandescent light made the visual instruments even more useful. High-frequency oscillating currents were introduced by Jacques-Arsène d'Arsonval in the late 1880s and were later used in diathermy. In 1893 Niels Finsen introduced light therapy for the treatment of skin diseases, and in 1896 he published the results of his work on the use of ultraviolet rays.

Perhaps no diagnostic method caused a greater revolution in medical practice and diagnosis than the discovery of the x-ray by Wilhelm Konrad Roentgen in 1895. The rapid application of this discovery to clinical medicine brought much information concerning the previously invisible organs of living patients. Correlation of the findings of photographic films or fluoroscopic screens with those at operations and postmortem examinations quickly demonstrated the tremendous usefulness of this method of diagnosis and rapidly established radiology as a separate medical specialty. The introduction of radiopaque substances into the gastrointestinal tract and bronchial tree and the selective excretion of radiopaque dyes by the liver into the gallbladder and by the kidneys into the urinary tract completely revolutionized the diagnostic capabilities of physicians in these fields. Introduction of air and occasionally of other contrast media into the cerebrospinal fluid spaces, into serous-lined cavities (peritoneum, pleura, pericardium, and joints) and, at times, into the retroperitoneal space offered more limited, but at times equally important, diagnostic aid.

The early hospital x-ray services were limited chiefly to the examination of the bony structures. The equipment was crude and its operation was hazardous

Roentgen-ray machine in use at the Philadelphia Polyclinic.

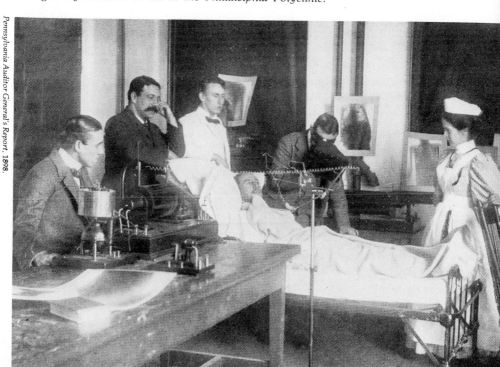

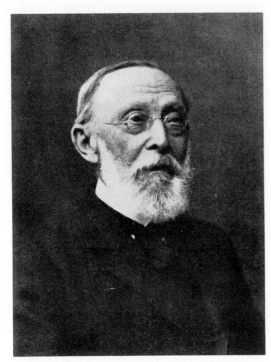

Courtesy National Library of Medicine.

Rudolf Virchow.

to both patient and roentgenologist. Crude as it was, the x-ray increased confidence in medical diagnosis and brought hundreds of additional patients to the hospital for treatment. Moreover, the first use of the x-ray marked too the beginning of medical care requiring equipment so elaborate that the average practitioner could not afford to install it for himself. The natural result was the founding of more community hospitals, in which local physicians could use such apparatus jointly.

Pathology, Microbiology, Medical Entomology, and Immunology

Modern pathology in this country found its inspiration in the German and Austrian universities of the mid-nineteenth century. At that time autopsy was used extensively in the study of disease, and most of the great advances in gross descriptive pathology had already been made. Much of the knowledge thus gained had been transferred to clinical practice, particularly in surgery. Probably the greatest pathologist of the day was Rudolf Virchow, director of the Pathological Institute of the University of Berlin. By the mid-1870s he had already completed his creative work, which left such an imprint on medicine. He had instituted the first modern journal in pathology, *Archiv fur Pathologische Anatomie und Physiologie,* and already 75 volumes had been printed. The new concepts of disease put forth in his book *Die Cellularpathologie*, published in 1858, had been made possible by use of the microscope in the study of diseased tissues. Experimental inquiry into the nature of pathologic phenomena was beginning, and applications to pathology of advances in physiology were being made.

From the standpoint of future developments in pathology in America, the influence of one of Virchow's pupils, Julius Cohnheim, was most important. Cohnheim's laboratory in Breslau was an active one in which the experimental approach to pathology was emphasized. His experiments on inflammation furnished the basis for current conceptions of this fundamental process. It was in Cohnheim's laboratory that William Henry Welch, often referred to as the dean of modern American medicine and as America's great pioneer pathologist, did his first experimental work. Welch's study, *On the Pathology of Lung Edema*, was published in 1878. Welch greatly valued his stimulating association with the Breslau laboratory. The dynamic concept of disease that he had studied in Breslau influenced future developments in this country, not only in pathology but in medical education and general medical thought as well.

In contrast to Europe, opportunities in this country for investigations in pathology were very limited. Before the 1890s there were no pathology laboratories, in the modern sense, in either medical schools or hospitals, and there were few, if any, medical men who devoted full time to pathology. The well-known pathologists of the day, such as Samuel D. Gross in Philadelphia and Francis A. Delafield in New York, were primarily clinicians who gave special attention to pathology. Yet despite many limitations, basic contributions to pathology were being made. In 1885 Francis A. Delafield and Theophile M. Prudden published the first modern textbook of pathology in this country.

Bacteriologists and their associates in pathology and medical microbiology stimulated widespread investigations. Before 1890 the causes of the following diseases were isolated: European relapsing fever (*Borrelia recurrentis,* by Otto Obermeier, 1873); leprosy (*M. leprae,* by G. Armauer Hansen, 1874); anthrax (*B. anthracis,* by Robert Koch, 1876); gonorrhea (*N. gonorrhoeae,* by Albert Neisser, 1879); typhoid fever (*E. typhosa,* by Karl Eberth, 1880); malaria (*P. malariae,* by Charles Laveran, 1880); lobar pneumonia (*D. pneumoniae,* by Louis Pasteur and George Sternberg, 1880); tuberculosis (*M. tuberculosis,* by Robert Koch, 1882); diphtheria (*C. diptheriae,* by Theodor Klebs, 1883); tetanus (*C. tetani,* by Arthur Nicolaier, 1884); cholera (*V. cholerae,* by Robert Koch, 1884); bacillus coli infection (*E. coli,* by Theodor Escherich, 1886); and Malta fever (*B. melitensis,* by David Bruce, 1887).

During this era of discoveries the foundation was laid for another new science: medical entomology. In 1877 Patrick Manson in Hong Kong showed that mosquitoes could carry the microfilaria of *M. bancrofti,* and in 1881 Carlos Finlay in Cuba believed that he had succeeded in transmitting yellow fever through Stegomyia mosquitoes. Eight years later Theobald Smith described the transmission of Texas cattle fever by ticks. Such a rich harvest of new scientific facts intensified interest in research and the medical revolution continued to gain momentum.

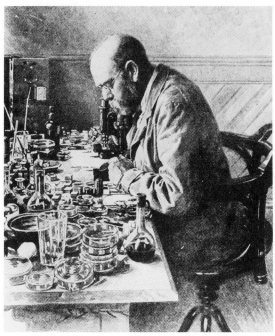

Courtesy National Library of Medicine.

Robert Koch.

The last seven years of the century were crowded with experimental activity, and still more organisms were discovered. These included the influenza bacillus (*H. influenza*, by Richard Pfeiffer, 1892); the Welch bacillus (*Cl. welchii*, by William H. Welch and George H. Nuttall, 1892); and the bacillus of plague (*Y. pestis*, by Alexandre Yersin and Shibasacuro Kitasato, 1894). In 1894 David Bruce began his work on anemia in Africa, which led to the incrimination of tsetse flies as vectors of trypanosomiasis. The same year, Patrick Manson suggested to Ronald Ross that the parasites of malaria might develop in the body of the mosquito and be transmitted from man to man in this way. In 1895 Ross went to India to test Manson's theory, and by 1897 he had shown that Anopheles mosquitoes could transmit human malaria. In 1898 Kiyoshi Shiga of Japan discovered the dysentery bacillus that bears his name.

Immunology developed almost hand in hand with bacteriology. In 1881 Louis Pasteur inoculated 25 sheep with weakened anthrax bacteria and left the same number unvaccinated. Later, all 50 were given a virulent form of the disease. The unvaccinated animals died, while the treated sheep remained well. With the establishment of the principle that the injection of a mild form of disease bacteria will cause the formation of antibodies that will prevent the inoculated person from getting the virulent form of the disease, the science of immunology was established on a firm footing. In 1890 Emil von Behring discovered the possibility of passive immunization against tetanus and diphtheria, which led to the concept of antitoxins. Prevention of smallpox by vaccination had long since been intro-

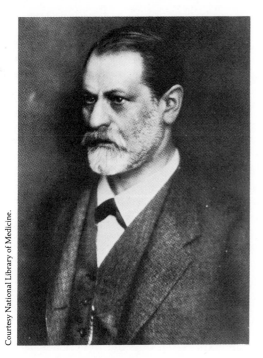

Courtesy National Library of Medicine.

Sigmund Freud, 1856–1939.

duced by Edward Jenner, to be followed by efforts to establish immunity against typhoid, rabies, whooping cough, typhus, and cholera.

Psychoanalysis

A most important advance toward an understanding of the mind was made by Viennese physician Sigmund Freud. In the last years of the nineteenth century he developed a technique, known as psychoanalysis, for dealing with emotional disturbances. From his clinical observations he gradually arrived at a radically novel explanation of the mechanism of human behavior. At the heart of his theory was the view that the conduct of the individual is vitally affected by irrational impulses, of which he is unaware because they are to a large extent subconscious. The repression of these instinctive drives, if severe enough, could lead to a psychological breakdown. More commonly it resulted in such maladjustments as phobias, compulsions, and complexes. Psychoanalysis proved valuable as a therapeutic technique in the treatment of emotional illness. Freud was also concerned with the question of man's motive force, the "libido," which he believed was rooted in the sexual urge. His concept of the Oedipus complex, whereby a child is strongly attached to the parent of the opposite sex and hostile to the other parent, brought world-wide attention. Although many of the theories advanced by its founder were eventually rejected even by his own disciples, in particular Carl C. Jung and Alfred Adler, psychoanalysis remained fundamental for an understanding of the disordered personality.

Gynecology and Obstetrics

Modern gynecology is a product almost entirely of the past century. Of his book *The Principles and Practices of Gynecology*, published in 1879, Thomas Addis Emmet wrote: "It was published, unfortunately, just before the full development or adoption of the aseptic treatment as applied to abdominal surgery" [1]. In other words, the principles and application of the aseptic techniques, prerequisite to successful operative gynecology, were just beginning to gain acceptance. Peritonitis was but poorly understood until 1880 when T. Gaillard Thomas clearly identified so-called "cellulitis" as peritonitis.

With the general employment of antiseptic and aseptic techniques, operative gynecology, along with abdominal surgery, had its real beginning, and the next few decades saw reports of countless new operative procedures. The first conditions addressed were naturally those which were most urgent, such as ruptured ectopic pregnancy. The progenitor of surgery in ectopic pregnancy was the great British gynecologist Lawson Tait, who first operated for this condition in 1883. Rapid progress was made: by 1891 Friedrich Schauta demonstrated that prompt surgery in ectopic pregnancy had reduced the mortality from 86.9 percent to 5.7 percent. With the advent of modern blood transfusion the death rate fell still lower.

Hysterectomy had its beginning in the epic struggle with myomata, an affliction characterized by fibrous, muscular tumors. Throughout the greater part of the nineteenth century, vast quantities of ergot (rye plant derivative) were taken by myoma victims in the futile hope that blood loss from these tumors could thus be stemmed. Although a few abdominal hysterectomies had been performed in the first half of the century, the mortality rate was extremely high because of hemorrhage and sepsis from the thick pedicle. In 1889 a general surgeon, Lewis A. Stimson, first suggested and practiced the systematic ligation of the ovarian and uterine arterial trunks as the cardinal principle of hysterectomy. This transformed the operation, which has since enjoyed many refinements in technique. Likewise, the whole field of female urology developed as the result of the invention of the air cystoscope by Howard A. Kelly in 1894. Surpassing these developments in operative gynecology in basic importance, if not in practical utility, were the vast array of advances made in knowledge of ovarian function, of the menstrual cycle, and of gynecologic pathology.

In the 1870s childbearing was a hazardous undertaking and any substantial deviation from the normal physiologic processes meant death. Throughout the greater part of the nineteenth century, cesarean section was the most fatal of surgical procedures. In Great Britain and Ireland in 1865 the maternal mortality rate from the operation had mounted to the appalling figure of 85 percent. In Paris, during the 90 years ending in 1876, not a single successful cesarean section had been performed. As late as 1887 Robert P. Harris reported in the *American Journal of Medical Science* that cesarean section was actually more successful when performed by the patient herself. He collected nine such cases from the literature, with five recoveries, and contrasted them with 12 cesarean sections, performed with only one recovery, in New York City during the same period. In the face of such results it is not surprising that many obstetricians of the nineteenth century doubted the wisdom of ever resorting to cesarean section and predicted that the operation would shortly become obsolete.

The turning point in the evolution of cesarean section was the appearance in 1882 of a monograph by Max Sanger, 28-year-old assistant to Karl Crede in the University Clinic at Leipzig. It was the purpose of this monograph to recommend the routine employment of carefully placed uterine sutures in cesarean section. Within a few years uterine suture was generally recognized as an indispensable step in cesarean section, and forthwith the modern operation came into being.

Pediatrics

The acceleration of scientific discovery at this time led to a veritable renaissance in medicine. Largely as a result of the unprecedented application of the scientific method to the study of clinical problems, in the laboratory as well as in the clinic, pediatrics finally emerged as a fledgling branch of scientific medicine during the waning decades of the century and proved itself to be a discipline less fettered by accumulated misinformation and more willing to adopt new concepts than were other long-established clinical specialties. In this atmosphere the American Pediatric Society was founded in 1888. During the same year, the first independent university department of pediatrics was organized for formal teaching of the subject at Harvard University.

The most spectacular reduction in the previously high mortality among children resulted from the discovery of the relationship between the contamination of water and food supplies, including milk, and the occurrence of enteric or diarrheal diseases. Since then, in no other major health-care area has cooperation among private practitioners, public health officials, and voluntary lay organizations accomplished so much as it accomplished in eliminating food and water contamination throughout communities.

Of the many advances made in the medical care of infants and young children, none were more important than those pertaining to malnutrition. The unsatisfactory results of artificial feeding of newborn infants, especially premature infants, were admitted by all physicians. A major portion of every pediatrician's practice until 1900 was devoted to the problems of artificial feeding and to the search for a formula that might be substituted for human milk.

"Wet nursing" registries and human milk stations were organized in the large population centers, but these were woefully inadequate even under the best conditions. Unmodified raw milk from other animal sources proved to "upset digestion," while highly diluted cow's milk formulas failed to produce acceptable weight gains. Thus elaborate milk modifications were devised, and sick infants were frequently shifted from one formula to another without benefit. Acute infection often ensued. Many babies had severe vomiting and diarrhea with attendant dehydration, exhaustion, and acidosis. Without adequate replacement of water and electrolytes lost in the course of such illness, mortality among these babies was extremely high.

The entire picture changed with the advent of greatly improved sanitation and the practice of boiling cow's milk formulas. Artificially fed babies began to thrive, and the mortality rates rapidly decreased to one-fourth their former levels as the serious dangers of infection, exhaustion, and vitamin deficiencies were eliminated. No longer were such disease entities as hypoproteinemic edema, scurvy, rickets, rachitic tetany, vitamin A deficiency, beriberi, pellagra, aribo-flavinosis, and iron-deficiency anemia inevitable in the child population.

America's First Center of Modern Medicine

The great developments in medicine during this period occurred principally in the university medical centers of Germany, Austria, France, and England. Just before the turn of the century, scientific methods in medicine came from the European countries to the United States; at the same time, a full-fledged university medical school was introduced here. Back in 1873, in the city of Baltimore, Johns Hopkins, bachelor merchant and financier, had willed his great fortune to found a hospital and a university within which a medical school was to be organized. While the University was getting under way, the trustees sought to build the hospital. Members of this board depended greatly on John Shaw Billings, whom they had chosen as their official adviser. Dr. Billings was a military physician and librarian attached to the Army Surgeon General's Office who had acquired wide hospital experience during the Civil War. Dr. Billings designed the Johns Hopkins Hospital buildings and assisted in preparing plans both for hospital management and for integration of the Hospital with the proposed medical school. He included plans for a school of nursing and for various supporting services, such as pharmacies.

On May 7, 1889, the doors of the Johns Hopkins Hospital and nursing school were formally opened, followed several years later by the medical school. Significantly, all faculty members who would be chosen for the Johns Hopkins University Medical School over the next few years would be comparatively young. The first to be named had been William H. Welch, as pathologist, in 1884. Then 34 years of age, Dr. Welch was to serve the University in various capacities for 50 years and was to become the most influential of the faculty members. Dr. Welch at once began to organize postgraduate courses in bacteriology and pathology for practicing physicians, using hospital facilities for teaching, since there was, as yet, no medical school. Much of the responsibility for selection of the rest of the Medical School faculty fell on Dr. Welch's shoulders.

Next to come, in 1888, was Canadian-born William Osler, called from his post at the University of Pennsylvania to become Physician-in-Chief at the Hospital and professor of the theory and practice of medicine at the University. Osler devoted much of his time to organizing the clinical staff. Organized upon the unit system, with a graded resident staff, as in German universities, the new medical school employed teaching methods similar to those used in Great Britain

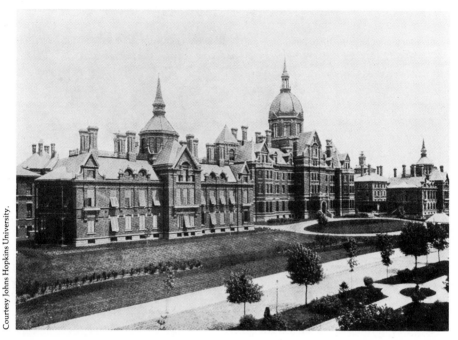

Johns Hopkins Hospital, 1889.

William Osler and a Johns Hopkins nurse at bedside, about 1895.

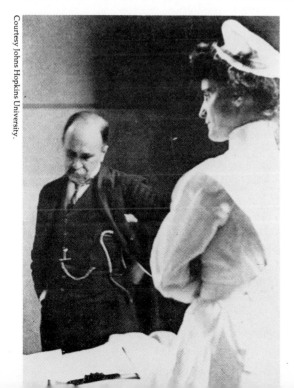

and France. The teaching program included instruction of small groups of students who served on the wards as clinical clerks and surgical dressers, in practical work in clinical laboratories, amphitheater clinics, and outpatient clinics.

A New York surgeon, William S. Halsted, working temporarily in Dr. Welch's laboratory, was made acting surgeon to the hospital, and Howard A. Kelly was called from the University of Pennsylvania to become staff gynecologist and obstetrician. As a team, these giants remade the face of American medical education. Bedside teaching and observation correlated with data obtained at the autopsy table and in the laboratory revolutionized medical education, medical practice, and medicine as a whole.

Hospital Usage Climbs

As pointed out earlier, general hospitals were slow in their development, and it was not until around 1900 that the use of hospitals for the care of all types of illness and all types of patients was widely accepted. By then the advances in medical science and the development of surgical x-ray and laboratory facilities in hospitals, coupled with the decrease in the size of houses (especially in the urban areas), the increase in families living in apartments, and the tendency to rely more and more upon agencies outside the home, made it increasingly difficult to care for the ill at home, particularly in serious cases. The result was a rapid increase in the number of hospitals. In all the nation's general hospitals in 1880 there were approximately 85,000 beds; in 1890 around 150,000; and in 1900 around 250,000. In 1872 the ratio was one hospital bed to 817 people. By 1900 the ratio was one bed to 304 people.

Sources of hospital revenue also began to change. Separate facilities for the private patients of staff physicians were added to the standard ward facilities. Patients began to pay an increasing proportion of the rising costs of hospital care. In accordance with the theory that the wealthy patients should be charged enough to provide funds for hospital care of the poor, the patients in the private rooms became not merely "pay patients" but often "overpay patients." However, in spite of the growth in income from patients, financing in voluntary hospitals still was based on deficit funding. The chief duty of the board of trustees in the early decades of the present century was to furnish or obtain philanthropic funds to make up the inevitable deficits. In 1900 the average cost per patient per day for all hospitals was estimated to be $2.00; total annual expenditures for hospital care were estimated to be $120 million. Payroll expenditures, including administration salaries, were estimated to be less than one-fourth of total expense.

The table on page 127 is made up from the official reports of 12 hospitals, in one large American city, which treated over 10,000 patients in 1900 [2]. The figures in this table reveal stark differences in per capita cost in the various hospitals.

Around the turn of the century there was a tendency to organize hospitals for specific diseases. Special hospitals were built for skin diseases, eye, ear, nose, and throat diseases, cancer, tuberculosis, fever, and diseases of the digestive tract. It was soon realized, however, that the hospital organized to treat

Hospital No.	In- Patients	Out- Patients	Total Patients	Total Running Expenses	Cost per Patient
A	1854	8197	10,051	$187,079.37	$10.65
B	1894	11,810	13,704	105,635.16	7.71
C	3850	12,559	16,409	83,410.06	5.08
D	901	11,433	12,334	53,787.05	4.36
E	3026	34,100	37,126	125,939.43	3.30
F	4079	30,860	34,939	116,790.30	3.34
G	4654	15,374	20,328	64,053.22	3.15
H	973	14,608	15,851	34,717.45	2.23
I	1266	24,011	25,217	53,392.86	2.12
J	745	23,666	24,411	45,813.40	1.87
K	2052	18,614	20,666	37,781.17	1.83
L	1898	34,281	36,179	63,378.79	1.75

only one type of disease was too limited in service, and the emphasis veered from hospitals organized for specific diseases to hospitals organized for certain age, sex, or occupational groups. Hospitals were built for maternity, orthopedic, isolation, industrial, incurable, convalescent, chronic, and cancer patients, and for children. Sanatoriums for convalescents, for patients with nervous and mental disorders, and for victims of drug addiction became hospitals when active surgical and medical clinics were added.

The original hospitals kept very few medical records. During the early part of the century most of them were satisfied to have a register of admission and discharges that contained a summary of the age, nationality, and condition of each patient, with a statement of the name of the disease and the condition at discharge. With advances in medical science, however, and with increase in the size of the medical staffs of hospitals, a system of casebooks grew in which were recorded the previous history of the patient, the course of his disease, a description of the operation performed (if any), and the condition of the patient upon his discharge from the hospital. These casebooks were generally bulky volumes, and routine notes on cases were made daily by clinical clerks appointed for that purpose. As the casebooks were inconvenient to handle and could not be carried to the wards, notes could not be easily made at bedside. Thus a modification of this system was adopted in all hospitals whereby notes were made at the bedside, on loose sheets of paper, and afterward collected, collated with charts, photographs, and graphic representations, and finally bound.

Every history of a patient's disease contained a full account of his condition prior to admission to the hospital. Inherited tendencies to disease were carefully noted along with previous illness, life-style, occupation, place of residence, exposure to unhealthful surroundings, and known addiction to alcohol or drugs. These and similar facts were scrupulously recorded. The state of the pa-

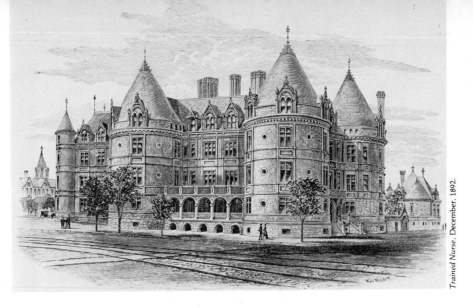

Trained Nurse, December, 1892.

The New York Cancer Hospital, about 1892.

tient upon admission was carefully described, and daily notes of his subjective and objective symptoms followed, together with the findings in the clinical and bacteriologic laboratories. If a surgical operation was done it was accurately described, and the pathologic changes in the tissue or tumor removed were recorded along with any information that had been obtained by the microscope. The termination of the disease was made a matter of similar record, and in the event of death a full protocol of the autopsy findings was added. Such histories were permanently bound and indexed for future reference. Cross-references were kept on index cards so that diseases might be grouped and all the clinical material of the hospital utilized for the description and further study of disease. In many hospitals this work was placed under the charge of a paid registrar who devoted his whole time to the preparation of casebooks and histories.

During the last quarter of the nineteenth century, great strides had been made in the science of medicine and in the improvement of hospitals. Better health was rapidly being attained. A baby born in 1875 had a life expectancy of only 28 to 40 years. In 1900 a child could be expected to live 47 years. Much remained to be done. In 1900 in the United States the principal causes of death were: (1) tuberculosis, (2) pneumonia, (3) diarrhea and enteretis, (4) heart disease, and (5) diseases of infancy and congenital malformations.

All the preceding developments and many others revolutionized medicine in the last quarter of the nineteenth century and probably yielded more progress toward the amelioration of human suffering than all the fumbling efforts of the preceding 1000 years. The implications of this revolution for nurses and nursing were very great. As physicians embraced the tenets of this new medicine, with its concomitant reliance on laboratory work, advanced surgery, and clinical diagnosis, many areas of their former domain—particularly those related to the so-called art of medicine—became the province of the nurse. As a result, the practice of nursing was markedly altered. The nurse not only stepped into the vacuum created by the physician's move into the world of scientific medicine but also began to participate in the more complicated medical and surgical procedures that were required for modern treatment. Most important, she faced new nursing care problems and unforeseen complications that came with the new methods of treatment.

Summary

Physicians of 1876 did their best to control the prevailing diseases, but treatment was directed primarily toward alleviation of symptoms rather than to the correction of underlying pathologic processes. The medical profession was still hampered by ignorance and superstition inherited from the past. Purging, bleeding, and use of extracts, tinctures, and mixtures of multiple drugs—many of them from substances now known to have little or no pharmacologic effect— were the common methods of treatment.

Major causes of death in the latter part of the nineteenth century were enteric disorders, malnutrition, and common respiratory and contagious diseases.

In the 1840s Ignaz Semmelweiss made a study of postmortem tissues of women who had died from puerperal fever in Vienna hospitals and concluded that it was spread by unclean hands, dirty clothes, and unsanitary hospital conditions. Between 1846 and 1848, through the simple expedient of cleanliness, he reduced the death rate in the maternity wards to one-tenth the previous rate.

French chemist Louis Pasteur demonstrated the scientific basis for Semmelweiss' theory by proving that bacteria were living microorganisms that increased through reproduction, not by spontaneous generation, and that they could be destroyed by heat and chemical action. Applying Pasteur's theory, Joseph Lister used carbolic acid sprays as an antiseptic in surgical operations after 1865 and thereby reduced the mortality rate in his hospital from 45 to 12 percent.

In 1876 Robert Koch published a paper on anthrax bacillus, showing for the first time that a specific infectious disease was caused by a specific microorganism, and in 1882 he announced his discovery of the tubercle bacillus. The fundamental science of bacteriology emerged from the work of Pasteur and Koch.

The success rate of surgery was greatly increased by two scientific advancements: (1) the use of ether as an anesthetic, beginning in the 1840s, which allowed surgeons to perform operations much more slowly and painstakingly, and (2) the discovery of the four blood groups, which made safe blood transfusions possible.

In the 1890s beside instruction and teaching in the wards were used for the education of medical students. The study of living patients and observations in the autopsy room and clinical laboratory, through the application of the scientific method, became of inestimable value in advancing medical knowledge.

Accuracy of diagnosis was greatly improved by Wilhelm Konrad Roentgen's discovery of x-rays in 1895. The introduction of modern medical equipment created the need for community hospitals, where local physicians could use the apparatus jointly.

By 1876 most of the great advances in gross descriptive pathology had already been made through the extensive use of autopsy. Before 1890 many organisms had been isolated as causes of specific diseases.

Improved diagnostic instruments as well as research findings emanating from the new sciences of pathology, microbiology, medical entomology, and immunology promoted the continued advancement of scientific medicine.

Advances in gynecology and obstetrics led to the development of new operative procedures and made childbearing much safer.

The most spectacular accomplishment in children's health resulted from the discovery that water, milk, and food could be contaminated by pathogenic microorganisms.

Advances in hospital care in the late nineteenth century included installation of new hospital facilities for the treatment of bacterial infection and for the promotion of antisepsis, founding of pathology laboratories, and establishment of a system of casebooks to record the patient's previous history and the course of his disease.

Progress in scientific medicine in the last quarter of the nineteenth century increased life expectancy from an estimated 28 to 40 years in 1876 to 47 years in 1900.

References
1. Thomas Addis Emmet, "Personal Reminiscences Associated with the Progress of Gynecology," *American Gynecological and Obstetrical Journal*, vol. 18, (May–June, 1900): 301–324.
2. "Some Hospital Statistics," *National Hospital Record*, vol. 5 (May, 1902): 13.

5
The Not-So-Gay Eighties and Nineties in Nurse Training Schools

The growth of nurse training schools had to await the acceleration of the general hospital movement in the United States. It was only when the concept of the community hospital became attractive to every major town and city throughout the country that these institutions began to acquire respectability, multiply, and elicit a much broader clientele. Let us examine just what the status of the hospital was as the nation moved into the 1880s and what conditions brought on the realization that trained nurses would be socially and economically useful in caring for the increasing hospital population.

Hospitals of the Late Nineteenth Century

The first complete census of hospitals in the United States was published in 1873, when the report of a survey of 178 institutions by the United States Bureau of Education appeared in *Transactions of the American Medical Association*. This report showed that 146,472 patients had been admitted to hospitals in 1872; that there were 35,604 beds; that 46 hospitals had between 100 and 200 beds, and 38 had between 200 and 400 beds; and that 18 had over 400 beds [1].

Fifteen of the hospitals were supported by cities, four by counties, seven by religious bodies, and 67 "by patients and other sources." Because several of the institutions established before that time were not named in this early survey, the statistics probably fall short of a complete account of existing hospital facilities, but they are full enough to establish a fair basis for comparison with the present.

The Civil War unquestionably did much to develop the hospitals of America, and certain features of hospital service were derived from the United States Army medical department. The most important of these was ambulance service, originated in New York City in 1868. In 1869 Dr. E. B. Dalton, who had served in the United States Army as a medical officer and had had considerable experience in the transportation of sick and wounded soldiers, divided New York City into districts in order to respond better to all calls for emergencies, accidents, and transfer of the sick from their homes to the various hospitals of the city.

Under his direction, ambulances with medicines, instruments, and other articles were built for the speedy and comfortable transportation of the sick and the

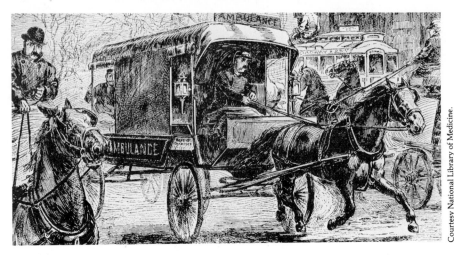

Hospital ambulance on an emergency call, about 1880.

Emily Dunning, America's first woman ambulance surgeon, was played by June Allyson in the 1952 biographical film, The Girl in White. *(From the MGM release* The Girl in White © *1952 Loew's Incorporated.)*

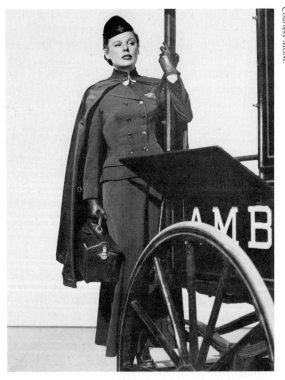

wounded. Arrangements were also made to have the vehicles accompanied by experienced surgeons who could give attention to the patients on the way to the hospital. Dr. Emily Dunning successfully challenged the conventions of male medicine in New York's Gouveneur Hospital in 1890 by becoming the first woman ambulance surgeon. By an order of the police department, ambulances were given right of way in the streets in order to prevent delay in the run between home and hospital.

The showcase of hospital architecture of the 1880s was the new 100-bed Presbyterian Hospital in New York City, which later opened its nurse training school in 1892. The hospital complex had been designed by Richard Hunt, at that time New York's most distinguished architect. The complex consisted of two major buildings, one for administration and the other for the hospital wards. Between them was a small structure that included the kitchen, laundry, and heating plants; another smaller one, the mortuary; and, lastly, one for the ambulance. The Hospital property comprised the block bounded by Manhattan's Seventieth and Seventy-first streets and Madison and Park avenues. Both the administration and hospital buildings sat upon the property lines of their respective streets and were connected by two long, covered corridors, the tops of which were used as roof gardens. The walls of both buildings were constructed of red brick and gray limestone.

The plan of the hospital building was simple. The first floor was devoted mainly to rooms for private patients. These rooms were of fair size and comfortably furnished; the charge for them was $30 to $50 a week. The surgical operating rooms, located on the third and fourth floors, were considered among the best of their day, although they were paneled with wood, less sanitary than tile. They

Presbyterian Hospital, New York City, 1872.

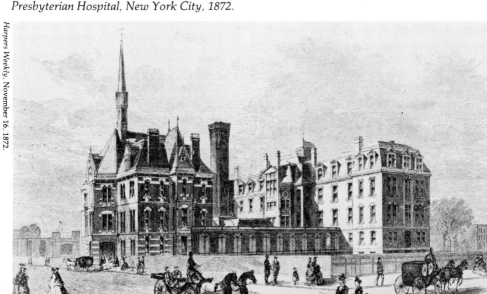

Harpers Weekly, November 16, 1872.

received excellent outside light and were conveniently equipped. The three upper floors were each divided equally into two wards of 12 beds. The ceilings were high, and the many windows of the wards were large enough to secure excellent ventilation. The walls were hard-finished and the floors were made of pitch pine to withstand heavy scrubbing. There were no passenger elevators: a staircase ran up through the center of the building.

Proliferation of Nursing Schools

To the planners of hospitals it was doubtful whether a successful hospital could be developed without an affiliated training school for nurses. This was not simply because the training school had proved to be the most economic means of providing nursing care, but because it was supposedly impossible to create the desired "home" atmosphere if graduates from various schools were employed. Each graduate nurse from outside would come with habits firmly fixed and with her own hospital traditions and ideas of service.

Consequently, after the founding of the first four schools of nursing in 1872 and 1873, other hospitals opened schools of their own, and by 1880 there were 15 schools, 323 students, and 157 graduates in the United States. Twenty years later these figures had soared to 432 schools, 11,164 students, and 3546 graduates. Irene Sutliffe, Superintendent of the Long Island College Hospital Training School for Nurses, and Isabel Hampton, Superintendent of the Johns Hopkins Training School for Nurses, warned against the premature organization of schools of nursing, but this warning was not heeded. New York State alone was responsible for the organization of 25 schools before 1890 and by 1902 had added 54 more of varying quality. By 1902 four states accounted for 230 of the 492 existing schools [2].

Nurse Training Schools, Public Schools, and Higher Education

If the nation's cultural level could be gauged by the status of the public school, then the latter part of the century showed a significant advance in American culture. The seven million pupils enrolled in the public schools in 1870 increased to 15,500,000 in 1900, the 300 public high schools of 1860 increased to over 6000, while the 12 state normal schools of 1860 increased to 175. At the end of the century there were almost 500 colleges—about double the number in 1860. Illiteracy declined from 17 percent in 1880 to less than 11 percent in 1900. By the end of the 1870s, most of the state universities had opened their gates to women. In the meantime, women's colleges on a par with the best schools for men had been founded: Vassar, opened in 1865 and supported by a rich brewer of Poughkeepsie; Mount Holyoke, transformed from a girls' seminary into a college; Smith, founded in 1871 through the vision of a country minister and the wealth of a village spinster; and Wellesley, created in 1875 through the largesse of a Boston lawyer. Women's colleges were added to the great universities: Barnard at Columbia in 1889, and Radcliffe at Harvard in 1894. More significant was that secondary schools as well as elementary schools were being taught largely by women by this time.

As compared with other professional schools or with colleges of the time, nurse training schools, despite their 7-day week, had an unprecedently long year. In the majority of schools the academic year took up 50 weeks of each year, with no Christmas, Easter, or Thanksgiving holidays and rarely a whole free Sunday. The annual vacation period was generally two weeks long, and although there were some schools allowing three weeks or even a month, there were others giving but 10 days of vacation annually. In all schools it was customary to require the student to make up to the hospital every day or half-day lost through illness or absence. Contrasted with the 50 weeks of the training school year were the 32 or 36 weeks of the academic year in the college or professional school.

Several months before entering a hospital training school, one prospective student nurse came across some stanzas entitled "Woman's Rights," one of which particularly impressed her:

The right to tread so softly beside the couch of pain,
To smooth with gentle fingers the tangled locks again,
To watch beside the dying in the still small hours of night,
And breathe a consecrating prayer as the spirit takes its flight [3].

This privilege to practice those "dearest rights of her sex" meant, in fact, the right to train and work under incredibly rigorous conditions, but that did not seem to discourage the young woman or a host of other new applicants.

Training School Applicants

The enormous number of applications received each year by the more famous training schools made it possible for them to attract students of a much higher caliber than had formerly been the case. The approximate number of applicants to the following training schools in 1905 substantiated their well-deserved reputations [4]:

Bellevue Hospital, New York	2000
Johns Hopkins Hospital, Baltimore	1400
St. Luke's Hospital, New York	1200
Presbyterian Hospital, New York	1100
New York Hospital, New York	1000
Illinois Training School, Chicago	1000
Boston City Hospital, Boston	1000
Massachusetts General Hospital, Boston	1000
Carney Hospital, Boston	900
Margaret Fahnestock Training School, New York	800
Lakeside Hospital, Cleveland	800

ILLINOIS TRAINING SCHOOL FOR NURSES

Connected .... With Cook County and Presbyterian Hospitals, Incorporated and Established 1880.

304 Honore Street, Chicago, Illinois.

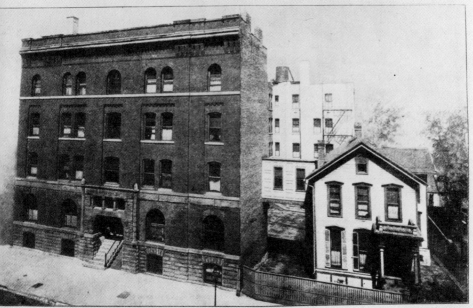

The Board of Directors offers a three years' course of training to women who desire to enter the profession of nursing. The course of training comprises practical work in the wards, theoretical work in class and lecture rooms, and cooking lessons; being divided into Junior, Middle and Senior years. The facilities for imparting theoretical and practical training to nurses are thorough and complete in all departments, including instruction by the ablest professors from different medical colleges, and the daily care of nearly one thousand patients in medical, surgical, obstetrical, gynecological, children's and contagious wards. Applications for admission must be made to the Superintendent, 304 Honore Street, Chicago, Illinois.

Trained Nurse, January, 1895.

Advertisement for the Illinois Training School for Nurses, 1895.

On the other end of the continuum were several hundred assorted schools that barely managed to attract enough students to allow the maintenance of even a skeleton student nursing staff. The enormous increase in the number of hospitals and sanitariums throughout the country and the consequent unrestricted development of training schools as a part of their working organizations led to a very large demand for students trained essentially for utilitarian purposes. Since the student supply was inadequate, training school standards were lowered or sacrificed to meet the current institutional staffing needs. Evidence was piling up as to the inferiority of many candidates. A school that could state honestly that it had 100 quality applicants annually was fortunate. The average large school of the time admitted a class of about 30 to 35 students each year.

Living Quarters

By the 1890s the leading schools of nursing generally maintained their own separate student residences adjacent to the hospital. The quality of these nurses' homes varied tremendously. Perhaps one of the finest facilities was built in conjunction with the new Johns Hopkins Hospital in Baltimore. The first floor of this structure included the superintendent and graduate nurses' quarters, a library, and a sitting room, while the students' rooms were on the upper floors. On the other

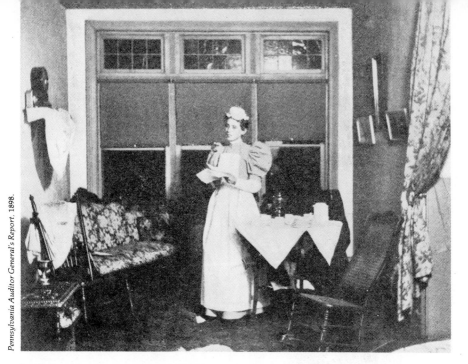

Student nurse's room at Meadville Hospital, Meadville, Pennsylvania, 1897.

hand, many schools still housed nurses in renovated hospital space, and the only place where students could meet guests was the office of the superintendent of nurses.

Student Characteristics

What were the students like? Nightingale standards dictated "good education; good character; good background; good health." Naturally, "good" meant what each hospital labeled as such. Eight years of prior schooling was an accepted educational standard, but often the required amount of preparatory education varied. Requirements concerning health and background differed as well. Although the minimum age varied, the students were typically older than young women enrolled in trade schools or colleges. Competition from other fields open to women soon put pressure on schools of nursing to take younger students in order to prevent them from drifting into other lines of work, and consequently the minimum age requirement of 25 was decreased to 21 or lower.

Of course one of the prevailing characteristics of nurse training school students was that they were all female. American nursing, based on Nightingale ideals, had no place for men except where physical strength was needed, and men attendants were used only in the care of alcoholics, insane and violent patients, and men with genitourinary diseases. In 1888, however, the training of male nurses for general patient care became a possibility with the establishment of

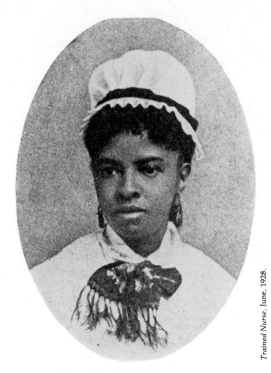

Trained Nurse, June, 1928.

Mary E. P. Mahoney, first black graduate nurse.

the Mills School of Nursing at Bellevue Hospital. A course comparable with that offered to the women students was developed, but this action was not widely emulated.

The first black nursing school graduate was Mary Eliza Mahoney. She attended the New England Hospital for Women and Children, completing her course of study, in 16 months, on August 1, 1879. The first separate school to educate black nurses was founded in 1886 at Spellman Seminary in Atlanta, Georgia, and two other similar institutions—Hampton Institute in Virginia and Providence Hospital in Chicago—opened their doors in 1891. Tuskegee Institute in Alabama started a school of nursing in 1892. As the twentieth century approached, the number of black students enrolled in schools of nursing—primarily in separate schools, but also in integrated ones—slowly increased.

Strict Discipline
During the Middle Ages nursing had been a function of religious orders, and the monastic ideals of asceticism, self-abnegation, and obedience to authority had survived as ideals deemed appropriate to nursing. In addition, the military influence upon nursing education was natural since the first hospital training schools had been built on the English model, which had closely followed Florence Night-

ingale's reorganization of the army medical service in the Crimea. Monastic and military traditions heavily influenced not only the actual workings of the schools of nursing but also the public's conception of them. It was expected that the nurse in training should yield to her superiors an obedience characteristic of a good soldier and that her actions should be governed by the dedication to duty derived from religious devotion. Hospital administrators shared these expectations. A leading hospital administration manual of the era warned: "Most of the women who enter the training school are only half-made women. They are but half-bridled in their moral and mental as well as their physical makeup" [5]. It was the duty of the superintendents of the training schools to mold the young women along proper lines, to teach them good morals, truthfulness, conscientiousness, devotion to duty, unselfishness, and to think less of themselves and of their pleasures and comforts and more of the happiness and comfort of others.

Any nurse probationer who in her early days showed a tendency to shirk distasteful tasks was declared unfit. Perhaps the most difficult problem came when a young woman, who had proved promising and worthwhile during her probation and had been subsequently advanced, unexpectedly developed undesirable qualities. She might have grumbled at extra-duty assignments or she might have regarded some rules as having been made to be broken; or perhaps she had developed a too-familiar attitude while dealing with men; or her records were untrustworthy; or she could not get along "sweetly" in all places she was assigned to; or she talked too much and openly criticized the doctors and head nurses. After having ignored a word of warning, such a borderline student would quickly be dismissed as a "troublemaker."

That strict discipline for student nurses was the order of the day was evidenced by one of the major questions at an early hospital association meeting: "Who has a successful method of disciplining pupils?" The participants had found it generally most satisfactory to give erring student nurses extra hours of duty, and it was maintained that discipline in the nursing school either made or broke a student's character. It was the task of the superintendent of nurses to decide whether or not a troublesome student was incorrigible or incapable of nursing. Those who went through the full nursing school course were expected to emerge from the experience with strong characters, disciplined wills, and a capacity for self-sacrifice.

Other authoritarian characteristics prevailed. In the dining room, there were separate tables for head nurses, seniors, juniors, and probationers. It was expected that a student who entered a hospital would readily accept that she would have no time for social activities and that she would be able to visit her friends at home only once or twice a year. Even then, it was recommended that friends allow her to rest when she was visiting them.

These rigid rules of conduct were difficult for young ladies of the era to tolerate. One student secretly complained:

Rules are necessary, of course, but surely we are subject to rather many. I have hitherto submitted meekly to every rule, but there are times when they chafe. Of late I have sometimes found myself longing to yield to the voice of an inward tempter that bids me defy

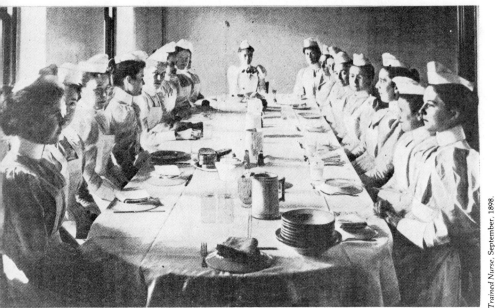

Trained Nurse, September, 1898.

Dinner at eight: student nurses at the Jefferson Medical College Hospital, Philadelphia, 1898.

The Florence Nightingale Pledge. (From the Warner Brothers release White Angel © *1936 Warner Bros. Pictures, Inc. Copyright renewed 1963.)*

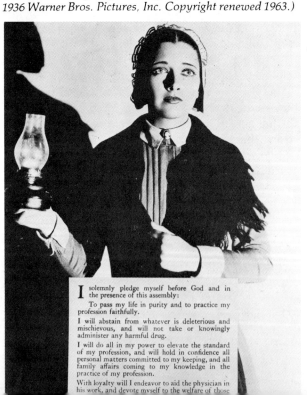

Courtesy Warner Brothers.

I solemnly pledge myself before God and in the presence of this assembly:

To pass my life in purity and to practice my profession faithfully.

I will abstain from whatever is deleterious and mischievous, and will not take or knowingly administer any harmful drug.

I will do all in my power to elevate the standard of my profession, and will hold in confidence all personal matters committed to my keeping, and all family affairs coming to my knowledge in the practice of my profession.

With loyalty will I endeavor to aid the physician in his work, and devote myself to the welfare of those red tape and regulations when it can be done without interfering with my duty to the patients. There are so many rules, such battalions of regulations, such miles and miles of red tape that to me seem totally unnecessary—the existence of some of them is a positive insult to the manners and discretion of the nurses. The idea of it being made compulsory for us to ask the lady superintendent's permission every time we want to go out on the street, even though we are off duty. It isn't as if we were very young girls. When a girl is fitted for a hospital nurse she is fitted to regulate her own conduct without the aid of a thousand rules. I think that when the rules of this training school were framed it was surely done upon the principle of making life as trying as it possibly could be made for the nurses. I fancy that the board must have sat down and made out a list of everything it seemed likely that young women would care to do for innocent pleasure and then passed a sweeping motion to the effect that they weren't to be allowed to do any of them [6].

No tolerance of student misconduct was allowed in the schools. Married and older women were generally excluded because, as one superintendent put it, "We see so few women past 30 who begin the career of a trained nurse, and who fall in with the life successfully, that we are constrained almost to take the broad ground that women over 30 are unfit for admission to a training school." She added that "of course it goes without saying that married women—divorced or separated from their husbands, with perhaps divorce in the background—are not proper probationers for a training school." Such women were "self-centered; their interests are elsewhere; in their own minds at least they have been abused, and they are unable to devote themselves to others to the exclusion of their personal affairs" [7].

The systematic hospital socialization of student nurses may best be understood as a concern with authority and self-control. Supervised by a trusted "director of nurses," surrounded by a tight wall of security, the school was intended to raise a plentiful supply of women nurses—respectful, obedient, cheerful, submissive, hard-working, loyal, passive, and religious. As workers on massive hospital wards, student nurses buried the Victorian stereotype of the woman-as-lady under a mountain of reality. Indeed it was difficult to argue that young women as a sex must be weak, timid, incompetent, fragile vessels of spirituality when thousands of them were exposed daily to a ritual of long hours, disease, death, human misery, and suffering.

The Florence Nightingale Pledge

Early in 1893 Lystra E. Gretter, Superintendent of Nursing at the Farrand Training School for Nurses at Harper Hospital in Detroit, became convinced that the fledgling nursing profession needed a code of ethics to guide the graduates in their work. Amid the trappings of surrounding Victorian America, Miss Gretter led a small committee of nurses to compose "The Florence Nightingale Pledge." A document with marked similarities to the Hippocratic Oath, and reflecting the idealism of the era, the pledge was first administered to the graduating class of Farrand Training School on April 25, 1893, as follows:

I solemnly pledge myself before God, and in the presence of this assembly: to pass my life in purity and to practice my profession faithfully. I will abstain from whatever is deleterious and mischievous, and will not take or knowingly administer any harmful drug. I will do all in my power to maintain and elevate the standard of my profession and will hold in confidence all personal matters committed to my keeping and all family affairs coming to my knowledge in the practice of my calling. With loyalty will I endeavor to aid the physician in his work and devote myself to the welfare of those committed to my care" [8].

Teachers and Textbooks

Who taught the students? Records of the early schools reveal that in the 1880s and 1890s the task of imparting nursing theory was borne by physicians while nursing practice was the province of the superintendent and her assistants. A few of the physician lecturers had some knowledge of educational methods, but most of them merely repeated to tired students notes that they themselves had taken in medical school classes. Sometimes even this poor formal instruction had to be modified when the pressure of ward work kept either the students or the teachers away and the class had to be canceled.

Lack of teaching materials and textbooks was also a serious problem. The leading schools developed their own instructional manuals of nursing arts, such as the *Hand-Book of Nursing for Family and General Use*, written by a committee of physicians and nurses connected with the Connecticut Training School at the New Haven Hospital and published by Lippincott in 1878. The committee felt that it was important that a summary of hospital nursing directions be given to each student nurse as well as to any graduate nurse who might be hired from another school. It was written in simple form to be easily understood, yet it was comprehensive enough to provide aid in the ordinary duties of the nurse. The table that follows shows the results of an 1883 survey of the characteristics of five leading schools of nursing and indicates textbooks in use at that time.

The manual was soon introduced for textbook use in other training schools. During the next two years, similar nursing manuals were published elsewhere. In 1885 Clara Weeks Shaw wrote *A Textbook of Nursing for the Use of Training Schools, Families and Private Students*. The title reveals that the level of presentation and content were designed for use by both nurses and the general public. Isabel Hampton's *Nursing: Its Principles and Practice for Hospital and Private Use*, appearing in 1893, was the first substantial nursing care text and was widely used in schools for the next 20 years. The first anatomy book for nurses was written in 1893 by Diana Kimber of the Charity Hospital School for Nurses in New York. Lavinia Dock, an 1886 Bellevue Hospital graduate, wrote *The Textbook on Materia Medica for Nurses* in 1890.

Five different journals for nurses were published before 1901. The first, *The Nightingale*, appeared in 1886 and was edited by a Bellevue graduate who was also a female physician. It died from lack of support in 1891. A second periodical, *The Trained Nurse and Hospital Review*, began business in August, 1888, and continued to appear monthly for more than 70 years. Two other journals, *The Nursing Record* and *The Nursing World*, appeared for several years during the

Gay Nineties before folding. In 1899, under the leadership of Mary E. P. Davis, a stock company was formed with about 550 cash subscriptions and a new journal, *The American Journal of Nursing*, managed entirely by nurses, made its debut in October, 1900, and continues to the present.

Theory Portion of Nurse Training

Although the theory portion of nurse training had been expanded somewhat since the late 1870s, when it had constituted less than 1 percent of the entire time spent in school, in the 1890s it still accounted for only about 2 percent of the total required hours. The other 98-to-99 percent was devoted to practice. Curricula of early days contained some anatomy and physiology, materia medica, and lectures on "special diseases."

In 1884–1885, at one of the better institutions of the time, the Farrand Training School for Nurses at Harper Hospital in Detroit, the students had two annual series of lectures, which constituted the total theory content of the 24-month course. The distribution and time devoted to the various subjects included anatomy (four hours), physiology (four hours), surgical emergencies (four hours), medical emergencies (four hours), dietetics (two hours), and hygiene (two hours). All lectures, including those on nursing, were given by physicians and were held from 8:00 P.M. to 9:00 P.M. for the months between October and March. During the remainder of the year, students provided service without the benefit of the formal classes.

The final examination questions at Evansville Sanitarium Training School in Evansville, Indiana, for the class of 1899 reveals the state of nursing theory of that time [9]:

SURGERY
How would you prepare for a celiotomy or a laparotomy at a patient's house?
How would you prepare for adjustment of a fracture of the forearm, and what would you do before the doctor came if he were long delayed? What is a simple fracture? A compound fracture? A comminuted fracture? A multiple fracture?
What means can you give for stopping hemorrhage?
What instruments should be prepared by curettage with repair of laceration of cervix and perineum?
What are the following operations: Ventral fixation? Alexander's operation? Vaginal puncture? Colpoperineoplasty? Colectomy? Hysterectomy? Paracentesis? Cholecystectomy? Nephrectomy? Gastroenterotomy?

MEDICINE
What is the temperature and pulse range in an average case of typhoid fever? What is a high temperature in this fever?
What is a relapse?

OBSTETRICS
If you were alone with a woman when she gives birth to a child, what would you do?
What does fever following delivery indicate?
What is puerperal eclampsia? What would you do for a case of it before the doctor came?

Results of a Survey of Hospital Superintendents Associated with Five Major Schools of Nursing in 1883.

	New York Training School At Bellevue Hospital	Connecticut Training School at New Haven State Hospital	Training School at Massachusetts General Hospital	Training School of the New York Hospital	Boston City Hospital Training School
Organized in:	1873	1873	1873	1877	1878
Admission Requirements:	Age 25-35, sound health, good moral character, and a knowledge of arithmetic, reading, penmanship, and English dictation.	Age 22-40, good health and character, and common school education.	Age 25-35, preferred, must be in sound health, and must present on application a certificate from some responsible person as to their good character.	Age 25-35, sound health, perfect senses, good moral character, and good common school education.	Age 21-35, preferred, good health and character.
Salary Paid Pupils:	$9 a month for the first year, $15 a month for the second year.	$170 for the term of eighteen months (average of $9.44 a month).	$10 a month for first year, $14 a month for second year.	$10, $13, $16 a month for the first, second, and third 6 months respectively; graduates, $25 a month.	$10 a month for first year, $14 a month for second year; graduate head nurses, $20-$30 a month.
*Textbooks Used: (By Number, See Below for Titles)	1, 4 and 7	4 and 6	2 and 3	4, 6, 7 and 8	3, 5, 7, 10 and 11
Number of nurses excluding Superintendent:	50	22	53	36	61
Average Number of Patients:	260	112	170	140	286
Average Patients Assigned per Nurse:	5	5	3	4	5
Does Hospital bear All Expenses of School?	Salaries and washing partly.	Board, lodging, and washing.	Board, lodging and washing, and part salaries.	Entire.	Entire expense.

Yearly average of Training School Salaries paid by Hospital:	$6,722.00	—	$8,527.33	$5,700.00	$8,820.00
Does the Superintendent of Hospital think the training school valuable to the Hospital?	"Certainly I do."	"I do."	"No Hospital of any size is complete without one."	"In all its developments and departments good and always good."	"Yes."
Does he know of any as good and cheaper plan?	"No."	"Not that I know of."	"Any other system inferior in every respect."	"No."	"The cheapest and best."
Length of Course:	1 year.	18 months.	2 years.	18 months.	2 years.

*(1) Bartholow, Robert. *A Practical Treatise on Materia Medica Therapeutics.* New York: D. Appleton, 1876; (2) Cutter, Calvin. *Second Book on Analytic Anatomy, Physiology and Hygiene.* Philadelphia: Lippincott, 1875; (3) Domville, Edward J. *A Manual for Hospital Nurses and Others Engaged in Attending on the Sick.* London: J & A Churchill, 1872; (4) Draper, John W. *Human Physiology.* New York: Harper, 1870; (5) Lees, Florence. *Handbook for Hospital Sisters* (ed. by H. W. Acland). London: W. Isbister & Co., 1874; (6) New Haven State Hospital, Connecticut Training School for Nurses. *Handbook of Nursing for Family and General Use.* Philadelphia: Lippincott, 1878; (7) New York Training School for Nurses Attached to Bellevue Hospital. *Manual of Nursing.* New York: The Hospital, 1878; (8) Nightingale, Florence. *Notes on Nursing: What It Is and What It Is Not.* New York: Appleton, 1860; (9) Smith, William R. *Lectures on Nursing.* London: J & A Churchill, 1875; (10) Williams, Rachel, and Fisher, Alice. *Hints for Hospital Nurses.* Edinburgh: Maclachlan and Stewart, 1877; (11) Woolsey, Abby H. *Handbook for Hospital Visitors.* New York: G. P. Putnam's Sons, 1877.

Source: W. B. Platt, "Table of Statistics of Several Training Schools for Nurses," *Medical News,* vol. 47 (June, 1885): 444.

With what would you feed the baby until the milk appeared? When does the milk appear? Is its advent accompanied by fever?

Give the stages of labor.

What is Crede's method?

PHYSIOLOGY AND HYGIENE

Give the difference between excretion and secretion.

Give systemic circulation; pulmonary circulation.

How would you ventilate a sickroom which had only one window and one door? What is natural ventilation? What is ventilation by extraction? Name three important rules in regard to ventilation.

How would you take care of the flush closets, stationary basins, and old dressings?

Give a thirty-line treatise on digestion.

ANATOMY

How many vertebrae are there? Name the divisions.

Name the bones of the head; of the face; of the leg.

Give the divisions of the alimentary canal. Of the region of the chest. Locate the heart, the liver, the spleen, and the kidneys.

Name five arteries; five nerves.

What kind of nerves are the fifth and seventh cranial nerves?

BACTERIOLOGY

Name five pyogenic germs which cause disease. How are they killed? What are the requirements for their growth?

What is aspesis? What is antisepsis?

MATERIA MEDICA AND THERAPUTICS

What is the dose of sulphate of atropia? Of sulfate of strychnia? Of hyoscine hydrobromate?

What would you do for a patient who had taken an overdose of opium, or morphine? What in poisons generally? What is a special antidote for carbolic acid poisoning?

In strychnine mixture with grs. II to 3VI of water, how much strychnine will be given to 3I dose?

How much morphia would you give to a child two years old? Four years old? Seven years old? How much strychnine sulphate to a child three years old? Eight years old? Twelve years old? Give the standard rule by which the dose for children is reduced.

CHEMISTRY

Give the meaning in reaction of urine, or acid, alkaline, and neutral. Give test for albumin and sugar and the normal specific gravity of urine.

How would you obtain a specimen of urine for examination? How is it often contaminated?

Write about one hundred words of general urinalysis.

How do you make saturated solution of boracic acid? Normal salt solution? Ten percent solution of nitrate of silver? How do you make bichloride solution 1-2000, 1-5000, 1-10,000?

Let us take a look at the work of an outstanding student in one of the schools of nursing with a large component of theory. In November, 1890, *Trained Nurse* announced the offer of "a prize of $10 cash for an essay upon the following subject: Give full particulars, with Notes, as to Temperature, Dietary, etc., of a Typhoid Fever Case, nursed by the Competitor herself, and describing, if possible, the Case from its commencement to its termination. Temperature and Diet-

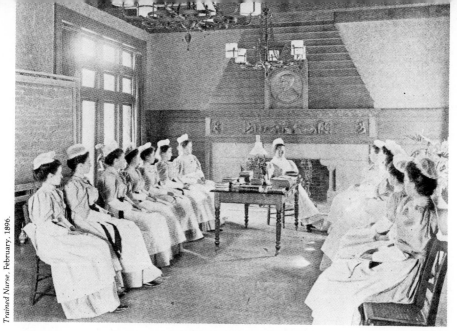

Class in session at the Henry W. Bishop Memorial Training School for Nurses, Pittsfield, Massachusetts, 1895.

Course of lectures for the 1884–1885 session at The Farrand Training School for Nurses, Detroit.

COURSE OF LECTURES 1884-5.

FARRAND TRAINING SCHOOL FOR NURSES.

ANATOMY,	Oct. 29, Nov. 12, Nov. 26, Dec. 10.
	DR. CARRIER.
PHYSIOLOGY,	Nov. 1, Nov. 14, Nov. 28, Dec. 12.
	DR. GILBERT.
SURGICAL EMERGENCIES,	November 15, November 19.
	DR. BOOK.
SURGICAL EMERGENCIES,	December 3, December 17.
	DR. WALKER.
MEDICAL EMERGENCIES,	November 17, November 20.
	DR. ANDREWS.
MEDICAL EMERGENCIES,	December 6, December 20.
	DR. CLELAND.
DIETETICS,	December 24, January 7.
	DR. FLINTERMANN.
HYGIENE,	December 27, January 10.
	DR. RUSSEL.
OBSTETRIC NURSING,	December 31, January 14.
	DR. DAVENDORF.
OBSTETRIC NURSING,	January 28, February. 28.
	DR. ANDREWS.
SICK ROOM NURSING,	January 3, January 17.
	DR. SHURLEY.
SICK ROOM NURSING.	January 31, February 14.
	DR. LYSTER.
GYNÆOCOLOGICAL NURSING,	January 21, February 4.
	DR. CARSTENS.
GYNÆOCOLOGICAL NURSING,	February 18, March 4.
	DR. LONGYEAR.
SURGICAL SICK ROOM NURSING,	January 24, February 7.
	DR. McGRAW.
SURGICAL SICK ROOM NURSING,	February 21, March 7.
	DR. MACLEAN.
NURSING CHILDREN,	March 14, January 21.
	DR. DOUGLASS.
NURSING CHILDREN,	March 18, February 25.
	DR. CLELAND.
EYE AND EAR,	February 25, March 11.
	DR. CONNOR.
NERVOUS DISEASES,	March 25, March 28.
	DR. EMERSON.

LECTURES FROM 8 TO 9 P. M.

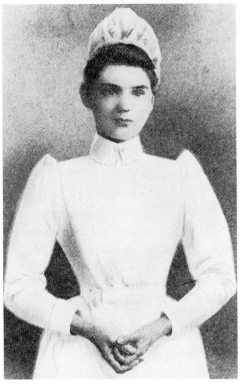

Adelaide Nutting as a Johns Hopkins student nurse in 1891.

Charts, etc., should accompany Essay, if possible." The journal's office was flooded with material from ambitious nurses eager to test their writing ability and their knowledge of clinical nursing. The winner was Mary Adelaide Nutting, a student at Johns Hopkins School of Nursing. Her "Notes of a Typhoid Fever Case" was awarded the first prize and appeared in the March, 1891, issue and documented the expert bedside observations she had made. In her record of the initial day of nursing care Miss Nutting noted:

> In order to follow satisfactorily the development of this case, it will be necessary to have some definite idea of the patient's surroundings and conditions previous to admission to the Hospital.
>
> The case had been reported to the Superintendent of the Hospital on December 18th, 1890, and a member of the staff was promptly sent out to investigate. In a locality amidst surroundings which were wretched in the extreme, and in quarters where poverty and filth held undisputed sway, this is what he found. On a sofa in the corner of a small room which was almost destitute of furniture, yet evidently served for kitchen, bedroom and living-room generally, the patient, a young man about twenty-one years of age, was discovered, lying in his clothes.

The room was already occupied by a woman and three small children, and the stench which pervaded the atmosphere was sickening to a degree, almost unendurable. The distress of abject poverty and accumulations of filth were visible everywhere. It was quite impossible to obtain accurate information concerning the first days and date of the patient's illness, but, from what could be gathered, it was now the beginning of the fourth week. For this length of time the poor creature had been lying in his clothes and was now in a state of neglect which beggars description. The first point to attract the attention was his mouth, in which not only the tongue but the lips and teeth and even the roof of the mouth were so covered with a thick, dry, dark, almost black crust that their original form and color were almost entirely lost. The cheeks and nose had a very peculiar dusky flush, and between the partially closed eyelids, the white of the eye only was visible. He was in a state of low muttering delirium and displayed a marked subsultus. His abdomen was found to be greatly distended, tense and tympantic, and it was discovered that involuntary movements of the bowels had been going on for some days, with the passage, also involuntary, of large quantities of urine. His pulse was irregular, intermittent and compressible, the respiration rapid and feeble, and it was questionable if he could live to reach the hospital. By exercise, however, of the very greatest care, they succeeded in removing him, and he was brought to the ward on the evening of December 18th at nine o'clock.

After admission his temperature was 102.5°, pulse 108, and very dicrotic, and respiration 42. An hour later the temperature rose to 103.6° and he was then given a tub bath, 70° F. of fifteen minutes duration, which brought it down to 98.6°. It was quite evident, however, that the temperature was not the great difficulty to overcome; the grave trouble lay in the extreme weakness of the heart, in which there was almost no impulse, the heart sounds indistinct, and the pulse thready and fluttering. Free stimulation was at once resorted to, brandy being administered in half ounce doses every two hours, and for a further cardiac stimulus was given 01. Terebinth M.v every three hours, for three doses. At 4 A.M. his temperature rose to 103.8° and he was given a second bath bringing it down to 99.8°; at this time his respiration had become 44, shallow and quivering, his pulse 124, still compressible and intermittent, and the cheeks showed a steadily deepening purplish flush. The lips and tongue were so dry, and the scabs so adherent, that it was with difficulty they could be removed, and then only with forceps and after repeated softening applications of glycerine and Boracic Acid Solution. With the utmost care that could be used they would bleed with every small portion that was removed and it was thought advisable to do only a very little at a time and vaseline was applied liberally after each attack.

Owing to his extreme weakness and prostration no attempt was made to give him the thorough cleansing bath he needed, but he was merely sponged off with tepid water, softened with Aromatic Spirits of Ammonia. At this point, 10 A.M., the application of Turpentine stupes to the abdomen was begun, applying them just as hot as could be borne, and changing every fifteen minutes when possible. For nourishment he had albumen, the whites of two eggs, every two hours, well beated, strained, diluted with cold water one-third, flavored a little with about two drachms of whisky and served with crushed ice. This he took easily, and never seemed to grow tired of. At 10 A.M. he was ordered Tr. Digitalis M.xv to be given every three hours, but this was discontinued after five doses (M.$lxxv$) had been given. At 10:39 the temperature had risen to 104.4°, and the bath which was given reduced it to 98°, and him to a condition which looked very much like collapse, for in addition to the subsultus, there was much tremor, coldness and blueness of the extremities, continuing for more than an hour, a feeble and fluttering pulse, a rapid and shallow respiration. He was able, however, to take both stimulant and nourishment very well, and drank water whenever it was brought him, most eagerly, this was generally done every hour, at regular intervals between nourishments. At 3 P.M. a bath was again due, the temperature being 103.6°, pulse 132, respiration 32, and the result was a reduction of temperature to 101.6°, pulse 132, respiration 44. At 10 P.M. it had risen again to 104, pulse 140, respiration 40, and was reduced to 98.2°, pulse 130, respiration 36, by a bath of seventeen minutes duration at 70°F. His condition after this was very much as described before, only with each feature more marked, and on this occasion, it was fully an hour and a half before the tremor ceased to be visible, while the pulse was extremely thready and fluttering, ranging from 132 to 140 and dropping a beat frequently. Later he became somnolent and remained in that state during the rest of the night. Although his temperature was 102.8°, above bathing point (which had been fixed at 102.5°), and remained there without moving for six hours, no baths were given, but he was roused every hour for stimulant and nourishment which came alternately, and the fomentations were steadily kept up. On the morning of the second day the tympanites was if anything increased, and as there had been about nineteen movements within twenty-four hours, it will be seen that the diarrhoea was not materially diminished. The movements were of course still involuntary as was also the passage of a really enormous quantity of urine. Later in the morning at 10 A.M. the baths were started once more, and the temperature from 102.8° was brought down to 99°, the effect after being that of the previous day. It was at this period that the pulmonary trouble began to be apparent, and dullness was noted at the left base, the exact cause of which was doubtful. A hypodermic puncture was made for diagnostic purposes, and a small syringe full of bloody pus was withdrawn. Aspiration was decided upon for the following day, and the diagnosis of pneumonia was made. Here I may say that upon aspirating the next day much to the surprise of everybody no fluid was found [10].

Physicians Attack Theory for Nurses

From the very first, debate was rampant over the proper mix of theory and practice in the education of the nurse. According to an 1875 paper by Dr. Samuel Howard, a professor of the theory and practice of medicine in Montreal, the new profession of nursing should require:

. . . a liberal preliminary education at least equal to that now required of the medical student, assigning, however, a first place to natural science and a lower one to the classics. And, second, a professional education extending over three full years, and embracing the following scheme of subjects: anatomy, physiology, chemistry, materia medica, pharmacy, dietetics, hygiene, and clinical instruction in nursing the sick and wounded, in dressing wounds, and applying splints, etc., for which education they would, of course, receive pay as medical students do [11].

Dr. Howard thought that nurses trained along these lines should receive a diploma, after an extensive examination, entitling them to practice nursing among the general public and to charge fees in rates proportionate to physicians. Such nurses would then not only be the helpmates of physicians but would also complement the work of the entire medical profession.

Such liberal ideas, however, were generally unwelcome. An opposing view voiced in a leading international medical journal warned of the dangers that would follow if such a course were to be pursued:

The principal argument in favour of the medical education of nurses is the necessity for their knowing the reason why in reference to all the details of management and treatment which fall under their cognisance . . . . To attempt to give nurses instruction as to the reason why . . . would be, in the majority of instances, to inflict a heavy task upon them and to lift them more or less out of their proper sphere, possibly at the risk of withdrawing them from due attention to their less intellectual but equally useful functions. To give them more than an insight into it is to demand for them complete education as medical practitioners and to transform them from nurses into doctors—a consummation assuredly not to be desired . . . . There are fashions in opinion as well as in dress, and there are enthusiasts in practical as well as in theoretical matters; and it is from time to time needful to show the folly or distortions of fashion and to put the curb upon such enthusiasm [12].

Twenty-five years later the opinion of the majority of physicians had not changed. During the early 1900s a Boston surgeon lecturing to a class of nurses surprised them by saying that, if he had to choose, he would prefer a nurse who knew a few ways of dressing hair to one well grounded in anatomy and physiology. Physicians repeatedly attacked attempts to increase the theoretical portion of nurse training. One claimed that if he was asked to state the function of the trained nurse he would answer: first, to care for the bodily needs of the patient; second, to carry out the orders of the physician; and, third, to record the "vital phenomena" of the patient. The entire scope of nursing practice should fall under one of these headings.

Yet in many proposed nurse training courses alarmed physicians discovered topics such as: mineral food and mineral waters; the amount of salt found in the body and its necessity in food; food value in heat, energy, and tissue-building; and the uses of calcium, sodium, phosphorus, magnesium, iron, sulfur, and potassium in the body. They were unhappy to see that, under the heading of practical work, nursing students were offered laboratory instruction in pipe analysis and were required to apply the flame test for sodium, potassium, calcium, and strontium on the Bunsen burner. Another lesson focused on sucrose, glucose, levulose, and lactose, comparing sources, preparations, composition, properties, and digestion. The pages of course outlines in such innovative curricula revealed lessons in chemistry and physiology that, according to some physicians of the day, had absolutely nothing to do with nursing the sick.

Physicians were quick to point out that if such "foolishness" continued, society would have a nurse with knowledge that would not be of the slightest use to her patient; at least two years of her time would have been wasted in the acquisition of theory that had no bearing on her work. Why should the nurse, they fumed, be taught urinalysis or the use of the microscope? Such objections as these kept the theory portion of nurse training at a very primitive level, and some curricula were restricted to less controversial content, such as how to make cranberry jelly, bake apples, and prepare peanut brittle.

Even in the early 1900s the complaints that nurses were overtrained continued. For example, a meeting of the Academy of Medicine in New York City was well filled on the evening of March 29, 1906, with an audience of physicians and nurses who had assembled for a symposium on the training of nurses. With one exception, the speakers voiced the opinion that nurses of the day were overtrained and that there was too much theory and too little practice in their training. Some of the public seemed to agree with the physicians on the matter. Indeed, an editorial that appeared in the *New York Evening Sun* of March 3, 1906, maintained:

Nurses nowadays are instructed in a great variety of topics, and it is a question whether the smattering of knowledge they acquire is not often more mischievous than useful. Some

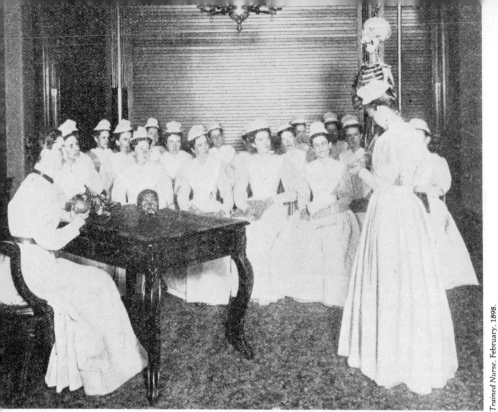

Lecture by the superintendent of nurses at the Mount Sinai Training School, New York City, about 1897.

Cooking class for nurses at the Presbyterian Hospital, New York City, about 1895.

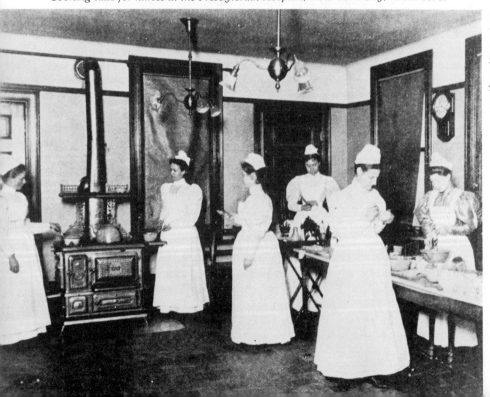

of them are too apt to think that their position entitles them to censure the work of the doctor and to carry out his orders or not as they see fit. Thus we have known of one who persuaded her patient that his surgeon was incompetent in having failed to remove some catgut sutures from a wound at the proper time; another, in a public hospital, who ignored the house physician's prescription of a narcotic in the case of a boy on the ground that "it was a shame to expose him to the danger of acquiring a drug habit." What we want in nurses is less theory and more practice. The place of the nurse is an honorable one, and every candid physician is glad to acknowledge that the successful issue in many cases, such as pneumonia and so on, depends at least as much on her services as on his. But to stuff her head with scraps of knowledge about a number of subjects which do not concern her duties at all would surely be foolish. A thoroughly trained nurse is indispensable. An overtrained and "learned" nurse is apt to be a nuisance [13].

Dr. W. Gilman Thompson made similar charges in a paper entitled "The Overtrained Nurse" in the April 28, 1908, issue of the *New York Medical Journal*. The editor noted that this paper "was read with huge enjoyment by physicians generally" as Thompson lashed out in measured prose:

Nursing is not, strictly speaking, a profession. A profession implies professed attainments in special knowledge as distinguished from mere skill; nursing is an honorable calling, nothing further, implying proficiency in certain more or less mechanical duties; it is not primarily designed to contribute to the sum of human knowledge or the advancement of science. The great and principal duty of a nurse is to make a patient comfortable in bed, something not always attained by the most bookish of nurses. Any intelligent, not necessarily educated woman can in a short time acquire the skill to carry out with implicit obedience the physician's directions [14].

The Practice Component

The better schools of nursing attempted to give a varied experience on all hospital nursing services, but if the hospital's need for personnel on a certain unit was acute, students would be assigned there regardless of their educational needs. Physicians also interfered with the distribution of experience. If a physician was being assisted by a student whose work he liked, he frequently used his influence to keep her on his service far beyond the stipulated length of time.

Very soon after schools of nursing came into being, some began to send students out as special private duty nurses and confiscated the money that the students earned. This development sprang from the premise that training in a hospital did not automatically fit a nurse to work in the home—the major kind of employment available after graduation. Thus, to overcome this deficiency, hospitals sent their students out into the community to nurse in homes, supposedly under school supervision. What resulted was a lucrative system of exploitation. A student might be kept on and on with a chronic or convalescent patient for reasons such as "The patient doesn't want to give her up," "The family can't pay a graduate," or, more openly, "The hospital wants the money," long after any teaching value remained in the experience. Even in shorter cases supervision was frequently inadequate, and the patient was left to the care of a partially trained student, who in the meantime missed the theory background and more balanced clinical experience she needed and deserved.

Income derived from this practice was supposed to go into the training school budget, but hospitals were supporting the schools, and the money for nursing service inevitably found its way into the hospital coffers. This encouraged several unethical 10- and 20-bed hospitals to recruit students from kitchens and restaurants, pay them $5 to $10 a month, and then, as quickly as the students were in uniform, send them out on special cases—for which the hospital received at least $21 per week. Physician stockholders of such proprietary hospitals might profit greatly by encouraging such practices. It was clear to progressive nurses of the day that nurse training schools could be exploited as important subsidiaries to dividend-paying businesses.

Even at better schools "specialing" was common. At the Illinois Training School for Nurses in Chicago the students brought in more than $2000 annually from such work. This amount was proudly mentioned as income in the school's annual reports, and regret was occasionally expressed that the press of work at the hospital had prevented more students from being available to answer the many calls for private-duty assignments.

A Probationer's Life

Much of the work required of the probationer was decidedly not nursing. Instead of being taught to care for the sick intelligently, the probationer was in many hospitals made to do the work of a chambermaid or scullion. She dusted, she

Medical ward of female patients, about 1897.

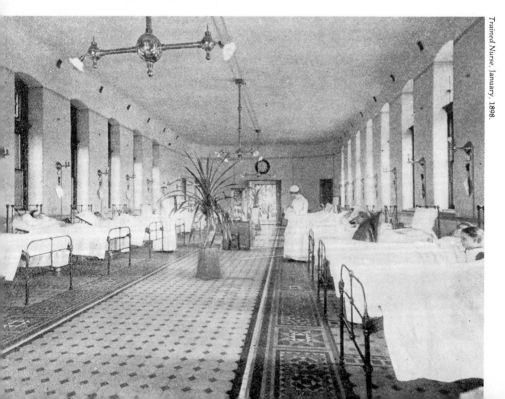

scrubbed, she washed dishes. Training for probationers of the 1890s usually meant working 14 hours a day, seven days a week. It meant each student being under continuous surveillance, with the superintendent at her heels, ready to pounce on her for the slightest mistake.

One might attempt to visualize the rigorous probationary period by hypothesizing a case for Miss X of 1893. The hospital Miss X entered required a probationary period of six weeks. She was certainly glad that her own probation was to be no longer than 42 days. She often wondered if the school was really going to keep her while she was scrubbing the floors, cleaning the windows, polishing the furniture, cleaning out the patient rooms and wards, and scouring the tubs and the copper "cookers" used in rheumatic cases. Probationers in her hospital, called "probies" for short, spent most of their time cleaning. "Well, if I'd ever had any idea that being a trained nurse was like this!" she moaned to a fellow student one day as they were polishing the "coppers." While she did not finish the sentence, it could easily be filled in: if she had known, she would have stayed home.

As a matter of fact, several girls who entered with Miss X did drop out before the six weeks were over. They were characterized as the type who had been attracted to nursing only for romantic reasons. They had pictured themselves in glossy white linen stooping to soothe the brow of a sick (but handsome) young man. Now they found themselves in blue chambray, bent over a kitchen floor, where sentiment could not even nudge them.

Miss X's experience was not isolated to her own school. The attrition rate among students was astonishingly high. For example, at the Farrand Training School at Harper Hospital in Detroit, about 100 applications were received in response to advertisements for admission to the January, 1884, class. Sixteen of these applicants were selected as probationers. Of this number, 12 probationers were soon rejected as not meeting the required standard of clinical performance, a mere four students were advanced to the status of "pupil nurse," and the same four were eventually graduated, for an attrition rate of 75 percent.

After the probationary period, the work of the students continued to be strenuous. Nursing demanded muscle and endurance. A student could generally count on being on her feet the whole time she spent on the wards, which contributed to the prevalence of the complaint known among student nurses as flat feet. In hospitals it was a law of etiquette that the nurse should never sit down while on the ward, even if she had the opportunity.

The intensity of the work varied greatly in different hospitals and depended much upon whether they were situated in busy urban centers or in quiet towns. In big city general hospitals, where patients were seriously ill and required much attention, student nurses were more effectively used and the greater part of the manual labor in the ward might be performed by ward maids and orderlies. In smaller rural hospitals or infirmaries, where the patients had mostly chronic illnesses, the proportion of students to patients was low, and all the time not spent giving nursing care was filled with scrubbing, sewing, washing bandages, and even cleaning windows. Thus the work of the nurse seemed to adjust itself to the circumstances at hand and essentially comprised whatever needed to be done.

All work, however, was governed by a strict set of rules. One student complained in her diary: "We are shown one certain way of performing each duty, and woe betide her who fails to adhere to the accepted method." Almost any attempt to experiment and find another, perhaps more efficient way of doing any task was discouraged. The elaborate procedure followed in the making of beds was a good example of the rigid attention to trifling details expected in the performance of all hospital duties. The sheets had to be placed just so, with their hemmed ends turned down in the prescribed fashion. The blankets also had to be placed with absolute accuracy, not a tenth of an inch farther down on one side than on the other, and the white coverlet had to be laid with geometric precision, its ends turned and folded in a certain way; the pillows were shaken up, beaten down, and flattened out and smoothed until they resembled padded boards. Finally, "one padded board was laid flat at the head of the bed and the other made to assume a bolt upright sentinel-like position on top of it. When with the head nurse's aid my first bed was completed, she drew me back a little distance and surveying it with pride desired me to observe the beautifully smooth, ornamental appearance it presented" [15].

To this particular student the bed looked like a shallow white box on slim legs, but smooth and even it certainly was, and she said so "with hast and eagerness, being in mortal fear lest the head nurse should discover some fancied flaw and insist upon my doing it all over again with the aid of a carpenter's square and spirit-level" [16]. Her private opinion was that, as long as the patients were clean and comfortable, it was not a matter of tremendous importance which hem, broad or narrow, happened to be tucked under the head of the mattress or whether the end of a white coverlet was a sixteenth of an inch lower or a full quarter of an inch higher than the prescribed line.

Long Hours and Seven-Day Work Weeks

Extremely long hours of service for student nurses continued to be the accepted pattern, and there was no improvement in this regard over the earlier practices in schools of nursing during the 1870s. In most hospitals the students on day duty rose at 5:30 A.M. to the sound of a loud bell, then dressed, made their beds, and cooked breakfast for themselves. At 6:45 A.M. another bell sent the students scurrying to the parlor to join their fellow nurses in a hymn, a Bible reading, and a prayer. They arrived on the wards at 7:00 A.M. and worked until 8:00 or 9:00 P.M., with about 75 minutes off for meals. In the large general city hospitals the hours "off duty" between sleep and work were generally two each day. When there were lectures for the students, they were held between 8:00 and 9:00 P.M. or later. Compulsory attendance at evening prayers often deprived students of an extra hour's rest in bed. Night duty hours were even longer, and most hospitals required a night duty of 12 hours per day, seven days a week, for a total of 84 hours.

A brief study made in 1895 of the hours of work at 111 schools throughout

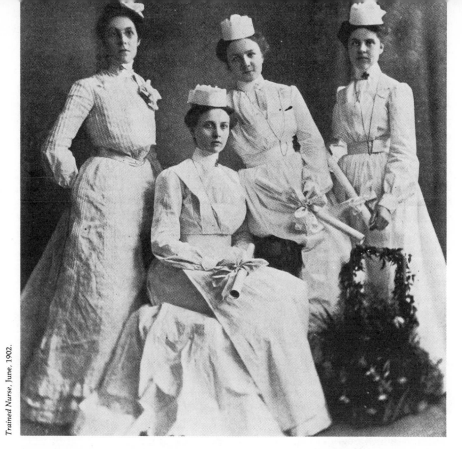

Graduating class of the City Hospital, Memphis, Tennessee, 1902.

the country showed that in about two-thirds of these training schools students were on duty for 10 hours or more daily. The hours of night duty were found to be 12 hours in 70 percent of the schools, and in the remaining hospitals they exceeded that number and ranged from 13 to 13.5 hours. In no instance were the night duty hours found to be under 12 daily. This first study of the working hours of students concluded that the hours were universally excessive and that such requirements were injurious to students' health and to the welfare of the patients and the hospital

A young woman who worked 10 to 12 hours a day was in no mental condition to profit by class instruction offered during the evenings. A common schedule of required hours per week in the 1890s was as follows:

Monday	9 hrs. work, 1 hr. class
Tuesday	10 hrs. work, 1 hr. class
Wednesday	5 hrs. day duty, 5 hrs. night duty
Thursday	12 hrs. night duty
Friday	11 hrs. night duty, 1 hr. class
Saturday	7 hrs. night duty, 5 hrs. private duty ("specialing")
Sunday	15 hrs. private duty in two shifts
Total:	82 hrs.

In 1896 a bill was introduced into the Massachusetts state legislature that aimed to limit the working hours of student nurses in private or public hospitals to 12 hours out of 24 and to supply them with sleeping apartments separate from those of the patients. The bill was strongly opposed by nurse administrators. Maria P. Brown, Superintendent of the Boston Training School for Nurses, attached to the Massachusetts General Hospital, said that it was impossible to regulate the work and daily lives of student nurses by any such arbitrary laws and that only those who were familiar with the needs, the variations, and the emergencies of the work could realize how impractical such rules would be. She claimed that a hospital was not like a workshop, which could have definite hours of work as a part of its operation. In the student nurse's life, she insisted, every day brought new demands, in that each patient constituted an individual requirement that called for some new and extra effort on the part of the nurse.

The rules governing the nurses at the Massachusetts General Hospital were similar to those at other institutions, Miss Brown explained. While to the superficial observer the hours seemed wearisome, they were, she pointed out, arranged with tact and a consideration for the nurses' welfare. The day nurses were on duty 13 hours, minus one hour for relaxation and mealtime. There was also the relief derived from turning from one kind of work to another—from the classroom to the ward and back to the lecture room. Students had an afternoon off every week and a part of every Sunday.

Of course, as Miss Brown noted, there were likely to be emergency calls at any time, which might elongate the ordinary hours. A day nurse might be called upon to do extra night duty in the case of a bad accident or other emergency, but the superintendent usually tried to select a nurse who had been given the afternoon off that day or one who was especially strong and well-fitted to bear the extra strain.

Although such extra calls came many times within some weeks, at other times they did not occur for long periods. When they did come, however, they had to be met, and it was thought that no regulations should hamper the hospital in carrying out its responsibilities to the patients. Miss Brown acknowledged that some smaller schools might need a degree of restraint in their practices, but, in her view, any state law would prove more of a hindrance than a help to nurses in their work. The main thing, she pointed out, was to have efficient graduate nurses in command of the schools and then to entrust to their judgment and discretion the direction and control of the students. The superintendent's rules would generally be found more efficient and practical than a direct and definite law passed by the legislature.

Despite such objections to outside regulation, it is clear that the long hours in schools of nursing were out of step with the times. Federal statistics show that the average hours per work week in all industrial establishments averaged 58.4 in 1890, 58.1 in 1895, 57.3 in 1900, and 55.7 in 1905. To expect 70 to 90 hours of work from a student nurse for a period of two or three years approached a form of slavery.

Excessive Illness among Students

It quickly became apparent that illness among student nurses greatly exceeded illness among other young women who worked for their living. A nurse of eight years' standing declared: "Doctor, there must be something wrong in the system which takes young women who are sound and healthy at the commencement of their training and graduates them three years later mostly wrecks." One student nurse poignantly testified:

I certainly cannot stand this much longer. I fainted last night for the first time in my life. Miss Gray said I must have eaten something that didn't agree with me and seemed to feel very much injured by my thoughtless action. She was greatly relieved when she found that I soon recovered sufficiently to continue my duty. I could stand the loss of sleep at night all right if I did not have to work so extremely hard. I think it a shame to have so few nurses on duty at night, when the work is the most trying. It oughtn't to be necessary to break down one's health in order to become a graduate nurse, but that is what it amounts to [17].

One investigator succeeded in obtaining from seven of the large hospitals of the city of New York data concerning the number of days of illness that kept student nurses from duty. His findings, ranging from a low of slightly less than 2 days to a high of nearly 22 days, were as follows:

Hospital A—Average number of patients, 173; number of nurses in training school, 41, being a little over four patients per nurse. Each nurse in this hospital averaged 1%10 days' illness of sufficient severity to keep her in her room. This was the best record of any of the seven hospitals.

Hospital B—Average number of patients, 178; student nurses, 99, being not quite two patients for a nurse. In this hospital, the average illness per annum per nurse, 4⅓ days.

Hospital C—Average number of patients, 110; student nurses, 51, a little over two patients for a nurse; average illness per annum per nurse, 6 days.

Hospital D—Average number of patients, 189; student nurses, 47; patients per nurse, 4; average illness per annum per nurse, 11½ days.

Hospital E— Average number of patients, 130; student nurses, 56; average patients per nurse, 2⅓; average illness, 11⅞ days per annum per nurse.

Hospital F— Average number of patients, 268; student nurses, 22; average patients per nurse, 12.5; average illness per annum per nurse, 21½ days. In this training school, more than 50 percent of the nurses were afflicted with flat and painful feet, and there was a high incidence of acute digestive disturbances (50 cases of two to three attacks each).

Hospital G—Average number of patients, 105; student nurses, 28; average patients per nurse, 3¾; average illness per annum per nurse, 11⅞ days [18].

It is illuminating to apply to other lines of work the system that had become characteristic of nurse training. One might speculate on the outcome of the growing stenographic field if every business or industry needing ten or more stenographers had said "We will have a stenographic school; we will have the president's secretary do the teaching (that will cost us nothing); the vice-president's and treasurer's secretaries will help (also without expense to us); we will keep our pupils three years and after the first six months expect them to work seven days a week, including some nights; we will give them room, board, and laundry; at the end of three years we will have a little celebration, perhaps in a church, and give each one a cheap gold pin; we will then take in a new group of students to do our work; we will recommend our graduates to people who need stenographers; of course, we will have no need to employ our own graduates, unless we can't get enough student stenographers."

An Added Year of Hard Labor

Although the course of nurse training up to the early 1890s was generally two years long, it was soon expanded to three years. Ten or more hours a day in addition to classwork and study might be endured for a period of two years, but the same hours extended to three years placed an even more serious strain upon the student's physical resources. Isabel Hampton, Superintendent of the Johns Hopkins Training School for Nurses, repeatedly pointed out the dangers of adopting the three-year course requirement unless shorter hours came with it. She insisted that superintendents of nurses should maintain their two-year courses unless they were prepared to limit practice to eight hours a day. In an 1895 paper on this subject, Miss Hampton warned:

I am sure that many of you have had some qualms of conscience at the way in which we are sometimes forced, I might almost say, to drive our pupil nurses through a two years' course. I assure you that I have had myself many anxious moments for the future of certain of my pupils as regards their health. It is well known that a combination of physical and mental labor is more exhausting than simple manual or simple mental occupation. It is true that for a time such a strain can be borne without producing any permanent injurious effects, and it is possible in most cases for women to stand the strain imposed upon them for two years, although I am afraid that not all of them come out of the trial unscathed. If, however, this high pressure is to be kept up for three years, I am sure that the health of the nurses will suffer. A woman who works physically over eight hours a day is in no mental condition to profit to any extent by class instruction or lectures. I maintain, therefore, that the three years' course must not be considered at all unless the hours of practical work are shortened, but if the two changes can be made together, then the preservation of the health of the nurse and the extension of her education and training will be insured. This again will result in an increase in her competency and consequently will be productive of greater benefits to the patients who come under her care during her training, and after she has graduated [19].

Founding of the First Nurses' Associations

The advance of the United States as a nation was vividly dramatized by a great spectacle, the World's Columbian Exposition, held in Chicago from May to October, 1893, to celebrate the four-hundredth anniversary of the discovery of America. The outstanding American architects, painters, and sculptors of the time joined in fashioning the gleaming and ornate "White City" that rose from the bogs and dunes along Lake Michigan. By the time the Exposition closed its gates, it had attracted more than 27 million visitors. Planned as a miniature of the ideal metropolis, the Chicago World's Fair boasted fine macadam roads, an excellent sanitation and water supply, underground telephone and telegraph wires, and ample hospital facilities. Its great dynamo showed that electricity was destined to displace steam as the prime mover of modern industrial civilization. The Chicago World's Fair symbolized a new stage in the development of an urban industrial society. It also marked the coming of age of nursing as a profession.

The exposition grounds were the meeting place of various congresses and conferences. Among many others, there was held an international congress of charities, correction, and philanthropy, with a section devoted to hospital care of the sick, to the training of nurses, to dispensary work, and to first aid to the injured, as well as a subsection on nursing. The chairman of this subsection was Isabel Hampton.

The nurses' meetings were held in the Hall of Columbus from June 15 to June 17, 1893. Attended by nurses from throughout the United States and Canada, the event marked the first time that nurses had met as a united body. Isabel Hampton read a paper, "Educational Standards for Nurses." Florence Nightingale, although not present, sent an address that was delivered before a large crowd. She wrote, in part: "Nursing proper can be taught only by the patient's bedside and in the sick room or ward. Neither can it be taught by books, though these are valuable accessories if used as such; otherwise what is in the book stays in the book."

"What is training?" she asked. "Training is to teach the nurse to help the patient to live. Nursing the sick is an art, and an art requiring an organized, practical, and scientific training, for nursing is the skilled servant of medicine, surgery, and hygiene." Miss Nightingale observed that a good nurse of 20 years before had not had to do one-twentieth of the work required by her physician or surgeon in 1893. The physician prescribed "for supplying the vital force, but the nurse supplies it," she concluded.

Lavinia L. Dock spoke on the relation of training schools to hospitals. She said that the training school idea did not originate within the hospital but had been grafted to it by the efforts of a few inspired women outside, who had seen the terrible needs of the sick, who knew the inadequacy of the care they received, and who bravely knocked at the hospital doors [20].

This meeting saw the birth of the first national nursing organization, the American Society of Superintendents of Training Schools of Nursing. This body had as its objectives: "(1) to promote fellowship of members, (2) to establish and maintain a universal standard of training, (3) to further the best interests of the nursing profession." At the first official meeting of the new society, in January, 1894, 44 superintendents were present.

There still remained the need for a national association of trained nurses. Isabel Hampton noted that the first alumnae association of nurses in the United States had been formed in 1889 by the graduates of the Bellevue Hospital Training

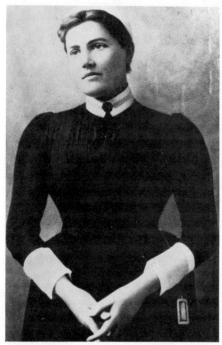

Courtesy Johns Hopkins University.

Isabel A. Hampton, first Superintendent of Nurses of the Johns Hopkins Hospital Training School for Nurses.

School, and that the next had been formed in 1890 at the Illinois Training School. By 1893 there were 21 such associations or clubs organized and in active operation and 10 in process of organization, all with the objective of advancing the interests of trained nurses and their role in society.

Three years later, in 1896, Miss Hampton's dream of one great official organization of trained nurses became a reality, at the third annual meeting of the American Society of Superintendents of Training Schools. A committee was appointed to prepare a constitution and bylaws for the proposed national organization and to meet with delegates from various alumnae associations in order to establish this association. The following year the constitution and bylaws prepared by the group were accepted, and the national nursing body completed its organization as the Nurses' Associated Alumnae of the United States and Canada.

Yet another group, the American Hospital Association—an international charitable and educational association of hospitals and hospital people—was originally organized as the Association of Hospital Superintendents, in 1899, with a membership of nine people. Its purpose was to "establish and maintain high standards of hospital service, to promote the efficient care of the sick, and to assist through its membership in the control and prevention of disease." Many nurses holding positions as hospital administrators played passive roles in the earlier years of the AHA, and this passivity cast a negative influence over nurse training standards [21].

The 1880s and the 1890s saw schools of nursing established by the hundreds in all parts of the nation as the financial advantages of the training system were fully exploited. This was a corollary to the rapid proliferation of general hospitals, and the two movements developed hand in hand. The initial skirmishes fought between physicians and nurses over the amount of theory instruction that students should be exposed to were but a prelude to a long-standing controversy. Giving focus to such matters, the professional nursing and hospital associations were founded and began to exert influence on the direction of nursing education and practice.

Summary

The concept of the community hospital became universal in the towns and cities of the United States toward the end of the nineteenth century, giving these institutions increasing respectibility among the public.

The Civil War had promoted the growth of hospitals, and certain new features of hospital service, such as ambulances, were derived from wartime developments in the medical department of the Union Army.

A nurse training school was considered an indispensable asset to a general hospital, both for economic reasons and because it was preferable to operate with a staff of uniformly instructed student nurses.

Schools multiplied without restraint during these decades. In 1880 there were 15 schools, 323 students, and 157 graduates; by 1900 there were 432 schools, 11,164 students, and 3456 graduates.

There were hundreds of applicants to the dozen best schools, while weaker schools struggled with recruitment.

The first school for men nurses was Mills School of Nursing at Bellevue Hospital, established in 1888. The first black nurse graduated in 1879 from the New England Hospital for Women and Children, and several schools for the education of black nurses were opened in the 1880s and 1890s.

Military and monastic nursing traditions stressing asceticism, duty, and the adherence to authority were major influences in the development of the nursing profession. Rigid rules of conduct prevailed in schools, and married or divorced women were considered unfit for nurse training.

Despite the ratio of more than 98 percent service to less than 2 percent theory in school of nursing curricula, physicians constantly complained that nurses were being overtrained.

Private duty nursing assignments were used as "field experience" for students in many schools, but this was generally a disguised form of economic exploitation. The hospital received payment for a student's special duty, which often continued for weeks at a time.

Students' long work days were filled with menial tasks, and days off were few. Illness was common among nurses in training, and the attrition rate in training schools was high.

There were a few unsuccessful attempts to improve working conditions, including a bill introduced into the Massachusetts state legislature to limit the working hours of nursing students.

Training programs were beginning to be expanded to three years. Isabel Hampton, the first superintendent of the Johns Hopkins Training School for Nurses, insisted that if the length of training was to be increased to three years, then a day's work of nursing practice should be limited to eight hours.

Nurses met as a united body for the first time at the 1893 World's Columbian Exposition in Chicago. The outcome was the first national nursing organization, the American Society of Superintendents of Training Schools—which was soon followed by a second organization, the Nurses' Associated Alumnae of the United States and Canada.

The American Hospital Association began in 1899 as the Association of Hospital Superintendents. The number of United States Hospitals grew from 178 in 1873 to more than 2500 at the turn of the century.

References

1. "Statistics of Hospitals in the United States 1872–73, Derived from Replies to Inquiries by the U.S. Bureau of Education," *Transactions of the American Medical Association,* 1873, 14:314–333.
2. U.S. Commissioner of Education, *Report of the U.S. Commissioner of Education for 1902* (Washington, D.C.: Government Printing Office, 1903), pp. 2043–2061.
3. "Night Duty," *Trained Nurse and Hospital Review,* vol. 41 (October, 1908):239–240.
4. U.S. Commissioner of Education, *Annual Report of the U.S. Commissioner of Education for 1906* (Washington, D.C.: Government Printing Office, 1907), p. 177.
5. A. J. Ochsner and M. J. Sturm, *The Organization, Construction and Management of Hospitals* (Chicago: Cleveland Press, 1907), pp. 92–95.
6. "The Journal of a Pupil Nurse," *Trained Nurse and Hospital Review,* vol. 40 (May, 1908):314.
7. "Training Schools," *Transactions of the American Hospital Association,* vol. 13 (October, 1911): 397–399.
8. Agnes G. Deans and Anne L. Austin, *The History of the Farrand Training School for Nurses* (Detroit: Alumnae Association of the Farrand Training School for Nurses, 1936), p. 58.
9. U.S. Commissioner of Education, "Final Examination Questions of the Evansville Sanitarium Training School for Nurses," *Annual Report of the U.S. Commissioner of Education for 1903* (Washington, D.C.: Government Printing Office, 1904), pp. 2231–2233.
10. M. Adelaide Nutting, "Notes of a Typhoid Fever Case," *Trained Nurse,* vol. 6 (March, 1891):121.
11. Samuel Howard, *The New Profession of Nursing* (Montreal: privately printed, 1875), p. 3.
12. "Nurses and Nursing," *British and Foreign Medico Chirurgical Review,* vol. 57 (April, 1876):283–301.

13. *New York Evening Sun,* March 3, 1906.
14. W. Gilman Thompson, "The Over-Trained Nurse," *New York Medical Journal,* vol. 83 (April 28, 1906):845–849.
15. "The Journal of a Pupil Nurse," *op. cit.,* vol. 42 (January, 1909):95–99.
16. *Ibid.,* p. 96.
17. *Ibid.,* vol. 40 (May, 1908):311–314.
18. A. T. Bristow, "Is the Present System of Training Fair to the Pupil Nurse?" *American Journal of Nursing,* vol. 7 (March, 1907):447–455.
19. Isabel Hampton, "Three Years Course of Training in Connection with the Eight-Hour System," *Transactions of the American Society of Superintendents of Training Schools for Nurses,* vol. 2 (1895):36.
20. J. S. Billings and H. M. Hurd, eds., *Hospitals, Dispensaries, and Nursing, International Congress of Charities, Correction and Philanthropy,* Sec. III (Baltimore: Johns Hopkins Press, 1894), pp. 86–98.
21. American Hospital Association, "Constitution and By-Laws," *Transactions of the American Hospital Association,* vol. 25 (October–November, 1923):605–606.

6
Gaslight and Shadow: The Practice of Nursing at the Turn of the Century

No large laboring or wage-earning class had developed in the United States before the Civil War. Although growing industries and other economic activities employed increasing millions of people, a substantial majority of the population were occupied in agriculture: as late as 1860, about 60 percent of the gainfully employed were farmers. But the rise of large-scale industry and big business during the period from 1870 to 1900 added millions of wage earners to the population.

One of the most important developments of the post-Civil War era was the rapid growth of cities. So swift was the transition that within a single generation the United States changed from a predominantly rural nation to one that was predominantly urban. In 1860 communities with populations of 2500 or more accounted for less than 21 percent of the total population; by 1900 this figure had grown to 39.9 percent.

Associated with increasing urbanism was the rapid growth of hospitals after the Civil War. Towns and cities sprouted up all across the United States. Cities, with their concentrated populations, new wealth, and numerous poor, offered a magnificent challenge to churches, religious orders, and enterprising physicians to found general hospitals. These groups looked for the sure thing, for opportunities to minimize costs and maximize services. Hospital administrators who could keep the books in the black and transfer a healthy surplus to the building fund became important and powerful figures.

Women in the Labor Force

The movement for increased rights for women was part of the Industrial Revolution and its consequent process of urbanization, and women advanced on various fronts during the 1880s and 1890s. A basic factor was the rapid increase in the number of jobs for women, amounting to a form of female emancipation. Even the conservative South dropped its severe restrictions upon remarriage after divorce. In 1882 New York courts allowed married women wider rights of property ownership and declared that wives could sue their husbands for damages incurred as the result of brutality. Gradually, most of the states conceded to wives their rights to own and to control their personal property, to retain their earnings, to sue, and to make contracts.

More employment alternatives for women opened up in the urban-industrialized society of the late century. Many career-minded ladies of the middle class still believed that elementary school teaching represented the chief form of employment for women, however. Philo Remington had started to mass-manufacture the typewriter, an invention that would open a new form of livelihood for women, and there were other new jobs for women as clerks and salespeople in the department stores and other merchandising establishments that had come into existence since the Civil War. Uneducated working women had been accepted long before into the first factories born of the Industrial Revolution, but now, for the first time, middle-class women in large numbers were moving from the home to industry and business. The number of female breadwinners rose from 2,500,000 in 1880 to 4,500,000 in 1890.

Opportunities for Graduate Nurses

Nursing did not fare well in comparison with many other lines of work that were opening up for women. After graduation from a school of nursing, a nurse

The "Gibson Girl," epitome of the ideal woman of the 1890s, as a hospital nurse.

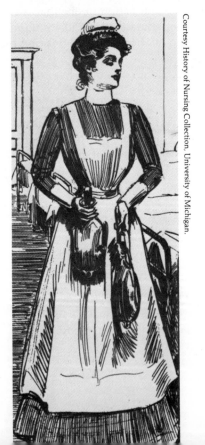

Courtesy History of Nursing Collection, University of Michigan.

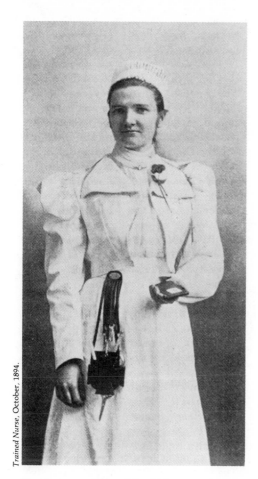

Trained Nurse, October, 1894.

Graduate nurse Josephine Osborn.

had two main career options: she could work in homes as a private duty nurse or she could serve in hospitals in the role of superintendent or head nurse. Opportunities for hospital work were slight for trained nurses. Even at the very best schools, few if any graduates were retained each year to fill the limited number of vacancies that occurred in the relatively permanent staffs of head nurses; as the size of the classes grew, the head nurse positions were usually turned over to students. At the Massachusetts General Hospital, the first class was graduated in 1875 with only three nurses. The second class numbered 11, the third class had five, the fourth class had 20 graduates, and the fifth class had just six. The Boston City Hospital Training School had a similar history, graduating its first class in 1880 and averaging 18 graduates annually until 1887.

It is of interest here to note what had become of the 300 graduates from these two schools by 1887 [1, 2]:

Remaining in the parent hospital	24
In other institutions	30
In district nursing	8
Total in institutional and public work	62
Private duty nursing	170
Total continuing in nursing	232
Married	37
Died	10
Studied medicine	1
Unknown as to abode and occupation	20
Total out of nursing	68

At the same time, trained nurses were beginning to make inroads against the untrained element: figures at the Registry for Nurses in Boston showed that 245 graduate female nurses were on the roll, as opposed to 408 nongraduate female nurses and 84 nongraduate male nurses. Untrained nurses, however, would still dominate nursing service for several more decades.

The Hospital Route

As the schools produced more nurses, new graduates began to migrate to other sections of the country without nursing schools. Emily L. Loveridge, a graduate of Bellevue Training School for Nurses, went west in 1890 to establish the first school of nursing in the Northwest at the Good Samaritan Hospital in Portland, Oregon. Her reminiscences vividly portray the challenges of those early nursing pioneers:

Coming to Oregon forty years ago to establish the first training school for nurses in the Northwest, I found myself one of three graduate nurses in a city of 70,000 people and entering a hospital of less than fifty beds. The Good Samaritan Hospital was a two-story frame building in those days, situated six blocks from the end of a street car line. The place looked small after the rambling buildings of Bellevue. I had plenty of courage but needed it. For six long months I was very homesick for the East.

In addition to being superintendent of nurses, I was the floor nurse and operating room supervisor, and in my leisure moments did any necessary work—sewing, cleaning, painting, etc.—that was to be done. We all worked and no one grumbled, not even at the end of a perfect day of twelve to sixteen hours of labor, for there were no hours off, and sometimes no afternoons off, in our schedule.

Our school of nursing, known at that time as the training school, started with five nurses, three of whom were on the hospital force at the time the school opened. All classes were held in the evenings.

Our first operating room had a double window at the end and single one at the side. Mrs. Wakeman conducted the first operation after my arrival, and my Bellevue training of even that period received a shock. She described an operation she witnessed in another hospital, where she was impressed with the convenient place used for the threaded surgical needles. They were stuck in the window shade! Our needles were run in a piece of bandage and boiled with the other instruments, or "carbolized."

The cold water used was boiled by the night nurse. Each kettle had to boil for fifteen minutes and was then emptied into a large covered granite can. The hot water was

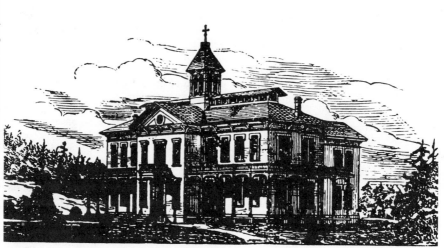

Good Samaritan Hospital, Portland, Oregon, 1892.

Operating room at the Oil City Hospital, Oil City, Pennsylvania, 1897.

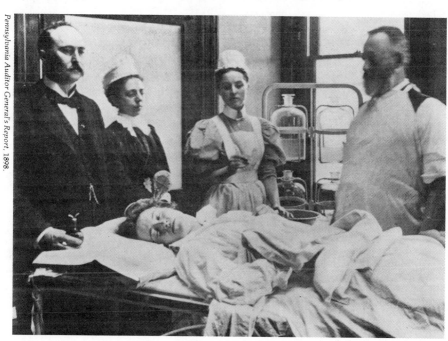

boiled in the diet kitchen and was carried in large porcelain pitchers covered with bichloride towels.

The field of operation was vigorously scrubbed and rinsed and washed in bichloride. We never felt that the patient's skin was properly cleansed until it was red from the scrubbing. After this the field was covered with towels soaked overnight in a 1/1000 bichloride solution and wrung as dry as possible. Every surgeon irrigated, using a rubber bag which had previously been sterilized by boiling. Not only the field of operation but all of the assistants at the operation were irrigated at the same time, and clothing and shoes had to be changed after a morning in the operating room.

At each operation one nurse was assigned as official brow wiper, for at that time the surgeons and assistants did not wear face masks. A few of the surgeons objected, preferring to let beads of perspiration fall when and where they would. One surgeon dropped his eye glasses into an abdominal cavity, but we irrigated more than usual and the wound healed by first intention.

Catgut was cut into yard lengths, wound on pieces of glass rods, put into glass jars, covered with alcohol, and boiled in water bath for four successive boilings at three day intervals. Preparing catgut was rather nervous work and there were several explosions during the time catgut was prepared in this manner.

When we bought our first operating gloves, only the surgeon operating wore them, then they were used by his assistant, and soon everyone used rubber gloves during an operation.

I recall the first abdominal operation performed. It took days to gather enough supplies and prepare them. . . . All went well during the operation until the ligature slipped from the pedicle and the patient died of internal hemorrhage. All of us were heartbroken.

Sunday was our busy day for operations. It was the only day that the doctors did not schedule for office hours—and there was no golf!

Our first ward beds had straw ticks, washed and refilled with straw during the interim between the discharge of one patient and the admission of another.

For ordinary heat we used stone jugs, bricks, and quart bottles, all in flannel covers. A few selected rubber bags were kept for abdominal application.

We had a diet kitchen in which each nurse in training served her allotted time. Here were made the softdiets, broths, etc. We sorted our milk in pans in the milk room. Some of these were skimmed for the cream and the thin milk was used for cooking.

In those days people frequently refused to come to the hospital—they were afraid of them—so the hospital went to the patient for operative work. All of the necessary paraphernalia was carried from the hospital. The kitchen table was frequently used as the operating table, and bedroom stands and marble top tables with the marble turned upside down were used for instrument and sponge tables. The operating room nurse usually went out a couple of hours previous to the operation and scrubbed everything. The tables were covered with bicholoride towels and hot water was kept in pans and kettles on the stove. Occasionally members of the family helped. It was better to keep them occupied and away from interfering with our surgical supplies [3].

Miss Loveridge found that Good Samaritan Hospital's management could function with relative simplicity. The annual report for 1891–1892 contained the following statistics regarding the services rendered:

Patients under treatment, May 31, 1891	73
Admitted during the year 1891–1892	907
Total	980

Died in hospital, 65; discharged, 846	911
Remaining under treatment June 1, 1892	69
Total	980

Of this number 234 were free or charity patients
   and 746 were paying patients.

Number of days of care given charity patients	4,793
Number of days of care given paying patients	23,551
Total number of days of care	28,344

Also included in the report were a classification of diseases treated, a note about the hospital's nurse training school, and a tabulation of patients according to religious belief.

Housekeeping Tasks

The practice of nursing at the turn of the century included many housekeeping tasks. The nurse of this time was occupied with maintaining an appropriate sickroom environment—room temperature, humidity, and ventilation—and preparing, cooking, and serving of food to the patients were included in the nurses' work. Every ward had its own kitchen. Scrubbing, cleaning, polishing, controlling insects, oiling furniture, washing clothes, folding linen, making bandages and rollers, and other similar duties were in the domain of the nurse, and many, many hours were spent on these lower-level duties.

The following job description of a hospital nurse during the 1880s vividly underlines just how arduous, task-oriented, and regimented nursing was:

In addition to caring for your 50 patients each bedside nurse will follow these regulations:

Daily sweep and mop the floors of your ward, dust the patients' furniture and window sills.

Maintain an even temperature in your ward by bringing in a scuttle of coal for the day's business.

Light is important to observe the patient's condition. Therefore, each day fill the kerosene lamps, clean chimneys and trim wicks. Wash the windows once a week.

The nurse's notes are important in aiding the physician's work. Make your pens carefully. You may whittle nibs to your individual taste.

Each nurse on day duty will report to duty every day at 7 A.M. and leave at 8 P.M., except on the Sabbath, on which day you will be off from 12 noon to 2 P.M.

Graduate nurses in good standing with the director of nurses will be given an evening off each week for courting purposes, or two evenings a week if they go to church regularly.

Each nurse should lay aside from each pay day a goodly sum of her earnings for her benefits during her declining years so that she will not be a burden. For example, if you earn $30 a month you should set aside $15.

Any nurse who smokes, uses liquor in any form, gets her hair done at a beauty shop, or frequents dance halls will give the director of nurses good reason to suspect her worth, intentions, and integrity.

The nurse who performs her labors and serves her patients and doctors faithfully and without fault for a period of five years will be given an increase by the hospital administration of five cents a day, providing there are no hospital debts that are outstanding [4].

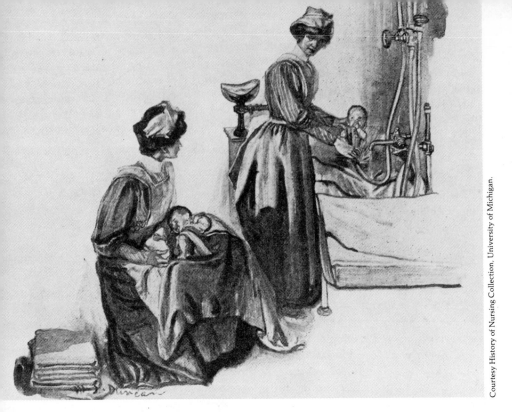

Washing babies with a sprinkling machine, 1890s.

In 1894, one nurse described the scrubbing duties in the ward lavatory as follows:

The nurses scrub a board about 2½ ft. long and 2 ft. wide, which usually lies on the tub, and is called a poultice-board . . . . It is always kept spotlessly white, and instead of feeling it a humiliation, one soon learns to take pride—and a great deal of pride, too, let me tell you—in seeing how white one can keep it . . . . One of the first things a nurse learns is that she must leave everything thoroughly "aseptic" . . . . You see, now, why it is that nurses do this part of the work instead of maids, who do not understand the importance of these things [5].

Nursing Care Responsibilities

Besides these housekeeping tasks the practice of nursing included making beds, giving baths, preventing and dressing bedsores, applying "friction to the body and extremities," giving enemas, inserting catheters, bandaging, dressing blisters, burns, sores, and wounds, and observing secretions, expectorations, pulse, skin, appetite, body temperature, consciousness, respirations, sleep, condition of wounds, skin eruptions, elimination, and the effect of diet, stimulants, and medications. Administering medications and treatments as ordered by the physician was another major responsibility of the nurse.

The degree of autonomy that the nurse could exercise in completing these tasks varied. In the early 1870s at the Woman's Hospital in Philadelphia, the temperature and the duration of the bath were ordered by the physician primarily because baths were used as a means of therapy. The "half-bath," for example, given in a long tub filled with six inches of cold or temperate water so that it covered only the legs and thighs, was used to treat selected cases of typhoid fever. One nurse, wetting her hands repeatedly with the bath water, rapidly rubbed the patient's shoulders, back, and chest while another nurse vigorously massaged the lower extremities and thighs. The patient splashed water on his own face. This procedure lasted three to four minutes and was repeated every six to eight hours. Other types of baths included the hot-air bath, the sheet-bath, the gelatin bath, the reducing or graduated bath, the vapor bath, the mud bath, the narcotic bath, the sand bath, the mustard bath, the sea bath, and many others.

Catheterization of male patients by female nurses was the source of considerable controversy in the late 1890s. The director of nurses at Saint Luke's Hospital in New York, Mrs. L. W. Quintard, read a paper on the subject at the Superintendents' Convention in 1896. She expressed grave concern about the practice

Hospital wheel carriage used during the 1890s.

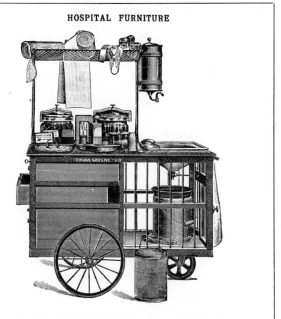

Sharp and Smith Medical Supply Catalog, 1895.

HOSPITAL FURNITURE

Fig. 1744. NECKER HOSPITAL WHEEL CARRIAGE.

Price, with wash bowl and slop bucket.....................................$100 00

These carriages are made from a model brought direct from Paris.   It is the pattern in use in each of the wards in Necker hospital.   After examining the patterns in use in most of the better equipped hospitals of the world, we selected this as being one of the most desirable.   They are well made from hardwood, have rubber-tired wheels on steel axles.   The bowl is of porcelain, while the upright rack for dressings is of wrought iron.   The whole apparatus combines many desirable features in the one appliance.

of using male orderlies to catheterize, bathe, and dress wounds or blisters in the pelvic region of men patients, because the men who were hired as orderlies in these hospitals tended to be careless and ignorant. Private duty nurses had no one to delegate such care to, and since most nurses did private nursing at one time or another, she believed that it was important for them to learn the procedure on "children and unconscious patients." Mrs. Quintard's suggestions were liberal for the Victorian times:

Is it wise to allow nurses to give a full massage or rubbing to male patients? When convalescence is once established such treatment should not be given by a male attendant . . . . In caring for the very sick we must, as far as possible, forget both sex and self. In their weakness men appeal to us as little children, and the motherliness inherent in every true woman's nature responds to their cry for help, and we give them what they need without any regard to our relation, except as patient and nurse [6].

Leeching

Among the more frequently administered treatments were applications of leeches, cups, poultices, counterirritants, and blisters. Leeches were used at that time to treat a wide variety of ailments, including meningitis and conjunctivitis (leech from the temples), otitis (leech from the mastoid area), and orchitis (leech from the perineum). Inflammations or engorgements were often treated by applying leeches to the affected area. Nurses were warned never to apply leeches near the eyelids or the scrotum.

The nurse's first step in administering this treatment was to wash and dry the part of the body to which the leeches would be applied. The leeches were dried in the folds of a soft towel and then applied by holding them in place with a wine glass or the top of a pillbox. They were never applied over a large vein. If they delayed taking hold, the nurse pricked her finger and put a drop of blood on the spot or a drop of sugar-and-water or milk. If the leech was applied to the mouth area of the person, it was put in a test tube or small bottle and held to the spot by the nurse. The leech would usually continue to draw blood until it was filled, then it would drop off. Each leech consumed about one teaspoon of blood. If the nurse wanted to remove the leech before it dropped off, she put a drop of water or some salt on its head to induce it to cease feeding. If, on the other hand, the bleeding had been insufficient, the application of warmth to the wound, particularly with a poultice, served to continue the bleeding and increase the depletion.

The number of leeches used varied with the patients' circumstances and the variety of the leech. Embarrassing accidents sometimes happened due to the migratory tendencies of the leeches, and caution was taken not to apply them too near a bodily orifice and to count every leech as it was applied and later when it was removed. If a leech was swallowed, salt water or port wine was given and followed, if necessary, by an emetic. If the leech entered the rectum, the salt water was given in an enema. It was possible to use a leech more than once, since it could be forced to disgorge the blood it had swallowed by drawing it, tail first, between the fingers, which acted to empty it by pressure. After detachment the leech was placed in clean water and left for later use.

Nursing Procedures Associated with the Use of Counterirritants

Counterirritants were agents used to irritate the surface of one part of the body in an attempt to relieve pathology in another part of the body. They were indicated for inflammation, congestion, and the absorption of "inflammatory products." They were also used for pain relief and as a stimulant in acute depression and narcotic overdose.

There was some dispute during the 1890s over why this treatment was effective. One theory that gained acceptance was that a counterirritant drew the blood supply away from the diseased part of the body. Another scientific explanation suggested that the irritation of peripheral nerves changed their molecular structure. This change was then communicated to the nerves in the affected organ. The choice of sites for application of counterirritants was frequently determined by the theory to which the practitioner subscribed. Milder forms of counterirritants, such as heat or friction, tended to be used more frequently and closer to the affected part of the body. Vigorous forms, such as blistering, were used more judiciously and farther away from the affected area. Counterirritants fell into four categories: rubefacients, vesicants, pustulants, and cauterants.

Rubefacients were agents that reddened the skin without destroying its integrity. The most common procedure used in the 1890s to achieve the rubefacient effect was dry cupping. Cupping was a treatment commonly performed by the nurse. This therapeutic procedure involved the application of a cup to the body's surface by means of a vacuum. This vacuum created local vascular congestion. The cup was made of rubber, glass, china, or metal. The objective was to establish a vacuum in one of these vessels, and this demanded elaborate procedures requiring considerable manual dexterity as the nurse burned paper in the cup and applied it to the patient's skin at the precise moment the paper was ready to extinguish. As the cup cooled, a vacuum was formed and local circulation increased. The nurse was admonished not to burn or bruise the skin.

Cupping was believed to temporarily relieve congested organs and tissues of surplus blood, thus affording relief to the patient during medical crises and was widely used in a variety of cases. As a rule, dyspnea due to cardiac disease and the pain and cough of acute pulmonary and pleural diseases were believed to be temporarily relieved by dry cups applied to the chest and back. Acute inflammation and congestion of the kidneys were treated with a large number of dry cups applied over the lumbar region, while intracranial congestion and inflammations were improved by cups applied to the nape of the neck or over the mastoid region.

A variation of dry-cupping, which was more akin to the use of leeches than counterirritants, was "wet-cupping." The skin was cupped. The cup was removed and a prick was made in the reddened area. Another cup was reapplied in the same area to suction out blood, creating a wet cup. This was an alternative to

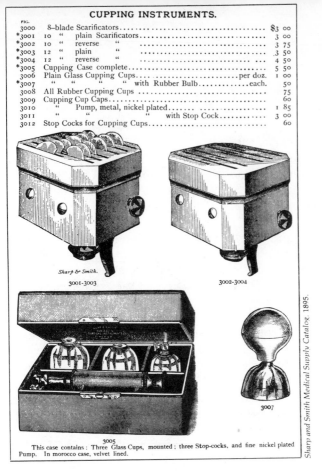

Sharp and Smith Medical Supply Catalog, 1895.

CUPPING INSTRUMENTS.

FIG.					
3000	8–blade Scarificators.....................................	$3 00
*3001	10 " plain Scarificators...........................	3 00
*3002	10 " reverse "	3 75
*3003	12 " plain "	.3 50
*3004	12 " reverse "	4 50
*3005	Cupping Case complete............................	5 50
3006	Plain Glass Cupping Cups.................. per doz.	1 00
*3007	" " " " with Rubber Bulb........... each.	50
3008	All Rubber Cupping Cups	75
3009	Cupping Cup Caps.................................	60
3010	" Pump, metal, nickel plated......	1 85
3011	" " " with Stop Cock...........	3 00
3012	Stop Cocks for Cupping Cups.....................	60

Sharp & Smith.

3001-3003

3002-3004

3007

3005

This case contains : Three Glass Cups, mounted ; three Stop-cocks, and fine nickel plated Pump. In morocco case, velvet lined.

Cupping instruments used in the 1890s.

the various methods of blood-letting and should not be confused with the use of "dry-cupping" as a counterirritant.

Poultices were also used extensively as rubefacients to allay pain and inflammation. They were moist substances applied externally in such a consistency that they adhered to the surface of the skin without spreading to adjacent areas and without becoming so thick that they stuck to the skin.

Poultices were made out of a variety of substances. Quite popular were linseed or flaxseed poultices, a mixture of linseed and boiling water gradually mixed by constant stirring until the correct consistency was achieved. Bread poultices were made from pulverized stale bread and hot water or hot milk, the latter being referred to as the "bread-and-milk" poultice. The disadvantages of bread poultices were that they cooled and dried quickly, crumbled, and became sour whereas linseed had oily mucilaginous characteristics. Indian-meal poultices were prepared from Indian corn meal and were believed to retain their heat longer than linseed poultices. Bran had the advantage of lightness. Powdered charcoal was added to flaxseed to treat "offensive ulcers." Similarly, warm yeast was smeared on the surface of bread poultices and placed near the fire to rise. An "iodide-of-starch" poultice, used to clean sloughing ulcers, was made with starch, boiling water, and liquor iodide. To eliminate "gaseous emanations from unhealthy sores," a chlorine poultice was applied. Poultices were also prepared with oatmeal, slippery elm, mashed potatoes, carrots boiled and mashed, starch, and wheat. Various medicines, such as opium, were added to the poultices for the rapid relief of pain.

The chief use of poultices was to relieve congestion and inflammation of internal organs, such as the lungs in cases of bronchitis, pleurisy, or pericarditis. Similarly, acute abdomens, lumbago, intestinal and hepatic "inflammations," and even peritonitis were believed to be alleviated with this treatment.

When the nurse applied the poultice, she followed a number of important steps. Because it was believed that pain extended beyond the inflamed part, a poultice large enough to cover the surrounding surface was made. The substance was spread from one-half inch to one inch thick on a heavy piece of cotton. The edges were made as thick as the middle so that the poultice would not dry too rapidly and be painful. The surface of the poultice was covered with a very thin gauze of muslin, mosquito net, or lace so that it would not stick to the surface and could later be removed in one piece. In applying it to the chest, the nurse was cautioned to avoid covering the nipples. The cloth on which the poultice was spread had to be large enough to double up around the four sides and up over the edges of the poultice in order to prevent it from oozing out. The nurse had everything prepared beforehand and the patient's clothing unfastened before she brought the poultice to the bed, and she applied it immediately, as hot as the patient could stand it. She covered it with oil silk or rubber sheeting and then with flannel to keep it warm for as long as possible. It was changed before it became cold, usually every two hours. During the poultice change the nurse was careful to keep the skin covered at all times and so prevent rapid loss of body heat. She was prompt in changing the poultices, due to the fact that, if left too long, they dried and adhered to the skin. A sleeveless poultice-jacket, made out of two layers of muslim sewed together at the edges, was devised to hold the poultice in its proper location.

Fomentations, or stupes, were warmed liquids applied to the surface of the body with absorbent material, usually a cloth. Sometimes an irritant, such as oil of turpentine, was added. The reasons for applying the fomentations were the same as for poultices, both treatments offering heat and moisture. But a fomentation lasted only a few minutes as compared with two hours for a poultice. Colic was treated with fomentations since a prompt, short action was required.

Another favorite rubefacient treatment was the mustard plaster. To apply a mustard plaster the nurse mixed ground mustard with boiling water into a thin paste, spread it on heavy paper or cloth, covered it with gauze or very thin cloth, and applied it to the patient's skin. It was removed after the skin became reddened. If a slower, milder, and continuous burning process was desired, she made a thick paste of Indian meal or flour and stirred in a tablespoon or more of ground mustard. This was applied and kept in place with a bandage. Mustard plasters were used to treat a variety of clinical problems. They were said to relieve pain when placed over an area of soreness. Colds and bronchitis responded remarkably well when mustard plasters were applied over the entire lateral surface of the affected lung or lungs. Diarrhea was treated with a plaster applied to the abdomen, nausea with one over the stomach, and migraine with one over the hepatic region.

Vesicants, agents that produced blisters, were used as a more vigorous form of counterirritant. The nurse was cautioned not to blister the skin's surface larger than a silver dollar. A number of small blisters seemed to be most effective. The agent used to blister the skin was most commonly cantharis, which could be used in ointment or oil, applied to paper, or dissolved in collodion. To apply a blister the nurse first washed and dried the location and then applied the blister agent to the area, holding it in place with strips of adhesive plaster or bandage. The time required for the blister to rise varied among patients. The nurse would examine it in three hours, then hourly, to determine when the blister appeared. The plaster came off easily when the blister had risen. The puffed skin was then snipped in several places with sharp-pointed scissors. The fluid that ran out was wiped away gently, an ointment was spread over the area, and a soft lint bandage was applied. Examples of specific diseases and the location of the blistering included: spinal meningitis (blister on nape of neck), headache due to intracranial lesions (blister over mastoid process), persistent nausea, gastric ulcer, colic (blister on abdomen), and neuralgia (blister over affected nerve existing from osseous canal).

The remaining two categories of counterirritants, pustulants and cauterants, were administered less frequently by nurses. Pustulants caused a pus-containing lesion on the skin, due to the use of agents such as croton oil or silver nitrate, or, more likely, to the introduction of bacteria through poor technique. The result of this kind of counterirritant was quite painful and difficult to heal. Cauterants were agents that burned and destroyed tissue. It was believed that a more powerful therapeutic effect was achieved with cauterants than by blistering, but without the pain of pustules. In this procedure the nurse passed white-hot metal over the skin but stopped short of actually searing the tissue, because this was not necessary to achieve the counterirritant effect.

Organization of Nursing Service

The method of dividing up the day's work varied from hospital to hospital according to the number of nurses, students, orderlies, and ward maids available and to the patient load. A pattern of functional nursing service was practiced. The following division of work was a typical one. The "temperature nurse" took temperatures and charted them, gave out medicines and kept the medicine closet in order, made out and gave to the head nurse the list of medicines for replenishment each day, served the meals and special nourishments to the patients, and took responsibility for the kitchen. In many hospitals this nurse also cooked the meals. The "right-side nurse" cared for the patients on the right side of the ward (exclusive of administering medicines, taking temperatures, and serving meals). This nurse bathed and ambulated these patients, made their beds, gave skin care, and maintained everything in good order on her side of the ward. She kept every bed in line and was responsible for the orderliness of the linen closet and for fold-

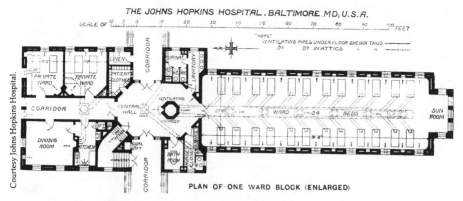

Typical ward at the Johns Hopkins Hospital, 1891.

ing the fresh linen. The "left-side nurse" had the same duties as the nurse on the right side but was responsible for the bathroom and lavatory instead of the linen closet. A fourth nurse took care of the special patients in the small private or semiprivate rooms off the ward and was responsible for taking care of the dressing carriage and preparing patients for surgery.

The probationers assisted in making beds, dusting, carbolizing the beds, cleaning mackintoshes, itemizing soiled clothes for the laundry lists, putting away new patients' clothes, and giving out meals. The ward maid, when available, assisted in the preparation of meals, washed dishes, scrubbed the stairs, woodwork, floors, closets, and lavatories, and cleaned the refrigerator, stove, and fireplaces. The orderly was usually hired for the male wards only, and there he was expected to ambulate and bathe the men as well as collect and wash urinals and sputum cups, give enemas, catheterize the patients, and assist in heavy lifting.

The head nurse, generally a senior nursing student, was held responsible for everything pertaining to her ward, including furniture, medicine chest, and linen. She was to make the rounds of the patients with the physicians during their visits, take down their orders, and see that those orders were faithfully carried out.

Care of the Surgical Patient

As the number of surgical operations increased, the student nurses took on new responsibilities. In the operating room of the 1890s the student nurse was responsible for making sure that everything connected with the operation was antiseptic. She prepared the room and scrubbed the floors, walls, and other surfaces with antiseptic solution. The surgical dressings were boiled, soaked, and wrapped in antiseptic towels or kept in large glass jars until needed. The nurse was also responsible for setting up the room with everything the surgeon might possibly need, such as hot water bottles, stimulants, clean towels, soft rags, lint, basins, pails, hot and cold water, ice, pins, needles, silk, scissors, petroleum jelly, soap, oil-silk, sponges, bran, sticking plaster, carbolized water, a rubber blanket, a

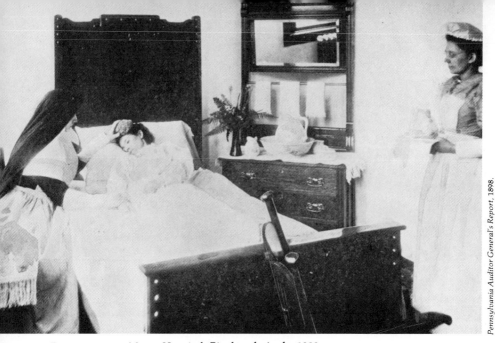

Pennsylvania Auditor General's Report, 1898.

Private room at Mercy Hospital, Pittsburgh, in the 1890s.

Physician-nurse relationships of the 1890s operated on strict authoritarian lines—nurses and physicians of the Bradford Hospital, Bradford, Pennsylvania, 1897.

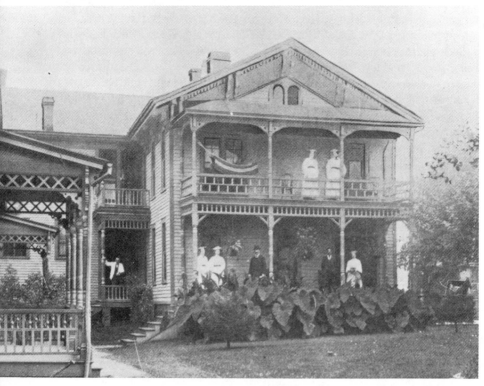

Pennsylvania Auditor General's Report, 1898.

pillow, and a sheet to cover the patient.

Preoperative preparation was done by the nurse, who bathed the patient, braided the hair for women, and dressed the patient in loose-fitting clothing. A pint of beef tea, or its equivalent in beef juice, was given four hours before the operation, along with an enema (especially if the surgery was to be in the region of the rectum or bladder).

After arranging the patient on the operating table, the student nurse had to be prepared for any emergency that might arise. She might help the physician to give the anesthetic, or in some cases she would administer it herself. Generally there were three nurses present at a surgical procedure of any importance: the head nurse and two others. The head nurse kept her eye on the surgeon and stood in a place where she could readily hand him hot towels, sponges, bowls of solution, or anything else he needed. The second nurse maintained the supply of hot towels, solutions, sponges, and hot and cold water, while the third nurse helped the person who was etherizing the patient. She also carried buckets of water, filled up empty pitchers, and wrung out sponges.

Physician Dominance

Wherever she worked, one of the first rules the student nurse had to remember was that the physician was always her director. She was told over and over that every good nurse was "wise as a serpent," quick to understand and obey whatever orders might be given, and "harmless as a dove" in remaining oblivious of any function of greater importance than that which the physician gave her to perform. According to medical dogma of the 1890s, there were few professions in which the scope of duties were more rigidly marked than nursing. Medicine, theology, art, music, law—all had unknown depths, and the student who drank at any one of these wells of knowledge could profit by the old quotation "Drink deep, or taste not." Only to the student nurse did the mandate apply: "Thus far shalt thou come, but no farther." Any nursing student who did not heed this advice was assured that she would fail miserably.

Illustrative of the child-like respect accorded 1890s physicians was a descriptive poem written by a nurse of the era, entitled "When Doctor's on the Floor":

Nurses moving quietly,
  Voices hushed in awe,
All things silent waiting,
  Obedient to the law
That we have heard so often,
  But I'll repeat once more:
"All things must be in order
  When Doctor's on the floor."

Soon a startled murmur
  Bursts upon the throng:
"Here's the Head Nurse for the rounds!"
  They'll be made ere long!

And now when long we've waited,
  As many a time before,
The rounds at last will soon be made,
  The Doctor's on the floor.

Quick I write a temperature
  Just as quick the spread,
Which hangs across a chair-back
  I put on baby's bed.
With my apron, quick I wipe
  The dust from off the door
Everything must be in state
  For Doctor's on the floor.

Nurses get their sleeves on,
  And straighten up their caps;
They gaze at spots on aprons,
  Which may be seen, perhaps.
The patients lie in silence,
  The babies cry no more;
They seem to know by instinct
  That Doctor's on the floor.

We nurses drop our quarrels
  And other little sins;
And when a breast is bandaged
  We share our safety-pins.
To wipe up water that in haste
  Is spilt from door to door,
Down goes a nurse upon her knees,
  When Doctor's on the floor.

If you pass the class-room
  On any lecture night,
You can hear the merry voices
  Each one talks with all her might.
But what a sudden silence comes
  If you approach the door,
And stop to whisper softly
  That Doctor's on the floor [7].

The chief reason for this attitude was the dependence of nursing upon the medical profession, in many respects nursing's progenitor. Yet nursing was supposedly a profession in itself. According to Victorian sentiments the cultured, educated, and "womanly woman" intuitively discovered and appreciated her limitations and did not venture beyond them. Once the student or graduate nurse overstepped the boundary of her prerogative, she was labeled a menace to society. Her intelligence, experience, and knowledge were considered to amount to nothing if she forgot the limitations of her training. The nurse was to read no medical books: if she had wished to be a physician, she should have gone to medical school, and then the field of medicine would have legitimately been open to her.

Medical Terms Illustrated

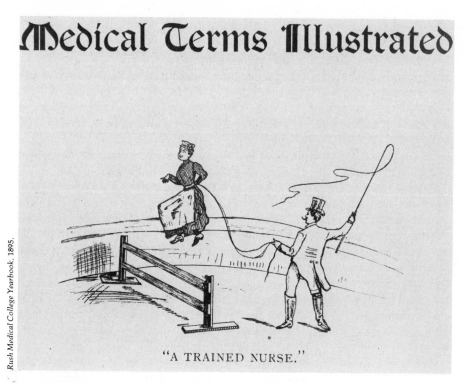

Rush Medical College Yearbook, 1895.

"A TRAINED NURSE."

A medical student's conception of "a trained nurse," 1895.

The consensus of physicians was that any nurse who read medical books and journals was overburdening her brain with useless knowledge that, in any case, she would probably not remember much longer than overnight. Such a nurse was apt to disgrace herself by daring to use obscure medical terms that only exposed her real ignorance and would quickly bring down the censure of the superintendent, the disgust of the physician, and the scorn of her patients.

In most situations the use of medical terms by a nurse was believed to be objectionable. If a physician asked a nurse, "Has this man had a nosebleed?" and she brashly answered, "Yes, doctor, he had quite an attack of epistaxis last evening," she would be scorned and probably accused behind her back of keeping "soiled medicine bottles in her ward closets" or of having "patients with long fingernails." Nursing textbooks stressed that physicians objected to the pedantic nurse. They would far rather have an ignorant "good, old-time Sairy Gamp," whom they could command and perhaps swear at a little and who would carry out their orders to the letter, out of ignorance. This pattern of interpersonal relations was carried into the social level, where interaction between nursing and medical staff was strictly prohibited. The reasons given were many and amusing. Some schools reported that it was for "disciplinary reasons," others said "professional," and several naively explained that "the nurses would lose respect for the doctors."

The World of the Private Duty Nurse

Private duty nursing took place in the patient's home, and the graduate nurse who undertook such a job was frequently expected to work 24 hours a day for as long as she was needed. The nurse's time was considered the property of anyone who employed her. She was ordinarily called into a private family when everyone was worn out and needed immediate relief from home nursing. For this reason the nurse did not expect to begin a case with an easy first night, even though she might arrive exhausted from a long carriage ride. The family was usually very anxious, and the nurse had to move quickly to shoulder the patient-care burden that they were too weary to carry a moment longer.

Entering the patient's room for the first time, she might give a pleasant look or a bow, since her first objective was to get acquainted with the patient and discern his needs. She did not sit where he could see her, and, although she was not to appear to be watching him, she would observe him constantly. The private duty nurse was to avoid whispered conversations and walking on tiptoe because such behavior caused the patient to strain to hear. She was to use a low, distinct tone when conversation was necessary and walk with light step. She was to avoid sitting on the bed, rattling newspapers, turning book pages, creaking a rocking chair, sewing, or clicking knitting needles. Neither was she to turn the gas lights up bright to improve the light for knitting or reading, because the gas burners were said to consume a large amount of the air needed by the patient.

The "good" nurse moved quietly, promptly putting things in their places. She anticipated the patient's wants and tried not to question him about his needs. If the patient was delirious, she was not to contradict him. The nurse listened attentively when the patient spoke, trying never to ask him to repeat. She never spoke to him from a distance or while standing behind him. She shut doors quickly and softly and oiled the hinges if they were rusty.

The private duty nurse of the 1890s had learned in her training school that a pleasant personal appearance would go far toward inspiring confidence. Therefore, she developed habits of extreme neatness in dress, always having clean handkerchiefs, collars, and stockings, spotless sleeves and aprons, starched caps, and a simple arrangement of the hair. Trailing skirts, flounces, hoop petticoats, frizzed or loose hair, rings, and all other jewelry were considered out of place in a sickroom. For her night use the nurse was to have warm slippers and a close-fitting dressing gown.

The nurse was careful to maintain her freshness with a daily bath. She accomplished this with a basin and towel by wringing out a rough cloth in soap and water and rubbing herself briskly from head to foot. She kept her nails scrupulously clean but never cleaned or pared her nails in front of the patient. She made a point not to use a toothpick or to arrange hairpins in public.

Because the private duty nurse literally moved in with the household, relationships with the family became important. If she was there for any length of time, she soon became a part of the inner family circle as interests hovered around the sickroom and private matters were openly discussed. According to the thinking of the day, the family had the right to expect a cheerful, helping disposition from

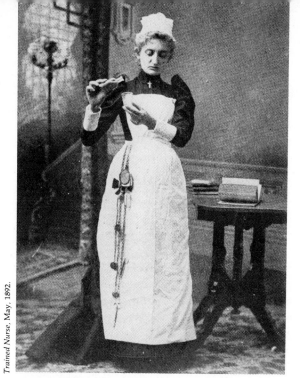

A private duty nurse of the 1890s.

Advertisement of an agency supplying private duty nurses.

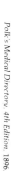

Telephone Call,
1406—38th St.

Calls responded to at any Hour,
Day or Night.

A. KREINBERG'S

Nurse ✚ Agency

904 SIXTH AVENUE,

Near 51st Street.

NEW YORK CITY.

My Staff of Trained Nurses Represents Graduates from the
Different Training Schools in the States.

Wet Nurses furnished between the hours of 10 A. M. and 4 P. M. This department is under the direction of a competent female attendant.

ARTHUR KREINBERG,

MASSAGE OPERATOR,

Cupper and Leecher,

904 Sixth Avenue.

the private duty nurse at all times. While she carried out the physician's orders and did what was essential for the patient, she was to readily accept suggestions from members of the family. She was to remember that she was responsible to the family as well as to the physician whose orders she followed.

Private duty nursing was strenuous work with low pay, often requiring weeks of continuous service. If the patient was dangerously ill, the nurse sat up all night and sometimes for more than a month had only two to six hours' sleep, snatched during daylight. Three weeks was the average length of a private duty engagement. The first 10 days of each case usually meant two hours of sleep out of 24, and the next 10 days might allow six hours of sleep per night. When the patient reached the convalescent stage, the nurse slept on a couch close by. If her patient was sleepless, the nurse was to stay awake to keep him comfortable. During the day, if the patient was not seriously ill, the nurse was expected to assist the family in sewing and other household chores.

There was not one hour of the long day and night that the private duty nurse could call her own except the time when she took her daily walk. Even that had to suit the convenience of everyone in the family. If no arrangements had been made with the family for the nurse to get some fresh air, she usually stated her case pleasantly and asked for relief—but she was never to show an unwillingness to attend to her patient, and she was never to let anyone see that she was tired or upset. After a case had been completed, the private duty nurse generally went home with a trunkful of soiled clothes, thoroughly exhausted.

Economics of Private Duty Nursing

In 1888 the Department of Labor investigated the weekly wages paid to women in 22 large cities. It found that average weekly wages varied from a high of $6.91 in San Francisco to a low of $3.93 in Richmond, while most women averaged from $4.00 to $6.00 a week. A govenment report noted that this was hardly enough to buy the necessities of life. Such inadequate wages, said the report, "must inevitably lead in many cases to the adoption of a life of immorality, and in fact there is no doubt that the low rate of wages paid to women is one of the frequent causes of prostitution" [8].

In 1890 it was claimed that nursing was one of the very best fields for women:

Trained nurses receive good pay in comparison with that of the ordinary employments of women, ranging from ten dollars per week upward to twenty, thirty, or even forty dollars, according to the difficulty of the case. While these prices are by no means higher than should reward a nurse who has given years in preparation for her profession and who works faithfully in it, they are yet burdensome to many families. A surgeon will sometimes refuse to take a case unless he can have the skilled nursing that he believes essential to success, and yet the pay of the nurse will take all the earnings of the father, on which the family rely for support [9].

On the other hand, it was not generally known by the public that a private duty nurse was overworked for some months yet idle for others. Consequently, an excellent nurse was very fortunate if she could gross $600 a year. Like all other independent practitioners in business for themselves, nurses found that sometimes they could not collect their fees. Instead, when the time came for settling the account, the family would offer her things such as food, old clothing, and trinkets, along with whatever small portion of her fee they might deem sufficient pay.

Despite difficulties in fee collection, some physicians charged that graduates of nurse training schools were overpaid. Dr. A. W. Catlin of Brooklyn, in December, 1894, publicly stated that the need for intelligent aid in the sickroom was apparent and that trained nurses were needed rather than ignorant Sairy Gamps. Yet the system of having trained nurses for private duty was fast becoming undesirable because of its exclusiveness. The private duty nurse was more and more of a luxury, he warned, and would soon be far beyond the means of the average family. He charged that schools of nursing taught students that upon graduation they should not take patients for less than $3.00 a day, and many schools stood firm on $25 a week as their unalterable fee. The wealthy could easily afford nurses, along with many other comforts, while people of moderate income had to deny themselves this service and, because of this denial, take additional risks on their lives.

Catlin's remarks outraged several private duty nurses who quickly refuted his charges in a series of letters to the *Brooklyn Eagle.* One commented that among the first principles she had been taught in training was loyalty to the physician, and she wondered why there should not be some loyalty given to the nurse by the physician. She had also been taught that by devoting two years of hard work to a hospital she would be given a diploma and then enter a profession that would enable her to make a living. Even the strongest nurses had to take a rest between patients, she noted, and it was often necessary to wait many weeks for calls— which brought the average nurse's income down to the price of unskilled labor. Private duty nurses were deprived of pleasures of every kind and spent their time in the sickroom, night and day for weeks and even months, without rest, giving their very lives for their patients. Could anyone think that it would be right to alter their charges so as to deny them regular prices, she asked, when all physicians in good standing were entitled to their standard fees?

Another nurse could not see why Dr. Catlin was so desirous of reducing a nurse's pay, although she knew that there were some physicians who preferred to have inexpensive nurses attending their patients in order to enable patients to pay the doctors' larger fees. Physicians knew, she continued, that where a good trained nurse was employed to care for a patient, it was unnecessary for the physician to make as many calls as otherwise would be required. Dr. Catlin, she thought, was no doubt getting at least $3 for one 15- or 20-minute house call, and yet he wanted a nurse to settle for $2 for working a 24-hour day for the same patient. She deplored the fact that any man would attempt to thwart a woman who was only trying to earn a decent living: "What right has Dr. Catlin to set salaries? No more right than the nurses have to say that his house calls are only worth 50 cents a visit." Dr. Catlin, she pointed out, wanted to know

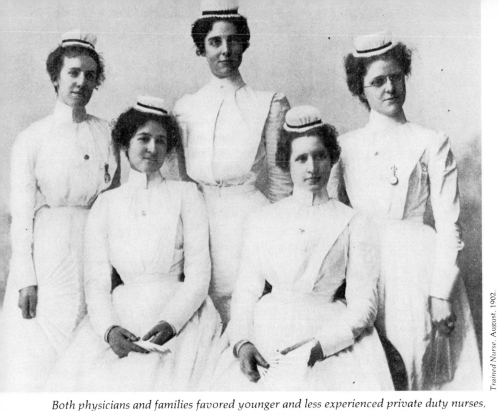

Trained Nurse, August, 1902.

Both physicians and families favored younger and less experienced private duty nurses, on the ground that they had much more physical vitality for demanding assignments: Graduating class, Bridgeton Hospital, Bridgeton, New Jersey, 1902.

Entrance to the Pan-American Exposition Hospital, where President McKinley was taken.

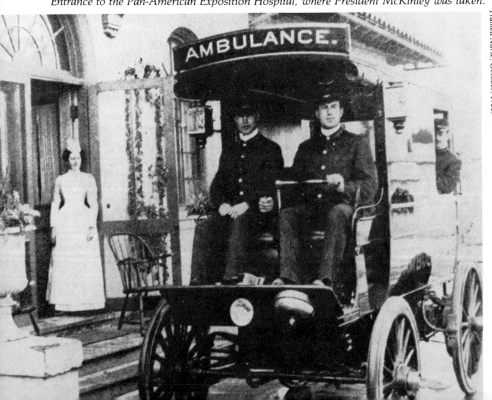

Trained Nurse, October, 1901.

who would join hands with him in building a home where he and several other medical men could teach 30 or 40 women to work cheaply as untrained nurses. Why not build a home for cheap physicians, this nurse retorted, assuring the newspaper readers that trained nurses would be willing to teach aspiring cheap physicians free of charge. What a beautiful memorial that would be for future generations, she speculated: a home where anyone could secure a physician for 50 cents a call. Trained nurses could then easily charge $30 a week [10].

It was not surprising that a nurse's practice began to wane soon after she reached age 40. Both physicians and families favored younger nurses. At one of the large training schools in New York, where many wealthy families requested names of graduates for private duty assignments, three-fourths of the requests were for nurses who were in their twenties. Private duty nurses with 10 or 20 years' experience behind them frequently lacked the physical vitality required for long night vigils and the hard work connected with demanding assignments. Although private duty nursing by trained nurses was still a young field, an increasing problem was how to provide for nurses over the age of 50. Occasionally, unmarried nurses achieved long careers by obtaining permanent positions in wealthy families, where they had duty no more arduous than in superintending other nurses under them. In one instance a trained nurse who had been sent from New York to Europe found that her sole work was to make sure that the daughter of a millionaire never went out in damp weather without overshoes.

Such nurses found that the very wealthy of this era were burdened with more money than they had time to use. They often spent it competitively to impress and surpass one another. They spent millions on huge mansions. Their parties, especially their masked balls, were spectacular functions to which the elite came by the hundreds, wearing costumes costing as much as $5000 each. Trained nurses, permanently hired, were an essential service component in the inner circle of fashionable families who wintered in Palm Beach, summered in Newport or Bar Harbor, and visited London and Paris as casually as could be. Such nurses found that they were often accepted as traveling companions and helped to manage the dozens of servants.

President McKinley and His Nurses

In September, 1901, President William McKinley was shot by an anarchist while visiting the Pan-American Exposition in Buffalo, New York. The nurses who were on duty in the emergency hospital on the Exposition grounds when President McKinley was carried in performed an active part in the historic event that was about to unfold. Though scarcely more than a first-aid station, the hospital had an operating room, and the President was at once laid on the table. He was in severe shock but conscious and entirely composed. As the nurses undressed him, a bullet fell from his underclothing. The first shot had richocheted off the breastbone, causing only an angry graze along the ribs, but the serious nature of an abdominal wound was immediately apparent to the physicians who gathered around the operating table. The President's lips were forming the words of the Lord's Prayer when ether was administered.

Adella Walters, superintendent of the hospital and a member of the first graduating class of the Buffalo General Hospital Nurse Training School in 1890, was at her post, and Miss Morris and Miss Barnes were the nurses on duty when the distinguished patient was brought in. The other nurses, Miss Simmons, Miss Dorchester, Miss Baron, and Miss Shannon, arrived soon afterward and assisted during surgery. The nurses "worked well, every one of them," said Miss Walters afterward. "I got all the things needed for the operation, for none of the nurses were as familiar with the places where the needed articles are kept as I, since the nurses change every month." Miss Simmons and Miss Barnes were the nurses who came in direct contact with the patient during the operation. They handled the instruments and dressings and prepared the President for the operation, Miss Simmons standing at the head of the table, fanning him.

In the spotless little operating room off the main hall on the first floor of the hospital, Miss Morris and Miss Barnes told reporters from throughout the nation of their services to President McKinley. "They brought him right here from the ambulance," said Miss Morris, placing her hand on the operating table, "and did not even lift him to remove the stretcher during the operation. I stood here and Miss Simmons stood over there"—indicating the opposite side of the table—"and Dr. Sasdin gave the anesthetic there," she said, pointing to the white-enameled stool at the head of the operating table. "He was the most admirable patient I ever saw," said Miss Barnes. "When we were taking care of him that first night, sick as he was, there was not the slightest service performed for him that he did not recognize in some way. If he could not speak, he would just give a little 'umph-umph,' just to let us know that he noticed what we were doing for him" [11]. Miss Barnes admitted that she was shocked to see whom the patient was: "I had no idea it was the President who was to be operated upon, when Miss Walters told me to get a hypodermic of morphia and strychnia. I looked at the face of the man on the table and said to myself: 'That looks like the President,' but it was some little time before I was quite sure about it" [12].

"It was so pathetic," said Miss Morris, "when he was on the table before the anesthetic was given. He seemed to feel so badly that anyone should shoot him because of a personal hatred. That seemed to be the thought that pained him most. He lay there, so white and still, never uttering a complaint, and seemed to be trying to comprehend what prompted his assailant to the deed. Once he said gently: 'He didn't know, poor fellow, what he was doing. He couldn't have known' " [13].

On opening the abdomen the surgeons found that the assassin's second shot had passed straight through the stomach, puncturing the front and rear walls. The operation consisted mainly of suturing those wounds and cleansing the peritoneal cavity. The bullet was not found. No use was made of a Roentgen-ray machine, even though one of them was on exhibition at the fair, and an attempt to probe was abandoned because of the patient's dangerously weak condition. The assisting physicians and nurses used a looking glass to reflect the rays of the setting sun on the surgeons' work and succeeded toward the end in rigging an electric light. The incision was finally closed, without drainage, and covered with an antiseptic dressing.

The President's improvement was remarkable, but it did not indicate recovery. Gangrene was creeping along the bullet's track through the stomach, the pancreas, and one kidney. After an eight-day battle to keep the President alive, he died, on September 14, 1901.

Summary

The rapid growth of hospitals following the Civil War was associated with increasing urbanization. Expanded urban career opportunities for women provided the impetus for continued emancipation that characterized the period between 1880 and 1890.

Trained nurses had two main options after graduation: private duty nursing in homes or in hospitals or hospital nursing in the roles of superintendent or sometimes that of head nurse. The vast proportion of hospital nursing service was carried out by students. Hospitals without schools of nursing generally used untrained attendants in place of students.

Student nurses of the 1890s were generally responsible for maintaining the environment of the wards (temperature and ventilation) and for housekeeping, food preparation, and laundry. It was argued that hospital maids did not understand the importance of aseptic conditions and therefore could not perform these tasks properly.

Treatments administered by the nurse included cupping, blistering, and applying leeches as well as preparing and applying poultices, fomentations, and mustard plasters.

The division of student labor on the hospital ward typically involved a "temperature nurse," a "right-side" and a "left-side" nurse for each half of the ward, a special assignment nurse, and a probationer, as well as the occasional services of a ward maid and an orderly for the male wards. These positions involved distinct tasks, and a pattern of <u>functional nursing was practiced</u>.

Nurses were responsible during surgery for maintaining antiseptic conditions, preparing the patients, and, in some cases, administering anesthetics.

The nurse was subject to domination by the physician, a situation rationalized by the Victorian ideal of women and maintained by the tacit injunction that the nurse avoid learning medicine or even reading medical books.

Private duty nursing required stamina and self-sacrifice. The nurse was expected to be always available to the patient, to maintain a constantly cheerful personality and to subordinate her personal desires to those of the family with whom she worked.

Average salaries for women were so low at this time—averaging from $4 to $6 per week in 1888—that nursing was reputed to be one of the best fields for women, with weekly salaries for private duty nurses falling in the range of $10 to $30 or more per week. Private duty engagements were occasional, however, and could usually yield only a modest annual income.

The assassination of President McKinley in 1901 demonstrated that not even the great resourcefulness and vigilance of nurses and physicians could compensate for the limited state of medicine at that time.

References

1. Massachusetts General Hospital, *Circular and Announcement by the Trustees of the Massachusetts General Hospital, of a Two Years' Course of Training in General Nursing* (Boston: The Hospital, 1889).
2. Boston City Hospital Training School for Nurses, *Circular of Information for Candidates and Probationers on the Necessary Outfit on Entering Service, Course of Training with a List of Questions to be Answered by the Candidate, and a Form of Agreement to Remain Two Years as a Pupil of the School* (Boston: City Hospital, 1889).
3. Emily L. Loveridge, "Reminiscences of Forty Years in Hospital Work," *Bulletin of the American Hospital Association*, vol. 4 (April, 1930):48–52.
4. Lutheran Hospital, Cleveland, "The Good Old Days," *Bright Corridors*, vol. 8 (January, 1963):1–4.
5. Mary Agnes Snively, "A Nurse's Day in a Hospital," *Trained Nurse*, vol. 13 (July, 1894):8–12.
6. L. W. Quintard, "Limitations of Pupil Nurses in Caring for Male Patients," *Proceedings of the American Society of Superintendents of Training Schools for Nurses*, 1896, 3:70.
7. "When Doctor's on the Floor," *Trained Nurse and Hospital Review*, vol. 16 (September, 1896):90.
8. U.S. Department of Commerce and Labor, *Report on the Condition of Woman and Child Wage-Earners in the United States* (Washington, D.C.:   Government Printing Office, 1911), vol. 9, pp. 24–25.
9. *New York Tribune*, February 18, 1890.
10. "Answering Dr. Catlin," *Trained Nurse*, vol. 16 (February, 1896):121.
11. *Buffalo Express*, September 8, 1901.
12. *Ibid.*
13. *Ibid.*

7
Nurses and the War with Spain

The *Spanish-American War* led to the emergence of the first large all-graduate nursing service and provided the first opportunity for incorporating the graduates of nearly 200 nurse training schools throughout the country into a single nursing corps. As a result of this war, trained nurses were accepted for the first time in miliary hospitals and thereby became forerunners of women in the armed forces.

The Spanish-American War, which began in April , 1898, and ended in August of the same year, was one of the last minor wars fought before the devastating, cataclysmic struggles of the twentieth century. The most important land fighting, which occurred in Cuba, lasted only a month. Enthusiastically reported by the press, this war produced enough heroes and slogans to supply a dozen larger ones. At the outbreak of hostilities, the Regular Army, only 28,000 men, was completely unprepared for war. There had been no brigade-sized formation of troops in the country for 30 years, and only a few officers had ever seen a unit as large as a regiment concentrated in one place. Because this force was inadequate for conducting a war against Spain, Congress authorized the President to increase the army to a standing force of more than 200,000 men.

The DAR Secures Nurses
Unable to supply hospital corpsmen for such vast numbers of soldiers, the War Department began to look elsewhere for assistance. When the National Society of the Daughters of the American Revolution offered to serve as an examining board for the military nurses, Surgeon General of the Army George M. Sternberg immediately accepted. Directing the committee appointed by the Daughters for this purpose was the young Dr. Anita Newcomb McGee.

Dr. McGee was born in Washington, D.C., on November 4, 1864, daughter of Simon Newcomb, one of the most eminent astronomers of his day. After attending private schools in Washington, she continued her education with three years of study and travel in Europe. Mrs. McGee was in her mid-twenties when she began studying medicine in the Medical Department of George Wash-

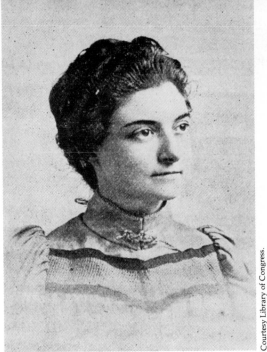

Dr. Anita Newcomb McGee.

ington University. In 1892, at the age of 28, she received her M.D. degree, which she later supplemented with a postgraduate course in gynecology at Johns Hopkins University. Afterwards she built up a large practice in Washington, D.C.

Since hundreds of applications for service with the Army were pouring in from trained and untrained nurses, they could not receive proper attention from the War Department, which was already overwhelmed with supervising the preparation of war material. By examining and screening this mass of applications from women nurses, Dr. McGee perceived that the DAR committee would be performing a valuable service for the government. Washington reporters raved that she was the ideal woman for the job because she was "young and charming, possessing unusual magnetism, vivacity, and a gift of language"[1].

The nurses of 1898 proved to be worthy successors to those of the Civil War. As the army grew in size, the sick rate rose in direct proportion, and the demand for nurses sharply increased. By working literally day and night the committee succeeded in examining nearly 5000 applications. In one of her reports Dr. McGee testified: "The work of separating the fit from the unfit was not so simple an accomplishment as it would appear, and the correspondence entailed was enormous. The visitors who made inquiries in person were also numerous. The officers were at their posts daily from 8 A.M. to 11 P.M."[2].

There were letters from eager, romantic young girls and from aged matrons who had served as nurses in the Civil War. Some appealed to the President, some to the Secretary of War. Some had enough knowledge to direct their applications to the Surgeon General, but their fitness for work ended there. A smaller number listed regular hospital training and service. Every one of these thousands of applications was examined, numbered, and filed in alphabetical order. Those applicants who had mentioned hospital training received the following letter in reply:

DEAR MADAM: Your application of recent date has been received. All applications from women for hospital positions, whether addressed to the Surgeon General or to the director of the D.A.R. hospital corps, are placed on file in this office.

The reserve list is composed, however, only of those who have had hospital training and who answer satisfactorily to the enclosed questions. Nurses who receive appointment in the army must be between thirty and fifty years of age. They will be paid railroad fare to the place of duty and $30 a month with board. If practicable, lodging will be given, but other expenses must be met by the nurse.

Women may later be appointed to shore duty in the navy, but no provisions have yet been made therefor.

Endorsements as to good character and general ability should accompany the application, and it is requested that, if possible, such endorsements should include one from some Daughter of the American Revolution [3].

A card was sent with the letter, requesting information such as age, state of health, and work experience. Significantly, the applicant was asked: "Have you had yellow fever?" and "Are you strong and healthy, and have you always been so?" Only graduates of training schools for nurses or of medical colleges were considered eligible. A physician's certificate that the applicant was in good health and strong enough for army duty was required. When the Surgeon General received a requisition for more nurses, he referred it to the DAR office, which in turn sent the nurse her contract, transportation, and orders. The first call for nurses was received from the Surgeon General of the Army on May 7, 1898, and within a few days four women nurses were on their way to the general hospital at Key West, Florida.

In addition to the contract nurses selected as above, Mrs. Namah Curtis, wife of Dr. Austin M. Curtis, Surgeon-in-Chief of Freedmen's Hospital in Washington, D.C., was sent on July 13 by the Surgeon General to New Orleans and other Southern cities to secure the services of immune black women as nurses for yellow fever patients. Mrs. Curtis was able to register 32 such nurses.

Sickness in the Camps

Of the more than 200,000 volunteers who enlisted in April and May of 1898, no more than 35,000 left the United States or were even assigned to expeditions during the war. The remaining soldiers sat out the war in military camps in the southern United States, where they spent many hours in target practice, drill, and large-scale combat maneuvers. In May about 6.75 percent of the men were sick. In June the sick rate climbed to almost 16 percent. By July this figure had risen to 20 percent of the Army's total strength of 203,350. The climax was fi-

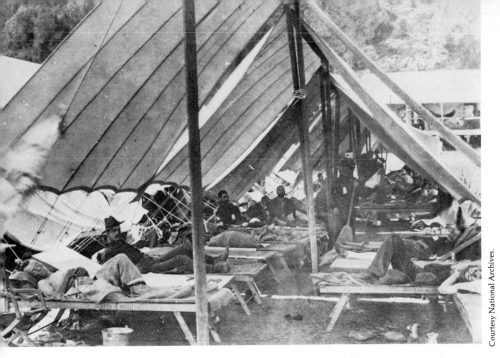

By July, 1898, 20 percent of the Army was suffering from disease.

nally reached in August, when the sick rate increased to 30 percent. Malaria, typhoid, dysentery, and diarrhea accounted for 60 percent of the sickness in July, August, and September of 1898. Eighty percent of all deaths were attributed to typhoid.

Meanwhile, Surgeon General Sternberg was downplaying the potential usefulness of female nurses on a large scale for the Army. On May 3, 1898, he made the following comments to the Secretary of War in regard to a joint resolution that had been introduced to authorize the greater use of trained women nurses in army general hospitals:

In my opinion this would be very unwise legislation. Trained female nurses are out of place as regular attendants of sick and wounded soldiers in the wards of a general hospital. They may be very useful for certain cases and especially in the preparation and serving of special diets to such an extent as may be necessary and desirable, but the passage of this bill would greatly embarrass me in the administration of our general hospitals[4].

Observers expressed their dismay at the pervasive filth in the military camps. Regiments often dug latrines and garbage pits within yards of their kitchens, hospitals, and living quarters. In rainy weather the shallow pits flooded and overflowed, spilling sewage throughout the camps. Regimental and company officers failed to enforce regulations controlling the use and maintenance of latrines, and the soldiers threw garbage on the ground near their tents and defecated in the surrounding woods. After viewing the camp of the Third United States Volunteer Cavalry at Camp Thomas, outside of the city of Chattanooga, Tennessee, an inspecting officer reported:

I have never seen so large an area of fecal-stained soil as that which we looked upon and walked over. This area was a checker board, marked with woody spots of irregular contour and open spaces, some of which had known cultivation. The woody lands were smeared with alvine discharges. As I have said, most of the soldiers had been removed before our arrival, but even then one could not walk under the trees without soiling one's shoes with human excrement. Behind every considerable tree it lay in heaped-up cones. The falling leaves and twigs did not suffice to hide it. The gentle winds had not wholly dispersed it; a hot September sun was drying it out. An occasional rain was sinking the pollution below the surface and down into the soil [5].

Failure of the Hospital Corps

To provide the male nurses preferred by Army surgeons at that time, the Medical Department tried to enlarge its small Hospital Corps. Strenuous efforts to attract civilian recruits and to persuade medically qualified volunteers to transfer from line regiments met with frustration. Even though the Hospital Corps had increased its ranks from a peacetime strength of 723 to almost 6000 men by August 31, 1898, it still had barely half the number required for the army of over 200,000, and most of its recruits lacked training and experience. In their search for nurses for the camp hospitals, commanders temporarily detailed squads of infantry to ward duty. These detail men, often the dregs of the units, were grossly unqualified to care for patients, and their neglect of elementary sanitary precautions helped spread diseases, such as typhoid, through the camps.

The low status attached to the soldiers of the Hospital Corps accounted for much of their low morale and incompetence. The male Army nurse, with his inadequate pay and enlisted rank, had little to expect but ingratitude from his fellow soldiers. The glory and distinction that might be gained on the battlefield was beyond the reach of the male nurse, although his duties were far more arduous and taxing than those of his comrades bearing arms. Since he was in constant contact with infectious diseases, he exposed himself to more danger than if he were on the battlefield.

A virulent outbreak of typhoid fever resulted in the more extensive use of women in the Army hospitals. Driven by despair to innovation, Surgeon General Sternberg for the first time in the Army's history employed large numbers of women nurses in military hospitals. Beginning in late July, typhoid cases increased the sick rate in every camp. The number of sick at Camp Thomas grew from about 2200 on July 25, to 3600 on August 8, and to 4400 on August 15. Typhoid patients sometimes lay in their own filth for as long as 24 hours because the hospitals lacked clean linen with which to change their beds. A medical officer at a Camp Thomas hospital wrote in panic [6]:

Leiter General Hospital   July 10, 1898
Chickamauga, Georgia
Dr. McGee D.A.R.

Dear Doctor:
   Miss Dunmise, the nurse I recommended, arrived this A.M. much to our delight and I am much obliged for sending her so promptly.

We are in terrible distress for nurses and can't understand the delay in sending them—there ought to be 50 good nurses in Washington willing and glad to come here. We have now in the hospital 150 cases of typhoid fever and six trained nurses to take care of these and there are 100 more cases waiting to come.

We need 30 trained nurses and cannot do with less.

I understand from the Surgeon General that the matter has been turned over to you and I trust you will at once relieve our distress. There are three good nurses at Providence Hospl. that I think you can get. I am glad to see the Daughters are taking so active a part. I am Vice Prest. S.A.R. of the District of Columbia, and hence have a fellow feeling with you in the good work you are doing.

I hope you will pardon me for speaking so plainly about this matter but only those in the field can know the exigencies of the occasion.

Yours truly,
J. W. Bayne
Major & Brigade Surg. U.S.V.

Battling Typhoid Fever

"It was certainly a most harrowing sight to see the long narrow cots filled with what had been strong, splendid men, hollow-eyed, emaciated, muttering in the delirium of fever," reported Anna Maxwell, on leave as Superintendent of Nurses at New York's Presbyterian Hospital, after viewing conditions at Sternberg Hospital at Camp Thomas. She noted that "some of the men's bones protruded through their skin, and bed sores several inches deep were not uncommonly found on hips, back, elbows, and often on the head and ears" [7]. All the energies and resources of the trained nurse were required to make the lives of these men less wretched and to restore them to health.

Ninety-one training schools from all parts of the United States were represented at the hospital. According to Harriet Lounsberry, who was on leave from her position as superintendent of nursing at Brooklyn Homeopathic Hospital, "it was curious and interesting to see representatives of so many training schools together." The nurses wore their own distinctive school uniforms during their work, for the military had made no effort to outfit them in a standard dress. Miss Lounsberry noticed that school badges, which reflected pride in one's alma mater, were prominently displayed. "Nothing would bring a nurse more quickly to a sense of her duty than to ask if in her training school she had never been instructed as regards this or that," she recalled [8].

Jean S. Edmunds of Rochester, New York, arrived at the Sternberg Hospital on August 17, along with 36 other nurses. She found that the nurses at Camp Thomas had been working day and night. As rapidly as tents were pitched and cots were placed within them, more ambulances with fever-stricken men arrived. "Hastily donning our uniforms," related Miss Edmunds, "but with skirts shortened and sleeves rolled up, we were each escorted to the tents where work had been assigned us by Miss Maxwell, who, while on the way thither, advised us of the need of strict discipline, as the eyes of America would be watching us" [9].

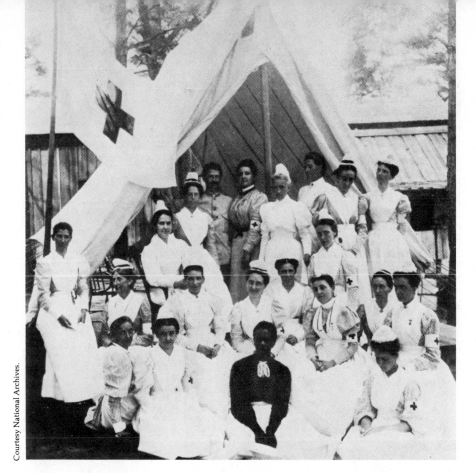

Nurses at Camp Thomas, Chickamauga Park, Georgia, August, 1898.

Experiences on Duty

The venerable Anna Maxwell constantly reminded the nurses that their work at Camp Thomas would forever speak for or against the women of America. During her first four weeks there, Miss Edmunds cared each day for 42 men sick with typhoid fever. The men presented a dreadful sight when they were first brought to her. "Their poor tongues were swollen and cracked," she noted, "their lips raw with the fever sores; often the back was one raw bed sore, for the fever was of the most virulent type, and they had received little or no care in the Camp and Division Hospitals" [10].

Each of these men required several ice baths daily, besides nourishment every two hours and all other care. Some of the more delirious ones had to be watched almost constantly. Despite all this work, Miss Edmunds had only one corpsman to assist her, and even he was replaced every few hours. Moreover, since each new aide had to be taught the fundamentals of caring for the sick, the nurses's capabilities were extraordinarily taxed. Unable to indulge in the luxury of tears, the nurses worked at a frantic pace. For the first four weeks their

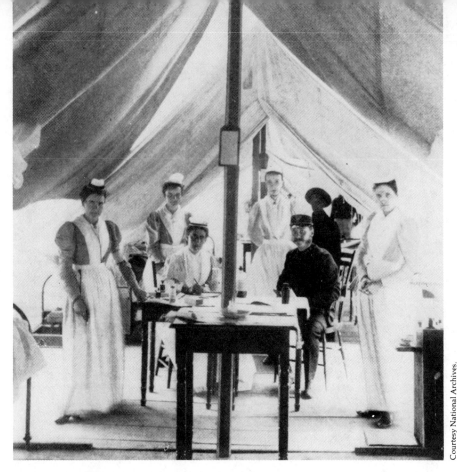

Interior of a hospital tent at Chickamauga Park, Georgia.

working day lasted from 7:00 A.M. until 9:00 P.M., with a mere 20-minute break for lunch and the same for supper.

Helen B. Schuler and Florence M. Kelly, contract nurses from New York City, concluded that it was only by the grace of God that anyone survived the primitive, unsanitary conditions at Chickamauga Park, Georgia, during the summer and fall of 1898. Sternberg Hospital consisted of 13 rough board huts, bare, cold, and unfinished. The windows, mere holes in the walls, without glass, provided the only means of ventilation and sunlight. Needless to say, these openings in the walls offered no protection against the hordes of flies and mosquitoes that were constantly streaming through. During a Georgia rainstorm the nurses were forced either to close these openings with wooden doors and endure the foul, humid air of an overcrowded, unventilated ward or to leave them open and contend with damp, flooded huts. The interior of these huts was absolutely primitive in every respect, and the uncertain light afforded by lanterns made medical treatment hazardous.

The heat, which could only be described as tropical, blanketed the nurses and their patients with "a suffocating pressure of steaming, smelly, deadening matter that passed for air." Attracted by all the sick men, the flies and mosquitoes multipled by the millions and spread infection between the sickbeds and the mess kitchen. The following passage illustrates a typical night:

Two hundred suffering patients, mostly all delirious, were brought to the Hospital. Every one of them previously had been given a dose of Calomel and Jalop. There was not a bed "Utensil" to be had and we, the nurses, suffered the consequences. The soiled clothing and bedding had to be taken care of and we had no way or equipment to handle it, so as to reduce to a minimum the danger of infection for us. We had no disinfectant whatsoever to use.
   There was not even one wash basin in these wards for the nurses to wash their hands.
   At one time there was a shortage of water for several days [and] we were requested "not to wash at all."
   The three toilets which were supposed to be adequate for the needs of the two hundred nurses, were over 500 feet away from their sleeping quarters. Every one of the nurses had contracted Dysentery and under these fearfully unsanitary conditions, consider how inevitable it was, that the majority of the nurses left Sternberg Hospital Service with an intestinal condition which soon became chronic and which we shall suffer from the effects of, until the end of our life [11].

Some of the nurses virtually worked themselves to death, as attested by a letter of August 18, 1898, from a Camp Thomas surgeon to Dr. McGee [12]:

I am sorry to trouble you again. Your nurses arrived and are hard at work. Owing to the large percentage of sickness among the nurses I felt obliged to keep all six that arrived here. Unless some are able to return to duty I shall be obliged to telegraph on Sunday morning for six or perhaps 10 more.
   Could not some of mine who can not stand this climate be transferred to Fortress Monroe or Long Island? These nurses are very zealous—they over-work themselves from the highest and best motives and many of them take it awfully to heart when they are stopped and to be invalided away is very bitter to them. Now I have to send a number to the Mountains every week to recuperate. Now if I could hold out to these unselfish women the prospect of similar work in a more bracing climate I am sure they would not be so distressed at having to go away. It is really a very serious matter with them.
Faithfully yours,
E. C. Carter
Major & Surgeon USV

Barbara U. Austin, a young nurse who had just finished her training, was assigned to Sternberg Hospital as one of the 166 women nurses on duty there during August of 1898. She recounted her experiences there as follows:

We were ordered to prepare the tents for the receptions of patients. I recall distinctly the blistering July day we were hemming woolen blankets for the beds. I can see the tent section on the hill side. Ten tents to a section and ten sections each having from four to six beds in a tent. It was a long trek from morning til night. Our beds were filled with typhoid cases, and all desperately sick. Carrying ice and nourishment up and down the hillside. Rain failed to dampen our ardor if it did our uniforms and frequently left us soaked all day. How grateful the boys were for these services. It made no difference to us that we were forty to fifty in a shack when off duty, just room enough to stand between the cots. One lantern banging in the middle of the building for light [13].

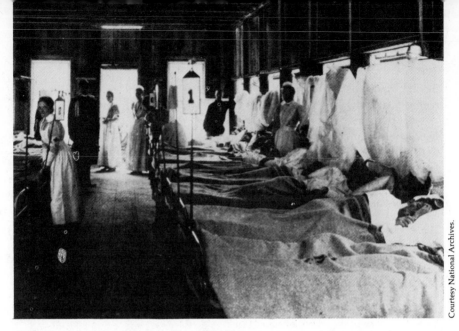

Army nurses caring for typhoid fever patients.

Sickness among the Nurses

One nurse who did not last long was Jane F. Riley of Boston. "When early in August, 1898, I read in the Boston papers that Miss Maxwell had sent out a call for nurses for Chickamauga Park . . . I immediately offered my services," remembered Miss Riley. Shortly thereafter, "about September 8th Miss Moore had to give up duty on account of sickness, and I on the 10th, several others had already taken sick, some having been sent to the Mountains, others sent North" [14]. They were not on a typhoid diet, but it did not matter, for these nurses wanted nothing to eat. Several doctors visited and examined them. The last physician, they were told, was Dr. Jesse Lazear from Cuba, an expert on tropical diseases. He decided that the sick nurses had typhoid. Because they could not be cared for at Sternberg Hospital, he recommended that they be sent north immediately. They left on September 13, in the charge of a Brooklyn nurse who had asked to be released, and were taken by ambulance to an awaiting hospital train.

Later, Miss Riley still remembered the jolting over the rough roads. Their destination was Boston City Hospital. Sick as they were when they left Sternberg Hospital, the nurses did not forget to ask for their discharge. The medical officer, however, informed them that he could not discharge nurses taken sick on duty but would grant them a furlough for an indefinite period and await the results of their illness. After they had been patients in the Boston City Hospital for some time, they were propped up in bed and asked to sign some papers, which, they presumed, were annulments of their contracts. Miss Riley was in the Boston City Hospital for 10 weeks, and for six months thereafter her weakened heart sapped her strength.

Harriet C. Lounsberry, who succeeded Miss Maxwell as chief nurse at Sternberg Hospital, kept a list of all the nurses who had departed from the hospital up until September 13, 1898, and recorded the reason why each had left. This information was tabulated as follows [15]:

Nurses leaving Sternberg Hospital from August 19 to September 13, 1898.

Number	From	Date of Arrival	Date of Departure	Reason for Departure
1	Boston, Mass.	Aug. 7	Sept. 10	Overworked
2	New York City	Aug. 7	Sept. 8	Diarrhea
3	New York City	Aug. 7	Sept. 8	Diarrhea
4	Newark, N.J.	Aug. 7	Aug. 19	Hysteria
5	Boston, Mass.	Aug. 17	Sept. 13	Typhoid fever
6	Rochester, N.Y.	Aug. 17	Sept. 7	Exhaustion
7	Brooklyn, N.Y.	Aug. 17	Sept. 7	Exhaustion
8	Brooklyn, N.Y.	Aug. 17	Aug. 30	Exhaustion
9	Boston, Mass.	Aug. 17	Sept. 7	Exhaustion
10	Brooklyn, N.Y.	Aug. 17	Sept. 13	
11	Pittsburgh, Pa.	Aug. 17	Sept. 7	High fever
12	Boston, Mass.	Aug. 17	Aug. 26	Broken down by night work
13	New York City	Aug. 17	Aug. 23	Diarrhea
14	New York City	Aug. 17	Aug. 30	Dismissed, not sick
15	New York City	Aug. 17	Sept. 6	Diarrhea
16	Rochester, N.Y.	Aug. 17	Sept. 11	Diarrhea and suspected typhoid
17	Cincinnati, Ohio	Aug. 25	Sept. 2	Typhoid fever
18	Wilkes-Barre, Pa.	Aug. 25	Sept. 13	Typhoid fever
19	Boston, Mass.	Aug. 26	Sept. 13	Typhoid fever
20	St. Louis, Mo.	Aug. 27	Sept. 6	High fever
21	Wilkes-Barre, Pa.	Aug. 19	Sept. 13	Rheumatism
22	Chicago, Ill.	Aug. 23	Sept. 13	Diarrhea and high fever
23	Chicago, Ill.	Aug. 25	Sept. 13	Diarrhea and high fever

Typhoid Investigation Commission

A team of medical officers, consisting of Major Walter Reed, Major Victor C. Vaughan, and Major Edward O. Shakespeare, was appointed by the Secretary of War on August 18, 1898, to investigate the cause of the prevalence of typhoid fever in the various military camps within the United States. Before it could begin compiling statistical data, the typhoid investigation commission had to determine the minimum period of incubation in typhoid fever.

The arrival of 50 trained women nurses from Chicago at Camp Thomas soon enabled the commission to obtain the desired information. The commissioners assumed that all the new arrivals were free from typhoid infection when they began their hospital work. They watched each nurse carefully, and when the first nurse came down with typhoid fever 10 days after her arrival, they concluded that the minimum period of incubation in typhoid fever was something less than 10 days. This finding was later confirmed repeatedly. Afterwards Vaughan wrote: "Of course with our present knowledge we would have vaccinated these girls and the probabilities are that all would have escaped the disease" [16].

The commission later concluded that, had a conscious effort been made to demonstrate the epidemiology of typhoid fever, it could hardly have been better staged than at Camp Thomas.

At first there were practically no trained nurses or hospital orderlies, either males or females. Before us every morning regiments were drawn up and so many men detailed from the ranks to serve in the hospitals as orderlies for the day. We followed these men to the hospitals and saw them handling bed pans in the awkward, ignorant way, often soiling their hands as well as the bedding, floors and the ground. At noon they went to lunch mostly without washing their hands, to say nothing of disinfecting them, handling their food, and passing it to their comrades. A like demonstration was repeated at supper. The next day a repetition of this cycle was re-enacted [17].

The 20,926 cases of typhoid in the Army during the Spanish-American War were precipitated by contaminated water supplies, infected food, and germ-carrying flies. The typical clinical picture was a disease of gradual onset, with vague anorexia and lassitude, low-grade headache, gastrointestinal upset, and pyrexia. Common specific symptoms, in order of frequency, were abdominal

Nurses with convalescent soldiers at Camp Thomas, Chickamauga Park, Georgia.

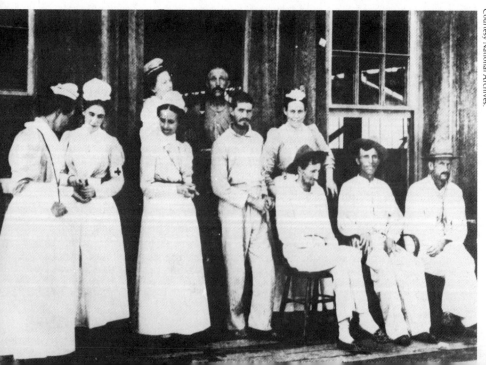

Courtesy National Archives.

discomfort, joint and back pains, diarrhea without blood, slight cough, and vomiting. Good nursing was absolutely essential, for the patients needed much rest, care of the skin and mouth, physiotherapy, and, most important, adequate fluid intake with a high-protein, low-roughage diet.

Observers quickly realized that the desperately ill soldiers, many of whom were also homesick, were acutely aware of how superior trained women nurses were to untrained male nurses. Under such circumstances the trained woman nurse was greeted as an angel of mercy in camp, on board ship, and in the hospital.

Adventures on a Hospital Ship

Realizing that military operations in Cuba would necessitate the evacuation of the sick and wounded by sea, the Surgeon General urged the fitting out of a hospital ship. The steamer *John Englis* was purchased on May 18, 1898, and rechristened the U.S.S. *Relief*. This ship was supplied with the more important medicines and dressings, along with enough equipment to outfit a 750-bed hospital for six months.

Esther V. Hasson of New London, Connecticut, who later became the first Superintendent of the Navy Nurse Corps, recalled that she experienced one of the greatest thrills of her life when she received a letter from Dr. McGee asking her to accept an assignment for surgical work aboard the *Relief*. A recent graduate of training school, she longed for something more exciting than private duty nursing. "Therefore, with youth and enthusiasm sufficient to counteract the rather depressing prospect of $30 per month [and] one ration in kind, I started out on the Great Adventure," she wrote [18].

It was July 3 before the *Relief* steamed out of Tampa harbor. The six women nurses aboard were immensely proud of their ship—beautiful in her fresh coat of white paint, with the green stripe of the Medical Corps encircling her hull, and flying the Stars and Stripes and the Red Cross flag. The space allotted to the hospital, on two of the upper decks, was divided into three large wards and one small ward of 30 beds, intended for officers but frequently used for overflow from the larger wards. The operating room directly to the right of the gangway was outfitted with the usual up-to-date equipment. Its crowning glory was the large x-ray machine lent by the Medical Museum in Washington.

Amidships, over the engine room, was a large pantry where the patients' food was served on trays carried to them by the hospital corpsmen. There were quarters in different parts of the ship for the medical officers, nurses, ship's officers, corpsmen, and crew. The six nurses occupied three small staterooms amidships, two in each room, on the upper of the two decks allotted to the hospital. Miss Hasson thought that it was "wonderful how much we managed to stow away in the two large drawers under the lower berths and in the tiny closet lockers in the hallway, or to use ship's language, gangway" [19].

"We made all possible speed to Cuba and upon arrival at Siboney, the hos-

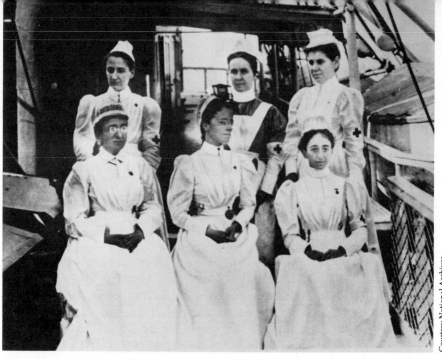

Esther Hasson and five of her nurses on board the hospital ship Relief *at Siboney, Cuba.*

Nurse and hospital corpsmen on Ward 3 of the U.S.S. Relief.

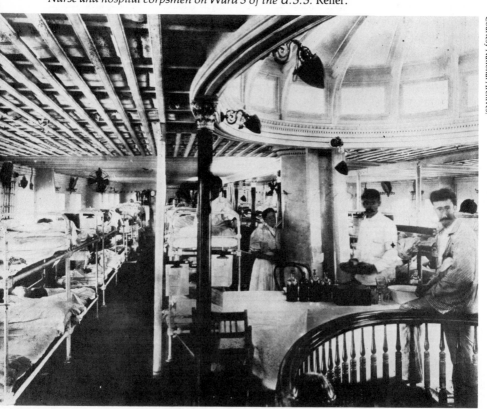

pital base of our army, were thrilled by the news of the naval battle [of Santiago Bay], which had taken place while we were at sea," related Miss Hasson[20]. On the morning of July 3 the Spanish squadron had steamed out of Santiago Bay, where they had been bottled up by the American fleet, and had turned sharply westward in a daring effort to escape. Since the commanders of all the American warships had specific orders concerning just such an escape attempt, they closed in upon the enemy vessels and forced them to hold their course near the shore, where maneuver was impossible. The *Brooklyn, Oregon,* and *Texas* were in the lead, and at the end of a 43-mile chase they had either destroyed or run aground the four enemy cruisers. The Spanish lost 323 killed and 151 wounded in this battle, while American casualties were only one killed and one wounded. Although battle losses were small, the rapidly deteriorating sanitary conditions were taking a toll. Yellow fever had broken out; malaria, typhoid, and dysentery were spreading. Hospital equipment and nourishment for the sick were in short supply, and incessant rain enveloped the nurses in seemingly endless vapor baths.

The *Relief* nurses began admitting patients at once. For several days thereafter, boatloads of wounded, sick, and exhausted soldiers were taken on board. Many had not removed their uniforms for days, and, since they had been too sick to care for themselves, they were in pitiful condition. After a bath, a clean bed, and sufficient nourishment, many regained enough strength to be shipped north on transports. Those who were in urgent need of medical or surgical attention remained on the hospital ship. During the two months from July 15 to September 15, 1898, the nurses aboard the *Relief* cared for 1234 sick, of whom 49 died, and for 251 wounded, of whom 16 died.

One old infantry sergeant whom Miss Hasson could never forget had been paralyzed from the neck down as a result of a gunshot wound in the head. In this condition he had lain in his wet uniform on a stretcher for several days. On his back was a bedsore that, to Miss Hasson's startled eyes, looked as big as a dinner plate, and there were others on his elbows and knees. He seldom spoke, and although he could not turn his head, his piercing gray eyes seemed to follow her everywhere. It was hoped that an operation might partially restore his physical capacities, but she never learned the outcome, for Miss Hasson lost track of him after he had been transferred to a hospital in New York.

On to Cuba

Meanwhile, the destruction of the Spanish naval squadron had completely demoralized the beleaguered Santiago garrison, which, unable to secure reinforcements, had no choice but to capitulate. After two weeks of negotiations, General William R. Shafter accepted the unconditional surrender of the Spanish forces on July 17. It occurred at an opportune moment, inasmuch as the American expeditionary was itself threatened with extermination by yellow fever, malaria, dysentery, and food poisoning. Ten days after the Spanish had surrendered, more than 4000 of Shafter's men were reported sick, and within a few more days Colonel Theodore Roosevelt stated that not even 10 percent of the men in his regiment were fit for active duty.

Physicians still had much to learn about the detection of yellow fever, malaria, and typhoid—the scourges that afflicted the Army in 1898. Secretary of War Russell Alger told General Shafter, on July 13 and 14, to begin shifting camps and quarantining yellow fever suspects. When new yellow fever cases quit developing among the regiment, Alger said, the troops could be shipped back to the United States. Alger did not anticipate an early return of the Army, which he thought should remain at Santiago "until the fever has had its run" [21].

In response to urgent pleas from Shafter, the War Department dispatched 65 physicians, 729 women nurses, and a large quantity of medical stores to Santiago. Among this contingent of nurses was Lillian Kratz from St. Louis, who described her arrival in Cuba as follows:

So under order, we embarked from New York Harbor, across the Atlantic, and steamed into Santiago Harbor, our battleship proud and defiant as we passed the fleet of battleships, dotted here and there in close proximity in the harbor. As we neared our destination, I think our brave hearts fluttered a bit at the great uncertainty that awaited all of us. When we anchored and got foot ashore, the sun was just sinking to rest, and on board of one of the battleships, we could hear the familiar strains of the Star Spangled Banner, and My Country 'Tis of Thee. To the right of us was the desolate battlefield, and as the sun gradually sank behind the horizon, casting the reflection of its rays in purple and gold on San Juan hill where our dead and dying still lay, and as the sun's glow became fainter and fainter, it seemed to cast a benediction over all, it seemed to say, "God be with you and with thy spirit—peace be to thy soul." And so we landed with this sombre setting on one side, while on the left we could see the huge palm trees [22].

Fighting Yellow Fever

Anna Turner, a nurse from New York City, was asked by some of her friends in the United States to describe the symptoms and treatment of the yellow fever victims for whom she was caring. She told them that the patients first complained of a severe aching of the whole body, much the same as in other acute diseases, but that the nausea and vomiting were much more pronounced. The patients' temperature, which did not run as high as in typhoid, rarely exceeded 104°. As it rose, the pulse usually became slower—another symptom that one looked for when making a diagnosis. Because of their intense suffering, the men afflicted with yellow fever were always very restless and rolled from one side to the other. In many cases it was necessary to put boards on the sides of their beds to prevent them from falling out.

The extreme nausea and vomiting continued until the crisis was past, a period of six or eight days. Hemorrhage was nearly always present, the most common form being the bleeding of the gums. Next came that of the stomach, which caused the "black vomit" so often referred to. Miss Turner had seen two cases of hemorrhage from the kidneys and a few in which the veins of the surface of the body ruptured and formed great knots under the skin. The kidneys were

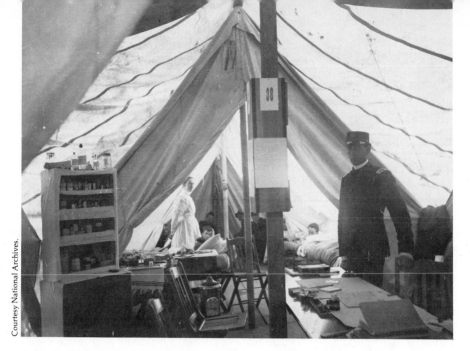

Yellow fever patients needed expert nursing care.

always affected, and the urine was loaded with albumin. The patients were always constipated and usually had jaundice. The fever also caused a distinctive odor found in no other disease. Since the Cubans never seemed to contract the disease, nearly all Miss Turner's patients were either Spaniards or Americans.

The general care was much the same as for other acute diseases. Because of the supposed contagion, all patients received a daily soap-and-water bath and a complete change of linen. Cold sponges were applied to reduce the high temperature and restlessness. The patients' mouths had to be cleansed thoroughly and frequently, due to the constant bleeding of the gums. Because they were unable to take or retain medicine, patients received two enemas of plain faucet water daily. No nourishment of any kind was given until all nausea and vomiting had ceased, a period of about one week. But due to the condition of the kidneys and the large amount of albumin present in the urine, water was forced day and night, regardless of the nausea and vomiting.

The quantity of water given to a patient was carefully gauged and recorded, as was the character and quantity of his vomitus. His urine was measured and saved for 24 hours. A rack of test tubes was kept on the stand for each patient. Every morning the oldest tube was removed from the rack and replaced by a new one containing a specimen from the previous 24-hour period. This latest specimen was boiled while the doctor was making rounds so that, after comparing it with the other tubes, he could note the increase or decrease in albumin. According to Miss Turner, some specimens were nearly solid after being boiled.

When the patients could safely ingest food, the nurses began by giving them milk, two drams every six hours. If there were no digestive disturbances, the quantity was slowly increased until the patients received four ounces every three hours. Then a dose of castor oil was administered. When they had recovered from its effects, they were ready for solid food. At first, when there were only a few patients on the hospital wards, Miss Turner cooked meals in addition to her other duties in the wards.

Three different buildings were used as wards: one for suspected cases of yellow fever, one for acute cases, and the third for convalescents. The extremely ill and dying patients had to be shifted constantly in order to keep them isolated. Because the orderlies were so expert in moving patients easily and quickly, the nurses going off duty were required to report the new location of the various patients. The nurses had 12-hour duty, which usually stretched into almost 13 hours, for, in addition to all their other work, they had to keep their charts in order. Every morning the night nurse had to total all the fluids taken in and excreted by the patients during the last 24 hours. Miss Turner then recorded these figures on charts.

Later, when a camp was established a few miles from the city of Havana for the study of yellow fever, Miss Turner was involved in the first experiments to prove or disprove that yellow fever was a contagious disease. The nurses were asked to put aside the sheets and pillow cases taken from the beds of their worst cases, and these were put on beds in screened tents. Uninfected men who had volunteered for the purpose were assigned to sleep in these tents. When no cases developed during a period of several weeks, it was proved that yellow fever was not contagious.

It was then decided to test the theory of Dr. Carlos Finley of Havana, who maintained that the disease was carried by a certain species of mosquito. The physicians came to the hospitals daily, armed with test tubes containing swarms of the suspected carriers. These were allowed to bite infected patients and then carefully released to bite uninfected volunteers, who shortly thereafter contracted the disease. These tests proved that yellow fever was a mosquito-borne disease transmitted by only one kind of mosquito. They also established the incubation period during which a mosquito that had bitten a yellow fever patient could transmit the infection to another man: mosquitoes that bit fevered patients after the third or fourth day of the patients' illness were no longer capable of carrying the infection. Upon this discovery new cases of yellow fever were soon kept in screened cages inside well-screened wards until the period of infection was over.

During these experiments nurses displayed a heroism and devotion to duty equal to that of any soldier or sailor in battle. Among these courageous nurses, the example set by 25-year old Clara Louise Maass of East Orange, New Jersey, deserves special mention. Moved by the suffering of her yellow fever patients and aware that scientific knowledge about the disease was pitifully inadequate, she volunteered to be bitten by a carrier mosquito in order to increase this knowledge. She was bitten on the hand, and when the subsequent attack of yellow fever was not considered sufficiently immunizing, she was bitten several more times. A martyr to science, she perished from these infections but helped prove that yellow fever was carried by mosquitoes.

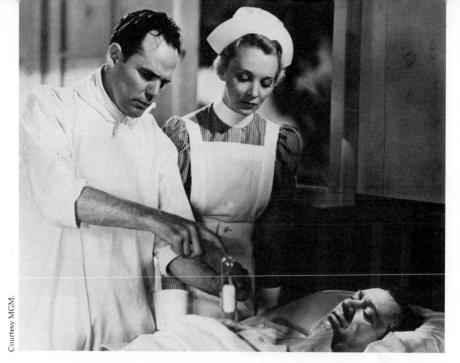

Battling yellow fever in Cuba. (From the MGM release Yellow Jack © *1938 Loew's Incorporated. Copyright renewed 1965 by Metro-Goldwyn-Mayer Inc.)*

Disease Drives the Army Home

Meanwhile, by August 1, the soldiers of the American expeditionary force were suffering more from disease than from Spanish bullets. Few precautions had been taken to safeguard the health of the men because the Medical Corps knew little about tropical diseases and because no effective measures had yet been developed to combat malaria and yellow fever. Theodore Roosevelt described the situation as

. . . horrible in every respect. I have over 100 men down with fever in my own camp out of my regiment of 400, 200 having previously died or having been sent to the rear hospitals. The mismanagement of the hospital's service in the rear has been such that my men will not leave the regiment if they can possibly help it; yet here we have nothing for them but hardtack, bacon, and . . . coffee without sugar [23].

On August 3, 1898, a group of volunteer officers of the V Corps assembled and drafted a round-robin letter describing the wretched plight of the Army. After this letter had been circulated and signed by all the divisional and brigade commanders, it was sent to General William R. Shafter, who forwarded it to Washington. Even before this document had reached Shafter, however, it had been leaked to the press, thanks largely to Theodore Roosevelt, now a brigade commander, who had been instrumental in composing it. The substance of this message was "This army must be moved at once or it will perish" [24]. Secretary of War Alger, who on the previous day had wired Shafter that there would be a considerable delay in moving troops from Cuba, quickly changed his mind on receipt of this news and ordered the immediate evacuation of the

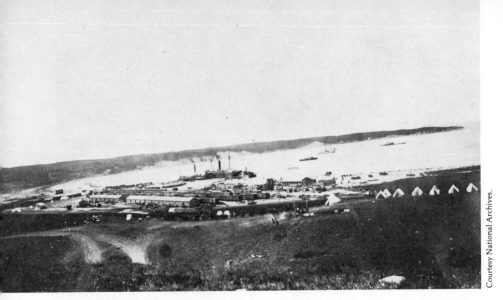

View of Camp Wikoff, late August, 1898.

expeditionary force to Montauk Point, Long Island. The first shipload of troops left Santiago on August 7, fleeing from the scene of their triumph as if the enemy were pursuing them.

On Surgeon General Sternberg's recommendation, Secretary Alger had selected 5000 acres of rolling ground at Montauk Point, on the eastern tip of Long Island, as the expedition's rest and recuperation camp. Christened Camp Wikoff, it was remote enough for effective quarantine, and troops arriving from Santiago could disembark there without passing through any of the port cities. When completed, the installation comprised a detention camp, where newly arrived regiments were to be quarantined until proved free of yellow fever, and a larger general camp, where the troops were to rest and recover their strength. Each camp was to have a large hospital.

When the regiments from Santiago began disembarking on August 14, four-fifths of the soldiers were ill and more than 10,000 required hospitalization. Most of the others were so enfeebled that they resembled walking scarecrows. Eighty-seven men had died aboard the transport ships, and about 200 more died after reaching the camp. Because the exhausted soldiers found no facilities ready for them, they were forced to sleep on the ground in tents without bedding. Sometimes they subsisted for days on short rations. In the half-completed, understaffed hospitals, sick men went untended for 24 hours at a time. Surgeon General Sternberg quickly authorized his subordinates at Wikoff to hire extra doctors and nurses without first having to send their requisitions to Washington for his approval.

Nightmare on a Long Island Beach

As a result of this poor preparation and lack of trained personnel, chaos reigned at Camp Wikoff. Nurse Kate M. Walsh reported that her white clothing was not suitable because there were no laundry facilities. According to her, the nurses should have worn canvas frocks. In two days she was "filthy-looking and distressed." The patients' beds, placed only a foot apart, had springs of wire mesh that protruded from all sides and tore the nurses' clothes to ribbons. Miss Walsh further stated that nurses "kept getting sick and some had to be sent away, some dying." One "convenience hut" was without a door for some time. Nurses fainted in this place and had to be carried away [25].

Miss Walsh confided that each night she felt that she could not stand another day: "The heat was intense and I perspired freely from long hours of overwork, heat and flies, together with my anguish that our dear sick men were not half cared for" [26]. In an attempt to relieve their overcrowded wards, surgeons at Montauk released hundreds of men prematurely, and sick, sometimes dying stragglers from Camp Wikoff collapsed in passenger cars and railroad stations across Long Island.

After this wretched beginning, conditions at Montauk slowly improved. The Medical Department enlarged its hospital facilities and brought in scores of contract surgeons along with about 300 women nurses. Numerous newspaper articles described the miserable conditions at the camp and mentioned the positive impact of women nurses on patient care. For example, a correspondent for *Harper's Weekly* wrote: "There is no exaggeration in the current stories of the starvation and utter neglect of these, our returning heroes." He further reported:

I saw the Eighth (regulars) arrive at their camp. They came from the detention camp in army wagons. When the wagons stopped, many of the men fell headlong in attempting to get down, and lay just where they fell. One, a bugler, stood a little while, swaying and dazed, and then fell in a heap by the roadside . . . . It remains only to say a word of appreciation of the self-sacrificing Red Cross nurses and Sisters of Charity, who are working night and day in the hospitals, and to hope and pray that the like of the shameful spectable of those poor famished lads gathered together after all their glory of achievement may never be witnessed in this country again [27].

Each ward in the camp hospitals consisted of seven-section tents, with board floors, placed end to end. Very soon there were 40 wards. Each ward was supposed to have four nurses and two orderlies on duty during the day and two nurses and two orderlies at night. Between the wards ran a boardwalk with kitchen and dining sheds at one end, where a large number of nurses, orderlies, and clergymen came for their meals.

At midnight a lunch was served for the night nurses, who took turns in going to the dining shed. Carrying lanterns, they would "follow along the boardwalk and watch the other lanterns flickering in the darkness, some coming, some going, and then in the none too well lighted shed we would eat our midnight meal." Miss Mary A. Quinn reported that her experience seemed a kind of dream, imaged by "the stream of faces coming in suddenly from the black night, the hurried meal, and the return to the darkness" [28].

By September 15 there were 281 nurses on duty at Camp Wikoff. There were at this time 43 hospital tents, each designed to hold 30 cots but often containing 50 patients. Surgeons soon transferred over 1000 of the camp's sick to hospitals in New York, Boston, Philadelphia, Providence, and other Northeastern cities. The shelter and care afforded to patients who remained at Montauk improved significantly. They were discharged as soon as possible, and by the end of October, 1898, the former hospital sites at Montauk Point had reverted to empty sand dunes. Despite reassuring statements from authorities that everything possible had been done, thousands of citizens who had visited or read about Camp Wikoff formed the unshakable conviction that the soldiers who had risked all for their country had been betrayed by the government.

A Government Investigation

On August 12, 1898, the Spaniards signed an armistice that brought the Spanish-American War to an end. During the calendar year May, 1898, through April, 1899, the Army suffered 968 battle casualties and 5438 deaths from disease. In stark contrast to the Civil War, in which 18 percent had fallen in battle, 15 percent had died of wounds, and 67 percent had died of disease, the Spanish-American War saw 10 percent slain in combat, 2 percent dead of wounds, and 88 percent killed by disease. These statistics provoked heavy criticism of the Medical Department.

On September 8, 1898, President McKinley, at the request of the Secretary of War, appointed a commission to investigate the conduct of the War Department during the War with Spain. This commission, headed by Grenville Dodge, held 109 meetings and heard a vast amount of testimony concerning the work of female nurses.

The Dodge Commission published the following conclusions and recommendations in regard to Army nursing: during the months of May, June, and July, the nursing force "was neither ample nor efficient, reasons for which may be found in the lack of proper volunteer hospital corps, due to the failure of Congress to authorize its establishment, and to the nonrecognition in the beginning of the value of women nurses and the extent to which their services could be secured." What was needed by the Medical Department in the future was a corps of selected trained women nurses "ready to serve when necessity shall arise, but, under ordinary circumstances, owing no duty to the War Department, except to report residence at determined intervals" [29].

The number of women Army nurses had reached a maximum of 1158 on September 15, 1898. After this date many nursing contracts were annulled, for the suppression of the typhoid epidemic and the mustering out of volunteer regiments rendered so large a nursing force unnecessary. Between the first appointments on May 10 and the close of 1898, the total number of contracted women nurses was 1563. They had worked on three ships and at 42 places, nine of the locations being camps that had contained several hospitals each.

Unwanted Women Army Nurses

The position of women nurses in the Army was precarious, however, as was indicated by a letter from Major L. M. Maus, Surgeon and commander of the U.S. Hospital at Fort Hamilton, New York, to Surgeon General Sternberg, dated June 3, 1899:

Should we expect to restore the Hospital Corps to that grade of efficiency that existed previous to the Spanish-American War, the employment of female nurses must be discontinued. As a result of the present state of affairs, the hospital private takes no interest in his duties as a nurse, nor can he be expected to, so long as he is brought in contact with the female nurse. There is a decided tendency on the part of the latter to ignore entirely the hospital corpsman's ability to care for his sick comrade, and to put him aside except for the menial duties of the ward.

Divested of any responsibility in the way of taking temperature, attending the serious cases, administering medicine, dressing wounds, etc., the private soon becomes a willing party to the arrangement, and hence his utter worthlessness as a nurse in the course of a very short time. It is practically impossible to divide the ward work equally between nurses so radically different in class. I also find it difficult to preserve good military discipline with this mixed personnel [30].

Especially severe was Major Maus' indictment against women nurses for "coddling" their patients:

The "coddling process," which is characteristic of the female nurse in caring for male patients, has become more accentuated in her treatment of the sick soldier, through some maudlin sentiment; as a consequence, I find that many men apply for treatment, who under normal conditions would never think of going to the hospital [31].

As a result of such hostile attitudes on the part of the military authorities, there were only 202 women nurses in Army service by July 1, 1899.

Movement to Establish an Army Nurse Corps

As early as December, 1898, a committee of influential women, many of whom were prominent nurses, advocated passage of legislation to establish a permanent Army Nurse Corps. Mrs. Winthrop Cowdin was the first chairman of this "Committee to Secure by Act of Congress the Employment of Women Nurses in the Hospital Service of the United States Army." Mrs. Whitelaw Reid, wife of the editor of the *New York Tribune,* contributed $500 in support of this movement, while others donated smaller sums. With the aid of these funds the committee was able to recruit a sizeable working force in Washington, D.C., secure able counsel, and open offices in both New York and Washington.

Adelaide Nutting, Principal of Johns Hopkins Training School for Nurses, was charged with informing the nursing groups of the importance of the proposed reform. A bill providing for the establishment of a permanent Army Nurse Corps was introduced into the House of Representatives on January 24 by Congressman Michael Griffin of Wisconsin. On January 25 it was presented to the Senate by Senator Julius C. Burrowes of Michigan and referred by each body to its Committee on Military Affairs.

A delegation of the bill's supporters appeared before the House Military Affairs Committee on February 3, 1899. The bill's virtues were outlined in detail by Margaret Chanler, a wealthy young aristocrat of the Astor family, who had been selected as speaker because of her "heroic service last summer" during the war with Spain. She was accompanied by Mrs. Bayard Cutting and Mrs. Winthrop Cowdin, "both exquisitely gowned," according to the report [32].

On the same day, at the Washington home of Mrs. John McLean, the wives of some senators and representatives held a meeting at which the nursing committee explained the full purpose of the bill. The lively discussion that ensued indicated that the nurses had many warm supporters among those present. The bill, reported on favorably by the Military Affairs Committee that same day, came before the House the following Monday, February 6. Although it passed by 40 votes, it lacked the full two-thirds majority necessary for it to be removed from the calendar. When the measure came before the Senate Committee on Military Affairs, it fell only one vote short of gaining approval.

In the belief that military medicine would derive much greater benefit from the services of graduate nurses than from those of the nonprofessional Hospital Corps, nursing leaders continued unrelentingly to agitate for a permanent Nurse Corps. Despite adverse opinions from several of his ranking officers, the once-reluctant Surgeon General finally accepted the idea of women nurses as a permanent component of the Medical Department.

Since there were already plans for a reorganization of the Army, Sternberg assigned Dr. Anita McGee the task of drafting a proposal for creating the Army Nurse Corps. This proposal, presented to Congress as part of a bill for a general Army reorganization, was written in the War Department and received the approval of both the Surgeon General and the Secretary of War. Before this bill was passed, the Senate added an amendment that the Superintendent of the Nurse Corps had to be a hospital school graduate. Since Dr. McGee was not, she was forced to resign from the Army when the Army Nurse Corps was established on February 2, 1901. Dita H. Kinney, Head Nurse of the United States Army Hospital at Fort Bayard, New Mexico, was appointed to succeed her as the Superintendent of the Army Nurse Corps.

The Navy Nurse Corps Is Born

During this time Surgeon General Presley M. Rixey of the Navy also became convinced that women nurses were by natural endowment and special aptitude superior to male nurses for much of the duty required in the care of sick and injured men. He was sure that their use would not conflict with the conditions arising from service in naval installations. Of course, the women nurses would have no place at sea except on hospital ships. But in the naval hospitals, where nine-tenths of the serious cases were treated, their exceptional capabilities for work in hospital wards and operating rooms made their services most desirable.

Trained Nurse, February, 1901.

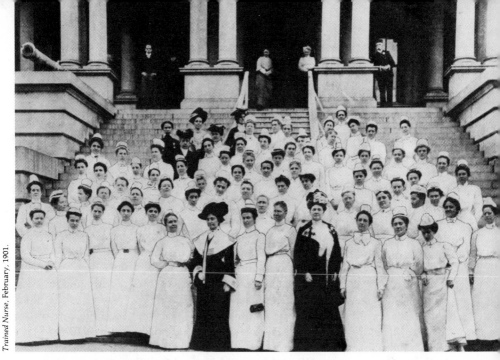

Dr. McGee (in dark coat, front row, left) and a group of Spanish-American War nurses on the steps of the War Department in Washington, D.C.

"The Sacred Twenty," the initial 20 members of the Navy Nurse Corps in 1908. Esther Hasson, the superintendent, stands in the front row, center.

Courtesy National Archives.

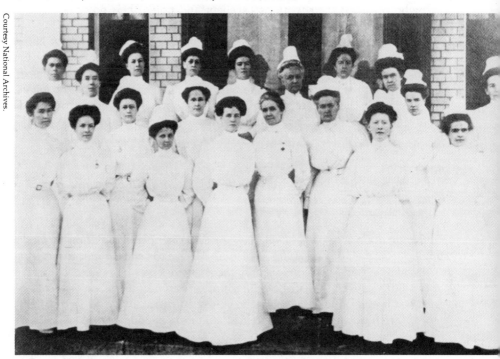

Congress was slow to act on the matter, and in his report for 1907 Surgeon General Rixey stated that he could not understand why it was so difficult to obtain Congressional approval for such a worthy measure. He recalled that the desirability of using trained women nurses in the medical branch of the naval service had been urged upon Congress for five years. The lack of female nurses was the most serious omission in the Medical Bureau.

His efforts finally bore fruit in 1908, when the Nurse Corps was established as an integral unit of the Navy. The first group of nurses assigned to the Naval Medical School Hospital in Washington, D.C., consisted of a superintendent, a chief nurse, and 18 staff nurses. Since the Navy did not provide quarters for these nurses, they had to rent a house and cook their own meals.

Esther Hasson was appointed the first superintendent of the Corps and served for three years. During her tenure the nurses proved their worth, and an additional 24 nurses were appointed. Early in 1909 nurses were sent to the naval hospitals in Annapolis and Brooklyn. Soon they were receiving orders for duty at Mare Island, California, and other naval hospitals. In 1910 the Navy sent its first nurses to the Philippines, and soon afterwards to Guam, Honolulu, Yokohama, Samoa, the Virgin Islands, Haiti, and Guantanamo Bay, Cuba.

As the only women in the Navy, the nurses were a unique group. By Congressional order they were designated as neither officers nor enlisted men, but they had military, as distinguished from civilian, status. Despite their nebulous rank, the nurses of the Navy earned the unqualified praise of the Surgeon General, who regarded their work as excellent and noted their positive effect in improving the level of nursing service in naval hospitals.

The official establishment of the Army Nurse Corps and the Navy Nurse Corps represented an important step in the professionalization of nursing. For the first time, two large nursing services were staffed entirely by graduate nurses. Student nurses, who represented the bulk of the work force in civil hospitals, had no place in this structure. Thus the military nursing services provided an opportunity for a unique demonstration in patient care.

Summary

The Spanish-American War led to wide-scale utilization of trained nurses in military hospitals and resulted in the emergence of the nation's first large, all-graduate nursing service.

The National Society of the Daughters of the American Revolution formed a committee headed by Dr. Anita Newcomb McGee to screen applications from nurses who wished to be employed by the Army as contract nurses. The applicants selected were graduates of either nurse training schools or medical colleges, had previous hospital experience, were between 30 and 50 years of age, were able to furnish character references, and were in good health.

Sanitary conditions in military camps, most of which lacked adequate garbage and sewage disposal systems, were exceedingly poor. Outbreaks of typhoid accounted for a high percentage of the sickness in military camps. Other prevalent diseases were malaria, dysentery, and diarrhea.

The number of untrained male nurses of the Hospital Corps rose from 723 to 6000. But since even more were sorely needed, unqualified infantrymen were often assigned ward duty, a practice that resulted in poor care and the spread of more disease.

Due to a virulent epidemic of typhoid fever, which struck more than 20,000 soldiers during the summer of 1898, Surgeon General Sternberg was forced to use women nurses much more extensively.

Primitive nursing conditions prevailed in the unfinished, shoddily constructed camp hospitals. Moreover, these poorly lighted, inadequately ventilated structures lacked sufficient space.

Many nurses contracted typhoid and other diseases and had to be transferred to hospitals in more favorable climates or sent home after having their contracts with the Army annulled.

The Army hospital ship U.S.S. Relief was staffed by six women nurses who cared for hundreds of sick and wounded soldiers being evacuated from Cuba.

The American expeditionary force, which suffered many more casualties from disease than in combat, was severely stricken by yellow fever, malaria, and dysentery, which necessitated the dispatch of several hundred women nurses to Cuba.

During an investigation to determine the cause and mode of transmission of yellow fever, specimens from patients so affected were analyzed daily, and symptoms indicating the progression of the disease were carefully observed. Three buildings were erected to isolate suspected cases of yellow fever from the acute and convalescent patients. Later, experiments conducted by Dr. Walter Reed and others demonstrated that the disease was not contagious but was transmitted by mosquitoes. Nurse Clara Maass gave her life as one of the study subjects.

American troops from Cuba were disembarked at Camp Wikoff on Montauk Point, Long Island, in order to identify soldiers who were carriers of disease and to care for these men in hastily erected isolation hospitals.

Four-fifths of the soldiers who arrived at Camp Wikoff, beginning August 14, 1898, were ill. By September 15, 1898, 281 trained nurses were serving in 43 hospital tents.

On September 8, 1898, the Dodge Commission was appointed to investigate the conduct of the War Department during the War with Spain. It found that the Army nursing force had been inadequate during the war because Congress had failed to authorize the establishment of a proper volunteer hospital corps and because the value of women nurses had not been sufficiently recognized.

The Commission therefore recommended the establishment of a corps of selected, trained women nurses.

As early as December, 1898, a group of influential women began advocating legislation to create a permanent Army Nurse Corps. Such a corps, headed by Dita H. Kinney, was finally established on February 2, 1901.

In 1908 the Navy Nurse Corps was established as an integral unit of the Navy, and the first 20 members began work at the Naval Hospital in Washington, D.C.

References

1. Unidentified newspaper clipping, May 17, 1898, National Archives, McGee Papers, RG 112.
2. Daughters of the American Revolution, *Second Report of the National Society of the Daughters of the American Revolution, October 11, 1897–October 11, 1898* (Washington, D.C.: Government Printing Office, 1900), Senate Document No. 425.
3. Application blank to applicants interested in nursing in the Army, National Archives, McGee Papers, RG 112.
4. Sternberg to Alger, May 3, 1898, National Archives, McGee Papers, RG 112.
5. V. C. Vaughan, *A Doctor's Memories* (Indianapolis: Bobbs-Merrill, 1926), pp. 385–386.
6. Bayne to McGee, July 10, 1898, National Archives, McGee Papers, RG 112.
7. A. C. Maxwell, "The Field Hospital at Chickamauga Park," *Trained Nurse and Hospital Review*, vol. 23 (July, 1899):3.
8. H. C. Lounsbery, "Some Reminiscences of Sternberg Hospital," *American Journal of Nursing*, vol. 3 (November, 1902):83.
9. J. S. Edmunds, *Leaves from a Nurse's Life's History, 1906*, manuscript in National Archives, McGee Papers, RG 112.
10. *Ibid.*
11. Helen B. Schuler and Florence M. Kelly, "Reminiscences," manuscript in National Archives, McGee Papers, RG 112.
12. Carter to McGee, August 19, 1898, National Archives, McGee Papers, RG 112.
13. Barbara U. Austin, "Conditions at Sternberg Hospital, Chickamauga, Georgia," undated manuscript in National Archives, McGee Papers RG 112.
14. Jane R. Riley, "Sternberg Hospital," undated manuscript in National Archives, McGee Papers, RG 112.
15. U.S. War Department, Typhoid Commission *Report (of board) on Origin and Spread of Typhoid Fever in the U.S. Military Camps during the Spanish War of 1898; by Walter Reed, Victor C. Vaughan, and Edward O. Shakespeare* (Washington, D.C.: Government Printing Office, 1904), vol. 1, p. 283.
16. Vaughan, *op. cit.*, pp. 386–387.
17. *Ibid.*, p. 385.
18. E. V. Hasson, "The First Trip of the Army Hospital Ship *Relief*," undated manuscript in National Archives, McGee Papers, RG 112.
19. *Ibid.*
20. *Ibid.*
21. War Investigation Commission, *Report of the Commission Appointed by the President to Investigate the Conduct of War Department in War with Spain* (Washington, D.C.: Government Printing Office, 1899), vol. 3, pp. 26–29.
22. L. Kratz, "Reminiscences of Santiago," undated manuscript in National Archives, McGee Papers, RG 112.

23. Henry Cabot Lodge, ed., *Selections from the Correspondence of Theodore Roosevelt and Henry Cabot Lodge, 1884–1918* (New York: Scribner's Sons, 1925), vol. 1, pp. 325–329, 331–334.
24. Russell A. Alger, *The Spanish-American War* (New York: Harper and Brothers, 1901), pp. 265–273.
25. K. M. Walsh, "Camp Wikoff, Montauk Point," undated manuscript in National Archives, McGee Papers, RG 112.
26. *Ibid.*
27. W. A. Rogers, "Camp Wikoff," *Harper's Weekly*, vol. 42 (September 10, 1898):890.
28. M. A. Quinn, "Montauk Point," undated manuscript in National Archives, McGee Papers, RG 112.
29. War Investigating Commission, *op. cit.*, pp. 395–396.
30. Maus to Sternberg, June 3, 1899, copy in National Archives, McGee Papers, RG 112.
31. *Ibid.*
32. A. N. McGee, "The Army Nurse Corps in 1899," *Trained Nurse and Hospital Review*, vol. 24 (February, 1900):119.

8
The Rise of Public Health Nursing

*A*s the United States approached the twentieth century, one of its most exciting developments was the rise of its cities. Their phenomenal growth eclipsed even the giant strides being made in industrialization. It was, of course, the rise of industry that made city growth possible, along with transportation improvements that enabled business to become national. Every city had its elegant mansions, the homes of fastidiously dressed socialites. In New York they lined Fifth Avenue. In Chicago they occupied two districts, the North Side and the South Side. The splendor carried over to monumental public buildings, formidable-looking banks, spacious churches, and luxurious hotels. Yet in every city the poor greatly outnumbered the well-to-do. Their hovels stood within a few blocks of the great mansions.

The Influx of Immigrants
Meanwhile, during the nine decades from 1820 to 1910, nearly 30 million immigrants were admitted to the United States; of these, 91 percent came from Europe. Until 1883, about 95 percent of the movement from Europe originated in the United Kingdom, Germany, Scandinavia, France, Belgium, Holland, and Switzerland. Even as late as 1882, these countries furnished 87 percent of the total immigration from Europe. Twenty-five years later, in 1907, however, 81 percent of the immigrants came from Austria-Hungary, Italy, Russia, Greece, Turkey, Spain, Portugal, Serbia, Rumania, Bulgaria, and Montenegro. Thus, in less than one generation, the principal sources of immigration had shifted drastically, and with this shift came a host of new social, economic, and health problems.

In 1893 the foreign-born population in the city of Baltimore was 16 percent of the total; in the slum district it was 40 percent. In Chicago, the total foreign-born in the entire city area constituted 41 percent of the population, while in the slum district it was 58 percent. In New York, the foreign-born made up 42 percent of the total population and 63 percent of the inhabitants of slum districts. In Philadelphia, the foreign-born constituted 26 percent of the total and 60 percent of the slum dwellers. These figures showed conclusively that the proportion of foreign-born was much higher in the slums of each city than in the total population pool.

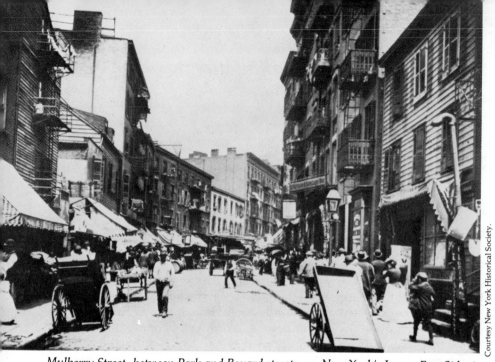

Mulberry Street, between Park and Bayard streets, on New York's Lower East Side, in the 1870s.

Mother and children on tenement house roof.

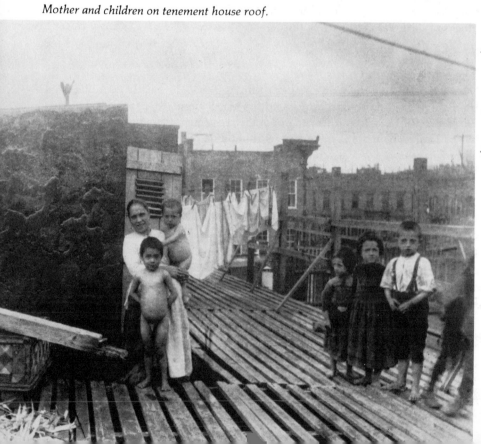

Of all the great cities, New York was perhaps the most intimately concerned with the problems of immigrants. By the late 1880s, foreigners from southern and eastern Europe had become a large element in the city's population. Italians had moved into the old Irish neighborhoods, driving out the earlier occupants. In 1890 Italians were found massed in the wards west of the Bowery. Russian and Polish Jews were packed to the east of the Bowery and were scattered up the east side of the city to Harlem. Hungarians, a considerable proportion of whom were Jews, were gathered in a large colony east of Avenue B, around Houston Street, and Bohemians centered on the Upper East Side, near the river, from about Fiftieth to Sixtieth streets.

The following is a description of New York's Italian colony in 1884:

In Jersey Street exist two courtyards. Six three-story houses are in each. These houses are old and long ago worn out. They are packed with tenants, rotten with age and decay, and so constructed as to have made them very undesirable for dwelling purposes [even] in their earliest infancy. The Italians who chiefly inhabit them are the scum of New York chiffoniers, and as such saturated with the filth inseparable from their business. The courtyard swarms with, in daytime, females in the picturesque attires of Genoa and Piedmont, moving between the dirty children. The abundant rags, paper, sacks, barrels, washtubs, dogs, and cats are all festooned overhead by clotheslines weighted with such garments as are only known in Italy. Sorting is chiefly done indoors, but at times a ragpicker may be seen at his work in any convenient spot to be had. In each yard live 24 families (nominally only, because lodgers here as elsewhere are always welcome), paying rents of from $6 to $9 monthly for two rooms, the inner one being subdivided by a partition consisting perhaps of a simple curtain, and measuring when so arranged about 5 by 6 feet each [1].

Tenement Houses

As space commanded more of a premium, tenement houses were constructed. An architectural design in 1879 had accelerated their erection and greatly contributed to the congestion. A New Yorker had devised a dumbbell-shaped floor plan that could pack an amazing number of occupants into a narrow six-story building. The "dumbbell" tenement soon became the standardized type. It was supposedly an improvement because an airshaft gave each room some slight exposure to the sun. Actually, by concentrating a minimum of 24 families in a six-story walk-up building on a narrow lot of 25 by 90 feet without any play yard, the dumbbell multiple dwelling, which sometimes housed as many as 36 families, made congestion, clutter, and dirt more acute.

The usefulness of the airshaft as a means of ventilation was subverted by its typical use as a garbage dump. It was said in the course of a tenement house investigation that, due to the rotting garbage, the airshaft could be called a "foul airshaft" or a "culture on a gigantic scale," and that it was simply a "stagnant well of foul air emptying into each of the rooms opening upon it." Many people testified that "the air from these shafts was so foul and the odor so vile that they had to close their windows opening into them, and in some cases the windows were permanently nailed up for this reason" [2].

By the mid-1890s about two-thirds of the 3,500,000 people living in New

York were packed into 90,000 tenement houses in districts without parks or recreation areas. In one New York block of tenements, 577 people were crowded into 96 rooms. In the Tenth Ward on Manhattan Island, the average population density was 747 people per acre. Boston developed its own characteristic form of "three-decker" wooden tenement. Slum colonies were found not only along the Eastern seaboard but also in interior cities like Cincinnati and Chicago. To make matters worse, immigrant families often converted their apartments into sweatshops, where garments or cigars were manufactured amid the most unsanitary conditions.

Such slums endangered health. In 1880 New York City, with a population of 1.2 million, had a death rate of more than 25 per thousand and an average of 16 people to a dwelling. London, a far larger city by comparison, with a population of 3.8 million, recorded a death rate of 21 per thousand and averaged fewer than eight persons to a dwelling. One especially crowded tract in New York had such a high death rate from tuberculosis that it was known as the "lung block." With vermin abundant and sanitary facilities inadequate and often out of order, diseases were inevitable. Any that were communicable had an excellent opportunity to spread, often with a strong likelihood of fatality. Slum dwellers were ravaged by epidemics of typhus, scarlet fever, smallpox, and typhoid fever, and many of them died or developed tuberculosis or other communicable diseases.

Establishment of Visiting Nursing

More than 20 years earlier, in Great Britain, the wife of William Rathbone, a wealthy citizen of Liverpool, died in 1859 after a long and painful illness. She had been attended during her illness by a very competent trained nurse, whose care had brought her great relief. Rathbone, a philanthropist, had long been interested in helping the Liverpool poor. He had concluded that if skilled nursing could do so much for his wife, who had already had everything that wealth could procure, how much more might it do for the poor, whose illnesses were aggravated by the misery of their surroundings. Rathbone was a man of action as well as of vision, and his kindly thoughts quickly crystallized into a concrete plan for helping the needy sick of Liverpool: nurses should be sent to their homes. To test the idea, Mary Robinson, the nurse who had attended his wife, was employed for a three-month term to visit the ailing poor of Liverpool.

Curiously enough, opposition to Rathbone's undertaking was based upon the very lack of comfort and the unsanitary conditions that were so often found in the homes of the poor. One contemporary physician had this to say about Rathbone's experiment:

It is evident that the essential conditions of rational and successful sick nursing such as good air, light, warmth, bedding, good food, etc., are altogether wanting in the homes of the poor. Of what use are the gratuitous supply and regular giving of medicines, if every necessity is wanting for ordinary healthy living? It is not that the nurse shrinks from the privations and injurious influences existing in the cottages and hovels, but it is the impossibility of being useful under such circumstances that renders home nursing unattainable for the poor. One can comfort them in their cottages, and give them food and medicine, but to nurse and heal them there with any prospect of success cannot be done [3].

The general belief was that home nursing for the poor was not practical. There were municipal and charity hospitals available for such care. If the poor were seriously ill, let them go to those hospitals.

Rathbone quickly countered such objections. He noted that many patients with serious illnesses were either unsuitable for or not admissable to a general hospital. Also, many sick persons objected to being taken to the hospital. Rathbone argued that "there are not enough and there never can be hospitals large enough and numerous enough to take in all cases of grave illness among the poor"; moreover, "the work done by district nursing is, in proportion to its results, far less costly than that done by the hospital". Rathbone's reasoning prevailed and funds were collected so that additional nurses could be employed. Thus visiting nursing was firmly established in Liverpool [4].

In the United States, visiting nursing began its development in 1877, when the Women's Branch of the New York City Mission sent its first trained nurses into the homes of the indigent. A little later the New York Ethical Society placed nurses in several city dispensaries and afterward, in 1883, sent a nurse to Chicago to begin similar work there. Three years later the Boston Instructive District Nursing Association was organized to promote health education. In 1890, 13 years after the first nurse had been sent out by the New York City Mission, there were 21 organizations in the United States engaged in the work of visiting nursing, most employing no more than one nurse each.

William Rathbone.

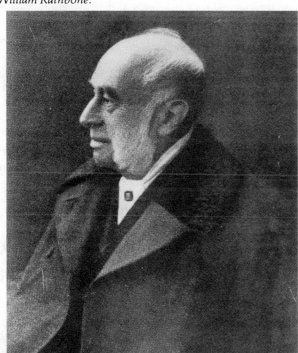

Lillian Wald

Full recognition of the widespread benefits that this new role might yield were
first recognized by Lillian Wald. Born in 1867, Lillian, when quite young,
moved with her family from Cincinnati to Rochester, where she spent her
growing years. She was properly educated in Miss Crittenden's English and
French Boarding and Day School for Young Ladies and Little Girls. Influenced
by relatives who were physicians, she went to New York City to become a nurse.

After three years of training at the New York Hospital School of Nursing,
from which she graduated in 1891, Lillian spent a year nursing at the New
York Juvenile Asylum. Unhappy with her scant medical knowledge, she entered
the Woman's Medical College in New York. While attending medical school,
she and a fellow nurse, Mary Brewster, were asked to go to New York's Lower
East Side to lecture to immigrant mothers on the care of the sick. What they
found there profoundly shocked them.

One morning in March, 1893, Miss Wald was showing a group of mothers
how to make a bed when a child came in asking for help. He led her to a foul
tenement, where nine pitifully undernourished people—most of them sleeping
on the floor and obviously in no need of lessons in bedmaking—were living in
two rooms. On a bed lay a helpless woman who, although seriously ill, had
not received care for two days. No one had ever told 26-year-old Lillian Wald
that such suffering existed. A self-respecting scrub woman might have fled,
nauseated, but as a nurse with a social conscience Miss Wald went to work,
bathed the woman, washed the linen, sent for a physician, and cleaned the
filthy room. She left hours later, visibly shaken by what she had seen. She resolved to leave medical school and join with Mary Brewster in embarking
upon a career of offering nursing care to such needy people. The two women
soon learned that there were thousands of similar cases in that same little neighborhood alone.

In order to implement their resolve, Lillian Wald and Mary Brewster set up a
nurses' settlement house in one of the slum sections of the Lower East Side to
serve as a focal point for a visiting nursing service for the poor. They readily
gave up a more comfortable living environment and moved into a little top-
floor tenement on Jefferson Street. The motives underlying the Settlement
were no more fully defined than to seek out the sick and nurse them.

Misses Wald and Brewster quickly established the concept of the nurse ready
to give her services in the home to all who needed them, making no distinction
between those who could pay and those who could not, allied with no religious
group, seeking to educate as well as to heal. They simply permitted it to be
known that their services were available to any of their neighbors who might
need them. At first, calls came almost entirely from families in which there
was sickness. In each case the nurses established communication with the physician, if one was already in attendance, and if not, they called one in. Sometimes hospital treatment appeared necessary, and the nurses arranged for admission. Often, among the very poor, bedding and other comforts were very

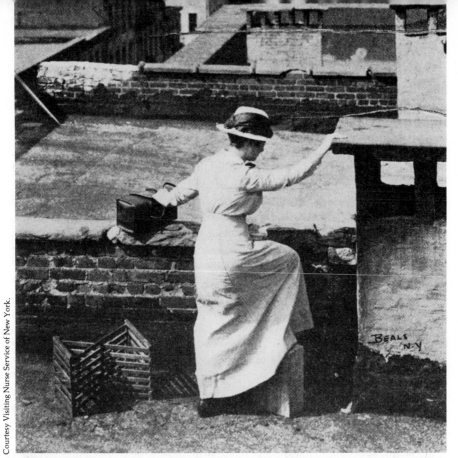

A Henry Street nurse traverses tenement roofs on her way from one family to another.

The Henry Street nurses in the late 1890s.

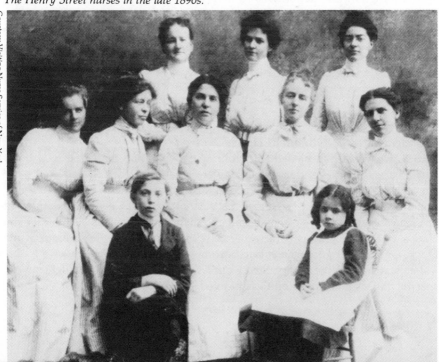

much needed, and the nurses met those needs with stores placed at their disposal by well-to-do friends.

Only during the first few days were the patients sought out. After that, calls for the nurses came by the hundreds. They became known and trusted by their neighbors as friends who did not draw back from contact, no matter how demanding the situation, and who were glad to place their education and skill at the service of all who needed them. Gradually, too, the nurses' work came to be valued by the physicians of the neighborhood and by those in charge of the various hospitals. Whereas at first practically all the calls came from families, a steadily increasing number of patients were referred by physicians. Lillian Wald and her associates brought basic nursing care into the streets. Neatly dressed in modest suits with black ties and spotless white blouses, they made daily calls wherever needed, often traveling over tenement house roofs as the shortest distance from patient to patient.

Illness was not new to Jewish, Italian, Greek, Polish, or Russian immigrants, but in the New World, traditional methods for treating the sick were not enough. Folk remedies were gradually abandoned, or at least combined with pills, ointments, diets, and bed rest made mandatory by the "nurse lady." Old superstitions did not die out altogether, however. A Jewish mother ensured the health of her growing children with fresh air, good diet, and regular milk—all the measures strongly recommended by the visiting nurse—but, just in case, she would also make sure that nobody inadvertently stepped over her child, an action which supposedly would stunt his growth.

From the beginning, one of the basic principles underlying Lillian Wald's work was that nursing care of the sick in their homes was to be the primary aim, and health instruction was to be secondary. Another guiding principle was that the visiting nursing service be analogous to the established system of private duty nursing. Thus the visiting nurse was to respond to calls from the people themselves, as well as from physicians, and to act with as little delay or red tape as possible.

The Henry Street Settlement House

Before two years had passed, the volume of work had increased to a point where larger facilities and more nurses were urgently needed. In 1895, with the aid of banker and philanthropist Jacob H. Schiff and others, Lillian Wald and Mary Brewster moved the Nurses' Settlement to larger accommodations at 265 Henry Street, where it then became known as the Henry Street Settlement House. Soon nine graduate nurses were living in the House, including Lavinia Dock, a vigorous figure who was to become a dynamic nursing leader.

The statistics of the Henry Street nurses' work for 1905 sheds light on the specific duties and responsibilities involved [5]:

Patients cared for in homes	5,032
Nursing visits	43,503
Friendly visits	4,372
First aid treatments	13,791

Cases reported by:	
Families	2,398
Physicians	1,881
Charitable agencies	753
Total	5,032

Disposition of cases:	
Cured	2,624
Hospital	740
Dispensary	598
Investigations	342
Died	312
Special nurse	165
Department of Health	69
Carried over into 1906	182
Total	5,032

Diagnosis of cases:	
Unclassified medical	1,735
Unclassified surgical	602
Pneumonia and bronchitis	956
Tuberculosis	296
Gynecological	212
Burns	197
Rheumatism	158
Obstetrical—normal and abnormal	155
Meningitis	123
Typhoid	122
Contagious	119
Ulcers	118
Cardiac	97
Eye diseases	90
Alcoholism	6
No illness	46
Total	5,032

By 1909 the Henry Street staff numbered 37 nurses, five of whom held administrative posts, with all the others providing direct nursing care. Of this group, the supervisors and 10 staff nurses lived in the Henry Street headquarters. A new nurse, except in case of emergency, began her work there and was assigned to one of the nearby districts. The work of the newcomer was very carefully supervised. Even if the novice Henry Street nurse had the status of a former nurse training school superintendent who, weary of administrative duties, desired to spend some time in direct bedside care, she still was asked to undergo the same careful initiation process, so that misunderstandings of immigrant families and their curious customs might be avoided.

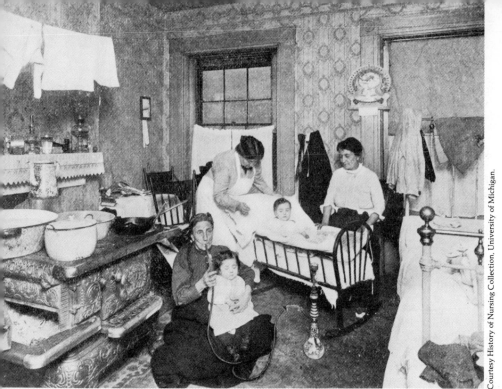

Visiting nurse assisting an immigrant family, about 1900.

At the door of a family in need.

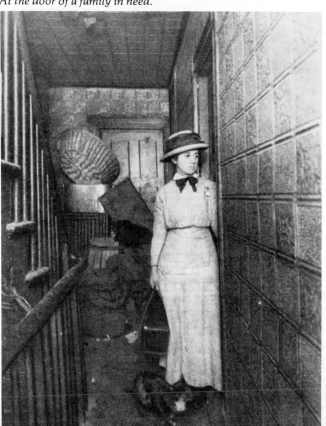

While there was no established period of probation, nurses were not considered permanent until at least three months' satisfactory service had been completed. Some nurses showed early aptitude for the work. To others, the Henry Street point of view, and understanding the people living under conditions and with traditions foreign to their own experience, dawned slowly. Only nurses who proved capable of delivering empathic nursing care were retained because the Settlement's leaders felt that their purpose was not merely to maintain a staff of nurses but also to seize the rare opportunity to demonstrate the value of truly understanding the condition and problems of the immigrant. In her daily work among the immigrants, each nurse kept two sets of records: one, a bedside chart with notes for the physician to review during his visits; the other, a record containing the main points of the nurse's work for the Henry Street superintendent of nurses.

The nature of the work varied somewhat, according to the nurse's district. Acute cases predominated in the crowded Lower East Side, where the Settlement had made its initial foothold among immigrant families from southern Europe, who were both distrustful of hospitals and less familiar with the other resources of the city. Pneumonia had the highest rate of incidence, followed by typhoid fever and meningitis. Many patients with severe pneumonia were cared for by the nurse, with only one or two visits made by a physician, who was kept informed of the patient's progress by the nurse's records. This was especially true when people were unable to pay for physician's visits.

First aid homes were established in several densely populated sections of the city, where a nurse was available daily for treating minor surgical cases, ear and eye problems, and other ailments. The majority of the patients, many of whom were schoolchildren, were sent to the nurses by dispensary physicians. Small but well-equipped surgical dressing rooms were maintained at the main Henry Street office and at several of the branches to accommodate patients who came to have surgical dressings changed. Unlike the typical visiting nursing association, Henry Street had a small obstetric service, with a separate staff, that attempted to uplift the level of practice of scores of immigrant midwives. A daily supply of certified milk was sent to the Settlement every morning, where it was bottled under aseptic conditions and sold at market price to patients who could afford to pay or was distributed free to indigent patients.

By 1909 the Henry Street Settlement had grown from two nurses living on the top floor of a tenement, nursing the sick, to a highly organized social enterprise with many departments. The residents included a staff of nurses and other men and women engaged in various social and civic efforts. Florence Kelley, General Secretary of the National Consumers' League, testified as one of the Henry Street staff:

I have lived 20 years at the bottom of the pit, first eight years at Hull House, Chicago, and now at The Nurses' Settlement in New York City. All these 20 years I have been increasingly depressed—putting it mildly—at the waste of the precious gifts that the young immigrants bring with them, the possibilities we crush out by the living conditions into which we allow the children to come, the lack of educational facilities, and the pressure under which they work. Sometime ago a little boy came to the First Aid room at the Settlement from the tenement house where he lived and said he was making paper bags. He said he could not make any more until his head stopped hurting. The nurse held him at a safe distance, sheared and cleansed his head, and told him to send all his sisters and brothers to her. He was put on the list of candidates for the truant officer. He said he did not think his mother could spare him to stop work and go to school.

A nurse followed him to his lair and found four brothers and a little girl five years old working with incredible rapidity turning out the little paper bags used for rolls and fruit and chestnuts, such bags as come from the grocer into the kitchens of all of us. The place in which this work was being done was a rear cellar bedroom. Not one of the children was tall enough to reach the window sill. They had lived there 18 months, and a charitable society paid their rent. Nobody had visited them but a series of doctors. The children had had the diseases of childhood. Different physicians had seen them through these, but no one had reported them to the truant officer. When the matter was taken up with the factory inspector, he said he never knew of any one occupying that room but had supposed their living place was a coal cellar.

These children were being robbed of all their school years. The oldest boy had once known how to read a little, and when he got into school the knowledge came back to him. Here was a perfectly dead waste, due to the civic negligence of the physicians who had pulled the children through their diseases and left everything as it was before. The family was never before brought to the attention of the truant officer and the truant officers are not allowed, under a series of judicial decisions, to go into a dwelling against the wish of the parent. The two persons who have access everywhere are the nurse and the doctor [6].

Beginnings of School Nursing

The success of establishing school nursing in America was also due to the efforts of Lillian Wald. In 1902 health conditions in the New York schools were so bad that an average of 15 to 20 children daily were sent home from each school. When 300 children were excluded from one school in a single day, however, the problem assumed massive proportions. Miss Wald suggested that placing nurses in the schools might help to solve the problem, since the nurses could effectively supplement the work of local physicians who examined the school children from time to time. This medical examination only excluded the child from school; the physician did not engage in any activities to prevent recurring cases of exclusion and did nothing in the way of following up the children during the period of exclusion. Lillian offered the services of Henry Street nurse Lina L. Rogers for one month as a demonstration of what could be done.

The experiment proved an unqualified success. During the month of September, 1902, 10,567 children had been sent home from the New York schools, while in September, 1903, with a school nurse in attendance, there were only 1101 exclusions. It was not difficult to account for this marked drop in the number of exclusions from schools. Many of exclusions had been for minor illnesses such as pediculosis, ringworm, scabies, and other problems that were easily curable and did not legitimately require the pupil to stay out of school.

Prior to the inception of school nursing, teachers and physicians often had

Public Health Nursing, March, 1934.

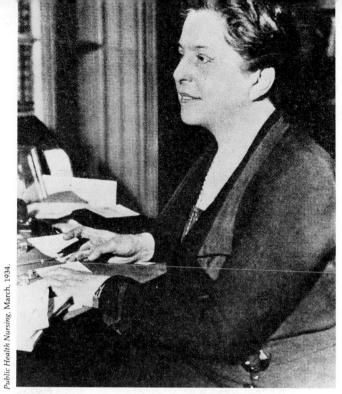

Lillian D. Wald.

School nurse at work, New York City, 1905.

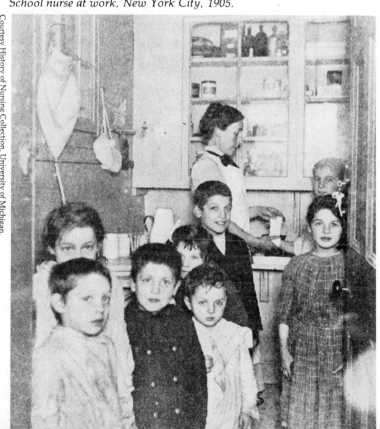

no choice but to send all children home who seemed physically unfit to associate with others. Indeed, in some cities such exclusions became an all-too-convenient method for easing the pressures of badly overcrowded classrooms. For example, the Henry Street Settlement nurse uncovered a boy of 12 who had never been to school because he had a tiny sore on his head. When this situation was investigated, it was found to be typical of many other children.

The New York Board of Health, realizing the value of the nurse in the school, soon appointed dozens of school nurses to assist in carrying out the work. Dr. John J. Cronin of New York City wrote: "When I state that in the city of New York, during the period of three months, out of 24,358 children who were actually excluded from school for longer or shorter periods, only 400 had serious diseases, imperiling their own lives, the others being more of the character of 'nuisances,' it will be seen what an advantage this system may prove from an educational point of view" [7].

School nursing, however, sometimes caused riots. In New York City on June 27, 1906, schools were stormed by excited mothers demanding their children. The cause of the riot was 83 adenoid operations that had been performed in the schools by three specialists, assisted by health inspectors and nurses. The rumor had got around the neighborhood that the children's "throats were being cut," and an excited mob demolished several windows and doors before the children could be dismissed.

A newspaper story of October 5, 1906, told of a similar riot in front of a public school near the Williamsburg Bridge in Brooklyn. According to the newspaper, the cause of this riot was the initiation of active measures in the school for the eradication of trachoma. About 1500 Italian women fought the police desperately and actually attempted to batter down the doors of the school building. Again, the trouble was based on a misapprehension.

Insight into some of the problems encountered by school nurses can be derived from letters received from parents [8]:

Miss Eichler:
We received the note from the Doctor and will say that we give him medical attention when he needs it. We know that George had headaches but when he comes home from school he complains of a boy in the 3rd grade by the name of Andrew Aimeck who knocks him down and jomps on him. I wish you would give this your attention. I know boys are all alike but this boy is mutch larger.

Very Respectfully Yours, S_____.

To Whom This May Concern:
I received your letter stating that Edna Ross (my Sister) is in need of glasses. It is utterly impossible for me to purchase her any as my husband is out of work and her father does not contribute one penny towards her support and I am obliged to share the little I have with her and have two infants of my own. Her mother is dead and the Father placed the child on my hands.

Yours Respectfully H_____.

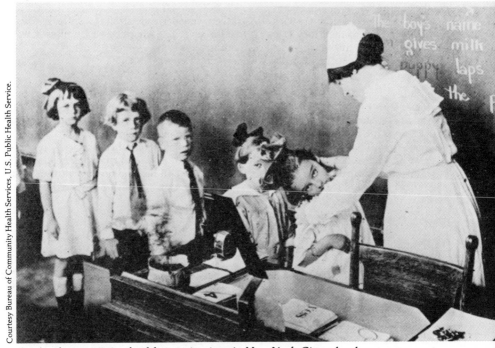

Courtesy Bureau of Community Health Services, U.S. Public Health Service.

A school nurse giving health examinations in New York City school.

Children waiting to be examined at a children's clinic in Harlem, 1912.

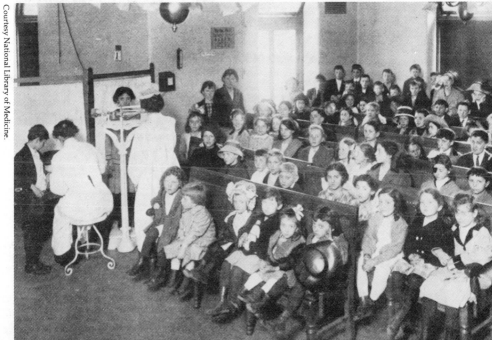

Courtesy National Library of Medicine.

To the Nurse:
Jennie was not born with here eyes crossed they were perfectly strait until after she was three years old and then they crossed. I could never tell what caused it unless it was from a fall down stairs which she got six months before.

Yours truly, S_____.

Miss Hill:
I received a note wich Martha brought home to instruct me to take her to a doctor now I want you to know that I or my can Judge wen Marth needs medical treatment if Martha is sick I keep her home. I send Martha to school to be instruction my wife has ask you to give Martha some lessons to bring home and my wife would instruct her you complain about Martha she keeps her mouth open well she does just as any other child would wen intrested or surprised it is more or less a habit with her and no catarrh she has a slight cold I will atmit but nothing more. So I hope you will give her some lesson to bring home and we will instruct her the best we can.

W_____.

One mother, upon being notified that her young son needed a bath, wrote: "teacher, Johnny aint no rose. Learn him; don't smell him." Another mother, upon receiving a notice that her boy suffered from *astigmatism*, wrote that she had whipped him soundly and hoped that he would not do it again [9].

Nurses of the Instructive District Nursing Association of Boston.

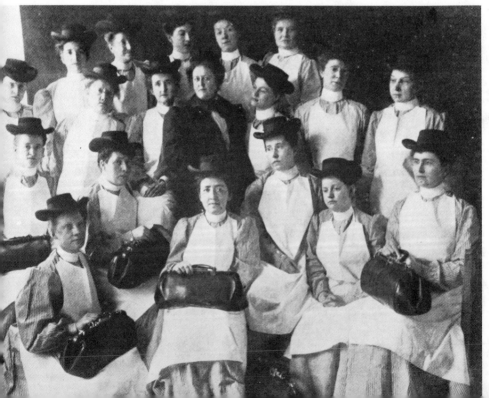

Metropolitan Life Employs Nurses

In June, 1901, at the suggestion of Lillian Wald, the Metropolitan Life Insurance Company organized the Visiting Nurse Department and entered into an agreement with the Henry Street Settlement in New York City, whereby the latter was to furnish the services of its visiting nurses to the company's industrial policyholders in a limited section of Manhattan. The service proved to be very satisfactory during the three-month trial and was extended to other parts of the city. Two months later it was introduced in Baltimore and in Washington, D.C. By the end of 1901, policyholders in Boston, Chicago, Cincinnati, Cleveland, Dover, Harrisburg, Philadelphia, St. Louis, Trenton, and Worcester were also given the privilege of this service. By the end of 1909 there were 14 Metropolitan nursing centers; by 1912 there were 589. Wherever possible, the company contracted with the local Visiting Nurse Association to furnish the nursing service at a certain rate per patient. Where that was impossible, the company hired its own nurses, under the direction of its field supervisors.

Standing Orders

The proper scope of nursing practice in the community was the subject of considerable debate among physicians and nurses. Visiting nurses experienced

Assessing the health status of an elderly patient.

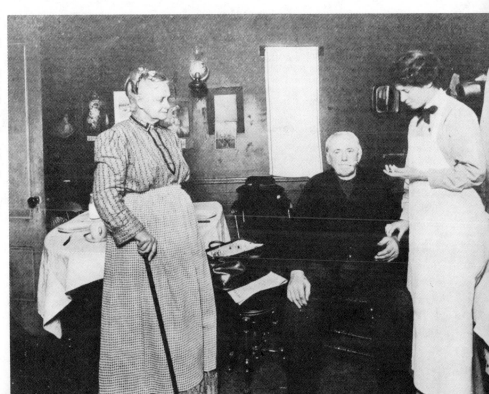

Annual Report, District Nursing Association, Boston, 1915.

more autonomy than their hospital nurse colleagues, yet the exact bounds of their responsibilities were not clearly defined. Some physicians thought the public health nurse should carry out numerous procedures that were thought to be traditionally medical, while others viewed the situation quite differently. A physician in a Massachusetts town complained bitterly that "the nurse took the temperature, pulse, and respiration, opened the windows and put the pneumonia patient on a milk diet, and left nothing for the doctor to do"; while a young surgeon in a nearby city told nursing students that "they should be prepared for any emergency . . . , even to giving an intravenous or to re-ligating slipped abdominal sutures" [10].

Because of these divergent approaches, in 1912 the Chicago Visiting Nurse Association prepared a list of standing orders for staff nurses. In this way they hoped that thorough and speedy care could be given to every patient. No medication, however, not even castor oil, was included in this list. Bath orders were included because many patients strenuously objected to taking a bath in cold weather. They were more likely to accept a bath philosophically when told that the physician had ordered it. The standing orders read as follows:

An Undiagnosed Case Running Temperature—Cleansing bath; liquid diet; low S.S. enema, P.R.N. when no abdominal pain or tenderness is present; sponge for R.T. 102.5°.

Sore Throat—Gargle and mouth-wash of baking-soda; liquid diet; children to be isolated if possible until physician sees case.

Colds—Cleansing bath; low S.S. enema, P.R.N.; liquid diet; for adults, plenty of hot water taken frequently.

Pneumonia—Cleansing bath; low S.S. enema, P.R.N.; sponge for R.T. 102.5°; liquid diet; cold-air treatment, if possible.

Typhoid Fever—Cleansing bath; low S.S. enema, P.R.N.; sponge for R.T. 102.5°; milk diet. Emphasize need for plenty of fresh air and cold drinking water (boiled if possible) and disinfection of stools.

Obstetrical Cases—For mother: cleansing bath; local cleansing with Lysol solution; abdominal binder; change pads; breast binder, P.R.N.; low S.S. enema, P.R.N. For the baby: alcohol dressing to cord; oiled and bathed.

Infants and Young Children (sick but not diagnosed)—Normal salt flushing, P.R.N.; diet, boiled water for twenty-four hours.

Infectious Diseases—Isolation; boric solution for eyes and nostrils, P.R.N.; Vaseline or cold cream for lips and nose, P.R.N.; oil rub, P.R.N. for all desquamating cases; liquid diet; sponge for R.T. 102.5°.

Pleurisy—Apply tight binder to chest.

Infantile Diarrhea—Normal salt flushing, P.R.N.; no food; boiled water for twenty-four hours.

Infantile Convulsions—Same orders as diarrhea.

Burn Cases—Remove clothing; apply normal salt or boric solution dressings; if severe burn, get into hospital as quickly as possible.

Chronic Ulcers—Clean with Lysol or boric solution; apply wet boric dressings and firm bandage.

Minor Dressings—For cuts, scratches, bruises and infected fingers, apply hot boric packs and refer to dispensary.

Discharging Ears—Cleanse the outer ear with moist boric solution swabs; do not irrigate; refer to dispensary [11].

Any or all of the above orders could be canceled or changed at any time by a physician who preferred to leave specific written orders. The standing orders were suggested as aids to both the nurse and the physician and were utilized when no other orders were given.

Early Efforts to Improve Maternal-Child Care

As a corollary to the visiting nursing movement, organized efforts to improve infant hygiene began. Early work concentrated on the improvement of milk and water supplies, such as the establishment by private agencies of milk stations for the distribution of clean, safe milk, or modified milk at a nominal cost for infant feeding, along with the passage of city ordinances controlling milk production, care, and distribution. The first milk station in the United States was established in New York City in 1893, and by 1910 similar stations existed in 30 other cities. From milk dispensaries, these stations often evolved into preventive health centers as the emphasis swung toward educational activity and physical examinations for preventive care.

In the early 1900s much innovative work was carried out in attacking maternal and infant mortality. For example, the Boston Lying-In Hospital's visiting nurses divided the city into four districts and cared for mothers in their homes. Five graduate nurses and two student nurses divided the workload into prenatal and postnatal cases. The nurse's first visit was devoted to assessing the social conditions of the patient's family. If the patient had sufficient money to pay for medical care, she would be referred to a neighborhood physician.

For those poorer mothers cared for by the visiting nurses of the Lying-In Hospital, the following plan of home care was implemented. First, the mother's general condition was appraised; if medical care was needed, the physician was notified. The mother was taught nutrition basics, with emphasis on milk-producing foods; because breast-feeding was highly encouraged. The second visit was used to review the necessary articles of clothing needed for the baby and the special supplies required by the physician for the delivery. The number of preparatory visits varied with the necessity for instruction, but three were typical. Postpartum visits involved care of both mother and baby. When the patients were discharged from the nurse's care, the mother was encouraged to attend well child care classes offered by the Milk and Baby Hygiene Association.

In spite of such efforts, however, the national rate of infant mortality remained distressingly high. It was estimated that 300,000 children under one year of age died each year in the United States, and that at least half of those deaths were preventable. A percentage breakdown of the cause of 154,373 infant deaths in the registration area of the United States in 1910 was as follows [12]:

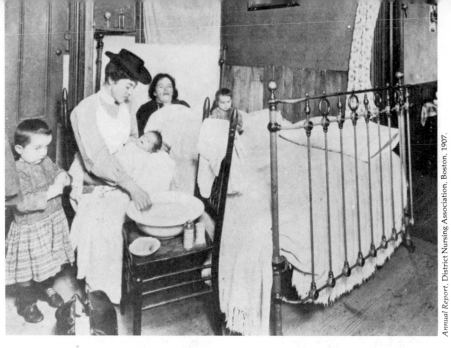

Annual Report, District Nursing Association, Boston, 1907.

Caring for a family of five children whose mother is suffering from tuberculosis and whose father is unemployed.

Preparing milk for infants in a milk laboratory, about 1914.

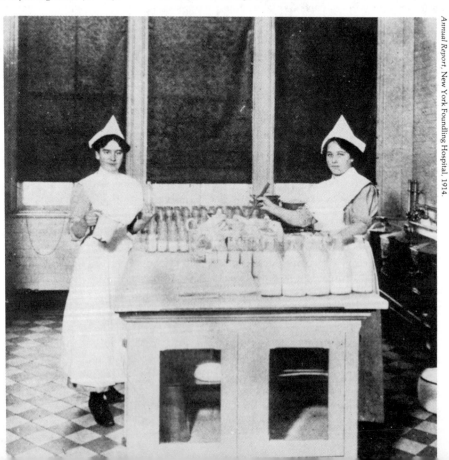

Annual Report, New York Founding Hospital, 1914.

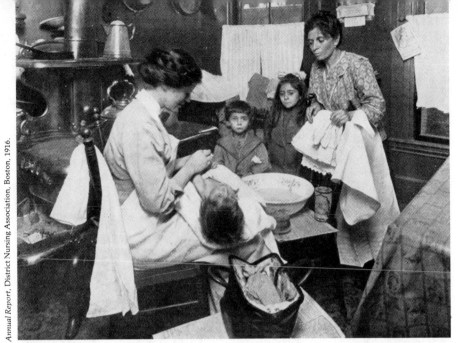

A public health nurse gives a lesson in caring for the baby.

A maternity nurse caring for a baby's eyes, as a means of preventing infection and blindness.

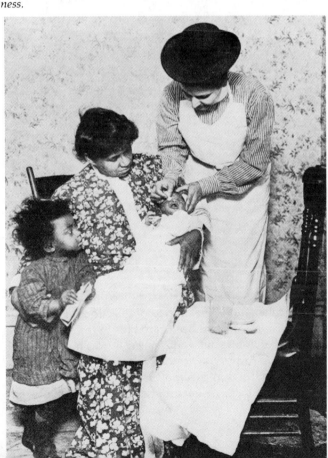

Diseases of the digestive system	32.1
Diseases of early infancy (including premature birth, 13.1 percent, congenital debility, 7.8, and injuries at birth, 2.4)	25.5
Diseases of the respiratory system (including broncho-pneumonia, 6.9, pneumonia, 5.5, and acute bronchitis, 2.7)	15.8
General diseases (including all forms of tuberculosis, 1.6, syphilis, 1.1, and whooping cough, measles, scarlet fever, diphtheria, and croup, 4.0)	9.2
Diseases of the nervous system (including convulsions, 2.6, and meningitis, 1.5)	5.5
Congenital malformations	4.9
All other causes	7.0
	100

The death rate per 1000 infants under one year of age in the larger cities of the registration area that same year revealed the following:

Oakland, Cal.	94.8	Dayton, Ohio	146.8
Seattle, Wash.	100.4	Cleveland, Ohio	147.2
Portland, Ore.	105.3	Cincinnati, Ohio	149.8
Los Angeles, Cal.	110.7	Jersey City, N.J.	153.2
San Francisco, Cal.	113.6	New Orleans, La.	154.9
Toledo, Ohio	125.0	Atlanta, Ga.	155.3
Cambridge, Mass.	126.1	Bridgeport, Conn.	155.5
St. Paul, Minn.	130.8	Philadelphia, Pa.	162.2
Birmingham, Ala.	133.0	Albany, N.Y.	162.9
Louisville, Ky.	134.0	Boston, Mass.	168.0
Denver, Col.	134.7	Worcester, Mass.	168.0
Grand Rapids, Mich.	134.8	Kansas City, Mo.	170.4
New Haven, Conn.	134.9	Milwaukee, Wis.	172.0
Nashville, Tenn.	135.1	Providence, R.I.	173.7
St. Louis, Mo.	135.8	Syracuse, N.Y.	176.4
Chicago, Ill.	139.5	Pittsburg, Pa.	179.6
Omaha, Neb.	140.0	Buffalo, N.Y.	180.9
Columbus, Ohio	140.4	Washington, D.C.	194.6
Spokane, Wash.	142.4	Detroit, Mich.	204.8
Indianapolis, Ind.	144.8	Baltimore, Md.	209.6
Newark, N.J.	145.8	Richmond, Va.	229.3
New York, N.Y.	146.2	Fall River, Mass.	259.5
Paterson, N.J.	146.7	Lowell, Mass.	261.0

The Attack on Tuberculosis

Through the nineteenth century the mortality rates showed that tuberculosis was perennially the leading killer among the myriad of infectious diseases. Although bedridden tuberculosis patients had been cared for by general visiting nurses from the beginning of the visiting nurse movement, it was not until 1899 that the first attempt was made to provide special home nursing service for tuberculosis patients. The first efforts in this movement were launched by a woman medical student who had been assigned to follow up tuberculosis pa-

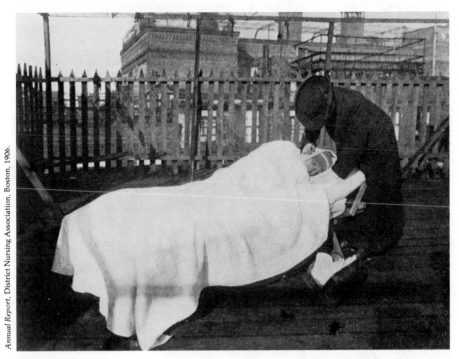

Annual Report, District Nursing Association, Boston, 1906.

Tuberculosis patient taking fresh air treatment on a roof.

tients from Johns Hopkins Hospital. She investigated and reported on the patients' living conditions and taught families the care and precautions necessary for treatment and prevention of the disease. Believing that the problem of tuberculosis was a home problem and therefore that it should be combated at home, Dr. William Osler of Johns Hopkins initiated the Laennec Society of Baltimore "to systematize and stimulate work in tuberculosis and diffuse in the profession and the public a knowledge of the disease" [13].

The first work of the Laennec Society was to investigate the social conditions of a group of 190 tuberculosis cases. This was the first study of its kind to be made, and it uncovered many tragic conditions. Patients in the last stages of tuberculosis were found to be living in one- or two-room apartments with half a dozen other people. Ventilation was poor or nonexistent. Often they slept in the same bed with one, two, and sometimes three others, and they always ate with the family, sharing the same utensils and often giving the children sips of coffee from their cups or bites of food from their forks. Obviously, the disease was rapidly being spread in such fashion, and the need for assistance to these patients and their families was urgent.

The publication of this study led to the appointment, in 1903, of a nurse who spent her full time following up tuberculosis patients in their homes. This nurse was instructed "to find 'lost patients' and get them back to the dispensary; to teach the doctrine of fresh air, good food, and rest; and not only report the

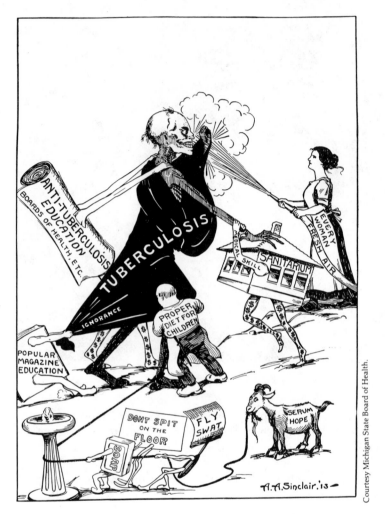

How to fight tuberculosis—the number one menace to the nation's health at the turn of the century.

home conditions, but to do all in her power with the help of relief agencies to improve them." She was also expected "to give bedside care to the sick and to establish the precautions necessary to avoid infection of others." In 1904, through contributions received from interested citizens, additional nurses were employed for tuberculosis work and were assigned for supervision to the Visiting Nurse Association of Baltimore [14].

As early as 1892 the Pennsylvania Tuberculosis Society, the first organization of its kind in the world, had been founded. Ten years later the Tuberculosis Committee of the New York Charity Organization Society was formed. In Chicago, Boston, Washington, Rochester, Buffalo, and a few other places, interest in organized tuberculosis work was strong. In 1903 Henry Phipps provided funds to establish a research institute in Philadelphia for the purpose of studying the disease, the first organization of its kind in America. In 1904 the National Tuberculosis Association was formed, uniting in one body these scattered groups and others interested in the subject. Antituberculosis associations in the United States had increased to 20 by 1905.

At this time there was still no general recognition of public responsibility in the control of tuberculosis. Leading health workers, as early as 1897, had put forth the principle that a city health department should take definite responsibility for the control of tuberculosis as a communicable disease, and the New York Health Department had made significant strides in that direction. In 1895 the Massachusetts legislature made an appropriation for the first state sanatorium for the treatment of tuberculosis in the United States. By 1905 there were 19 public sanatoriums or hospitals for tuberculosis, including three federal, four state, four county, and eight municipal institutions. All these institutions hired at least a few graduate nurses, and several began nurse training schools to assist in staffing rather than hire a large number of untrained attendants.

Red Cross Nursing

Another growing movement was Red Cross nursing. The idea that led to the birth of the Red Cross had originated in June, 1859, three years after Florence Nightingale had returned from the Crimea. An investment banker from Geneva, Switzerland, J. Henri Dunant, went to Italy with the intention of securing a meeting with Napoleon III of France, then on campaign, but instead found himself at Solferino, in the midst of the bloodiest battle of the war between France and Austria. Horrified to learn that some 6000 wounded men were being attended by only two physicians, he organized a makeshift nursing service and successfully persuaded the local people to bring water, bandages, and food to the men. Three years later, in his famous *Recollections of Solferino*, Dunant proposed the establishment of a permanent international relief society that could take immediate action in time of war. This idea was incorporated into the Geneva Convention guidelines, signed by 12 governments on August 22, 1864. On that day the International Red Cross was born.

It was not until 1881, however, that the American Red Cross was first organized, through the efforts of Clara Barton, a former New England school teacher who had found a psychological outlet by attacking vast social burdens. In 1854 she had been appointed to a clerkship in the Patent Office in Washington, D.C., and this was perhaps the first time a government position was held by a woman. During the Civil War Miss Barton independently directed a large-scale war relief operation, arranging for huge quantities of supplies to be furnished to the Army and the hospitals. On occasion, she also did personal nursing, and during this time she had ample opportunity to determine the need for an organization like the Red Cross.

In 1870 Miss Barton served with the German Red Cross during the Franco-

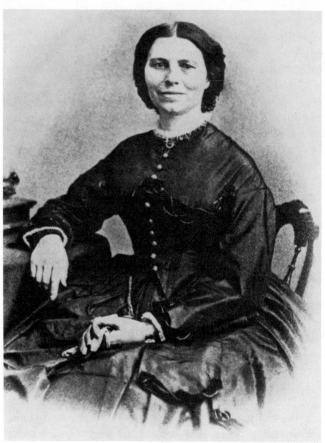

Courtesy Library of Congress.

Clara Barton, founder of the American Red Cross.

Prussian war; after her return to the United States, she organized the American Red Cross. She was instrumental in persuading Congress, in 1882, to ratify the Treaty of Geneva, so that in times of peace the Red Cross Society could continue to engage in humanitarian work. The charter stated that the Red Cross was dedicated "to continue and carry on a system of national and international relief in time of peace and to apply the same in mitigating the sufferings caused by pestilence, famine, fire, floods, and other national calamities, and to devise and carry measure for preventing the same" [15].

Miss Barton served in relief work with the Red Cross during a number of disasters, including the yellow fever epidemic in Florida in 1888 and the Johnstown flood of 1889. During the half-century following 1882 Red Cross nurses gave assistance in more than 1000 disasters in the United States, at a cost of $53 million. These disasters included 271 cyclones, tornadoes, hurricanes, and other storms, 152 floods, and 139 fires. In addition, there were mine cave-ins, explosions, epidemics, forest fires, steamboat wrecks, train wrecks, and numerous other types of catastrophes.

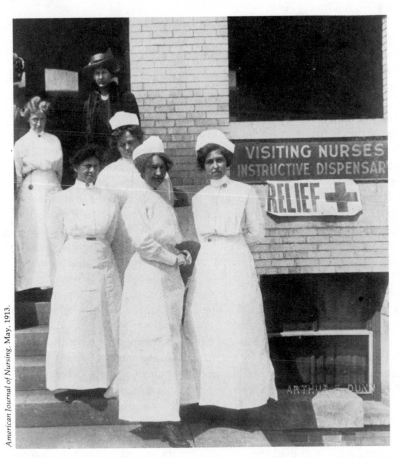

American Journal of Nursing, May, 1913.

Red Cross nurses at a relief station following the Omaha Tornado of 1913.

The Town and Country Nursing Service

Rural public health nursing progressed slowly. With few exceptions, there was practically no nursing service available for the great mass of people living on farms or in lonely country districts. At the second annual meeting of the Association for the Prevention of Infant Mortality, held in 1911, Lillian Wald gave an address on rural problems. She reviewed the terrible health care conditions found in rural districts—the high prevalence of tuberculosis, hookworm, and fevers, the gross inadequacies in maternity care, and the extraordinarily high infant and maternal mortality rates. She compared the different attitudes in the United States with the work going on in Great Britain, Canada, and Australia, where nation-wide nursing services for rural populations were provided. Miss Wald asked: "Why should not our National Red Cross Society, with all its splendid organization and resources, support, direct and operate such a national service during the intervals of time in which there is no need for its emergency duty?" [16].

In 1912 the Red Cross did indeed undertake to establish a rural nursing service, which provided nurses to care for the sick, to give instruction in sanitation and hygiene in the homes of the rural people, and to attempt to improve living conditions in little villages and on lonely farms. The organization of the Red Cross Rural Nursing Services was made possible by a generous gift of $100,000 from New York financier Jacob H. Schiff, together with $1000 annually from Mrs. Whitelaw Reid, wife of the editor of the *New York Tribune.* Both gifts were secured through the efforts of Lillian Wald.

This money was used for administrative and supervisory expenses, but the salaries of the nurses were paid for by the communities that they served. A superintendent of nurses was appointed, and headquarters were opened in Washington, D.C. In the following year the name was changed from Rural Nursing Service to the Town and Country Nursing Service, in order to include the small towns where no visiting service was found. Although this effort in extending nursing service met a great need, it grew slowly. With a typical disdain for national supervision over what might be considered local affairs, many communities hesitated to call in the aid of the National Red Cross. Others could not raise the money for the nurses' salaries. Consequently, up to 1915, only 40 or 50 Red Cross public health nurses were employed throughout the nation.

Due to the vast unmet rural health care needs, it was necessary in the town and country districts to make certain restrictions on the visiting nurses' work. Almost invariably the nurses reported the prevailing diseases to be tuberculosis, pneumonia, and typhoid. Other common ailments were grippe, rheumatism, gonorrhea, hookworm, pellagra, cholera infantum, malaria, and epidemics of measles, scarlet fever, tonsillitis, smallpox, and typhus, together with all the contagious diseases of children occurring in some form in nearly every community. Among miners and in foreign settlements, grippe, pneumonia, and other pulmonary diseases were conspicuous. In order to prevent epidemics, nurses engaged in setting up quarantine and enforcing the laws for smallpox vaccination. In only a few communities were contagious cases sent to hospitals. Under the jurisdiction of the local health authority, they were usually quarantined at home, in vacant houses, or sometimes even in tents.

An interesting phase of the rural nurse's work was the remarkable degree of resourcefulness she had to develop out of pure necessity. Very few nurses had adequate stocks of medical supplies; many of those that she had taken for granted during her training were nonexistent now, and it was up to her to contrive substitutes. Examples of such improvisations included using hot bricks, salt, or sandbags in place of hot water bottles, making bedrests out of chairs, soaping windows to give opaque light for surgical operations, fashioning a protective cradle out of three barrel hoops wound with strips of muslin, using wooden blocks for raising low beds, and constructing a stretcher out of boards padded with quilts. Sometimes the rural nurse had to make long trips for drinking water or perhaps melt snow in order to secure water to bathe patients. Boiled water was carried in fruit cans to maternity and surgical cases.

Early rural nurses recommended many practices that yielded improved living conditions, such as the screening of houses, the fumigation and whitewashing of rooms after tuberculosis patients had occupied them, the reporting of bad conditions in outhouses and the careless disposal of garbage, and the improvement of sanitation ordinances. Nurses also instituted vigorous action against flies by promoting practices such as keeping garbage pails covered, emptying them more frequently, and discouraging the practice of throwing potato peelings out into the yard. In many homes, heavy, dirty, unwashable bed quilts were either replaced by new ones or kept covered with clean sheets. As a result, areas served by rural nurses showed decreases in infant mortality and the general death rate and overall improvements in cleanliness, nutrition, and sanitation.

The Birth of Industrial Nursing

Industrial establishments also made use of early visiting nurses. In 1895, in Vermont, Fletcher D. Proctor, son of a governor and himself one-time governor of that state, introduced "district nursing" into several villages whose residents were mostly employees of his Vermont Marble Company. As president of this company, Proctor demonstrated unusual interest in the welfare of his employees. After observing the work of visiting nurses in several cities, he selected 24-year-old Ada Mayo Stewart, an 1894 graduate of the Waltham (Massachusetts) Training School, to do visiting nursing among the families of his workers at Proctor. A few months later, Ada's sister Harriet was hired to care for the company's employees and their families in the village of West Rutland and Rutland Center.

In this early form of industrial nursing, little emphasis was placed on the care of injuries. It was essentially a home visiting service with patient referrals coming from physicians. Records were not kept for the first year, but the figures for 1896 through 1898 showed that obstetric patients topped Miss Stewart's workload, with medical cases coming a close second, followed by a few surgical patients. Service was free to employees of the Vermont Marble Company and their families and to other townspeople who were unable to pay for medical care.

Formation of the National Organization of Public Health Nursing

Although the decade from 1900 to 1910 witnessed a rapid expansion and extension of visiting nursing, there had been no effort to organize and standardize this type of care and there were no recognized requirements for being employed as a visiting nurse. But on June 7, 1912, a handful of visiting nurses, who unofficially represented 2500 poorly prepared and unsupervised colleagues in 900 agencies, formed the National Organization for Public Health Nursing. This was an organization of nurses and lay people engaged in the actual work of public health nursing and in the organization, management, and support of such work. Leading organizers included Lillian D. Wald, Ella Phillips Crandall,

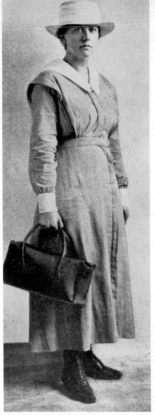

The Red Cross Town and Country nurse in her plain blue gingham dress and panama hat.

Ada Mayo Stewart (left) was the first industrial nurse.

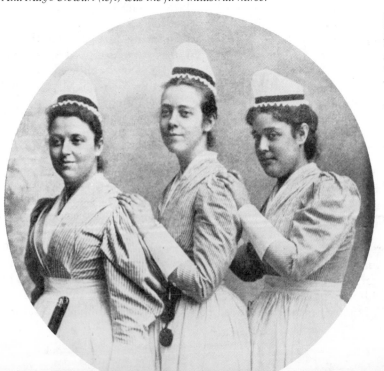

Mary Beard, Mary Lent, Edna Foley, Lystra Gretter, and Elizabeth G. Fox. Favoring the term *public health nurse* as more inclusive than *visiting nurse*, the founders declared that "the experience data available emphasized the urgency and practical necessity for the extension of public health nursing service to a much larger proportion of wage-earners and people of moderate means than now have the benefit of the same" [17]. Lillian Wald was chosen as the first president of the NOPHN.

In 1909 an unpretentious little magazine entitled *The Visiting Nurse Quarterly,* the first American publication to deal exclusively with the subject of public health nursing, was initiated by the Cleveland Visiting Nurse Association. Three years later the Cleveland Association offered this quarterly to the National Organization for Public Health Nursing, on the very day the Organization was founded. Under the new title *The Public Health Nurse Quarterly,* it quickly proved to be a valuable means of communication among the membership.

NOPHN founders soon noted that mortality statistics for the first 14 years of the twentieth century showed an overall decline in the death rate, a development that was attributed to improved water supply, better methods of sewage disposal, cleaner streets, better housing laws, and more stringent regulation of food and dairy products, as well as to recent discoveries in medical science, the work of visiting nurses, and an improved awareness among the public regarding the importance of health. The decline in the following most prevalent diseases, per 100,000 people, is shown in the figures below [18]:

	1900	1905	1910	1914
Typhoid fever	35.9	27.8	23.5	15.4
Diphtheria and croup	43.3	23.6	21.4	17.9
Tuberculosis of all forms	201.9	92.3	160.3	146.8
Pneumonia	180.5	148.8	147.7	127.0
Diarrhea and enteritis under two years [of age]	108.8	97.0	100.8	66.0

Certain other diseases were on the increase:

	1900	1905	1910	1914
Cancer	63.0	71.4	76.2	79.4
Organic heart disease	123.1	143.8	150.4	150.8
Cerebral hemorrhage	67.5	71.6	73.7	77.7
Nephritis	89.0	103.4	99.0	102.4

Also in 1912, the United States Children's Bureau, a longstanding dream of Lillian Wald, was created by act of Congress as part of the Department of Commerce and Labor. Several years earlier she had helped found the National

Child Labor Committee to fight the ruthless exploitation of child labor. To ensure that all aspects of child health and welfare be promoted, Lillian had repeatedly suggested to the government the need for such an agency and had been summoned to Washington by President Roosevelt in 1905 to explain her plan in detail. Four years later the legislation passed, and Julia C. Lathrop, M.D., a resident of the Hull House settlement in Chicago, was chosen by President Taft to head the new Bureau. Nursing was related to most of the aspects of the Children's Bureau functions, which included investigating and reporting on all matters pertaining to child welfare.

By 1912 the rapidly expanding public health nursing movement could look back nearly 20 years to the Nurses' Settlement on Henry Street, knowing that from humble beginnings a humanitarian ideal had grown into a substantial force, which was effectively attacking much human suffering and need. The noticeable decline in tuberculosis, diarrheal diseases of children, and typhoid fever—campaigns in which public health nurses had taken so active a part—inspired the confidence that still better results were within reach.

Summary

In the 1880s and 1890s immigrants poured into New York City by the hundreds of thousands, taking up residence in grossly overcrowded tenement houses. The congestion and poor living conditions in these tenements resulted in a New York City death rate of more than 25 per thousand in 1880.

The concept of visiting nursing was first put into practice by the efforts of William Rathbone of Liverpool, England, who in 1859 sent a trained nurse into the homes of the needy sick of the city.

The first American organization to send trained nurses into the homes of the sick poor was the Women's Branch of the New York City Mission in 1877. Other visiting nurse agencies soon developed.

A major forward thrust for the visiting nurse movement came in 1893 when Lillian Wald and a nurse colleague, Mary Brewster, were exposed to the wretched health conditions of New York's Lower East Side. Appalled by what they saw, Lillian and Mary set up a nurses' settlement house, later moved to Henry Street. Here they lived among the tenement dwellers they served, offering nursing care in the homes of the sick and health instruction to all who requested it.

Lillian Wald was also the driving force behind the establishment of school nursing in America. In New York City, thousands of children were excluded from school each month due to health problems. Lillian offered the services of a Henry Street nurse for one month as a demonstration. The experiment was an unqualified success, with a drop from 10,567 exclusions in September, 1902, to only 1101 in September of the following year. This led to the employment of school nurses throughout the New York City schools.

In 1901, at the suggestion of Lillian Wald, the Metropolitan Life Insurance Company introduced a visiting nurse service for its industrial policyholders. The first service, operated in a limited section of Manhattan, was so successful that the program rapidly expanded. By 1912 there were 589 Metropolitan nursing centers throughout the country.

Although visiting nursing, by its very nature, entailed somewhat more autonomy than hospital nursing, many physicians were reluctant to relinquish any control of patient treatment, while others expected the public health nurse to make medical judgments when she was alone in the home. This dichotomy created problems that were attacked, with varying degrees of success, through the promulgation of standing orders.

In the early 1900s, efforts to improve infant and maternal health that were associated with the visiting nurse movement included establishing milk stations for the distribution of safe milk, working for the passage of city ordinances regulating the milk supply process, and providing maternity home care for mothers and new babies.

Antituberculosis associations employed nurses to care for patients at home, to engage in case finding, and to identify networks of probable infection, especially within the family unit itself.

Movements devoted to organized tuberculosis work helped draw attention to this disease as a major health problem. State and city governments began assuming responsibility for tuberculosis control by making funds available to build sanatoriums, some of which developed their own nurse training schools.

The International Red Cross was formed in 1864, largely through the efforts of J. Henri Dunant of Switzerland, who had organized a relief nursing force during the war between France and Austria.

Similarly, in 1881, the American Red Cross was organized through the efforts of Clara Barton, who had directed a large war relief operation during the Civil War. Nurses played the central role in most aspects of Red Cross work, especially in time of disaster.

Red Cross Town and Country Nurses, faced with conditions of overwhelming need and limitations of scarce health resources in the rural areas of the nation, were unable to make the positive impact that was originally sought.

Another new type of service, industrial nursing, began in 1895 in Vermont, where Fletcher D. Proctor, president of the Vermont Marble Company, introduced "district nursing" into several Vermont villages whose residents were employed mainly by the company.

In 1912 the National Organization for Public Health Nursing was established, bringing together nurses and lay people engaged in the service and support of public health nursing. Lillian Wald, who had pioneered many of the public health nursing services, was chosen as the first NOPHN president.

The overall decline in the death rate between 1900 and 1914 was attributed to improved water and sanitation conditions, new medical discoveries, and the work of public health nurses.

Lillian Wald, who first put forth the idea of a federal bureau to promote child health and welfare in 1905, saw her dream fulfilled seven years later when Congress established the United States Children's Bureau.

References

1. New York Association for Improving the Condition of the Poor, *Annual Report for 1884* (New York: The Association, 1884), p. 43.
2. New York Tenement House Commission, *Report of the Tenement House Commission for 1900* (New York: The Commission, 1900), p. 17.
3. W. Rathbone, *History and Progress of District Nursing* (New York: Macmillan Co., 1890), p. 7.
4. *Ibid.*
5. Henry Street Settlement, *Annual Report of the Henry Street Settlement for 1905* (New York: The Settlement, 1906), pp. 3–14.
6. Florence Kelley, *Medical Problems of Immigration* (Easton, Pennsylvania: American Academy of Medicine Press, 1913), pp. 6–7.
7. Allen G. Rice, *Medical Inspection of Schools* (Providence: Snow & Farnham Co., 1912), pp. 48–49.
8. U.S. Children's Bureau, unpublished letters in Bureau records, National Archives, RG 102.
9. *Ibid.*
10. Edna L. Foley, "Standing Orders," *American Journal of Nursing*, vol. 13 (March, 1913): 451.
11. *Ibid.*, pp. 451–453.
12. U.S. Department of Commerce and Labor, Bureau of the Census, *Mortality Statistics, 1910:   General Death Rates; Specific and Standardized Death Rates; Infant and Child Mortality; Causes of Death* (Washington, D.C.:   Government Printing Office, 1913), pp. 1–142.
13. Ellen N. LaMotte, *The Tuberculosis Nurse: Her Function and Her Qualifications* (New York: G. P. Putnam's Sons, 1915), pp. 33–35.
14. *Ibid.*, pp. 36–38.
15. J. E. Pilcher, "The Red Cross," *Military Surgeon*, vol. 20 (April, 1907): 230–237.
16. Mabel T. Boardman, "Rural Nursing Service of the Red Cross," *American Journal of Nursing*, vol. 13 (September, 1913): 937–939.
17. Mary Sewall Gardner, "The National Organization for Public Health Nursing," *Visiting Nurse Quarterly*, vol. 4 (July, 1912): 13–18.
18. U.S. Department of Commerce, Bureau of the Census, *Mortality Statistics 1914* (Washington, D.C.:   Government Printing Office, 1916), pp. 9–23.

9
In Quest of Reform, 1909–1917

The progressive era was a time of political, economic, and social reform in the cities, the states, and the nation. It gained its first impetus at the local level in the 1890s, reached the national scene with the succession of Theodore Roosevelt as President in 1901, and lasted until 1917, when the United States entered the First World War. As a reform impulse, progessivism was primarily an urban, middle-class response to the abuses and evils that had sprung up in the wake of uncontrolled industrialization and metropolitan expansion after the Civil War.

The Crusade for Registration
Within nursing, reform was also needed. A large proportion of those who were practicing as "nurses" had never received any training, yet there were no legal restrictions against their presenting themselves to the public as fully trained graduates. Legislation to control the practice of nursing and the importance of having well-organized state associations to help secure it was recognized by the growing number of trained nurses. The idea of nurse registration to separate trained from untrained nurses was not a new one. It had been instituted in South Africa in 1891, and other countries had adopted it, in the following order: Natal (1899), New Zealand (1901), and Great Britain (1902). For the United States, however, such legislation would have to be handled on the state rather than the federal level.

In 1898 Sophia Palmer made the first public statement on the subject of nurse licensure in a paper read before the New York State Federation of Women's Clubs. As a result, the Federation passed a resolution favoring the establishment of a board of examiners chosen by the state society of nurses and recommending the inclusion of nursing in the list of professions supervised by the Board of Regents of the State University of New York.

An event that emphasized the need for immediate action by nurses to secure nurse registration occurred in 1900 when the Philadelphia County Medical Society and the College of Physicians of Philadelphia boldly announced that they were launching a school of nursing that would fully prepare students in only 10 weeks. At the same time, several correspondence schools began operations on

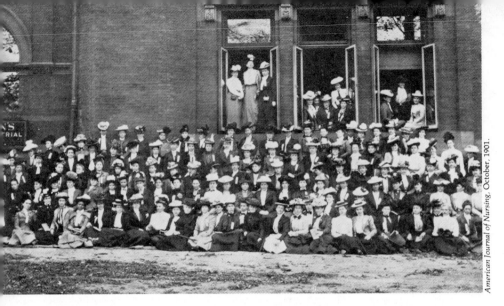

Delegates and visitors to the International Congress of Nurses, Buffalo, September, 1901.

a wide scale, advertising extensively with such promises as: "You can become a trained nurse by study at home. Send ten cents for handsome catalogue to the National Correspondence School of Health and Hygiene, 41 Telephone Building, Detroit, Michigan" [1]. The advertisement was illustrated with a nurse's cap, apron, badge, bottle, and spoon. The ten cent-fee quickly bought eager applicants the "handsome catalogue," which stated that for about $13 and a few "extras," anyone, regardless of age or physical condition, could become a trained nurse by a mere few months' "study at home." Every graduate would receive an impressive-looking diploma—that would often fool the public and discredit legitimate schools of nursing.

In September, 1901, the first meeting of the newly founded International Council of Nurses was held in Buffalo. Nurses in attendance were strongly encouraged to launch an effort to elevate and maintain the highest possible nursing standards. At one of the sessions, with many hundreds of nurses present, the following resolution in favor of state registration of nurses was proposed from the chair by Mrs. Bedford Fenwick of Great Britain, president of the Council:

Whereas the nursing of the sick is a matter closely affecting all classes of the community in every land; Whereas to be efficient workers, nurses should be carefully educated in the important duties which are now allotted to them; Whereas at the present time there is no generally accepted term or standard of training nor system of education nor examination for nurses in any country; Whereas there is no method, except in South Africa, of enabling the public to discriminate easily between trained nurses and ignorant persons who assume that title; and Whereas this is a fruitful source of injury to the sick and of discredit to the nursing profession, it is the opinion of this international congress of nurses, in general meeting assembled, that it is the duty of the nursing profession of every country to work for suitable legislative enactment regulating the education of nurses and protecting the interests of the public, by securing State examinations and public registration, with the proper penalties for enforcing the same [2].

Following the ICN congress, the introduction of nurse registration bills in the various state legislatures was generally preceded by the formation of state nurses' associations composed either of individuals or of individuals and organizations, such as alumnae associations. In North Carolina and New York, strong, widely representative graduate nurses' associations already in existence spearheaded the drive to gain passage of the legislation. North Carolina's was the first state nurses' association to present a bill before its legislature. The North Carolina nurse registration bill passed the State House of Representatives on January 20, 1903, with very little alteration. In the Senate a few weeks later, however, it met with strong opposition from the lobby of the state medical society, and finally a bill with much weaker provisions was substituted, which was passed in March of the same year. As signed by the governor, completion of a nurse training course was not required for registration. Any applicant, regardless of training or experience, who passed a state-administered examination was entitled to a certificate and a license to practice. The responsibility for developing the examinations and issuing licenses was assigned to a new board of nurse examiners, composed of two physicians and three nurses.

Among the initial state registration laws, New York State's legislation was

The nurse registration movement sends Sairy Gamp packing.

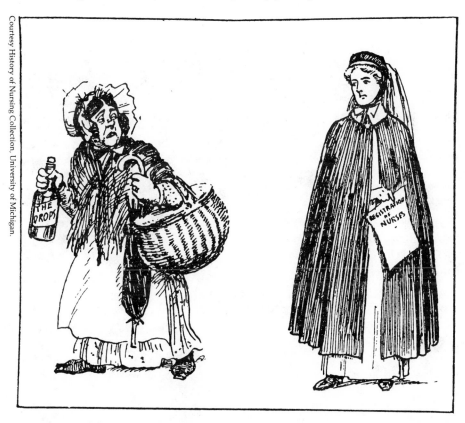

considered the most progressive. To be eligible for registration in New York, nurses had to be graduates of training schools approved by the Regents of the State University. Nurses who had been trained outside the state and who were engaged in institutional, private, or visiting nursing in New York were required to register in accordance with the law in order to continue their in-state work. Thus, schools from many of the other states in which these nurses had been trained soon applied to the Board of Regents for registration. In some instances they altered their methods of teaching and expanded their curricula in order to conform to New York State requirements.

These requirements, as defined by the State Board of Nurse Examiners, established the minimum amount of practice and theory instruction in subjects considered essential to developing professional knowledge. A course in obstetrics, not offered by many nurse training schools, was early made a curricular requirement by the State Board—bringing about new obstetrical nursing courses throughout the East. One large hospital that had met all New York requirements except experience in the nursing of sick children opened a children's ward to enable its students to receive state approval. As the result of a hard-fought battle with New York medical societies, the nurse examining board in New York was composed entirely of nurses.

Graduating class at St. Joseph's Hospital School of Nursing, Syracuse, New York, February, 1902.

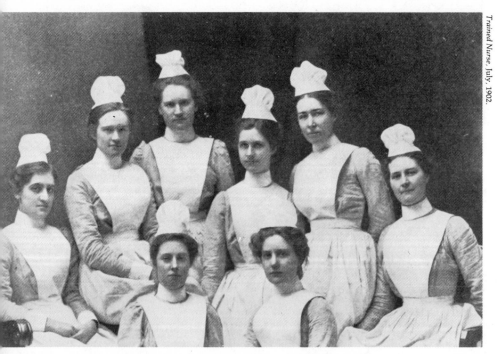

Trained Nurse, July, 1902.

But even this law was not fully satisfactory. The need for tightening up the registration laws was glaringly apparent. In New York in 1909, for example, there were registered nurses who had completed three-year courses, others who had finished two-year courses, and some who had received no formal nurse training at all, registering under a grandfather clause in the nurse registration act. Until the carry-over of nurses from preregistration days slowly ran through the active labor force, the effectiveness of the registration laws was dulled.

Postgraduate Problems

A second area of nursing in need of reform involved the nebulous concept of postgraduate training. The term *postgraduate* was applied indiscriminately to many clinical courses that were offered to diploma-holding nurses as substitutes for advanced nursing education. The level of achievement attained through many of these so-called postgraduate clinical courses could just as well have been gained through general staff nursing experience in a hospital offering good clinical experience together with an effective in-service staff education program. Most of these so-called postgraduate courses were characterized by service. The nurse went on duty at 7:00 A.M. and stayed until 7:00 P.M., completing the ward-scrubbing in addition to caring for the patients. She was often used, for the benefit of the hospital, to fill in gaps or to help out during vacations.

There was a tremendous lack of uniformity in the postgraduate courses conducted by various hospitals. In one 1905 postgraduate course, there was no allowance, while in another, $20 per month was offered. In still another, no provision was made for classwork, no lectures were given, no examinations were administered, yet certificates were awarded. A 1902 postgraduate course offered by the Woman's Hospital and Infant Home in Detroit included lectures by the specialists of the medical staff and classroom work with demonstrations given by the supervising nurse once a week. In addition, postgraduate students were allowed to attend the Farrand Training School lectures with the undergraduates.

An article entitled "My Impressions as a Postgraduate," published in the *American Journal of Nursing* in 1904, disclosed that:

There were classes and clinics both medical and surgical that we were privileged to attend. I went to a good many and liked going, but very often was too tired even when I had the time . . . . Could it not be possible to shorten the hours of graduates, giving them more time for study and making it compulsory to attend certain classes and clinics? To partly cover the expenses I would suggest that an entrance fee be charged [3].

The results of a 1905 survey of postgraduate courses in 114 general hospitals and 20 special hospitals revealed that, among general hospitals of 100 beds or more, 26 gave a supplementary postgraduate course, only three of which made

. . . any provision for a regular course of lectures and class work. The others permit the graduates to attend the lectures and classes of the pupil nurses, but as many of the schools

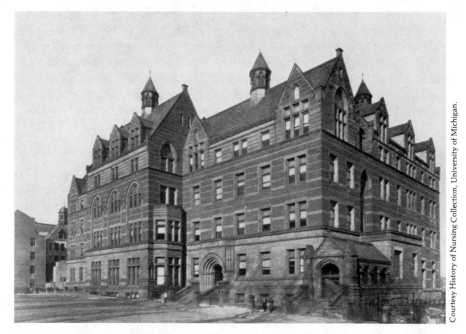

Teachers College, Columbia University, in 1899 established a course to prepare superintendents of nurse training schools.

admit graduate nurses only during the vacation season, there are no lectures and classes to attend . . . In one, a fee is charged of one dollar per day, while in others we find allowances given of varying amounts to as much as twenty dollars a month [4].

Nurse training school superintendents who were finding it difficult to secure competent assistants and head nurses felt that postgraduate courses in which the nurse could secure expertise in the art of hospital housekeeping were absolutely essential. An ideal course would include information about the various hospital departments: kitchen and laundry, storerooms and linen rooms, as well as details such as cutting and making hospital garments, ordering supplies, and learning the business management of hospitals. Such training would allow hospitals to fill their nursing administration positions with qualified graduate nurses.

In 1899, as a result of this obvious need, a course in hospital economy was established at Teachers College, Columbia University, through the efforts of the American Society of Superintendents of Training Schools for Nurses, for the purpose of preparing graduate nurses to become teachers in training schools and superintendents of nursing in hospitals. Its eventual aim was to attain uniformity in training school methods so that nurses graduating from a school connected with any general hospital would be similarly trained.

The Society appointed a board of examiners, whose duty was to select all candidates for the Teachers College course. The board required the aspiring superintendent to enter Teachers College for a full term of eight months. It also stipulated that either before or after this term she was to spend from three to four months in private duty nursing. After this year of extra education and experience, and if she passed the required final examinations, the nurse received a certificate, signed by the Dean of Teachers College, Columbia University, attesting to her qualifications as a superintendent for either a training school for nurses or a hospital.

The general supervision of this course was in the hands of Anna L. Alline, instructor of hospital economics, who supplemented the work of the special lecturers and conducted excursions and field work in various hospitals and health agencies. The course covered subjects such as the preparation of culture media, the isolation and culture of bacteria, and the preparation of antitoxins. Visits were made to laboratories preparing modified, sterilized, and pasteurized milk. A survey of various types of hospitals, including general, private, and special hospitals, mental institutions, and others, identified the unique nursing service demands of each. Special lectures were given on the following topics: hospital construction, four lectures by Eva Allerton of the Rochester Homeopathic Hospital; the history of hospitals, three lectures by Adelaide Nutting of Johns Hopkins Hospital; a study of hospital administration, six lectures by Maud Banfield of the Polyclinic Hospital in Philadelphia; and a practical exposition of training school administration, eight lectures offered jointly by Isabel Hampton Robb of Cleveland and Lucy Walker of the Pennsylvania Hospital.

In 1910 a $150,000 endowment by Helen Hartley Jenkins, a trustee of Teachers College, allowed the postgraduate course to be expanded in length and quality. This gift marked the first substantial financial provision for any part of the education of nurses. A new department of nursing and health was created at Teachers College, embracing three main divisions of work and preparing nurses for teaching and supervision in nurse training schools, for administration in hospitals and training schools, and for work in the social and preventive branches of nursing. Adelaide Nutting, former superintendent of nurses and principal of the Training School for Nurses at Johns Hopkins Hospital from 1894 to 1907, who had come to Teachers College three years earlier as professor of hospital economics, was now appointed to head the new department of nursing and health. Under her leadership the nursing program at Teachers College soon became the world leader in preparing nurse educators.

Reform of Medical Education

Criticism of the low standards prevailing in the field of medical education had also been heard, but no one fully realized how shoddy conditions were until Abraham Flexner, with the support of a grant from the Carnegie Foundation, began a nation-wide investigation. After a preliminary period of careful study and preparation, Flexner proceeded on a swift tour of medical schools in the United States and Canada. He had no fixed pattern and used no questionnaire in his investigation, yet he personally visited every one of the 155 schools and talked, in each instance, with medical school faculty members and their students.

Flexner soon came to realize that five points were conclusive in judging the quality and value of a medical school, all of which were just as pertinent for nursing education:

First, the entrance requirements. What are they? Are they enforced?

Second, the size and training of the faculty.

Third, the sum available from endowment and fees for the support of the institution, and what becomes of it.

Fourth, the quality and adequacy of the laboratories provided for the instruction of the first two years and the qualifications and training of the teachers of the so-called preclinical branches.

Fifth, the relation between medical schools and hospitals, particularly including freedom of access to beds and freedom in the appointment by the school of the hospital physicians and surgeons who automatically should become clinical teachers [5].

The conditions depicted by Flexner in his 1910 report were shocking, and he pulled no punches in applying words such as "disgraceful" and "shameful." For example, the city of Chicago, with its 14 medical schools, was described as "the plague spot of the country." He found that entrance requirements were enforced in only 10 of the 155 medical schools in the United States and Canada. Libraries were inadequate or nonexistent in 140 of the schools, and laboratory courses for the first and second years were deplorably equipped and poorly conducted in 139 of the schools.

Part II of the report lashed out at specific abuses found in each school:

California Medical College (Los Angeles)—This school had led a roving and precarious existence . . . a disgrace to the state whose laws permit its existence.

Georgetown University School of Medicine—There is no library accessible to students, no museum, and no pharmacological laboratory.

Georgia College of Eclectic Medicine and Surgery (Atlanta)—Its anatomy room, containing a single cadaver, is indescribably foul . . . . Nothing more disgraceful calling itself a medical school can be found anywhere.

Kansas Medical College (Topeka)—The dissecting room is indescribably filthy; it contained, in addition to necessary tables, a single, badly hacked cadaver and was simultaneously used as a chicken yard.

Maryland Medical College (Baltimore)—The school building is wretchedly dirty . . . one neglected and filthy room is set aside for bacteriology, pathology, and histology: a few dirty test-tubes stand around in pans and old cigar-boxes.

St. Louis College of Physicians and Surgeons—The school is one of the worst in the country.

Pulte Medical College (Cincinnati)—Anything more woe-begone than the laboratories of this institution would be difficult to imagine. The dissecting room is a dark apartment in the basement.

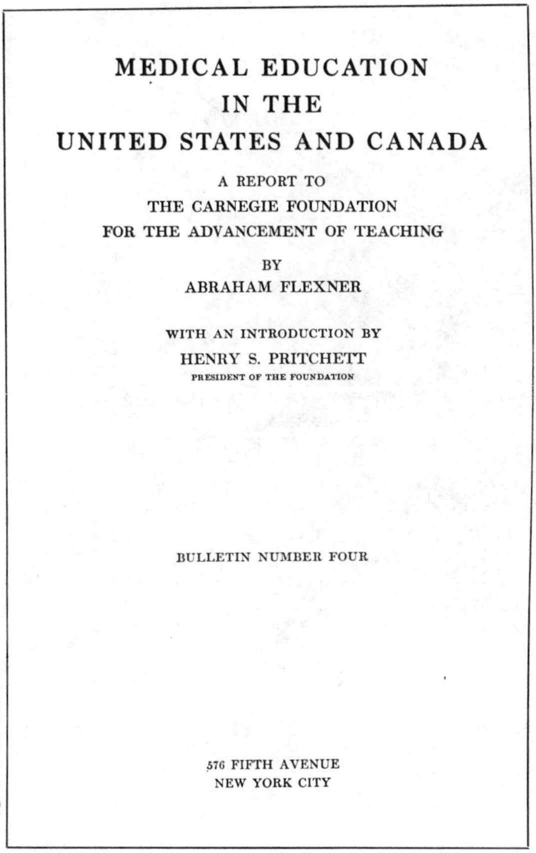

MEDICAL EDUCATION
IN THE
UNITED STATES AND CANADA

A REPORT TO
THE CARNEGIE FOUNDATION
FOR THE ADVANCEMENT OF TEACHING

BY
ABRAHAM FLEXNER

WITH AN INTRODUCTION BY
HENRY S. PRITCHETT
PRESIDENT OF THE FOUNDATION

BULLETIN NUMBER FOUR

576 FIFTH AVENUE
NEW YORK CITY

Carnegie Foundation, 1910.

The Flexner Report wrought a revolution in medical education standards.

Flexner's report contained such candid and drastic criticism of the defects of medical education in North America that the weaker schools were unable to continue. Of the recognized schools that survived, some merged for mutual strengthening, and most secured university connections. All became nonprofit institutions. In his preface to the Flexner report, Henry S. Pritchett, president of the Carnegie Foundation, anticipated such changes when he stated that "progress for the future would seem to require a very much smaller number of medical schools, better equipped and better conducted than our schools now as a rule are; and the needs of the public would equally require that we have fewer physicians graduated each year, but that these should be better educated and better trained" [6].

The decade from 1910 to 1920 saw the establishment of medical education as a university discipline with definite educational standards, but only the better-financed and better-led schools were able to develop adequate laboratories and hospital affiliations in order to achieve the requisite quality of medical education. The number of inferior schools quickly dwindled.

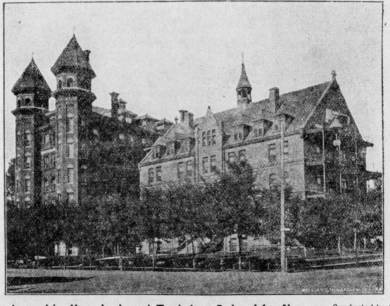

Advertisement for St. Joseph's Hospital and Training School for Nurses, Denver, about 1910.

A Flexner Report for Nursing?

Leading nurse educators were enthusiastic for a similar comprehensive survey of schools of nursing to be made. In 1911 the American Society of Superintendents of Training Schools for Nurses presented a proposal for such a study to the Carnegie Foundation in hopes of securing assistance. Adelaide Nutting reported the results of this effort in a report at the annual convention of the superintendents in 1912. She related to the group that President Pritchett "seemed much interested in the matter, but stated that the Foundation was at the time unable to take the question up [as] all of its energies were centered in work in other directions."

The following year Miss Nutting told the assembled nurse educators: "Realizing the enormous benefit to medical education resulting from such an investigation of medical schools by the Carnegie Foundation, the Committee is confident that similar benefits must result from such an investigation of our much more complicated educational problems" [7]. Meanwhile, Pritchett directed a considerable amount of Carnegie Foundation funds into "Flexner-like" studies of dental, legal, and teacher education and passively ignored the pleas of nurses.

Training School Life in the Progressive Era

According to the second edition of the *American Medical Directory*, by 1909 the number of general hospitals in the United States had increased to 4359, 1006 of which operated nurse training schools. In addition, 90 mental institutions ran schools. A typical hospital school of nursing in a smaller city of the era required two years of high school for admission along with evidence of "careful home training" and a "definite knowledge of housekeeping duties." Students were admitted between the ages of 18 and 35.

When a candidate made application for training, she was sent the usual application blank and physician's certificate form. If her responses to these, together with the required references, were satisfactory, arrangements were made for a personal interview. When a class of probationers entered training, all entrance credentials, application blanks, references, and entrance examination papers were filed, each set in its own large envelope. With the exception of maintenance, textbooks, and uniforms, the probationers received no financial compensation during the first year. The second year they received a monthly allowance of $7.50, and the third year it was raised to $15. The school had found that the absence of any allowance during the entire first year did much to discourage those who might have entered nursing for financial reasons.

Two classes of probationers were admitted yearly, one entering September 1, and the other February 1. The superintendent always met a new class of probationers personally and gave them an informal word of welcome and encouragement. This was followed by a weekly class in ethics, which covered many important and necessary dos and don'ts.

In the first two weeks after admission, probationers were not allowed to be on the wards for more than one or two hours a day. This orientation period was only long enough to permit them to become somewhat familiar with hospital customs. During this time they were not assigned to care for patients but were shown how to keep a ward in order, how to care for flowers and patients' belongings, and other minor details. Their hours and duties on the ward were gradually increased during the next two months, until, at the end of their third month, they were in the wards from six to seven hours daily. During this time they attended classes in nursing and were taken by the assistant superintendent into the wards, where they were taught to put the latest lesson into practice.

During their third month, the head nurse, who was a third-year nursing student, supervised the work of these new students, as directed by the assistant superintendent. At the end of their third month, an examination was held on all subjects taught up to that time. If this was passed satisfactorily, and if her clinical performance and personality were also considered satisfactory, the probationer was accepted as a student nurse.

The school gave a three-year course of training, which included three months of probation, although the entire first six months were considered to be a preparatory course. The curriculum of this typical school was as follows [8]:

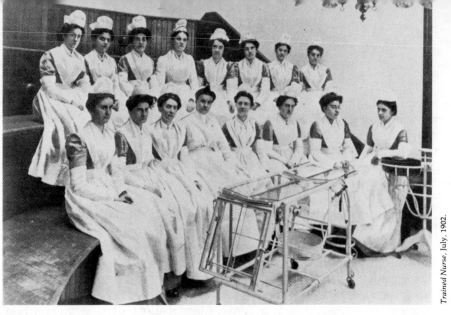

A class in session at the Newark City Hospital School of Nursing, about 1902.

Preparatory Class
Anatomy and Physiology	15 hours
Solutions	7 hours
Practical Nursing	24 hours
Theoretical Nursing	24 hours
Preparatory Materia Medica	6 hours
Nursing Ethics and Hygiene	10 hours
Principles of Cookery and Dietetics	20 hours
Bacteriology and Urinalysis	12 hours

Junior Class
Anatomy and Physiology continued	20 hours
Principles of Cookery and Dietetics	20 hours
Surgical Nursing and Bandaging	16 hours
Obstetrical Nursing	6 hours

Intermediate Class
Medical Diseases and Contagion	7 lectures
Surgery	10 lectures
Obstetrics	12 lectures
Gynecology	4 lectures
Pediatrics	5 lectures
Eye, Ear, Nose, and Throat	5 lectures
Materia Medica, Regular	12 lectures

Senior Class
Massage, Hydrotherapy	20 hours
Advanced Nursing, with lectures on nursing, topics of day and current events	12 hours

The course of instruction was taught according to the following arrangement:

Nursing Ethics
Hygiene
History of Nursing, with lectures on   } Superintendent
   special nursing topics and current events

Theoretical Nursing
Practical Nursing
Solutions   } Assistant
Preliminary Materia Medica   Superintendent
Practical Obstetrical Nursing
Practical Ward Surgery

Surgical Technic
Bandaging   } Surgical Supervisor

Massage and Hydrotherapy   Special Hydrotherapy Nurse

Dietetics—chemistry of food
Cookery—preparing of invalid diet   } Instructor from the Manual Training School

Anatomy and Physiology
Materia Medica—regular and homeopathic
Medical Diseases
Contagious Diseases
Surgery
Gynecology   } Physician's Lectures
Obstetrics
Bacteriology
Urinalysis
Eye, Ear, Nose, and Throat

   The staff of the training school consisted of the superintendent of nursing for the hospital and training school, the surgical supervisor, and the night superintendent—all registered nurses—and one graduate dietitian. The school's enrollment averaged about 22 student nurses. There were no full-time teachers. The larger part of the teaching and actual nursing supervision was in the hands of the assistant superintendent. An authoritarian atmosphere was insured by assigning one of the graduate nurses to be in charge of the students at all times. In the operating room, the instruction in surgical technique was given by the surgical supervisor, and while on night duty the nurses were entirely responsible to the night superintendent, receiving all necessary instructions from her.

   The hospital utilized a nine-hour day, but the nurses were on actual duty 56 hours per week, each nurse being allowed three hours for meals and rest daily, a half-day off on Sunday, and an additional half-day off during the week. A student nurse assigned to a special patient was always given eight consecutive hours of rest daily and one day off for every seven days on the case. Required night duty amounted to six weeks of continuous duty for juniors, with three days off when the service was terminated, and eight continuous weeks for seniors, with a four-day rest upon completion.

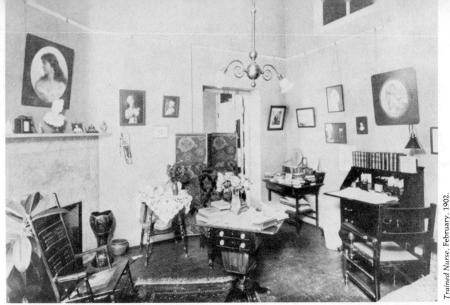

Superintendent Nurse's Room, Margaret Fahnestock Training School, New York Post-graduate Hospital.

In common with all other training schools, this institution had a strict set of rules, which were read to the probationers during their first week of training. So far as possible, the hospital superintendent tried to make the school self-governing. One of the first things she told a class of probationers was that every nurse in the school was on her honor—if it was found that a nurse could not or would not voluntarily act in an honorable manner, she would be expelled. There was also a special set of rules for the guidance of advanced students, who functioned in the role of head nurses:

The head nurse is to be on duty promptly at 7:00 A.M. and immediately to assign morning work to senior and junior nurses.

To take report from night nurse and see that charting room and lavatory are in order, and fresh towels ready for doctor's use, nurse's table in order, etc.

At 7:15 take charge of diet kitchen and at all times to *personally supervise and assist* in serving trays, making sure that all food is hot, nicely cooked and served, and that each patient is getting correct diet as prescribed by doctor; to carefully instruct juniors in proper tray service and to see that all helpless patients are fed; to make a room-to-room trip after trays are served to see that patients have eaten and enjoyed meals.

To give all medication occurring before and to 9:00 A.M. inclusive.

To take all T.P.R.'s up through that hour.

To make up all drug lists, requisition lists, etc.

To write up all charts to 9:00 A.M. inclusive.

To be entirely responsible for cleanliness of drug closet.

To prepare surgical trays and take charge of surgical dressings.

To make rounds with doctors and superintendent, reporting carefully about patients.

To see that all doctors' orders are carried out at the earliest possible moment, and to carefully supervise and direct nurses doing same, and to assume care of certain patients whenever necessary.

The head nurse is absolutely responsible for the comfort and welfare of all patients entrusted to her care.

She is to practice and to insist upon the greatest care and economy in the use of all hospital supplies.

She is to report any failure to carry out doctors' orders, with any reasons for same, at the earliest possible moment; also any sudden change in patients' condition or any high temperature to house surgeon and superintendent.

To inspect all beds and backs of all bed patients at least once daily.

To *immediately* report any accident happening to any patient under her charge to house surgeon and superintendent.

To write up night orders and diet slips.

To give personal supervision to all work done by nurses and orderlies or ward maids; to see that work is arranged so that day nurses can get off duty promptly at 7:00 P.M., and never go off duty, unless told to do so by supervisor.

To report to dietitian immediately any unsatisfactory diet, shortage, etc., and, in the event of repeated trouble, to report to supervisor; to make out all diet lists, ordering only the probable amount of extras needed, and practice judgment and economy in ordering of food and supplies.

To get a signed order from superintendent for any rush or special work from laundry.

To see that linen is carefully used and to have all torn or ragged articles placed in a bag for repair or to be replaced; to see that all private room patients are bathed every day and ward patients twice a week; bed patients given alcohol rub every night.

In absence of the senior nurse, her duties are to be assumed or arranged for her by the head nurse.

One of the most important duties of the head nurse is to keep the assistant superintendent informed at all times about any matter of interest or importance on her floor; any reports or complaints from patients or doctors must *always* be immediately referred to assistant superintendent; also any shortages of working materials, medicines, linen, supplies, etc.

The head nurse is to insist upon order and quiet at all times, and must eliminate all unnecessary noises, such as loud talking, rattling of dishes, utensils, etc. The head nurse should stand out as a leader, from the standpoint of efficiency, ethics, and good breeding, by her own personal example and precept.

The duties of the senior nurse were somewhat less responsible than those of the head nurse, but still very demanding:

The senior nurse is to assume duties and responsibilities of head nurse when she is absent or off duty.

To take charge of the most ill patients as assigned by head nurse. (Probably three, in emergencies, four.)

To take all T.P.R's except those previous to 9:00 A.M.

To assist when necessary in making rounds with doctors and in preparing dressings, trays, and doing surgical dressings.

To give all unusual or special treatments.

To prepare patients for operation, and take them to operating room when necessary.

To be responsible for caring for work of juniors when they are off duty.

To see that all charting after 9:00 A.M. is kept up at all hours of the day.

To keep dressing trays set up and look after all surgical instruments and supplies, and see that all such supplies are left ready for the night nurse.

The juniors were charged with the following duties, which reflected the decreasing degree of authority:

The juniors will be responsible for any of the senior work during absence of senior, or any other work arranged by head nurse.

To care for patients as assigned by head nurse; to do work thoroughly and quickly, and have patients comfortable and well cared for at all times; also to have private rooms and wards in strictest order.

When two juniors are on a floor, one shall be responsible for the diet kitchen and linen closet, and the other for the bathrooms and utensils.

To give any medication or treatment directed by head nurse and, if directed to do so, to keep up patient's charge after 9:00 A.M.

To keep head nurse carefully informed as to patient's condition at all times. If any bed patient shows the least tendency to bed sores, same to be immediately reported to head nurse.

The lowly duties of the probationers demanded a strong back and very little thinking:

Probationers are to dust rooms, arrange flowers, put empty beds and rooms in order, and care for bathrooms, diet kitchen, linen closets, and chart rooms; also to have such other duties concerning the personal care and treatment of patients as arranged for by superintendent with head nurse for the application of the principles of nursing as taught [9].

The school taught the students to be prompt and careful in carrying out physicians' orders. The head nurse or senior on the ward made the rounds with the various members of the medical staff, waiting on them as necessary. Before leaving the floor, the physician wrote his own orders in the order book or requested the house physician to do so. The nurse who carried out the order initialed it in red ink and also noted the hour. By means of this simple plan it could be immediately ascertained, should any question arise, which nurse had carried out the order.

Complaints from physicians were generally made personally to the superintendent or her assistant. When a patient's complaint reached the head nurse, it was immediately reported for investigation; when a complaint concerned a

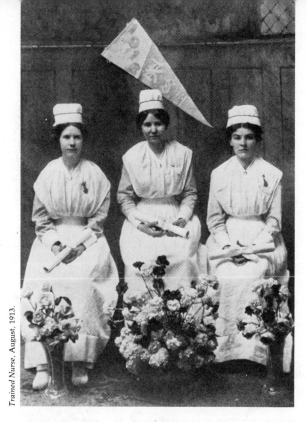

The black band on the caps of head nurses was worn proudly—Graduating Class, Kane Summit Hospital, Kane, Pennsylvania, 1913.

specific nurse, she was requested to reply in writing. If the mistake made was of a serious nature, the nurse was removed from duty by the superintendent until the matter had been fully investigated. In the third year of training, the students were given black bands for their caps, designating them as head nurses, and the greatest punishment that could possibly befall a third-year nurse was to have her black band taken away. The most common method of discipline for any serious misdemeanor was to extend the nurses' period of service from two to four weeks.

Waste of the Nurse's Energy

A great deal of unnecessary energy was expended by nurses on ward duty. In 1913 one enterpising physician attacked what he called a lack of cooperation on the part of training school authorities in implementing conservation of energy on hospital wards, especially in matters concerning the comfort of patients. He placed pedometers on nurses in several hospitals and discovered that in a single day one of the nurses walked seven and one-half miles while the average nurse walked some five and one-half miles.

In one hospital, this investigator discovered that a ward was so long that the farthest bed was 120 feet from the ward kitchen. Worse still, hospital custom required that trays be carried individually to and from each bed three times a day. He added up the unnecessary walking required of the ward nurse and found that it amounted to about two miles a day. The food trays and their contents were found to weigh 15 pounds. Thus the nurse had to haul considerable weight for two extra miles. When he suggested that wheel trucks be used to carry all the trays at one time, the objection was that the food would reach the patients cold. Similarly, the bedscreens weighed 31 pounds, and, since it took three screens to surround a bed when a patient used the bedpan, the nurse had to carry 93 pounds to and from his bed and then, of course, carry the bedpan back and forth, walking a total distance of 480 feet.

A Walk around the Wards

Let us walk the wards of a big city hospital with one of the nurses of this period by leafing through the pages of her diary.

February 10—Monday—My funny Irish woman, Mrs. Maloney, is much dissatisfied with the nurses and doctors. She says they ought to be middle-aged people. We had a horrid afternoon, a rushing, tumbling kind. I had to fly to get around, yet the patients were unusually kind. Bridget encouraged me in her rough way. Poor Alice had a sinking spell and was so sick.

February 11—Tuesday—A probationer was put into our ward and under my special care. I am having good times teaching her, for she is so nice and quick to learn. We have a patient poisoned with carbolic acid, who is doing nicely. Alice is better.

February 12—Wednesay—Chaos, rushing, and weariness! Another case of attempted suicide.

February 13—Thursday—A little negro girl, one of my patients, died this morning. She had only been in a day and was very sick, poor child. She had told me while I was trying to clean her nails, against her express desire, that I was not a good nurse, being too determined. A new stretcher case was brought in. It is the worst morning we have had. Poor Miss Dunstan gave up and cried.

February 14—Friday—Miss Thayer is back, and we are so glad. Things will go better now. Our nice little probationer has patients of her own and is doing beautifully. Poor Nellie is very much worse. I have had such a fancy for the child ever since she came in, and she has wanted me to do everything for her. She is delirious now, and knows no one; I do hope she will get well. I bathed five and one-half people this morning. One woman I fixed had a double nail on one toe and she told me she used to have six toes on her left foot, but one had been amputated.

February 15—Saturday—We didn't half get through our work. We had four new cases, one on a stretcher and two in wheelchairs. Seven of the patients have to sleep on the floor. We have over sixty.

February 16—Sunday—Was on in the morning and the work went beautifully.

February 17—Monday—Alice gave me fifty cents to spend for her, and asked me to get two envelopes, two sheets of paper, two stamps, a can of honey, and some gingersnaps. Nellie knew me for the first time in ever so long, but she is no better.

February 18—Tuesday—Miss Thayer called the nurses together and told us we *must* finish our work on time. Then she divided it differently and gave me two private rooms and four patients in the ward. That gives me ten patients in all; six are typhoids, and all are very sick. Nellie is my patient now, but is too sick to know it. I have a homesick little Bohemian, and a repulsive paralyzed woman. Two of my patients have bedsores that have to be dressed every day.

February 19—Wednesday—We watched all day a threatened case of abortion, but it didn't come off before we came away.

February 20—Thursday—Miss Dunstan, our senior nurse, is sick, so I have the senior work—medicines, temperatures, and the private rooms. Our ward is so full that eight sick patients have to sleep on the floor. We had to send away two of our best help, the night woman and the kitchen woman, because they fight so. Our case of abortion still hangs on.

February 21—Friday—I have Annie to care for now, and she is funnier than ever. She is a little delirious yet, and when she does anything horrid and I talk to her about it, she opens her big black eyes and says, "Forgive me, nurse." Miss Drake telephoned to Miss Thayer, who was taking her half day, that she must come back, and she did. Finally, Miss Fife appeared on the scene with uplifted hands and a look of horror, saying, "Really, Miss Thayer, Ward E will drive me distracted." When they had gone, we laughed, for we didn't feel a bit guilty; we had worked so hard and every necessary thing was done, though things did look horrid.

Washington's Birthday—Saturday—I was on the morning and spent most of my time over Frances, giving her stimulants and hypodermic injections. We have sixty-five patients now. An extra row of beds has been put down the middle of the ward.

February 23—Sunday—I was on in the morning again and had a terrific time getting through. I had to keep up poultices and fomentations, besides fixing fourteen patients. Poor Frances died last night.

February 24—Monday—They have moved two very sick patients from the ward into my rooms and my hands are full. They have to have turpentine stupes kept up day and night. Nellie got out of bed today under the delusion that she had to move to Broadway. I had to tie her in bed after that. I tied one foot to the foot of the bed. Some time after, I found her looking sadly at the foot, and she said to me, "Nurse, won't you please release this prisoner? He has been tried and has proved himself clear; he was only one of a gang." It is very odd that though she is all the time delirious, she knows me, and though she won't answer one of my questions sensibly, she will take anything I give her, and makes a great fuss with any one else. Our abortion woman departed in pretty good health today.

February 25—Tuesday—A horrid, vile day. I was so tired my legs wouldn't walk, and my arms wouldn't work, and I had so much to do. In the afternoon Miss Thayer asked me to print some labels, and then when I started, she sent me on errands everywhere, and each time I went through the ward half a dozen patients would shout at me for something.

February 26—Wednesday—Poor little 43, a Swedish girl, with golden hair and blue eyes, is getting worse so fast. I have to give her milk every fifteen minutes and a stupe every hour; 41 is very sick too.

February 27—Thursday—41 died last night. I feel so sorry that I ever pulled her hair. It used to get so tangled I could hardly help it. The little Swedish girl is dying. Her doctor does not believe in stimulants, so we have just had to watch her grow worse and worse without doing anything for her. It does seem wicked. The two patients in my middle room always amuse me so much—Nellie, and Bohemian Mary. I made some lemonade for them today, and they were perfectly delighted. I used to think Mary was very stupid, but she talks a little now in her broken English and says I am "awfoo good," which makes me as happy as anything I have ever heard. She has a dreadful bed-sore.

February 28—Friday—Nellie grows more amusing every day. She begs me every morning to make her some "clarimot," which is as near as she can get to lemonade. She asked Miss Gault today to bring her a few squirts of water. Mary is ever so much better, but her back is dreadful. She says it is "no good." Sophie went away today; she has been one of my favorite patients, so pretty and timid and willing. She scrubbed my tables and chairs for me before she went. Annie was funny, too, today. When she did something she ought not and I said, "Oh, Annie!" she replied, "Poor little Annie's got to die." While I was changing the sheets, she tried to console me by throwing kisses.

I did not half finish my work today, but the patients have been so nice to me. One woman in the ward never fails to smile when I go by, because when she first came I would not let them cut her hair, which was fearfully tangled, but after a half hour's tug got it smooth [10].

The Rise of Women's Rights

Student nurses were classed as employees by the Bureau of the Census. According to the Bureau, in 1909, 20.6 percent of the nation's 6,615,046 wage earners were female. Of the total work force, about 2.1 percent were children under 16 years of age. The number of women engaged in gainful occupations had increased rather steadily since 1870. In that year, only 13 percent of the gainfully employed workers were female, but by 1910 the number had increased to over 20 percent. More than half the workers in 12 of the nation's 88 leading industries were women, and nursing was almost entirely in the hands of women. Large numbers of women were also employed in various aspects of the textile industry, in canning and preserving, in confectionary, and in the manufacture of tobacco products.

The fact that divorce had increased from 27 to 86 per 100,000 population from 1867 to 1906 reflected the liberalization of divorce laws. There had been fewer than 10,000 divorces in 1867, when divorce had meant social ostracism. By 1907 over 72,000 divorces were granted in the United States—more than in all the rest of the Christian world. In part, this trend reflected the loosening of economic and religious bonds and the sharp increase in careers open to women who chafed against the restraints of unhappy marriages. The growing insistence on a single moral standard led legislatures to relax the procedural requirements of having to establish adultery, as well as desertion and cruelty, as grounds for divorce. The waiting period for divorces was usually a year, although ordinances in Reno, Nevada, cut this in half during the early 1900s. Divorces were most frequent in the individualistic, newer sections of the country, such as the West and the large cities.

Conservative churches, among them the Roman Catholic and Lutheran, tried to check the official divorce rate, but they could not halt the sensational increase in desertion, "the poor man's divorce." Desertion—at least four times more common than divorce—seemed to thrive in the unstable social environments of unemployed or migratory factory hands and broken immigrant homes.

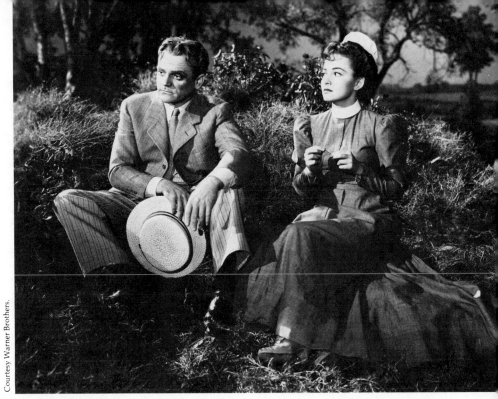

"A nurse! Twenty-three skidoo!" In the early 1900s the matrimonial prospects of nurses were inordinately low, a theme brilliantly reflected in James Cagney's initial lack of interest in Oliva De Havilland in the 1941 film The Strawberry Blonde. *(From the Warner Brothers release* The Strawberry Blonde © *1941 Warner Bros. Pictures, Inc. Copyright renewed 1968.)*

Many regarded increased divorce as evidence that unhappiness in marriage was greater than ever before. Others asserted that there had always been a great many unhappy marriages, and that the high divorce rate meant only that more people were taking the legal way out of an unfortunate situation.

Matrimony and the Nurse

Whenever a nurse and her patient married, newspapers were inclined to treat the incident as a romance, and the reading public, forgetting that the atypical was always more newsworthy, often came to regard matrimony as the ultimate goal of all trained nurses. The reverse was true, according to a 1916 investigation published in the *Journal of Heredity*, which found that fewer than half of the graduates of the best nurse training schools had married. The lowest number of married graduates, 21 percent, was reported at the training school of Washington University in Saint Louis, while the highest, 52 percent, was recorded at Saint Luke's Hospital Nurse Training School in New York.

The *Journal of Heredity* investigator observed that no amount of optimism could bring one to conclude that the marriage rate of trained nurses—or at least of the graduates of the best training schools—was even reasonably high. Ironically, it was generally felt that the education of a nurse prepared her admirably for homemaking and motherhood. While the investigator postulated that nurses should have been in great demand as wives, the extraordinary infrequency of marriages suggested that men did not use good judgment in selecting mates. It was possible that there was something in a nurse's education to which men objected; it was also possible that many nurses preferred to remain single. It was thought that their remaining single could not be largely due to a lack of opportunities to meet men, for, indeed, such opportunities appeared to be plentiful.

Any attempt to analyze the causes of this low marriage rate were considered futile until more solid data were available; however, there was one simple cause suspected—age. Ten or 15 years before this report, the age of admission to good training schools had often been from 21 to 25 years. The average age of nurses at graduation was certainly not less than 25. Nurses who graduated in classes before 1902 were already, therefore, well toward the end of the most marriageable period of a woman's life. More recently, training schools had been reducing the age standards, 20 perhaps being an average minimum, while many schools had begun to admit students at the age of 19. The average age of graduates at the time of the *Journal of Heredity* investigation was about 23. It was thought that this lowering of age alone would soon tend to increase the marriage rate of the more recent graduates.

The Progressive Impact on Nursing

There were implications for nursing in the 1908 Supreme Court case of *Muller* v. *Oregon*, which involved a state law limiting women factory workers to a 10-hour day. The case was notable for the presentation made by Louis D. Brandeis of a heavily documented brief that forcefully argued from factual evidence rather than from legal deduction that long hours of work were detrimental to both the health of women and the general welfare. The "Brandeis Brief" became a landmark in the practical application of "sociological jurisprudence." The Court upheld the Oregon law and, by accepting the Brandeis Brief, gave judicial cognizance to a type of concrete presentation that other progressive lawyers learned to use to good effect.

Much of the data for the Brandeis Brief had been gathered by Josephine Goldmark, Brandeis' sister-in-law. Josephine, along with another sister, Pauline, did important work with Florence Kelley in the National Consumers' League, staying on to eventually become chairman of the League's committee on the legal defense of labor laws. Miss Goldmark's book, *Fatigue and Efficiency*, based on this experience and written in collaboration with Brandeis, was destined to become a source book of great value in framing protective legislation for women. The decision in *Muller* v. *Oregon* opened the way to a surge of protective legislation. Between 1908 and 1917, 39 states either passed new laws or strengthened old ones regulating the hours of women's work.

In 1910 a special federal investigation of occupations that were "morally dangerous" for women concluded that nursing was a job entailing moral risk.

Five types of morally dangerous work were assigned by different social and rescue workers: domestic service, the work of hotel or restaurant waitresses, the lowgrade factory trades, trained nursing, and the less desirable stenographic positions. The report expressed some surprise at having found trained nursing to be a calling in which women were especially likely to "go wrong," but it had been so identified in several places, all large cities. The investigators had therefore concluded that there seemed to be good reason to look at nursing as a somewhat dangerous pursuit.

The nurse was subjected to periods of long and exhausting mental strain along with a great amount of hard physical work. Her position made it convenient for her to secure drugs and liquors, and the nature of her work created a special demand for stimulants or restoratives. It was easy for her "to become a hard drinker or a drug fiend, and when a woman adopts either habit the chances of her going wrong in other ways are much increased." Also, the nurse, like the domestic servant, was "in a position which makes it easy for men to essay advances toward her if they have any desire in that direction." She did not have the protection of working in public that was afforded by the factory or the department store, and, when she was nursing a man, "opportunities for complications are evident" [11]. In light of this kind of reputation it was no wonder that the pendulum of morality swung to a nearly monastic extreme in many training schools.

California Leads the Way

Although progressive states attempted to minimize the most outrageous and indefensible forms of exploitation of the working population, they largely bypassed the hospitals. One notable exception to this indifference took place in California. In 1911 a bill was passed in the California legislature that was known as the "Eight-Hour Law for Women." This bill, which in the course of time became law, limited the working hours of women employed in any mercantile, mechanical, or manufacturing establishment or office to eight hours a day for six days in the week.

Early in 1912 the first indications of a movement to extend to student nurses the protection of the eight-hour law were revealed in certain communications between California progressives and several state nursing organizations. Such an amendment was introduced in the legislature in 1913 on behalf of the California Bureau of Labor. Investigation revealed that in many California hospitals the hours of student nurses were excessive because it was general practice to use students as special private duty nurses. It was said that the income of certain proprietary hospitals accrued almost entirely from this practice. For the benefit of the student nurse herself, as well as for the good of the patient, it seemed essential that these young women have the same protection as that given to almost all other working women in California.

The bill was fought bitterly by commercial hospitals in the state. Even the Nurses' Association of Southern California sent a petition against its passage.

In addition, hospitals submitted petitions signed by hundreds of undergraduate nurses opposing the measure. A small group of graduate nurses in San Francisco and Alameda counties provided the only visible support that proponents of the bill could garner from the nursing profession.

One reason for this was the argument, voiced by many hospital physicians, that the nursing profession would be debased by its inclusion in a law that could be enforced by the State Bureau of Labor. Many nurses agreed and were honestly incensed by the Bureau's action. The bill had the support of a few progressive physicians, but for the most part the medical profession vigorously opposed the measure.

The bill was introduced in the California Senate by Henry H. Lyon of Los Angeles and in the House by Assemblyman Walter McDonald of San Francisco. Debate in the Senate was heated, and the bill was impeded in its progress by a phalanx of opposition members. Senator Lyon, who championed the bill, reviewed the situation in the hospitals of the state, pointing out the long hours of labor required by student nurses, the money earned by them for their institution, and the pittance, barely enough to cover the cost of uniforms and books, paid to them. He urged speedy passage of the bill but was blocked at the outset by an amendment proposing that hospitals be exempted from the operation of the law. From that time, the fight centered on the amendment.

The spirited Lyon was followed by one of the Northern senators, who read

California hospitals were cited as grossly exploiting the labor of students such as these at the California Hospital, Los Angeles.

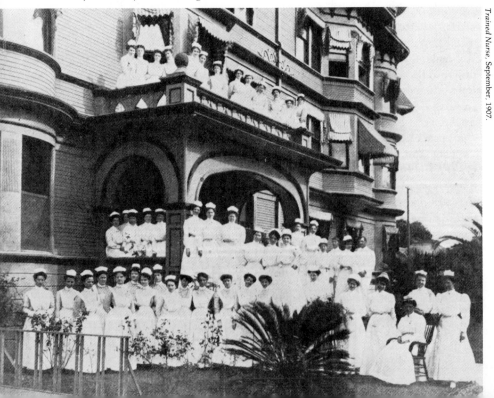

several letters from prominent people asserting the critical need among student nurses for the protection of the eight-hour law. Senator Anthony Caminetti also made a vigorous objection to the amendment, pleading that the eight-hour legislation be backed by every man who had the cause of humanity at heart:

We took a great step forward two years ago when we passed the Eight-Hour Law, and I don't know a man who fought against it at that time who would change it now. We cannot go backward. We must go forward. Our parties have pledged themselves to the uplifting of humanity; it was the slogan of our last campaign, and there can be no better example of putting into practice than by passing this bill by an almost unanimous vote [12].

That evening Senator Caminetti spoke again in support of the eight-hour bill, introducing statistics showing the detrimental effects of overwork. Despite vehement objections and an avalanche of opposing telegrams, the bill passed. The Senate chambers and galleries had been crowded all day with women interested in the passage of the bill. Many of the wives of assemblymen, some of whom had been student nurses, stayed on until passage of the bill was assured.

To provide for possible referendum, the bill was required to wait 90 days before final passage into law. There was a great deal of agitation on the part of hospital owners for such a referendum. Many errors of fact were circulated in an attempt to provoke such action, the most preposterous of which claimed that all graduate nurses would be included under the law, and that families in need of private duty nurses would have to circulate three nurses over 24 hours— an impossible financial burden for most people. What is more, the state hospital association sent delegates to the governor asking him to withhold his signature, thereby scuttling the bill. When the governor looked over the room filled with physicians and hospital representatives, he asked, "Where are the people in favor of this law?" Bessie Beatty of the *San Francisco Bulletin* told him that the people in favor of the law were the young women in hospitals caring for the sick who were unable to get away to present their claims. The governor signed the bill.

On October 14, 1913, in an attempt to halt enforcement of the new law, the trustees of the Associated Hospital Workers of Southern California filed a petition in the United States District Court for a restraining order. Two months later, however, the United States Court of Appeals upheld the California eight-hour law for student nurses as being constitutional and in no way impairing the right of contract guaranteed by the Fourteenth Amendment. Oakland's Merritt Hospital then took the law to the Supreme Court for decision.

In the case of *California* v. *Merritt Hospital* the argument for the defense was presented by the attorney for the hospital, who attacked the constitutionality of the eight-hour law, while two briefs were presented by the representative of the labor organization defending the law. A decision was rendered on February 23, 1915, which held that "the same restriction as to the hours of employment of student nurses in hospitals is not an unconstitutional violation of the freedom of contract, as these persons, upon whom rests the burden of immediate attendance upon and nursing of the patients in hospitals, are also pupils engaged in a course of study, and the propriety of legislative protection of women undergoing such a discipline is not open to question" [13].

From the viewpoint of California hospital administrators, there was little to be said in favor of the new law. It forced a larger payroll and bigger housing and operating expenditures because additional graduate nurses were required to supplement the work of the students. After passage of the law, these expenses were offset in the private institutions by an increase in rates and in the endowed institutions by a decrease in charitable work. According to the critics, an increased management burden fell on the hospital administrators, while greater expenses fell on the taxpayers, for the maintenance of public institutions, and upon the patients themselves, for the maintenance of private hospitals. The law also caused a decrease in the dividends of commercial hospitals.

The decrease in outside income generated by sending students into homes for private duty work seriously affected the finances of some hospitals. In a paper on this subject read before the American Nurses' Association in April, 1914, Lila Pickhardt, Superintendent of Nurses of the Pasadena Hospital, reflected: "Just how great this revenue was may be estimated when we have reason to believe that in some institutions 40 percent of the student nurses were on special cases. Frequently, probationers were assigned to special duty, and some have estimated that two-thirds of the time while enrolled as a student nurse was given to special duty" [14].

The following extract from the letter of a California superintendent of nurses to a friend expresses the reactionary view of the establishment at that time:

The eight-hour law is still a heavy burden, really the most cruel thing they have ever done in the nursing profession; I don't know when it is going to end. Patients are complaining, head nurses work day and night doing the student nurses' work, while the latter are constantly grumbling and in a state of discontent at not getting all the experience they should have; that is, the conscientious ones, while the others are running around, attending picture shows, theatres, etc., tiring themselves out before they begin their work. . . . I worked out a system of instruction—it worked beautifully, but the eight-hour law has smashed it all up, crippled us, for every time a head nurse wants to teach a student anything, she is off duty, and I have to form classes at night to give instruction that should be learned in the wards. The patients also complain of the constant change of nurses—the doctors, also, as orders are frequently overlooked or not properly attended to. We cannot keep a nurse on half-an-hour longer today and make it up tomorrow, even if it is in the middle of an operation or obstetric case she must drop everything and go. . . . The eight hours has compelled us to increase the number of nurses threefold, which also means more head nurses, maids, cooks, waiters, etc., etc. [15].

Anne A. Williamson, Superintendent of Nurses at the California Hospital, Los Angeles, complained that a young woman gave up three of the best years of her life to learning her profession, and it was unjust to deprive her of the work to which she was entitled. According to Miss Williamson, nursing was a profession that belonged exclusively to women; it called for the highest in character and education; and it could not succeed without perseverance, deter-

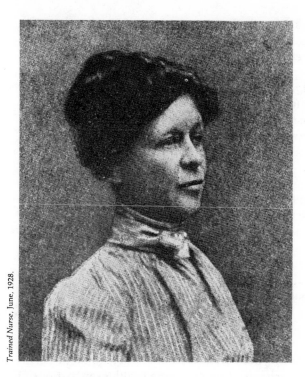

Lavinia L. Dock.

mination, and self-sacrifice. But how could hospital schools instill those principles into the minds of their pupils when the first lesson they had to teach was
the self-centered eight-hour law?

The Elements of Sacrifice

Neither fresh ideas nor nurses who had them were welcome in the places where
elderly, respectable superintendents of nursing held the levers of authority,
harkening only to the wishes of hospital authority figures. The idea of labor
control in hospital training schools was repugnant to most graduate nurses.
They saw a grave danger in the entrance of labor laws into nursing and hospital affairs, for once the wedge was entered, no one could guess how deep it
would go. The demand might be for eight hours one year, but who could guarantee that it would not be six hours next year, and something else the year
after?

Physicians generally agreed. Dr. Antonio D. Young, in a paper "The Nurse's
Duty to Herself," claimed: "The element of sacrifice is always present in true
service. The service that costs no pangs, no sacrifice, is without virtue, and
usually without value." On the other hand, a reform nurse, Lavinia Dock, argued: "I think nurses should stand together solidly and resist the dictation of

the medical profession in this as in all other things. Many M.D.'s have a purely commercial spirit toward nurses (have private hospitals of their own, etc.) and would readily overwork them." She added: "If necessary, do not hesitate to make alliances with the labor vote, for organized labor has quite as much of an 'ideal' as the M.D.'s have, if not more" [16].

In the October, 1913, issue of *Ladies' Home Journal,* the editor published a scathing criticism of the manner in which hospitals fed their student nurses. The editor noted that hospital superintendents all across the nation were voicing concern over the decreasing numbers of nurse-training applications and the slipping personal standards of those who did apply. Yet how could administrators expect "women of better education and finer feelings" to come to a place where they would be "asked to sit down to rations of a kind and quality only a remove better than what we might place before a beggar?" The way the nurses at the average hospital were fed "was nothing short of an outrage upon womanhood," and this outrageous condition could be found in seven out of every 10 hospitals. Indeed, it was a common remark among resident doctors in hospitals that "they would not stand the stuff that is put before the nurses to eat." There was not "one scintilla of doubt that if those nurses were men the present order of things would soon change by compulsion," concluded the *Journal* editor [17]. Little complaint came from the student nurses, however, as such would be grounds for expulsion.

Recognizing that only healthy young women would be able to do the strenuous work required of them, schools of nursing gave health examinations to entering students as a matter of routine. At the time of entrance, careful health records were taken, and only the physically fit were admitted. Theoretically, the health training that was given the student should have placed her in a better situation to avoid infection. However, administrators of schools of nursing knew that the health of the average student did not improve during the years spent in the hospital; on the contrary, it tended to deteriorate.

In training hospitals that admitted tuberculosis patients, it was well known that the majority of students who entered with negative tuberculins would have developed positive tuberculins upon finishing their training. In the average general hospital carrying a tuberculosis service, approximately 80 percent of the student group graduated with positive tuberculins. Two investigators found that the frequency of tuberculosis infections contracted by student nurses in three general hospitals in Minnesota was five times greater than the frequency among girls who were attending regular colleges in the same communities.

Progressive nurses had begun agitating for educational reforms. Adelaide Nutting expressed this move forcibly in addressing the Superintendents' Society in 1911:

From ecclesiastical control . . . nursing has by degrees passed over into the control of the hospital and the medical profession, quite as distinct a hierarchy as any ecclesiastical organization that ever existed. Under the control nursing has prospered in certain ways and has done valuable service, but that service has been strictly subordinated to hospital and medical needs [18].

Obstacles to Nursing Reform

The obstacles to reform in nursing were largely a product of the vested interests of hospital boards of trustees and medical societies who wanted to maintain the existing nursing conditions. At the 1912 meeting of the American Hospital Association, Dr. Henry M. Hurd, Secretary of the Board of Trustees of Johns Hopkins Hospital, stated:

The hospitals of the United States and Canada find themselves without adequate funds for the increased cost of operation because of the growing need of expensive apparatus for the diagnosis and treatment of disease; for the greater cost of all food supplies due to the high cost of living; for the increased cost of service in every department; for the increased scope of hospital service; for the need of doing more for the education of nurses and the training and education of physicians and hospital administrators; for more departments, better operating service, and better equipped hospital wards; and lastly, for ample resources to carry on social service and preventive work [19].

Although more than 10,000 trained nurses were being graduated each year, health care for the majority of the population was inadequate. When a worker or one of his family got sick, the medical and nursing services available were few and comparatively simple. Illnesses viewed as minor were still treated with home remedies and patent medicines. For severe illnesses the family physician was called in. Among families with moderate and lower incomes, even this was not done without serious consideration of the cost involved and a determination as to whether the family resources could be stretched to cover the bill or whether the physician could be asked to wait for his fee.

Often, calling the physician was delayed until it was too late, especially in cases of childhood diseases. The wife still handled the nursing duties with what help she could obtain from relatives and neighbors. When she was ill, the family and friends did as much as they could, or a practical nurse was called in. In childbirth, untrained midwives often took the place of both physician and nurse. Although the dangers of this action were recognized and frequently publicized, this practice continued, particularly among families of recent immigrants and unskilled native-born laborers.

Hospitalization was still the exception among all groups. Aside from their high cost of treatment, many hospitals retained the stigma of the pesthouse. As to cost factors, George P. Ludlam, Superintendent of New York Hospital, observed:

It is, I think, an acknowledged fact that the per-diem cost of patients per capita is constantly increasing. Also, I think it will be admitted that this increase is not wholly due to advances in the market cost of supplies. It is due in large measure to the advance and development of medical and surgical science which has revolutionized old methods and introduced such as are unquestionably more costly. To this fact may be added the other patent one that constant familiarity with these methods engenders a spirit of extravagance which permeates the whole establishment and which it is exceedingly difficult to check or control. I do not mean deliberate intentional waste. I suspect that does not exist. But the generous, liberal, and even extravagant use of supplies of all kinds leads to precisely the same results in the matter of the cost of maintenance, and this habit is, undoubtedly, prevalent in a controlling degree [20].

The editor of *The Modern Hospital* deplored the presence of "disreputable hospitals" in a ringing 1914 editorial:

There are many hospitals in this country that are a disgrace to everybody connected with them. Some are immoral in one way, some in another, and some of them are immoral in their very essence and in every way. Some are notorious abortion "parlors," some of them have a reputation for the immorality of the training school, some are distinguished by a reputation for shady transactions in their financial dealings [21].

Uplift of Hospital Conditions

Gradually a few enlightened administrators began to see the necessity of adapting hospital service to community needs. The Administrator of Johns Hopkins Hospital in Baltimore in 1916 declared:

We need to study and to understand the broader relationship of the hospital to the community. That we have begun to appreciate this broader usefulness is evidenced by the inauguration of social service work, indicating that we are no longer content to ignore the relationship of the individual to his family, to previous environment, to the community, and to post-hospital environment and opportunities . . . . In the great public health movement the hospital, with its trained clinicians and investigators and its many points of contact with the community, occupies an important, indeed a strategic, position [22].

There was an awareness of the need for properly trained hospital administrators. A speaker at the 1916 Conference of the American Hospital Association said:

Whatever may have sufficed in the past, the institution for the sick, small or large, of the future, will need apparently for its administration an educator, a scientist, a sociologist, and a good businessman or woman, or one whose business it is to be a composite of all [23].

One of the first considerations in maintaining high efficiency of personnel was to allocate duties properly. The complaint voiced in the following 1916 editorial was commonplace:

Serious difficulties in hospital administration are often due to the lack of a proper differentiation of the regular duties of the several departments. Nurses, for example, sometimes cannot resist the impulse to regulate the kitchen or laundry. Matrons occasionally are found who have overwhelming desire to assume the responsibility and direction of the nursing work, to the neglect of their own duties. Physicians sometimes long to undertake the distribution of pupil nurses in ward duty, and seek to instruct them and some times to discipline them . . . . The watchword of every large institution should be departmental independence, coordinated through the office of the head of the hospital [24].

The hospital's physical environment was generally bleak and uninviting for patients as well as nurses. In 1916 an architect said in an address at Johns Hopkins Hospital that:

While the medical profession and the hospital people consider it highly necessary that the sick should be surrounded by pleasant odors as against the older offensive smells of ether and iodoform, and while it is considered necessary that there be quiet in the hospital, yet no consideration is given to the patient's sense of sight. Glaring white walls, severely simple furniture, and absence of draperies and curtains and the little incidentals of home comfort certainly impress the mind of the sick. Why would not pleasing sights and harmonious colors and agreeable forms serve to shorten the stay of the sick and influence their recovery [25]?

During this period, hospitals in America were administered haphazardly. There was no real organization and the management had no standard to follow. Some hospitals gained a good reputation because of the presence of a superior surgeon who required better organization, but such hospitals were looked upon as unusual and no effort was made to copy them.

When the American College of Surgeons was founded in 1913, its organizers understood the necessity for hospital improvement. In its earliest program of activities this organization published its intention to study hospitals and to encourage improvements. By 1918 considerable analytical work had been done, and the College was ready to embark on a program of hospital standardization. During 1918 and 1919 field representatives visited 671 hospitals of 100 beds or more in the United States and Canada; of these, 89 in the first year and 198 in the second year were approved as meeting the minimum standard, and further progress was soon effected on many fronts. The 10 fundamental requirements of the "Minimum Standard for Hospitals" were:

A modern physical plant, properly equipped for the comfort and scientific care of the patient.

Clearly stated constitution, by-laws, rules and regulations setting forth organization, duties, responsibilities, and relations.

A carefully selected governing board having complete and supreme authority for the management of the institution.

A competent, well-trained executive officer or superintendent with authority and responsibility to carry out the policies of the institution as authorized by the governing board.

An adequate number of efficient personnel, properly organized and under competent supervision.

An organized medical staff of ethical, competent physicians for the carrying out of the professional policies of the hospital, subject to the approval of the governing board.

Adequate diagnostic and therapeutic facilities with efficient technical service under competent medical supervision.

Accurate and complete medical records, promptly written and filed in an accessible manner so as to be available for study, reference, follow-up, and research.

Group conferences of the administrative staff and of the medical staff to review regularly

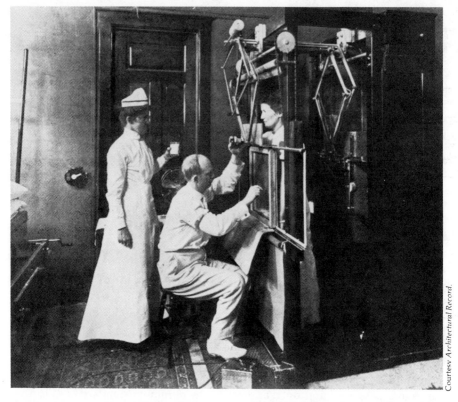

Courtesy Architectural Record.

By 1917 the fluoroscope had become an important diagnostic instrument in hospitals. From Edward F. Stevens, The American Hospital of the Twentieth Century *(New York: The Architectural Record Company, 1921), p. 320.*

and thoroughly their respective activities in order to keep the service and the scientific work on the highest plane of efficiency.

A humanitarian spirit in which the best care of the patient is always the primary consideration [26].

National Health Status in 1920

What was the state of the nation's health by the end of the second decade of the twentieth century? While in 1901–1902 the average life expectancy of a white male child at birth was 48.23 years, it rose to 50.23 years in 1909–1910 and to 54.05 years in 1919–1920. As seen from the table below, the improvement in longevity held true until one reached the age of 40. After that age, the chances of increased longevity actually fell somewhat below the expectations of 20 years before. The same was true, to a smaller extent, for women. At the age of 40, the premature development of degenerative diseases of middle age set in, carrying Americans off much more rapidly than Britons, Swedes, Norwegians, Danes, Dutchmen, or Australians.

Comparison of Changes in the Expectation of Life, 1890–1920 [27].

Age	Massachusetts	Original Registration States		
	1890 (Males)	1901–1902 (White Males)	1909–1910 (White Males)	1919–1920 (White Males)
0	42.50	48.23	50.23	54.05
7	51.15	53.76	53.85	55.34
12	47.64	49.72	49.56	51.02
22	39.97	41.44	41.13	42.69
32	33.39	34.15	33.33	34.93
42	26.70	27.03	25.99	27.32
52	20.09	20.08	19.02	19.91
62	41.15	13.76	12.85	13.38
72	8.88	8.56	7.95	8.17
82	5.08	4.81	4.56	4.53
92	2.37	2.69	2.70	2.10

When in 1917, amid preparations for war, the Progressive Era in American history came to a close, perceptive nurses could see that the reform movement for nursing had largely been muted. The unique external constraints imposed upon student and graduate nurses had prevented any large-scale alteration of either the educational or the work environment. Nevertheless, nurses of that era had achieved some important early insights into the developing conflict between nursing's professional idealism and the reactionary tendencies of the hospital and medical establishment.

Summary

After the turn of the century the need for nurse registration became increasingly apparent. In September, 1901, at the first meeting of the International Council of Nurses, a resolution was passed in favor of uniform registration.

As a rule, the presentation of nurse registration bills in the various state legislatures was preceded by the formation of a state nurses' association. While North Carolina, in 1903, was first to enact a nurse registration law, the New York registration law, which followed shortly thereafter, was considered the more progressive.

Postgraduate education, a term loosely applied, generally consisted of nothing more than routine hospital service, and there was no uniformity in fees, allowances, curriculum, or certification.

A course in hospital economy established through the efforts of the American Society of Superintendents of Training Schools for Nurses at Teachers College, Columbia University, in 1899 was aimed at preparing nurses for teaching and supervisory positions.

In 1910 Abraham Flexner, after touring the 155 medical schools in the United States and Canada, prepared a report that shocked the sponsoring Carnegie Foundation and brought about the closure of some schools and abrupt reform in many others. Most of the schools that survived this critical scrutiny secured university connections and became nonprofit institutions.

A request made by Adelaide Nutting for Carnegie Foundation funds to support a Flexner-type study of schools of nursing was turned down, although similar investigations of the education of dentists, lawyers, and teachers were being funded by the Foundation.

The typical hospital school of nursing of 1910 was still characterized by a highly authoritarian atmosphere, a set of strict rules that governed the students' activities in all spheres of life and work, and long hours of task-oriented practice.

A great deal of energy was wasted by nurses in excessive walking and unnecessary lifting of heavy objects and as a result of inefficient arrangement of hospital wards.

A flurry of protective legislation to limit the working hours of women was evident in many states between 1908 and 1917. Meanwhile, nursing was cited in a federal investigation of women's work in 1910 as an occupation that was not only very strenuous but also "morally dangerous" for women.

The only state to legislate against excessive exploitation of student nurse labor was California, which, in 1913, after an emotional legislative fight, limited students to eight hours of work daily.

Many graduate nurses opposed the idea of government legislation of hours of hospital labor because they viewed nursing as a self-sacrificing service that could not be regulated by the time clock.

In the early 1900s health care for the majority of Americans outside the wealthy classes was woefully inadequate. Lack of money to pay for medical care and fear of hospitals rendered millions of people unable or unwilling to consult a family physician in times of illness, and untrained midwives were often relied upon for care during childbirth.

A growing realization of the need to adapt hospital service to community requirements caused hospital administrators to focus on improved methods of business management and provisions for a broader array of services. Environmental considerations formerly considered peripheral, such as the impact of bleak interiors on patient welfare, began to receive attention. Generally, however, hospitals were run haphazardly, and, in order to help effect needed reform, the American College of Surgeons developed a minimum standard for hospitals, which eventually wrought a revolution in hospital conditions.

References
1. *New York Tribune,* April 16, 1900.
2. Lavinia L. Dock, "Secretary's Report of the Meeting of the International Council of Nurses, Buffalo, New York, September 16, 1901," *American Journal of Nursing,* vol. 2 (October, 1901):51–54.
3. Mary Allenson, "My Impressions as a Post-Graduate," *American Journal of Nursing,* vol. 5 (November, 1904):100–103.
4. Clara Noyes, "Postgraduate Study for Nurses," *Proceedings of the Annual Meeting of American Society of Superintendents of Training Schools for Nurses,* vol. 11 (June, 1905):121–129.
5. A. Flexner, *Medical Education in the United States and Canada* (New York: The Carnegie Foundation for the Advancement of Teaching, 1910), pp. 3–185, *passim.*
6. *Ibid.,* pp. vii–xvii, 185–319, *passim.*
7. M. Adelaide Nutting, "Report of the Committee on Education," *Proceedings of the Convention of the National League of Nursing Education,* vol. 19 (June, 1913):76–77.
8. Elizabeth A. Greener, "Organization and Administration of the Nursing Department," *Modern Hospital,* vol. 2 (March, 1914):163–164.
9. *Ibid.,* pp. 166–167.
10. Katharine DeWitt, "Hospital Sketches," *American Journal of Nursing* vol. 6 (April, 1906):455–459.
11. U.S. Department of Commerce and Labor, *Report on the Condition of Woman and Child Wage-Earners in the United States* (Washington, D.C.: Government Printing Office, 1911), vol. 15, pp. 87–89.
12. *San Francisco Chronicle,* May 2, 1913.
13. *San Francisco Examiner,* February 24, 1915.
14. Lila Pickhardt, "Recent Legislation Governing Hours of Duty of Pupil Nurses in Hospitals," *Proceedings of the 20th Convention of the National League of Nursing Education,* vol. 20 (June, 1914):106–111.
15. "The Eight-Hour Day for Nurses," *Trained Nurse and Hospital Review,* vol. 53 (July, 1914):37–38.
16. "Nurses and Labor Laws," *Trained Nurse and Hospital Review,* vol. 52 (January, 1914):37–38.
17. "Are Nurses in Hospitals Underfed?" *Trained Nurse and Hospital Review,* vol. 51 (December, 1913):364–365.
18. M. Adelaide Nutting, Address, *Proceedings of the Annual Convention of the American Society of Superintendents of Training Schools for Nurses,* vol. 17 (June, 1911):18–22.
19. Henry M. Hurd, President's Address, *Transactions of the American Hospital Association,* vol. 14 (September, 1912):88–89.
20. *New York Times,* March 3, 1913.
21. Henry M. Hurd, "Disreputable Hospitals," *Modern Hospital,* vol. 2 (May, 1914):296.
22. Winford H. Smith, "The Educational Function of the Hospital," *Modern Hospital,* vol. 6 (January, 1916):1–4.
23. Annie W. Goodrich, "How Shall the Superintendents of Small Hospitals Be Trained?" *Transactions of the American Hospital Association,* vol. 18 (September, 1916):359.
24. Henry M. Hurd, "Another Source of Friction in Hospital Administration," *Modern Hospital,* vol. 6 (February, 1916):112.
25. Charles F. Neergaard, "Some Glaring Faults in Hospital Construction," *Modern Hospital,* vol. 6 (June, 1916):408–410.
26. American College of Surgeons, *Manual of Hospital Standardization: History, Development and Progress of Hospital Standardization; Detailed Explanation of the Minimum Requirements* (Chicago: The College, 1938), pp. 61–67.

27. U.S. Department of Commerce, Bureau of the Census, *United States Life Tables, 1901–02, 1909–10, 1919–20* (Washington, D.C.: Government Printing Office, 1923), pp. 16, 48, 62.

10
Days of Triumph:
Nursing in World War I

On June 28, 1914, a shot fired in Sarajevo, in Serbia, set off a sequence of events that brought almost all Europe, and subsequently most of the world, into a long and terrible war destined to cost millions of lives and do incalculable damage. The United States was to enter it a little less than three years later, after a long struggle to maintain neutrality, and the nation's nurses were to be an important part of this involvement. They had already read of the execution of nurse Edith Cavell before a German firing squad on October 12, 1915. Miss Cavell, the superintendent of a nurse training school in Brussels, Belgium, had been charged with harboring British and French soldiers and assisting them in escaping from Belgium. Miss Cavell, who had nursed both German and Allied soldiers, could herself have escaped, but she stayed at her post until she was apprehended and sentenced to death.

The United States had never been in a war like the one it was entering in April, 1917, but few nurses realized this. It was a global conflict that set one coalition of nations against another. Much more so than either the Civil War or the Spanish-American War, it was a war of material, calling for the expenditure of vast amounts for supplies and demanding the organization of all the nation's resources for military purposes. It was also total in its impact upon society, compelling the government to mobilize men, women, money, material, and even public opinion.

Nurses Join the Fight

An American army of three and a half million men was assembled, and over two million of this force were transported to France. At the same time, the size of the Army Nurse Corps was rapidly expanded and soon began to approach a strength of 20,000. The Navy Nurse Corps expanded too, but since fighting was primarily on land, it grew much more slowly. Applicants for appointment for both military nursing services had to be between 25 and 35 years of age, unmarried, and graduates of training schools for nurses that offered solid theoretic and practical courses and were attached to general hospitals of at least 100 beds. As the war continued, however, graduates of schools connected with

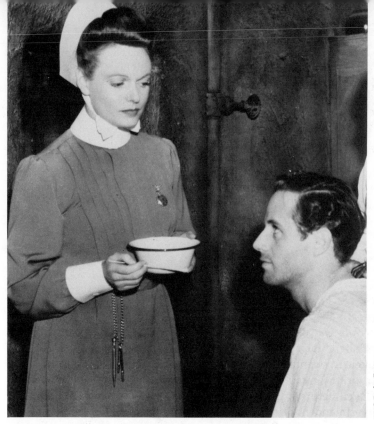

English actress Anna Neagle brilliantly played the title role in the 1939 film biography Nurse Edith Cavell, *which depicted the idealism and sacrifice of this British nurse.*

hospitals not meeting the 100-bed requirement were also accepted.

To determine an applicant's qualifications the Army and Navy requested certification of the nurse's moral character and professional qualifications from the superintendent of her school. Married nurses were unacceptable for appointment, and those who married while on active duty were dishonorably discharged.

Among the women of the United States, interest in nursing quickly began to rise after war was declared. Society girls and others with romantic notions—but without training—who were eager to go overseas to serve as nursing aides at their own expense quickly enrolled in intensive Red Cross courses. On April 8, 1917, Clara Noyes, director of the new Red Cross Bureau of Nursing, wrote to Adelaide Nutting in desperation:

Surely we need your prayers. There are moments when I wonder whether we can stem the tide and control the hysterical desire on the part of thousands, literally thousands, to get into nursing or their hands upon it.

Tell Annie [Goodrich] of Albany that if I were not convinced before, I should be now that the most vital thing in the life of our profession is the protection of the use of the word nurse. Everyone seems to have gone mad. I talk until I am hoarse, dictating letters to doctors and women who want to be Red Cross nurses in a few minutes, not knowing the meaning of the word nurse and what a Red Cross nurse is [1].

Nurse educators were horrified that Army nursing might fall into the hands of aristocratic socialites, as it had done under the auspices of the Red Cross in most European countries. Such women, including those of royal families, lusted to be near the glory of battle, confident that they could fully carry out the "angel of mercy" role merely by dispensing large quantities of morphine to the wounded.

Nursing Resources and the War

Consequently, Adelaide Nutting, Annie Goodrich, and Lillian Wald met on June 24, 1917, to determine ways of avoiding some of the mistakes in providing nursing service to the military that had been made by other countries already in the war. Headed by Miss Nutting, the Committee on Nursing also included Jane Delano, chairman of the American Red Cross Nursing Service, Lillian Clayton, president of the National League of Nursing Education, Dora Thompson, superintendent of the Army Nurse Corps, Dr. Winford H. Smith, president of the American Hospital Association, and several others. The announced purpose of the group was to devise "the wisest methods of meeting the present problems connected with the care of the sick and injured in hospitals and homes; the educational problems of nursing; and the extraordinary emergencies as they arise" [2].

Ten weeks later, on August 2, 1917, the Committee on Nursing was attached to the General Medical Board of the United States Council of National Defense, and was granted federal status and backing. The government provided space for an office, secretarial service, and a few other items, but most of the committee's work was financed from funds contributed by friends of nursing and nurses themselves.

The committee estimated that there were about 200,000 active "nurses," both trained and untrained, in the nation in 1917. Some 115,000 (98,000 registered and 17,000 unregistered) were fully trained nurses, while 85,000 untrained and partially trained nurses made up the remainder. The only field that had a reasonable supply of nurses was private duty nursing, which comprised approximately 150,000 or 75 percent of the total active number. In addition to this mixed pool of 200,000, there were about 45,000 student nurses in training. The challenge at hand was to maintain a steady supply of trained nurses for the care of acutely sick patients from both the military and civilian sectors. This was a tremendous undertaking, inasmuch as the original request for 10,000 nurses for the Army soon rose to 20,000, then to 30,000, and finally to 35,000. Civilian needs also became acute, especially in industrial centers and in towns and cities adjacent to military installations.

The United States, starting almost from scratch, swung into the war effort. A general conscription act was passed, after much opposition, on May 18, 1917, more than a month after the declaration of war. Housing and training this vast number of draftees required building 32 camps, each able to shelter over 40,000

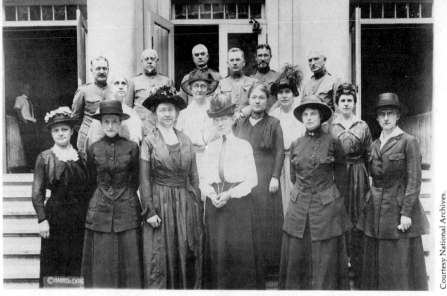

The Committee on Nursing of the United States Council of National Defense, including Annie Goodrich (front row, second from left) and Adelaide Nutting (front row, fourth from left).

Propaganda poster aimed at showing the supposedly inhumane conduct of German nurses.

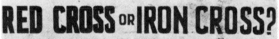

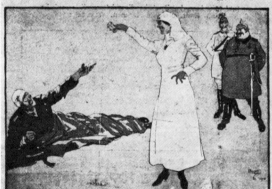

men. In spite of great difficulties in supplying and equipping them, the camps soon came to resemble small cities, with running water, electric light, amusement centers, libraries, and hospitals. After six months of preliminary training, the troops went abroad for further instruction before being sent to the front. To motivate people at home to fully support the war effort, a massive propaganda drive was waged by the Committee on Public Information, established by Congress. Motion pictures, pamphlets, and posters proclaimed that Germans were depraved. Even German nurses were depicted as inhumane and cruel.

Over There

Six months after the United States had entered the war, nearly 1100 nurses were overseas, about half of them stationed in six British general hospitals. American troops were close on their heels. Vera Brittain, who served as a nurse behind the British lines, described her first sight of American troops:

I was leaving quarters to go back to my ward when I had to wait to let a large contingent of troops march past . . . though the sight of soldiers marching was now too familiar to arouse curiosity, an unusual quality of bold vigour in their swift stride caused me to stare at them with puzzled interest.

They looked larger than ordinary men; their tall, straight figures were in vivid contrast to the undersized armies of pale recruits to which we had become accustomed . . . . Had yet another regiment been conjured out of our depleted Dominions?

Then I heard an excited exclamation from a group of Sisters behind me.

"Look! Look! Here are the Americans!"

The coming of relief made me realize how long and how intolerable had been the tension, and with the knowledge that we were not, after all, defeated I found myself beginning to cry [3].

Nurses enrolled in the American Red Cross constituted the unofficial reserve of the Army Nurse Corps for service in time of war or other emergency. Consequently, when an increased number of nurses was needed, the Red Cross was called upon to furnish them. In addition, entire medical and nursing forces were organized at many of the large medical centers in the United States. On May 7, 1917, the first base hospital unit, the Lakeside of Cleveland, with Grace E. Allison as Chief Nurse, sailed for Europe. This was quickly followed by the Peter Bent Brigham Unit of Boston, with Carrie M. Hall as Chief Nurse, and by the Presbyterian Hospital unit of New York, with Janet B. Christie as Chief Nurse. Two weeks later, three more base hospital units sailed—the Saint Louis, with Julia C. Stimson as Chief Nurse; the Pennsylvania of Philadelphia, with Margaret A. Dunlop as Chief Nurse, and the Northwestern of Chicago, with Daisy D. Urch as Chief Nurse. Then came an interval of almost three weeks, and on June 9, 1917, the Johns Hopkins Unit of Baltimore, with Bessie Baker as Chief Nurse, sailed.

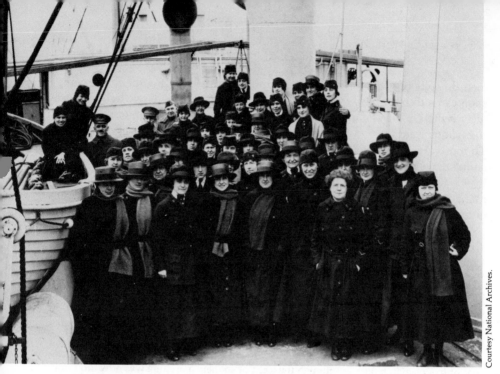

The U.S.S. Cartago carried these Army nurses to France in 1918.

Americans were repeatedly reminded of the importance of nurses in World War I.

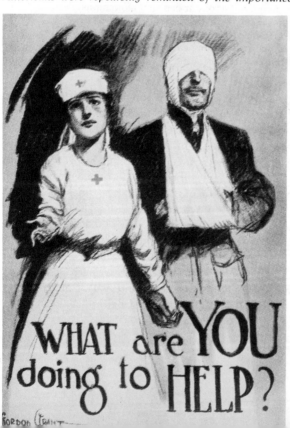

WHAT are YOU doing to HELP?

Shortages at Home

Every nurse who enrolled in the Army Nurse Corps might be taken away from a community where she was urgently needed. An increasing problem, therefore, was how to answer the demand for service abroad with the Army and, at the same time, fill the hundreds of vacant places at home. It would be disastrous if the nation were to let civilian hospitals suffer from lack of competent nurses, particularly for lack of superintendents, supervisors, and teachers. It would also be a very short-sighted policy to allow nurse supply in the public health organizations to run down when there was an increasing number of dependent families to care for and when the wartime situation made conditions favorable for the spread of disease.

Stepped-Up Recruiting Activities

The next challenge was to increase the actual supply of student nurses. The General Medical Board Committee sent out a torrent of posters, motion pictures, photographs, speeches, and pamphlets aimed at making America nurse-conscious and creating a positive attitude toward the nursing profession. More than 70,000 copies of the 15-page pamphlet *Nursing—A National Service* appealed to the young women of America to prepare for nursing. It stressed the need for student recruits, outlined the opportunities for service during and after the war, and listed the kinds of training available and the way to get in touch with good nursing schools. Additionally, 55,000 impressions of the four-page brochure *State Sources of Advice and Information on Nursing* presented a list of names and addresses of nursing representatives in all the states, from whom information regarding nursing schools and other local nursing matters could be secured.

In addition to these direct measures, a widespread campaign of newspaper publicity was waged, and arrangements were made for magazine articles on nursing. Toward this end, the *Ladies' Home Journal*, with former President William H. Taft as editor, urged women to help "the boys over there" by enrolling in schools of nursing. Entitled "A Distinct Call to Women," the editorial asked:

Have you felt that you could best answer the war's appeal to you by entering the nursing service? Then this is the day of your opportunity, provided you are in earnest and wish to set your patriotic impulses free in the place where they will do the most good.

That place is in a regular nurses' training school, such as is conducted in nearly every hospital in America. Many women, untrained in nursing, have been disappointed to learn that their services were not wanted on the field of battle, nor even in a base hospital.

It is the professional nurse only who has been called and accepted, and more than a thousand of her are now in active service. More thousands will follow soon. They are the finest of their profession, and they go gladly; but do you realize that each one is leaving behind her important work in civil life, which must now be done by someone else?

We have no right to expect—though we may hope for—a short war. We must put away makeshift methods and think of a year from now, two years, perhaps even three years. The woman who enters training today is the woman who a little later will be prepared to take the place at home of the nurse who has gone, or even to follow her to the Front.

The Red Cross earnestly hopes that many young women, particularly those with the advantages of a good education, will let their desire to be of service take a most practical form and prepare to enter a profession which has been called upon to do so noble a work [4].

Having done everything in its power to attract educated young women to enroll in schools of nursing, the General Medical Board Committee next appealed to the 700 leading nursing schools throughout the country to enlarge their schools immediately to the limit of their capacities, resources, and clinical facilities. To this end they were requested to secure additional nursing dormitories and more supervisors and instructors and to shorten the lengthy working hours that had so long been an impediment to the entrance of more middle-class women into nursing. Where they were unable to find additional quarters, it was suggested that temporary arrangements be made to permit local students to live at home during at least part of their training.

As a result of these measures the number of students entering schools of nursing during the year 1917–1918 increased by about 25 percent. This meant that instead of a yearly output of 12,000 to 15,000 graduate nurses, the nation would have 15,000 to 18,000 available in 1919 and 1920. By April, 1918, approximately 7000 applicants over and above the normal 15,000 admitted annually were enrolled in nursing schools. The wartime publicity campaign for student nurses was the first to be organized on any large scale, and its effectiveness was due in large measure to its patriotic wartime appeal.

Nursing's Image among High School Students
Helpful relations were established with the Women's Committee of the Council on National Defense, which, through its state and local committees, publicized the importance of assisting hospitals in their recruiting efforts. Some outstanding work was done on the local level. For example, a women's group in Cleveland became eager to measure the average high school girl's interest in nursing as a possible vocation. With the help of the city's high school teachers a regional survey was conducted.

The questionnaire was designed to yield a comparison between the amount of interest displayed toward a possible future college arts and science degree and a possible future course in a school of nursing. Chief among the objections to a nursing career that were raised by 1139 high school graduates were the long hours, hard work, severe discipline, lack of recreation and pleasure, and low quality of education. Among the objections and difficulties voiced were: "I can't stand it physically"; "It is a life of drudgery"; "The work is too strenuous"; "When you get old, nobody wants you"; "The nervous strain is too great"; "Too much scrubbing"; and "Too much standing on one's feet." Over 73 percent did not know of any positions that a graduate nurse could fill.

It was significant that although nearly one-half of the respondents had previously talked with a member of the nursing profession, fewer than one-fifth considered nursing as a career possibility. Undoubtedly, school of nursing alumnae were not giving very glowing reports of their schools and of their work. A massive national effort was obviously needed to lessen hours of duty, decrease drudgery, and elevate nursing educational standards by expanding the theoretic portion of the curricula and by hiring full-time instructors and lecturers.

Many nursing schools did not have facilities for even a modest educational program, and their living and working conditions were nearly intolerable. Complaints soon began to reach the Committee on Nursing from some of the beginning students. To try to improve poor nursing school conditions, a circular letter was sent by the Women's Committee of the Council of National Defense to the 12,000 state and local committees of the Women's Committee, urging them to follow up the young women who had been placed in nursing schools in their vicinity, to take an interest in them, and try to see that they secured their training under satisfactory conditions. They were especially asked to investigate students who had been admitted to low-quality nursing programs. Enclosed with this letter was a memorandum prepared by the Committee on Nursing entitled *What Is a Good Training School of Nurses?*

Tapping the College Woman

The urgent need for a greater number of better-educated women in many areas of nursing led to an informal effort by the Committee on Nursing to see if some of the leading schools of nursing would be willing, in the national emergency, to reduce the term of three years for college graduates with satisfactory backgrounds in science. Most schools were willing to allow credit for eight to nine months of the usual three-year course, and some would allow a full year. Other schools were more cautious, however, and some openly skeptical. Superintendents wanted to know what evidence existed to show that college graduates would make good nurses or that a longer period of academic education would be any special asset in the training of a nurse.

Using these reactions as a basis, the Committee proceeded in a bold attempt to attract female college graduates into nursing through an experimental program at Vassar College. The objective was to utilize the plant and resources of Vassar College in an effort to interest numerous college women in nursing service by providing an intensive preparatory course of three months on the Vassar campus. A vigorous recruiting campaign was organized by the Vassar alumnae to secure enrollment.

The summer school for nurses at Vassar opened auspiciously with 439 college graduates selected from a large number of applicants. They ranged in age from 19 to 40 and represented 115 of the nation's colleges. Over half the women had been teachers, some with excellent positions. The next largest group comprised students entering directly from college, but a number of secretaries, social workers, newspaper women, librarians, and others were also in attendance.

There were two terms, with classes six days a week and a half-holiday on Saturday. The expenses amounted to $25 for tuition and $70 for room and board. All the usual preparatory subjects were covered, including courses in anatomy and physiology (60 hours), bacteriology (48 hours), chemistry (48 hours), hygiene and sanitation (30 hours), elementary materia medica (24 hours), nutrition and cooking (60 hours), elementary nursing and hospital economy (60 hours), and history of nursing (10 hours). In addition, all students who had not yet had psychology and social economy took a 30-hour course in each of these subjects.

At the end of the summer the students chose from a list of 33 cooperating hospitals a school of nursing in which the balance of their training would be completed in two years and three months. It was impressive that 418 of the 439 college graduates completed the Vassar course, and 399 of these entered the 33 affiliated schools, each of which had promised to admit a certain number of these students and to carry them through the remainder of the program. Fifty-seven went to Bellevue Hospital in New York, 21 to City Hospital, New York, 17 to Boston City Hospital, and 13 to the University of Michigan Hospital. Eventually, Vassar Training Camp graduates would help fill key leadership roles for the next four decades.

Soon, five other universities (Western Reserve in Cleveland, the University of Cincinnati, the University of Iowa, the University of Colorado, and the University of California) set up similar courses, to which high school students were also admitted. The prenursing or preparatory course that was given at Vassar College and at other universities during the summer of 1918 showed what might be done on a large scale in the way of cooperating with higher educational institutions for a part of nurses' training. The standard of teaching was much higher than that available in the great majority of nursing schools. It seemed to many nurse educators that even if the special incentives of the war period were eliminated there would still be an advantage in having prenursing work conducted under the auspices of a recognized college or university.

Increased War Demands
Meanwhile, since the declaration of war against Germany on April 6, 1917, the United States had been exerting a stupendous national effort in carrying out its responsibilities to the Allied cause. Eventually, the total strength of the United States Army would reach 3,685,458 men. Of these, approximately two million would be equipped for combat, preliminarily trained, and transported to France to form the American Expeditionary Force. They would not participate in military action in Europe until the late spring of 1918—just in time to help stem the great German offensive. Then, they would serve in camps and in the field, and fight great battles, from Château-Thierry in July to Saint-Mihiel in September, and the Meuse-Argonne offensive from September 26 to the Armistice on November 11, 1918.

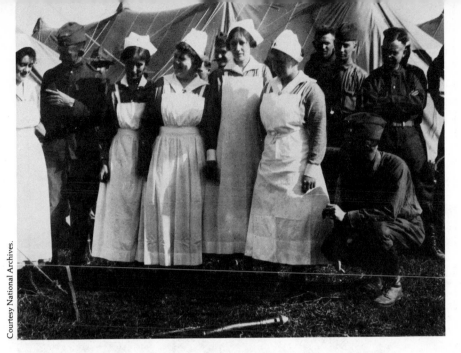

German aerial bomb dropped on the night of August 12, 1918, within 15 feet of a ward tent containing about 50 wounded American soldiers. The nurses in the picture are Jennie Conn, Blanche Feister, Lucy Raeter, May Conyard, and Mary Swain.

Since only graduate nurses were eligible for military service, by the winter of 1917–1918 the country's civilian nurse supply was seriously depleted. In European nations the solution to the problem had been found in accepting as military nurses women who had undergone a short period of training as aides. For the United States the question of Red Cross nurses' aides versus trained nurses for the military was full of emotion and controversy. Although members of the nursing profession eagerly sought financial and moral support from women of the leisure classes, they did not want to turn their profession over to those who hungered for tinsel glory.

Trained nurses were forced to fight large and highly vocal groups of society women anxious to serve as nurses but hesitant to enroll when a definite period of training was suggested. These lay women clung to the belief that the war had created a demand for a reduced standard of nursing service, which they themselves would be unwilling to accept in times of peace. They seemed to feel that there was something especially patriotic in serving as a volunteer free-lance rather than as a regularly enlisted member of the Army Nurse Corps. These socialites pointed to the huge numbers of amateurs who had served in hospitals abroad, and they clamored for an opportunity to show their patriotism and devotion in a similar way.

Although both Dora Thompson, Superintendent of the Army Nurse Corps, and Jane Delano of the Red Cross Nursing Service urged the use of nurses' aides to conserve the supply of graduate nurses in civilian hospitals, military personnel returning from overseas for War Department conferences encouraged Surgeon General William C. Gorgas to take a firm stand against use of the aide

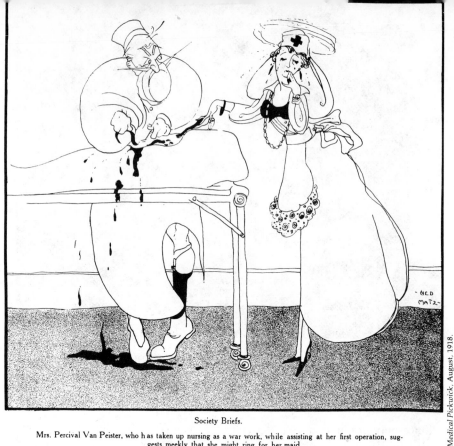

Society Briefs.

Mrs. Percival Van Peister, who h as taken up nursing as a war work, while assisting at her first operation, suggests meekly that she might ring for her maid.

Medical Pickwick, August, 1918.

Society women clamored for war nursing duties despite their lack of training.

group. As the pace of war increased, Secretary of War Newton D. Baker asked the Surgeon General to take a "long look ahead" in order to relieve the personnel situation. Somewhat alarmed, Surgeon General Gorgas temporarily abandoned his earlier opposition to aides and notified the Red Cross on February 9, 1918, that it could proceed with its nurses' aides plan. Such aides would be selected from applicants who had completed a four-week course in elementary hygiene and home care of the sick, supplemented by a short practical training course of not less than one month.

Personnel so trained would be utilized as civilian employees of the Medical Department, paid a salary of $30 a month, and be granted quarters, subsistence, laundering of uniforms, and travel expenses when under orders. The Superintendent of the Army Nurse Corps was in agreement with this program and planned to assign aides to convalescent patients only, thus freeing graduate nurses to care for the seriously ill. Adelaide Nutting, however, sharply disapproved of the nurses' aides plan. She complained that wounded and dying men should not be left to the care of inexperienced nurses. She quoted President Wilson's statement that war was not a job for amateurs.

After receiving reports critical of nursing conditions in American military camps, the Committee on Nursing asked that the Surgeon General appoint

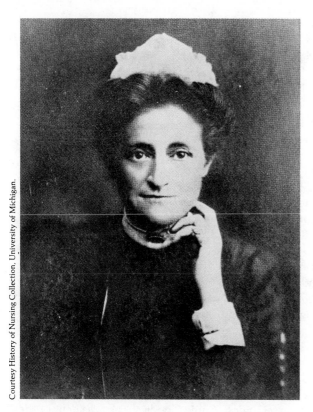

Courtesy History of Nursing Collection, University of Michigan.

Annie W. Goodrich.

Annie W. Goodrich to evaluate the quality of nursing service in military hospitals. Shortly thereafter, Miss Goodrich, president of the American Nurses' Association and an assistant professor in the Department of Nursing and Health at Teachers College, Columbia University, received an appointment as Chief Inspecting Nurse of the Army hospitals at home and abroad. She reported for duty at the War Department on February 18, 1918. Miss Goodrich was considered especially well suited to this position because of her varied experience, including much experience in inspection of training schools. Assisting her was Elizabeth C. Burgess, the Inspector of Training Schools of New York State.

On March 24, 1918, upon completion of their tour of inspection, both Miss Goodrich and Miss Burgess reported that the military base hospitals presented a sharply negative contrast to the best civilian hospitals. In civilian hospitals the bedside care of the patient was given by a carefully selected group of student nurses under the constant supervision of highly qualified instructors and supervisors. In military hospitals the trained nurses were unable to handle all the bedside care; much of their work was delegated to the continually changing hospital corpsmen, who, as enlisted men, did not approach the task with any desire to excel. Meanwhile the patient struggled to help himself or to help others, in order to relieve both the nurses and the corpsmen.

Controversy over an "Army School of Nursing"

The unfavorable report on nursing conditions in the Army was accompanied by a formal proposal on March 24, 1918, to establish an Army school of nursing, which would provide for patients in Army hospitals the kind of student care that was furnished in civilian hospitals. Miss Goodrich recommended that the Committee on Nursing of the Council of National Defense act as an advisory group to the proposed school.

The Army School of Nursing was to be centralized in the Surgeon General's Office, under the supervision of a dean, with training units and teaching staffs in many camp hospitals. More than a mere effort to circumvent the Red Cross training program for aides, the plan represented Annie Goodrich's determination to implement an educational pattern totally new in nursing education. The school faculty would determine all aspects of instruction, administration, and professional training of students at the Army camp hospitals. Each hospital would be an individual unit, with its own staff, supervision, and teaching equipment. Miss Goodrich believed that the care given by Army student nurses under expert instruction and supervision would far surpass that given by hastily trained aides. New units would be opened as needed, each offering a three-year diploma course and meeting requirements for state registration.

Early in May, 1918, the second joint annual meeting of the National League of Nursing Education, the American Nurses' Association, and the National Organization for Public Health Nursing was held in Cleveland. The Germans had already struck their second blow on the Western Front at this time and were preparing for the third major offensive. Now, Cleveland became the battleground for the dispute over nurses' aides. Annie Goodrich, as president of the American Nurses' Association, welcomed the group with a ringing proclamation: "We have come together in the most momentous period not in the history of this country, but in the history of the world, to consecrate ourselves anew to the service of humanity through our chosen profession" [5].

The two convention addresses of greatest importance were those presented by Colonel Winford H. Smith, which outlined plans for the Army School of Nursing, and by Dr. S. S. Goldwater, which advocated, under the title "A Nursing Crisis," the employment of nurses' aides. Colonel Smith's paper represented Miss Goodrich's ideas. He told the audience:

Under this plan, it is proposed to enroll young women between the ages of 21 and 35, who have received the equivalent of a high school education, and to assign them to the schools in military hospitals . . . .

We believe that the requirements of 21 to 35 age limits and the equivalent of a high school education will interfere less with civil hospitals than [would] a lower standard or acceptance of candidates for short courses. It will likewise guarantee to us a type mentally and morally best fitted to our service, and if we are to place these young women in our camps, they must work under and live under close supervision and control, and no better system can be devised than that which the civil hospital has found successful after years of experience. Recognize please that what we propose is, in our opinion, a better protection to the civil hospital training school than the short course system for nurses' aides [6].

On the other hand, Dr. Goldwater's argument was that the nation could not spare the necessary number of trained nurses from the civilian sector. He claimed that the proposed Army school would divert large numbers of applicants from civilian nursing schools, that standards in civilian hospitals would very seriously suffer, and that an Army school of nursing would leave the United States with a huge surplus of nurses at the close of the war. He asserted that women of the leisure classes were the only significant labor reserve of the country, that they were willing and eager to serve, and that they should be permitted to do so.

I come finally to what appears to me to be the safest and best way out—in fact, the only way out; namely, the training of a large number of non-professional, voluntary war nursing aides, enlisted for the period of the war only and composed of a class which will not take up nursing professionally under any circumstances, but which is willing to give gratuitous hospital service during the emergency. Such women can be obtained quickly, in large numbers. Among the 1500 training schools of the country, there should be no difficulty in finding 300 which are capable of training and which can be trusted to train 12 nursing aides or nurses' assistants per month, or say, 150 per annum. With the moral support of the Army, the hospitals of the country can easily obtain and turn out 25,000 nurses' assistants before the end of the present year, or 40,000 by July, 1919 [7].

A lively discussion followed in which Frances Payne Bolton, a wealthy and influential citizen of Cleveland, supported Miss Goodrich's plan for the Army school. Adelaide Nutting then rose from her chair and strongly endorsed acceptance of the Army school plan. When a vote was taken, the three nursing organizations backed the establishment of an Army school of nursing.

Before the close of the convention in Cleveland, however, Annie Goodrich received an official telegram from the Surgeon General's Office stating that the plan for an Army school of nursing had been rejected by the General Staff of the War Department. The boards of the three national nursing organizations held an emergency meeting and appointed a committee to go to Washington and appeal to Secretary of War Baker to override the decision of the General Staff. Recognizing the value of lay support, they named only one nurse to the committee, Annie Goodrich. The two other members were Florence Linden Brewster and Frances Payne Bolton.

The Secretary of War granted a special hearing on the proposed Army school of nursing on May 25, 1918. By courtesy of the Surgeon General, Mrs. Bolton, Mrs. Brewster, and Miss Goodrich were admitted to Baker's office, where they waited some hours for the weary Secretary of War to return from a long session on Capitol Hill. Many years later Mrs. Bolton shed some light on the circumstances of the meeting:

At the time that the nursing situation in this country was exceedingly serious and some of us had joined with a number of the top nurses in the American Nurses' Association to establish an Army School of Nursing, we found nurses faced with formidable opposition. Secretary Newton Baker was very much inclined to the Army School, but it was apparent to all of us that someone, some organization, some group stood very much in the way . . . . There was no question in any of our minds that a few weeks or even a very few months of aide "training" could not take the place of skilled nursing care. Fortunately for our boys, the Secretary saw the wisdom of making possible transportation of our skilled women and the establishment of the Army School of Nursing [8].

Indeed, at the May 25 meeting, Baker agreed to approve the Army School of Nursing and nullify the action of the Army General Staff. His consent came following assurances by Mrs. Brewster that the Council of National Defense Women's Committee volunteers would exert every effort to recruit students for civilian nurse training schools, thus saving them from depletion at the hands of the Army school.

Seeking Applicants for the Army School of Nursing

The Committee on Nursing of the Council of National Defense set out in the summer of 1918 to recruit 25,000 women for the Army School of Nursing and other training schools, thus to provide an adequate supply of student nurses. The first literature concerning the Army School, issued on June 7, 1918, announced that it offered to women desiring to care for sick and wounded soldiers a course leading to a diploma in nursing. Candidates had to be between 21 and 35 years of age, in good physical condition, and of good moral character. They were also required to be graduates of recognized high schools or present evidence of an educational equivalent.

Within 10 days after the first official announcement in the press, 981 letters of inquiry were received; eight months later, over 10,000 applications had arrived in the Surgeon General's Office. When the first year's campaign ended, 14,000 applications had been received. Of these, 5380 applicants were admitted to the Army School and 5185 were enrolled for entrance into civilian schools of nursing. The rest were put on a waiting list.

Annie Goodrich was appointed Dean of the Army School of Nursing. She and her assistants carried on their activities from the Army Surgeon General's Office. She saw in the Army School plan an opportunity to establish an outstanding demonstration school in which the accepted principles of organization, administration, and teaching would be effectively applied. No tuition was required. The students were provided with board, lodging, laundry, and required textbooks. They had to provide themselves with indoor uniforms for the probationary period and, upon its successful completion, with an outdoor uniform and such additional indoor uniforms as were required during their residence in the school. A monthly allowance of $15 to meet these and other school expenses was provided, except during a period of affiliation.

The three-year course was based on the new *Standard Curriculum for Schools of Nursing*, published by the National League of Nursing Education in 1917. The time allotted to the various subjects was divided between lectures and demonstrations by members of the medical staff, or among special lectures and classes, quizzes, and laboratory work under qualified nurses and other instructors. The hours of duty on the ward were arranged to accommodate required classwork. Unlike the schedule in most civilian hospital schools, duty hours

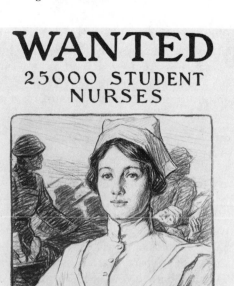

World War I student nurse recruitment poster.

A group of Army School of Nursing students at Camp Grant, Illinois, in 1918.

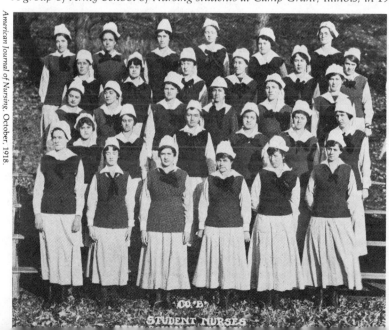

during the probationary period did not exceed six daily; after that, eight hours daily was the maximum. The military hospitals provided experience in surgical nursing, including orthopedic, eye, ear, nose, and throat, and medical nursing, including communicable, nervous, and mental diseases. Experience in the diseases of children, gynecology, obstetrics, and public health nursing was provided through affiliations in the second or third year.

At the Front

Meanwhile, on the front, contrary to expectations, the war offered no heroic glamour. The firepower generated by modern artillery was so devastating that armies could no longer stay on the surface of the battlefield. Consequently, trenches hundreds of miles long were dug. Then, in order to secure the trenches from surprise attack, each side spun hundreds of thousands of miles of barbed wire before its entrenchments. The art of offensive warfare shifted to wallowing, defensive action amid mudholes and barbed wire. Armies became cannon fodder as the glory of war disappeared in the mire of eastern France.

Military nurses soon saw the devastating effects of modern artillery fire. Fragmentation shells burst into a hail of small, deadly splinters that caused extensive, deep, and ragged wounds highly favorable to infection. The great lacerations due to explosive projectiles required expert surgical specialists and good nursing. Shrapnel (consisting of jagged pieces of iron) often cut across different organs of the trunk or abdomen and produced multiple injuries at a single impact. High-explosive blast concussion alone could destroy several parts of the body at once. Shrapnel caused deep, penetrating wounds that were ready culture for infections and demanded the most careful nursing care. "The wounds which you will be called upon to handle and dress are such that you have never imagined it possible for a human being to be so fearfully hurt and yet to be alive," exclaimed one nurse.

The soil of France and Belgium, manured and cultivated for centuries, was found to be heavily laden with pathogenic germs. Long periods of duty in the muddy, often filthy trenches made the soldier's skin, as well as his uniform, dirty and germ-laden, so that bits of the soil driven into a wound almost inevitably produced infection. Consequently, nurses on the Western Front soon discovered that there was no such thing as a sterile gunshot wound.

These women also saw the effects of the new steel-jacketed bullets. Impact reduced soft body tissues to a devitalized pulp that quickly necrotized and was an ideal medium for the growth of pathogenic bacteria. Surgical asepsis under such conditions was impossible, and it became necessary to regress to fundamental listerism or antisepsis. It was soon found, however, that strong antiseptics applied to deep, infected wounds would not sterilize them. An added difficulty was that strong antiseptics were likely to kill both the infectious organism and the surrounding healthy tissue.

Medical researchers attempted to find a substance that would kill the germs without causing injury to tissue. An answer to this problem was found by sur-

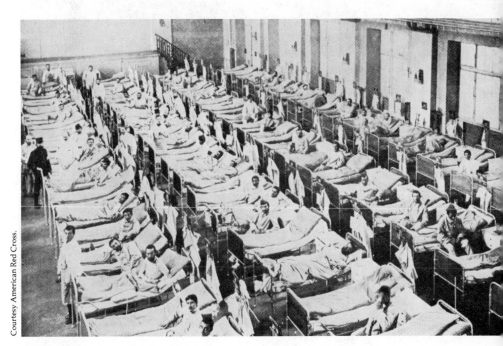

A crowded European Army hospital.

geon Alexis Carrel and chemist Henry Dakin, who developed an effective method of disinfecting wounds by using a weak chlorine solution in continuous irrigation. Continuous irrigation was secured by Carrel's device of inserting into the wound a series of rubber supply tubes through which was fed the chlorine solution. In this way it became possible to disinfect a wound and thus permit more rapid healing. After use of continuous irrigations, the progress of the wound was checked biologically by the laboratory as to the kind and number of bacteria. When the dangerous kinds had disappeared and the ordinary types were present in very small numbers, the surgeon practiced what was called secondary suture, and healing progressed with a new rapidity.

Superhuman Demands

Given the new challenges of patient care, it was not uncommon for nurses to work 14 to 18 hours a day for weeks at a time, and some hospitals had only 70 or 80 nurses caring for up to 2100 patients. One hospital reached a patient load of 5000, with only 70 nurses to furnish patient care. There were many other hospitals with equally disproportionate figures. A nurse at Crézancy described her situation:

About 2 o'clock Monday morning the journey's end was reached. No place to lie down. All lay down with suits, coats and raincoats on, with gas masks and helmets near at hand, and in spite of the soft drizzle of rain slept, forgetting the war, until 8 A.M. That

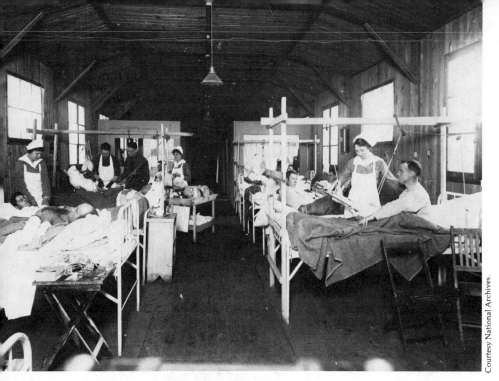

Army nurses at work at U.S. Base Hospital No. 52 at Rimaucourt, Haute Mare, France, early 1918.

The struggle to save a life in one of the operating rooms.

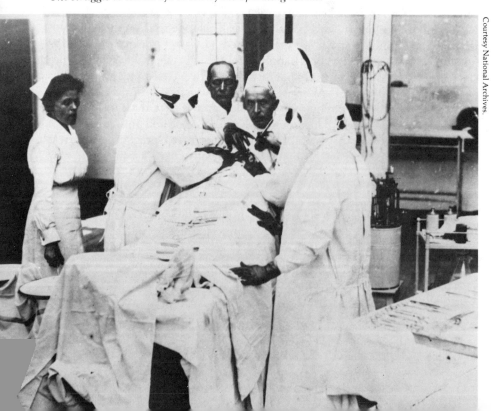

day several nurses appropriated a tiny house by the side of the road; and others got a cot in barracks or little tents. Later, marquise tents were provided for all of the nurses.

The drive was on, the wounded poured in, the nurses forgot themselves in a combined effort to do their share to check the crimson tide which was so terrible at this place. The nurses with operating teams as well as those attached to the hospital worked, not caring how hard nor how long the hours. The object of all was to save.

The dead about Crézancy were still unburied, and the flies and yellow jackets were too terrible for description. Many of the nurses were ill. Sanitary conditions here were most pitiful.

The weather was extremely hot—especially were the tents extremely hot—the blazing sun beat down on the tents at day. The combined smell of ether, blood, stale air and heavy atmosphere from the steam sterilizers is one to be not easily forgotten after fifteen or eighteen hours of work [9].

The work of the Army nurse was exceedingly strenuous. Emma Quandt, a nurse from Chicago, wrote:

A hypodermic of morphine was given the patient so that he would rest until morning, provided his condition or the nature of the wound did not need surgical attention in the operating theatre. I shall never forget my first convoy of wounded soldiers, twenty-seven stretcher cases, almost every one had to have an amputation of some member of the body. A number of my patients died from exposure in the trenches, because it had been about thirty-six hours before any aid could reach them. It was a pitiful sight to see these strong, healthy, young men, blind or crippled for life [10].

The 8587 nurses with the 184,000 wounded and sick American soldiers in the 153 base hospitals, 66 camps, and 12 convalescent hospitals in Europe in mid-1918 became familiar with many dramatic scenes. As the wounded were brought in, their packs, gas masks, and helmets were thrown on the salvage heap to be carted away at any slack hour. There was no time to remove the clothing from the men. The wounds were hurriedly fluoroscoped, and places where shell fragments or bullets were lodged were marked with a cross in indelible pencil as a guide to the surgeons. The stretchers were placed directly on the operating room table to save time, and the clothing cut away from around the wound. As the patient was given chloroform and ether, the wound was cleansed with gasoline, then iodine was applied. Each wound was laid open and the injured tissue cut away—an operation called a débridement.

Experiences in War

One nurse described the scene at a large allied hospital in France as follows:

Eleven P.M. The whistle sounds three times. Six newcomers.

"This leg is bleeding badly. Don't jolt him. Take him carefully to the operating room. Hurry."

"Your wound is in the head, I see. Doctor, to which ward shall he go?"

"Wash him and warm him. Then let them take him to Salle III. It is Nourier's turn tomorrow. He will operate."

"And this one, ma soeur?"

"A bullet in the abdomen; hardly any pulse and he has been vomiting."

"When was he wounded? Twenty-four hours ago? It is a scandal. We must operate at once. You say that none of them have had antitetanus serum? What criminal neglect. An inquiry must be set afoot. Such things cannot be allowed to pass. Where is he from?"

"From Bosinghe."

"Our section. How can they expect us to save them if they keep them so long before sending them on? What with poisoned ammunition and exposure, the odds are all against them."

"This man, doctor, is wounded in the neck. His card says the bullet went through the neck and is probably lodged in the base of the skull or in the spine."

"When was your last dressing done, mon ami? I can hardly hear what you say—two hours ago? Two? (Holding up two fingers.) You have come all that way with your head over the end of the stretcher like that? I see, you could not breathe with it otherwise? Get him warm, nurse, and send him to the operating room. Then we will see."

"How terrifyingly blue his face is. Such a nice face, too. He has hardly any pulse."

"Here, my friend, let me put this cushion under your head and raise it a little. And the hot-water bottles will soon make you feel better. Thank you for that smile."

All bad cases tonight.

In the operating room the boy with a bullet in the abdomen lies on his stretcher on the floor, apparently dead. They do all they can to bring him round. He revives. They chloroform him, open the abdominal cavity. Floods of dark blood well out.

We are too late.

"If they could only send us these abdominal cases at once. A fine, handsome young chap like that, too."

"Yes, appalling. It's war. Now for that leg; it cannot wait" [11].

Shirley Millard was assigned to a field hospital in France. The carnage was on a scale beyond anything she had imagined. "Day after day we cut down stinking bandages and expose wounds that destroy the whole original plan of the body. One man had both buttocks blown off, one arm had been amputated at the elbow, and he had a host of smaller wounds from flying metal. Another lay propped on sphagnum moss to absorb the discharge from two large holes in each thigh" [12]. Like other healthy young women, she felt somehow guilty in the presence of so much suffering and such majestic pain:

No matter what we did, how hard we worked, it did not seem to be fast enough or hard enough. More came. It took me several days to steel my emotions against the stabbing cries of pain. The crowded, twisted bodies, the screams and groans, made one think of the old engravings in Dante's Inferno. More came, and still more . . . .

My hands tremble as I pull at sodden boots and uniforms. The weather is cold and wet and most of their garments are caked with mud from head to foot, so that to get the things off without causing excruciating pain is almost impossible. "Leave me alone, will you," they scream wildly and resist my ministrations. Many of them have nothing on their wounds but a strip of coat sleeve or an old muffler or a muddy legging wrapped on quickly by a comrade in the field. Some have only newspaper tied on with a bootlace. I remove blood-and-mud-soaked bandages and find an arm hanging by a tendon. . . .

Gashes from bayonets. Eyes torn by shrapnel. Faces half shot away. Eyes seared by gas; one here with no eyes at all. I can see down into the back of his head. Here is a boy with a gray, set face. He is hanging on . . . too far gone to make a sound. His stomach is blown wide open and only held together by a few bands of sopping gauze which I must

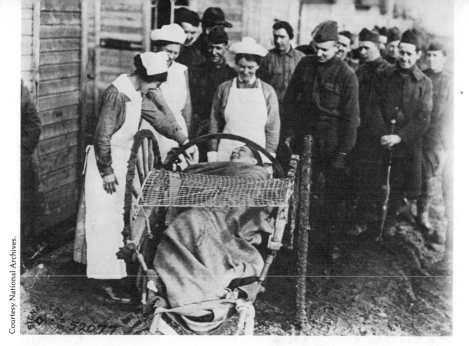

Nurses of Ward 4, Base Hospital 52 say goodbye to a soldier who has had much of his lower body shot away.

Army nurse preparing for a poison gas attack.

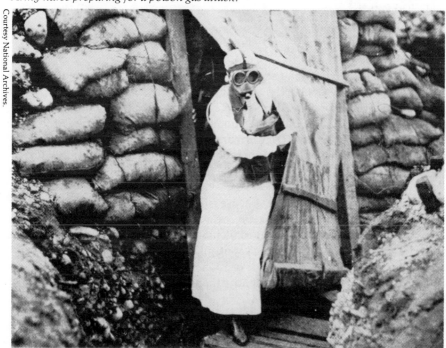

. pull away. I do so, gently as I can. The odor is sickening; the gauze is a greenish yellow. Gangrene. He was wounded days ago and has been waiting on the grounds. He will die [13].

The high-speed butchery of the operating theaters after a battle had its own horrors. The leg that one of the nurses was holding came off with a jerk, and she fell down still clasping the foot. She stuffed the leg into the dressing pail beside the other arms and legs. The emergency was so great that surgery was performed right on the wards, and amputated legs were stuck in buckets in the corridors outside. Still the casualties kept coming:

Here is an unconscious lad with his head completely bandaged. The gauze is stiff with blood and dirt. I cut carefully and remove it, glad he is unconscious; much easier to work when they cannot feel the pain. As the last band comes off, a sickening mass spills out of the wide gash at the side of his skull. Brains. I am stunned. I cannot think what to do. No time to ask questions. Everyone around me is occupied with similar problems. Boldly I wrap my hand in sterile gauze and thrust the slippery mass back as best I can, holding the wound closed while I awkwardly tie a clean bandage around the head. It does not occur to me until afterwards that he must have been dead.
　A boy from Idaho, a big round boy, had his head all bound up and the tag around his neck, put on at a dressing station, said: "Eyes shot away and both feet gone." I talked to him and patted him on the shoulder, assuring him that everything would be all right now. He moaned through the bandages that his head was splitting with pain. I gave him morphine. Suddenly aware of the fact that he had other wounds, he asked: "Sa-ay, what's the matter with my legs?" Reaching down to feel his legs before I could stop him, he uttered a heartbreaking scream. I held his hands firmly until the drug I had given him took effect [14].

A New Weapon—Gas

As if wounds from bullets and shrapnel were not enough, an even more terrifying and gruesome weapon of war emerged with cataclysmic results—poison gas. Its first use had occurred on April 22, 1915, in the vicinity of Langemark, near Ypres. On that fatal day, after bombarding the French forces with high explosives at early morning, the Germans halted their fire about two hours before sunset. Then they opened more than 500 cylinders containing 168 tons of pressurized chlorine gas and waited as the light wind bore it steadily toward the opposing forces. The effect was devastating—chlorine, a greenish-yellow gas with a sharp, acrid smell, causes intense irritation of the lungs; if inhaled in a concentration of more than 1:10,000 for a minute or two, death ensues. The same concentration is incapacitating if inhaled for only a few seconds. The Germans had released the gas over a four-mile front upon an enemy totally unprepared for this kind of attack. All resistance was eliminated on the front to a depth of several miles. There were more than 15,000 casualties, including 5000 fatalities.
　Even more feared was dichloroethylsulphide, better known as mustard gas, from the odor of its impure, liquid form, first used by the Germans in July, 1917. Like many of the toxic "gases," mustard is liquid at ordinary tempera-

tures, boiling at 217°C. It evaporated slowly; and, when collected in the soil, it took weeks to evaporate completely. The liquid itself was harmful, quickly penetrating clothing and causing severe, deep burns on the skin, which were difficult to heal. The effects themselves took a few hours to appear but were often widespread. The eyes became inflamed and the lungs irritated. Large doses caused severe vomiting, nausea, fever, and side effects, among them shock, which resulted from the severe trauma to the human body. Even diluted to 1:100,000, the gas still produced its effects after only one or two minutes' exposure. These began to appear about an hour after contact and would be fully developed after perhaps five hours.

It was easy enough for the nurses at the base hospitals to see why mustard gas was so effective. It was practically colorless, and its garlic or mustard smell lasted only a few minutes. Provided that the means by which the gas was delivered was not discovered, there was no reason why it would be detected until the effects had begun to appear some hours later. By this time massive doses would have been received. Furthermore, the liquid and vapor would linger, making any position that had been attacked by mustard gas untenable for some time. During the last year of the war it accounted for 16 percent of the British casualties and 33 percent of the American ones.

Margaret Dunlop, Chief Nurse of the Pennsylvania Hospital Unit, recalled that their first hard experience in nursing came shortly after their arrival in France when the field hospital received an exceedingly large convoy of mustard gas victims.

These patients were horribly gassed and were pictures of misery and intense suffering. They poured upon us in great numbers—600 in less than forty-eight hours—and their sufferings were pitiful to see, but their bravery, unselfishness, and fortitude were impressed upon us very fully. The nurses worked hard and faithfully during this short period, but the awfulness and immensity of suffering and cruel barbarity of war upon the individual were a soul-harrowing experience to them all. It was a tremendous strain on mind, heart, and body, being untrained to the handling of such large numbers and not yet inured to the immensity of the work. During that summer of 1917, we had our baptism of horror and work, but after a few months the whole Unit settled down to the inevitable, and as the handling of large numbers of severely wounded was efficiently expedited, the fear of not being equal to the task gradually disappeared [15].

After a gas attack the burned and sightless eyes made all the faces look like a ghastly row of masks, and the utter silence completed the illusion of one's being surrounded by puppets:

November 8th, 1918

More and more Americans in the death ward. Gas cases are terrible. They cannot breathe lying down or sitting up. They just struggle for breath, but nothing can be done . . . their lungs are gone . . . literally burnt out. Some with their eyes and faces entirely eaten away by the gas, and bodies covered with first degree burns. We try to relieve them by pouring oil on them. They cannot be bandaged or even touched. We cover them with a tent of propped-up sheets. Gas burns must be agonizing because usually the other cases invar-

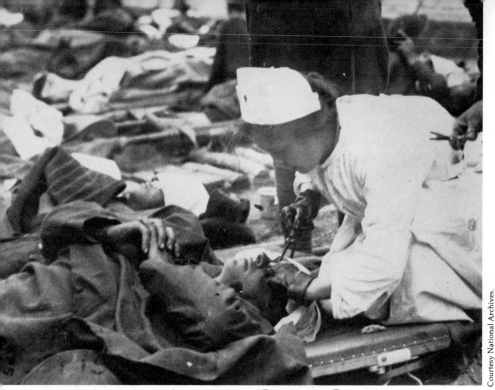

Nurse bathing the eyes of gas patients near Royaumeiux, France, in 1918.

Nurse and physician caring for a patient suffering from Spanish influenza, December, 1918.

A nurse, wearing a mask as a protection against influenza, fills a pitcher from a water hydrant.

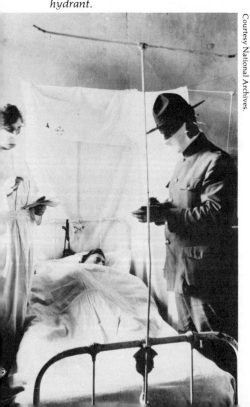

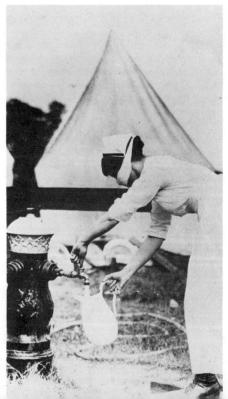

iably are beyond endurance and they cannot help crying out.

One boy today, screaming to die. The entire top layer of skin burned from his face and body. I gave him an injection of morphine. He was wheeled out just before I came off duty [16].

Shock, hemorrhage, infected wounds, and the care of gassed patients challenged the powers of observation and the technical skills of nurses. Barbara Thompson recalled:

Gas was very disastrous in this war. I went on night duty during an artillery barrage, and I prepared morphine shots for twelve hours to ease the severe pain of the wounded. These patients suffered severe shock and pain and many died before first aid could be given. Working conditions were primitive. Not at all like the conditions in the operating rooms in the U.S. I was on night duty during the Château-Thierry drive. One night as I was giving a soldier an anesthetic when almost under he yelled, "I am the strongest man in America," and off the table he went with me hanging fast to his chin with the ether mask over his face [17].

The Great Influenza Epidemic of 1918–1919

Meanwhile another insidious force was at work. This phenomenon, a massive influenza epidemic that would cause many more deaths than did the fighting, burst upon the nation and the world without warning. The continual movement of the troops created avenues of travel for the disease, and the mingling of people from home and abroad was probably the facilitating element in the development of the highly virulent strain of influenza that emerged. Soldiers and civilians alike faced an unseen and unconquerable enemy, a microscopic virus—not photographed until 1933—in many ways more formidable an adversary than the armies themselves.

During this great epidemic, from September, 1918, to August, 1919, the United States experienced the highest excess death rate in its history. Ninety-two percent of all the excess deaths were directly attributable to influenza and its colleague in death, pneumonia. When it was over, incomplete data revealed that the death toll in the United States alone for the last four months of 1918 and the first six months of 1919 was 548,452—five times greater than total World War I American military deaths.

Nurses were expected to perform the more everyday chores of caring for influenza patients and to deal with situations of life and death. Often physicians were unavailable, and in the final analysis the nurses were the heroines of the fight of hundreds of thousands of human bodies against the epidemic. Shockingly, estimates of the number of influenza deaths world-wide ranged from a "low" of 15 million to a high of 30 million, with most estimates running around 22 million.

The influenza epidemic in America was in full force by the time news of the Armistice came. On November 11, 1918, there were 193,000 patients in hospitals in France and 70,000 patients in Army hospitals at home. The larger hospital centers in France, such as Allerey, Bazoilles, Toul, Mesves, Mars, and Savenay were originally 1000-bed units but in times of heavy casualties had become huge installations with an emergency capacity of 10,000 to 40,000 beds. For example, the Mesves Hospital Center had, in November, 1918, 25,000 beds, with 20,186 patients and 394 nurses.

A Summing Up

Though the ideal ratio was one nurse to every 10 patients, records show that at one time the Army hospital in Savenay, France, had 59.5 patients to every nurse. In another hospital, 150 women were caring for 9000 wounded. During the great Meuse-Argonne drive, all the hospitals in France were shorthanded, while the demands due to the great influenza epidemic in the United States were even more serious. Often the nurses worked until they themselves became patients, sometimes with fatal results. American nurses also helped staff the hospitals of United States' Allies, who continually asked for more of them.

In all, nearly 300 military nurses laid down their lives. None were killed in action, though three were wounded by enemy fire. Two lost their lives and one was seriously wounded in a premature explosion during target practice at sea on an American transport. One hundred others narrowly escaped with their lives when their transport collided and sank in New York harbor. More than two-thirds of the nurse casualties resulted from pneumonia and influenza, induced largely by overwork, exhaustion, and poor living conditions.

The war gave the Navy Nurse Corps its first major opportunity to impress upon any remaining skeptics its importance to the Navy. Assigned to hospitals in England, Ireland, and Scotland, and on the French coast, Navy nurses firmly established their value through devotion to duty, high-quality patient care, and effective instruction of hospital corpsmen. The demands of World War I upon the Medical Department of the Navy were reflected in the strength of the Nurse Corps, which increased its ranks to a peak strength of nearly 1500.

After the Armistice most of the nurses returned to their homes and to civilian nursing or married. But for many of those who had witnessed the carnage of battle, life would never be quite the same. The vivid images of the destruction caused by war and by the influenza epidemic lived on in their minds, and many of the nurses probably felt as did Dante in the *Inferno*—that the multiple horrors they had beheld defied description:

Who even in unrhymed words
Could ever fully tell in many narrations
Of the blood and the wounds I now saw?

Every tongue certainly would fail
Because our language and our memories
Are insufficient to contain so much [18].

Although nurses would never forget the nightmare of treating mass casualties

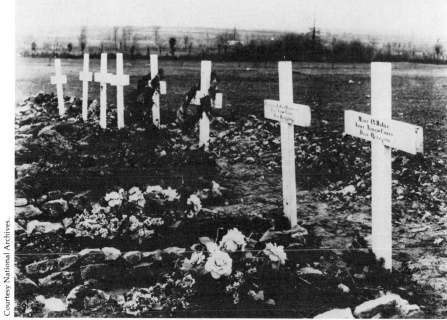

Graves of American military nurses who died in service near Mars-Sur-Allier, Nievre, France.

Wedding bells for an Army nurse and an officer, somewhere in France.

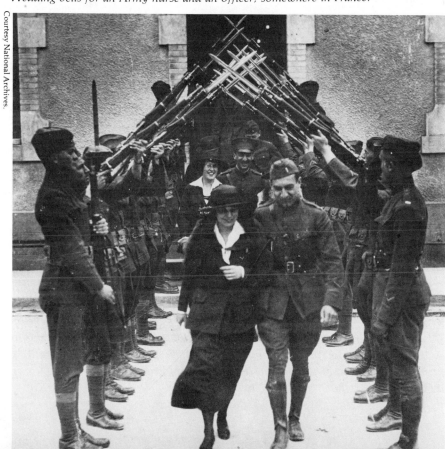

of the fighting and the accompanying diseases of World War I, they would remember with pride their own crucial and dramatic battles to save endangered lives and to lighten the toll of war and pestilence.

Summary

As America entered World War I, nurses faced the enormous challenge of providing nurse manpower for both the military and the civilian populations.

Although the Army Nurse Corps and the Navy Nurse Corps were expanded greatly in strength, the military need was not fully met and the drain on civilian nursing grew increasingly more serious.

Following the pattern set in European countries, American society women and other untrained persons expressed great interest in providing nursing care on the battlefields. Nurse leaders, horrified at this prospect, formed an emergency committee (the Committee on Nursing) to develop a plan to deal with the crisis.

Schools were called upon to increase their facilities to accommodate more students. Consequently, admissions to schools of nursing during 1917–1918 increased by about 25 percent.

A drive was made to interest college women in nursing, since they were needed for leadership roles. Schools were asked to reduce the three-year requirement for those college women with satisfactory backgrounds in science, but many administrators were hesitant to cooperate.

Consequently, a highly successful experimental program, known as the Vassar Training Camp, was developed, in which female college graduates enrolled in a three-month intensive preparatory course at Vassar and then entered a regular school of nursing for the balance of their training.

As civilian nurse supply reached the danger level and the quality of nursing service in Army hospitals deteriorated, it became evident that massive reform was needed. Annie Goodrich proposed that an Army school of nursing be established, to provide patients in Army hospitals with the same standard of student nurse care available in civilian general hospitals.

After a period of emotional debate and a dramatic plea by Frances Payne Bolton and others to Secretary of War Newton D. Baker, asking him to overturn the negative report of the Army general staff, the Army School of Nursing was approved and implemented.

Annie Goodrich, the school's dean, saw the venture as an opportunity to develop an exemplary nurse-preparation program based on sound educational principles. The response to the Army School of Nursing was overwhelmingly positive, and it attracted many more qualified applicants than could be accommodated.

The types of wounds received from the modern artillery and exploding projectiles of World War I mandated new nursing skills. Wound infection became a nearly overwhelming problem.

In late 1918 a massive influenza and associated pneumonia epidemic spread throughout America and the world. Soldiers acted as vectors of the disease, and a highly virulent strain emerged, killing more than 548,000 Americans and an estimated 22 million people worldwide.

In all, nearly 300 military nurses died in World War I, more than two-thirds as a result of influenza and pneumonia. Those who survived carried vivid memories of the terrifying carnage of battle back into civilian life.

References

1. Noyes to Nutting, April 8, 1917, Nursing Archives, Teachers College, Columbia University.
2. U.S. Council of National Defense, *First Annual Report of the Council of National Defense, Fiscal Year 1917* (Washington, D.C.: Government Printing Office, 1917), pp. 1–5.
3. Vera Brittain, *Testament of Youth: An Autobiographical Study of the Years 1900–1925* (New York: Macmillan Co., 1933), pp. 420–421.
4. William Howard Taft, "A Distinct Call to Women," *Ladies' Home Journal*, vol. 34 (July, 1918):22.
5. Annie W. Goodrich, "Report of the Survey of the Nursing Resources of the Country," *American Journal of Nursing*, vol. 18 (August, 1918): 959–961.
6. Winford H. Smith, "How Nurses are Meeting the Present Needs," *American Journal of Nursing*, vol. 18 (August, 1918):979–986.
7. *Ibid.*, pp. 983–986.
8. Interview with Frances Payne Bolton, Cleveland, Ohio, July 31, 1972.
9. "A War Nurse's Diary," *Trained Nurse and Hospital Review*, vol. 60 (February, 1918):90–91.
10. Emma Quandt, "Active Service on the Western Front," *American Journal of Nursing*, vol. 18 (March, 1918):454–455.
11. Maud Mortimer, *A Green Tent in Flanders* (New York: Doubleday, 1918), pp. 173–174.
12. Shirley Millard, *I Saw Them Die: Diary and Recollections of Shirley Millard* (New York: Harcourt, Brace, & Co., 1936), p. 12.
13. *Ibid.*, pp. 14–15.
14. *Ibid.*, pp. 15–16.
15. Margaret A. Dunlop, "History of the Nursing Corps of Base Hospital No. 10, U.S.A." *History of the Pennsylvania Hospital Unit in the Great War* (New York: Paul B. Hoeber, 1921), p. 85.
16. Millard, *op cit.*, p. 108.
17. Statement by Barbara Thompson Sharpless, World War I nurse, in an interview, Ventura, California, July 31, 1973.
18. Dante Alighieri, trans. H. R. Huse, *The Divine Comedy* (New York: Henry Holt & Co., 1954), p. 133.

11
Boom and Bust, 1920–1933

As the 1920s dawned, the nation's nursing staffs were still disorganized and depleted. Hospitals had not yet recovered from the double strain of war and influenza. Many graduate and student nurses had died in the epidemic, and the long-term effects of the disease forced many more to give up their work. The entire educational program in most schools of nursing had been suspended for weeks because of the absence of instructors and the critical situation in hospitals.

Shortage of Students
During the war, applications to nursing schools had greatly increased, and, in response to appeals from the Committee on Nursing, extra classes had been admitted to help meet wartime needs. As a consequence, it was estimated that in the 1755 schools of nursing in the United States, several thousand of the 54,953 student nurse enrollees would not have been attracted to nursing without the war-induced stimulation. A fairly large proportion of these young women had been drawn from other occupations and had patriotically entered the schools "for the duration of the war." Most young women with such motivation who were physically fit remained through the influenza epidemic. Shortly afterward, however, they felt their war service was over, and large numbers dropped out of the schools.

There was an approximate shortage of 55,000 trained nurses in the United States in 1920. In the Public Health Service, which was temporarily handling all the hospitalization for war veterans, there was a need for 10,000 more nurses than could be recruited. According to statistics compiled by the National Organization for Public Health Nursing, 70,000 American babies died in 1920 because their mothers did not have proper prenatal or postnatal care. Of those deaths, 5000 occurred in New York City. Physicians everywhere complained that they were greatly handicapped because they could not get competent nurses for serious cases. Hospitals were unable to provide adequate nursing service for their patients for this same reason.

Schools of nursing could not recruit enough students to fill their classes. In Connecticut the schools were short 700 student nurses. In New York State the roster was 2500 short. At the Lenox Hill Hospital, New York City, where the

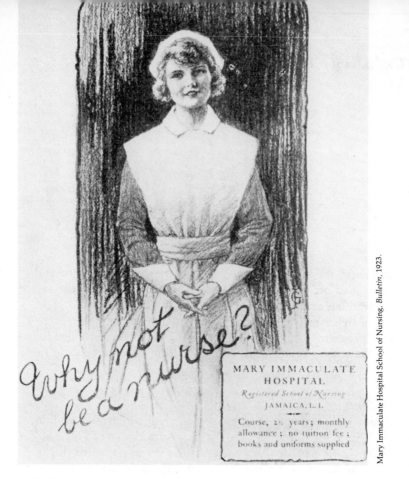

Inside the advertisement:

MARY IMMACULATE
HOSPITAL.
Registered School of Nursing
JAMAICA, L. I.

Course, 2½ years; monthly
allowance ; no tuition fee ;
books and uniforms supplied

Why not be a nurse?

Early 1920s nurse recruitment advertisement.

quota of nursing students was 125, the classes totaled only 56. Recruitment prospects had grown so hopeless in Indiana that some hospitals in the smaller towns were closing their doors.

The Impact of World War I

In 1921 Isabel Stewart, Assistant Professor, Department of Nursing and Health, Teachers College, Columbia University, summed up the impact of the war years on the nursing profession in a separate bulletin issued by the United States Bureau of Education, *Developments in Nursing Education Since 1918*. She observed that through widespread publicity the number of young women entering nursing schools during 1917 and 1918 had been increased by 25 percent. Every effort had been made to attract the more serious and better-educated women for this service, and as a result the average educational level of entering students had increased noticeably. In spite of the disruptions caused by the war, the epidemic, and the disorganization of teaching and supervisory staffs in hospitals, the educational status of nursing schools was in certain ways better at the end of the war than it had been at the beginning. Miss Stewart concluded:

Probably the greatest contribution of the war experience to nursing lies in the fact that the whole system of nursing education was shaken for a little while out of its well-worn ruts and brought out of its comparative seclusion into the light of public discussion and criticism. When so many lives hung on the supply of nurses, people were aroused to a new sense of their dependence on the products of nursing schools, and many of them learned for the first time of the hopelessly limited resources which nursing educators have had to work with in the training of these indispensable public servants. Whatever the future may bring it is unlikely that nursing schools will willingly sink back again into their old isolation, or that they will accept unquestionably the financial status which the older system imposed on them [1].

The Image Problem

From the point of view of the hospital administrators of the 1920s, student nurses were a necessity and could be secured only by an apprenticeship system of education. Financially, the institutions were well repaid, since student nurses furnished nursing care at very low cost. As a result, numerous additional schools were established, as the figures surged from 1755 in 1920, to 1964 in 1923, and to 2286 in 1927. During the same span of years student enrollments soared from 54,953 in 1920 to 77,768 in 1927. Too many nurses were soon being graduated, many without adequate training. From the student nurses' point of view, their own exploitation was rarely considered, since an overriding consecration to service was taken for granted among those who entered the profession.

Following the glamour of service in the war, the overall prestige of nursing declined sharply. Nursing's lower prestige was in part related to the fact that 95 percent of the active nurses in the nation were women. In a culture that was

Main hospital building and nurses' home at Saint Francis Hospital, Peoria, Illinois, 1924.

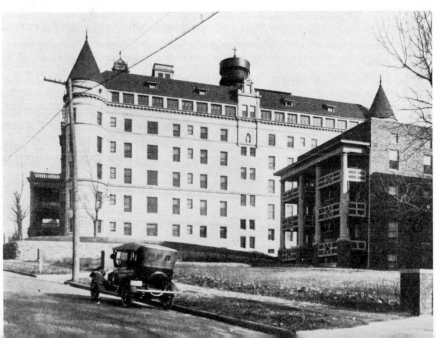

predominantly "a man's world," any occupation made up primarily of women was considered to be feminine, and therefore inferior. Added to this was the social phenomenon that a great majority of nurse leaders were unmarried; therefore they lacked the social prestige that marriage brought in the society of the time.

An unforgettable picture of middle-class American sex-typing was clearly presented in the sociological study *Middletown*, by Robert S. Lynd and Helen M. Lynd. Here, as depicted in 1924, men and women belonged to two different subcultures: the man's world involved professional leadership, while the woman's involved the care and training of small children. Male authority always loomed in the background. This role differentiation was based on an assumption that men and women were different kinds of people. Men were portrayed as stronger, bolder, more logical, and more reasonable, but in need of coddling and reassurance from women. Women, although more delicate physically, were considered stronger morally and more refined, sympathetic, and sensitive. What held in *Middletown* was postulated as true of the nation as a whole.

The fast-growing motion picture industry, with its myriad depictions of nurses on the screen in such productions as *Goodnight Nurse* and *When a Woman Sins*, was of little help to hospitals in stimulating nurse recruitment. In 1921 Edwin P. Haworth, Superintendent of Wilcrest Hospital and Willows Sanitarium, Kansas City, Missouri, noted that "nursing life" had always been looked upon by the laity "as a Florence Nightingale or Clara Barton sort of life—something ideal, with a purpose" [2]. It was the model profession for the humanitarian, one that might often be enhanced by altruistic or religious commitments. It was a nonwordly profession. For the non-Catholic world, nursing was the substitute for the Sisters of Charity, an opportunity to give one's life in service to society. As such, nursing had had its own distinct and lofty appeal.

"Why do movies have such unreal stuff when they attempt to present a drama of nursing or hospital life?" Haworth asked. He had just seen Mary Miles Minter in the 1920 film, *Nurse Marjorie*. Miss Minter skillfully acted the part she had to play, but it was clear that she was not a nurse. "No nurse would do the things she did," Haworth complained. No hospital of standing would tolerate the actions of such a nurse. It was not typical of nursing or hospital life [3].

He worried that with the film presenting the nurse and her profession in this light, the nursing standards of earlier years would not be preserved for the eyes of the world. He perceived that movies were beginning to elicit school of nursing applicants who came with the "wrong ideals." In the meantime, young women with the proper ideals were not choosing nursing in the proportion they once did. Haworth concluded:

Perhaps I am wrong in thinking the movies are treating the nursing profession worse than other kinds of life. Perhaps it is merely the unusual and farfetched method of handling all lines of life and thought. If so, so much the worse for the movies. If they are as abnormal and unrealistic as that, then they are a more demoralizing influence for civilization than I

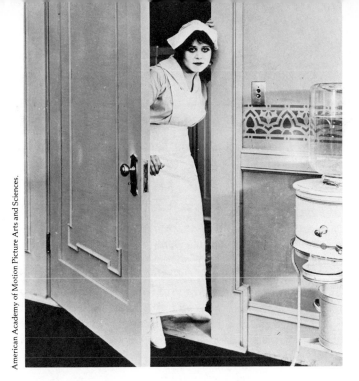

Theda Bara played a nurse in When a Woman Sins.

Mary Miles Minter as Nurse Marjorie in the 1920 motion picture based on the 1906 play by Israel Zangwill.

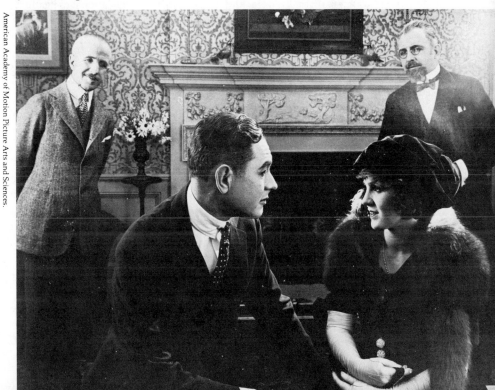

had thought. But the life of the nurse, pupil and graduate, is subject to worthwhile dramatization if presented faithfully. There are details in her life that appeal to the imagination and show her to be a character worth spending an hour with in the movies. Why can't we see the real nurse on the screen, instead of the movie-actress, play-nurse! Both the personality and the dramatic motive would then be improved, much to the advantage of our ideals, and the future of the nursing profession [4].

Inadequate Financial Support

According to Isabel Stewart, there was no hope for any substantial advancement in nursing education until nursing schools were removed from hospitals and placed on a separate standing. This did not mean that pupils should not be trained in hospitals but that the nursing school, "like the medical school, should have an independent financial status and the power to work out its own system of education, unhampered by the complicated and often crushing demands of the hospital" [5]. She maintained that if some form of endowment could not be found for nursing schools, they should be supported by state or municipal funds. Miss Stewart boldly put her finger on the core of the problem:

The plain facts are that nursing schools are being starved and always have been starved for lack of funds to build up any kind of substantial educational structure. As someone has recently said, the nursing school has been literally buried in the hospital, and few people have been aware of its existence. It has fed on the crumbs that fell from the hospital table—a very frugal table, as everyone knows. The educational interests of the school have had no chance whatever against the pressing economic interests of the hospital, and it is probable that even if the hospital recognized its educational obligations, which it has never done, it would find considerable difficulty in meeting them as they should be met [6].

The Goldmark Report

In 1918 Adelaide Nutting had approached officials of the Rockefeller Foundation in an attempt to secure an endowment for her alma mater, the Johns Hopkins School of Nursing. During the interview she stressed the need for improvements in the education of public health nurses. This meeting resulted in the appointment, in January, 1919, of the Committee for the Study of Nursing Education, which was to investigate "the proper training of the public health nurse." Financial support was provided by the Rockefeller Foundation [7]. The committee of 19 chaired by C. E. A. Winslow, a professor of public health at Yale University, included six nurses: Adelaide Nutting, Annie Goodrich, Lillian Wald, S. Lillian Clayton, Mary Beard, and Helen Wood.

Also included were 10 physicians, among whom were two hospital superintendents. Two lay representatives, Julia C. Lathrop of the United States Children's Bureau, and Mrs. John Lowman completed the committee membership. It soon became obvious to the committee that the fundamental problem in public health nursing education was the condition of hospital training schools. Therefore, the scope of committee inquiry was broadened to a study of nursing

NURSING AND
NURSING EDUCATION
IN THE UNITED STATES

REPORT OF THE

COMMITTEE FOR THE STUDY OF NURSING EDUCATION

C.-E. A. WINSLOW, Dr.P.H., *Chairman*

MARY BEARD, R.N.	MRS. JOHN LOWMAN
H. M. BIGGS, M.D.	M. ADELAIDE NUTTING, R.N.
S. LILLIAN CLAYTON, R.N.	C. G. PARNALL, M.D.
LEWIS A. CONNER, M.D.	THOMAS W. SALMON, M.D.
DAVID L. EDSALL, M.D.	WINFORD H. SMITH, M.D.
LIVINGSTON FARRAND, M.D.	E. G. STILLMAN, M.D.
ANNIE W. GOODRICH, R.N.	LILLIAN D. WALD, R.N.
L. EMMETT HOLT, M.D.	W. H. WELCH, M.D.
JULIA C. LATHROP	HELEN WOOD, R.N.

JOSEPHINE GOLDMARK, *Secretary*

and

REPORT OF A SURVEY

by

JOSEPHINE GOLDMARK, *Secretary*

New York

THE MACMILLAN COMPANY

1923

Title page of the famous "Goldmark Report."

education in general.

The committee secretary was social worker and author, Josephine Goldmark, best known for her 1912 study of the relationship between fatigue and industrial efficiency, who was placed in charge of the survey research. Under her direction, opinions from leading nurse educators were gathered and synthesized. In addition, surveys were made through scientific sampling of representative conditions in schools of nursing and in public health and private duty nursing. An extensive survey of the more than 1800 hospital training schools in the United States was obviously beyond the resources of the committee. It was therefore decided to select a small group of schools for intensive study. Twenty-three such schools were finally chosen, representing large and small, public and private, general and special hospitals in various sections of the United States. These schools were undoubtedly well above the medium grade, and their average could be taken as fairly representative of the highest standards of nursing education. Each school was studied in detail by two special investigators, one a practical expert in nursing education and the other an experienced educator from outside the nursing field. The investigation of these schools covered the records of 2406 students.

After the release of the general findings in 1922, the exhaustive 500-page study by Josephine Goldmark, upon which the conclusions of the Committee were based, was at last made public in 1923 to form the initial landmark in the evaluation of nursing education. Entitled *Nursing and Nursing Education in the United States*, this document emphasized the desirability of establishing university schools of nursing to train nurse leaders. It pointed out the fundamental faults in hospital training schools and identified the primary obstacle to higher standards as the lack of funds set apart specifically for nursing education.

The Committee concluded that while training schools for nurses had made remarkable progress, and while the best schools reached a high level of educational attainment, the average hospital training school was not organized on a solid enough basis to be compared favorably with the standards required in other professions. Formal instruction in schools of nursing was too casual and uncorrelated, and the educational needs and the health and strength of students were often sacrificed to hospital service demands.

"From our field study of the nurse in public health nursing, in private duty, and as instructor and supervisor in hospitals," said Miss Goldmark, "it is clear that there is need of a basic undergraduate training for all nurses alike, which should lead to a nursing diploma." She concluded that postgraduate training in any one of the three above nursing specialties should be given after the completion of basic undergraduate courses and should lead to an advanced diploma or degree [8].

The reasons for the failure of some schools of nursing and the factors contributing to those failures were reported, including:

Tradition

Continuance of the apprenticeship system

Needs of sick predominate; the needs of education must yield thereto.

Lack of a paid group of graduate nurses to meet the hospital need, relieving the student body of non-nursing duties.

Irregular assignments.

Failure to extend the education promised in catalogue.

Failure of superintendent to show the board the impossible nature of task.

No training school committee.

School remains as a department of the hospital.

Many schools accept low educational entrance standards.

Failure to include all services, such as communicable and mental and nervous.

Understaffing of wards.

Lack of adequate supervision.

Careless techniques.

Lack of sufficient and proper affiliations.

Need of appointment of full-time instructors.

Poor planning, in that instruction does not precede technique.

Theory and practice often taught by different women, differently trained, without conferences.

Lack of well-qualified teachers.

Neglect of suitable laboratory instruction and equipment.

Insufficient allowance of time for study.

Overcrowded character of courses.

Waste of student's time.

Lack of endowments.

Lack of graded training.

Use of students as head nurses.

Lack of conferences.

Lack of adequate records.

Lack of correlation between practice and theory.

Failure to use dispensary and clinics as teaching field.

Too much stress placed upon curative medicine to the detriment of preventive medicine.

Psychology, public health and social service not included in curriculum.

Excessive length of hours on duty.

Classwork in evening hours.

Lack of recreational facilities for students.

Failure to provide students with one day's rest in seven and to notify students of days off.

Assignments of night duty service disproportionately long and too close together.

Class hours interrupt sleep, when on night duty [9].

In commenting on several of these problems, the report stated that in most hospitals the major services—medical, surgical, obstetric, pediatric, and communicable—were too often staffed by students who lacked instruction in the diseases or conditions of patients committed to their care, other than for nursing procedures that were given by the clinical instructor. After her preliminary period of four months, the student nurse was usually assigned to one of the main hospital services, either medical or surgical. It was obviously important that the medical and surgical lectures be given during this period. Yet in 75 percent of the small and medium-sized hospitals the students nursed medical and surgical patients after only four months of preliminary instruction; they received instruction in medical and surgical diseases during the second and third

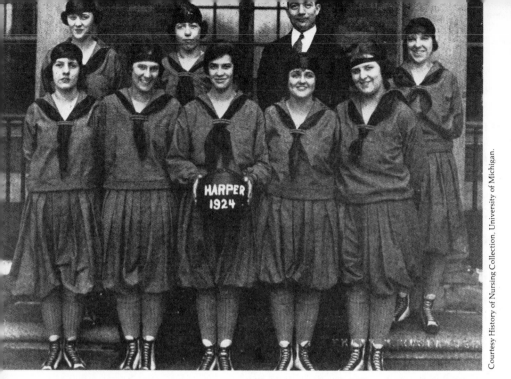

Recreation for students was not neglected at Harper Hospital School of Nursing, Detroit, where basketball was a highly popular sport.

Bath time at the Jewish Maternity Hospital, Philadelphia. A typical scene in the nursery any morning at 9:30.

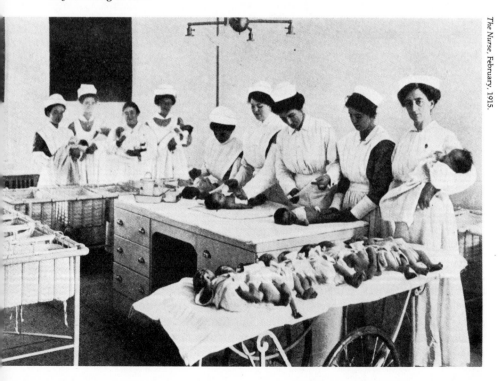

years. These students were assigned to night duty after only six months. They cared for critically ill patients both during the daytime and at night, without adequate teaching or supervision.

Too often the pressure of "getting the work done" removed any possibility of either good teaching or good supervision. It was determined that in most schools:

The sciences and the theory and the practice of nursing were frequently being taught by unprepared instructors in poorly equipped basement classrooms.

Hospitals controlled the total teaching hours or reduced the ground covered to the barest outline or might omit some subjects entirely.

Lectures were often given to students at night after a day of hard work.

The student's practical experience was usually limited to those services which were found in the hospital. The student learned to nurse those patients for whom the hospital cared.

The practical experience might be under the direction and guidance of graduate nurses who had neither preparation nor time to teach [10].

The survey made by the Goldmark Committee yielded the basic conclusion that the training of nurses was a serious educational business that must be directed by those who were primarily committed to quality nursing education. The Goldmark Committee emphasized the fundamental need to recognize the hospital school as a separate educational department, dedicated to giving students not a course of training but a thorough liberal education in nursing.

The First University Schools of Nursing

In 1909 Richard Olding Beard had successfully maneuvered to have the new nurse training school at the University of Minnesota organized as an integral part of that institution. Though it was subsumed under the college of medicine and offered only a three-year diploma, the Minnesota program was still a great step forward. Prior to this time, schools of nursing on college campuses had functioned as mere offshoots of the university hospitals and had been in no way part of the academic organization.

In 1916 Annie W. Goodrich reported that 16 colleges and universities maintained schools, departments, or courses in nursing education. A growing development in several universities was the combined academic and professional course of four to five years, leading to a nursing diploma and a bachelor of science degree. The usual arrangement was to admit the student upon completion of her high school course for two years of preliminary work in the university and then to give her two years of nurse training in the hospital, followed by a year of clinical work and study during which she would specialize in some particular branch of nursing.

By the early 1920s Simmons College, Northwestern University, Columbia University, and the universities of Cincinnati, Minnesota, Michigan, California, Colorado, Indiana, and Washington had introduced courses of this type. Only a few students took the longer course leading to a degree, although it was open to any who could meet the requirements. By 1926, although there were 25 colleges and universities conducting nurse training schools that granted A.B. or B.S. degrees in nursing, the enrollment in these schools was only 368. The small number of students in these courses attested to the continued dependence of the affiliated university hospitals upon the student body for the nursing care of its patients and the necessity of stressing the three-year course for almost all of the students. It was not surprising, therefore, that the findings of the Goldmark study concerning the influence of the university relationship in raising the standards of nursing education were disappointing.

The prenursing or preparatory course that had been given at Vassar College and at several universities during the summer of 1918 had demonstrated what might be done in the way of working with colleges and universities for at least a portion of the nurses' training. The standard of teaching at Vassar had been much higher than that which prevailed in the great majority of nursing schools. It was thought, however, that the great weakness of such detached courses was the absence of any organic connection with the hospital in which the student acquired her clinical experience and subsequent training.

Yale School of Nursing: First Autonomous Collegiate School

Shortly after the Goldmark Report was released, the Rockefeller Foundation, prodded by the Committee for the Study of Nursing Education, awarded a five-year grant to Yale University to establish a truly collegiate school of nursing. Founded as an experimental and pioneering venture, this school was epoch-making in that, for the first time in the history of nurse training, the financial means were provided whereby the content of nurse education might be developed according to curative and preventive needs. The grant was contingent upon the University's implementation of a course which would consolidate nursing theory and practice in the shortest feasible curriculum and eliminate traditional nonnursing assignments. Nursing theory was to be correlated with practical experience, and emphasis throughout the course was to be placed on the preventive aspects.

The Yale School of Nursing, opened in February, 1924, was the first in the world to be established as a separate university department with an independent budget and its own dean—Annie W. Goodrich. Hospital affiliation was arranged with the New Haven Hospital, which discontinued operation of the venerable Connecticut Training School for Nurses. Undertaken on an experimental basis, the Yale program demonstrated its effectiveness so markedly that in 1929 the Rockefeller Foundation assured the permanency of the School by awarding it an endowment of $1 million. The 28-month course led to the degree of Bachelor of Nursing, followed a definite educational plan, and included public health, community work, and hospital service. Applicants for the course had to have completed at least two years of work in a college of established standing, and their credits had to show at least 15 hours of academic work per week in relevant subjects of study, including courses in elementary chemistry, psychology, and the biologic sciences.

The professional training of the student in the actual care of the sick was strengthened by in-depth exposure to the underlying theory of disease as well as to the social, psychological, and physical aspects of patient welfare. Courses in the various hospital services were supplemented by observation and assistance in the dispensary clinics and follow-up work through the local visiting nurse association and other health and welfare groups. The program of clinical experience was designated as the "case assignment method," with the students assigned to the care of one or more patients rather than to a series of hypothetical nursing procedures. By employing this approach it was believed possible for the student not only to master the required skills but also to attain an intelligent understanding of the patient and his mental and physical needs. Such an approach fostered attainment of a high degree of technical skill and an understanding of the underlying principles of the required procedures, together with an insight into the social and economic forces that inevitably bore heavily upon any given patient.

Every student received a balanced curriculum, something very rare in the traditional school of nursing. The carefully planned clinical experience, whether surgical, medical, pediatric, or obstetric, included all aspects of the particular subject. For example, the course in medical nursing included periods in the general medical, tuberculosis, syphilis, and skin clinics of the outpatient department, in the wards for communicable diseases, and in the general mental disease wards at the Butler Hospital in Providence, Rhode Island. Included in the comprehensive course in pediatrics was brief but intensive study in a nursery school directed by child psychologists, allowing the students to observe the development of the well child as compared to that of the ill child.

The Yale School of Nursing won quick success, five years later elevating its admission requirements to demand a bachelor's degree in arts, science, or philosophy and offering a 30-month course leading to a Master of Nursing degree. The 128 women nursing students, plus 300 other coeds, were surrounded by nearly 5000 male students.

Opposition to the Collegiate Nursing Movement

Widespread emulation of the Yale program was not forthcoming, although there were a few other positive developments. In 1923 a collegiate school of nursing that later offered the M.N. degree and B.S. in Nursing degree was endowed by Frances Payne Bolton at Western Reserve University. Seven years later the hospital school of nursing at Vanderbilt University was upgraded to a full-fledged academic unit of the University with the aid of a $1 million endowment from the Rockefeller Foundation and additional assistance from the Carnegie Foundation and the Commonwealth Fund. In 1925 the University of

Chicago founded a nursing school, absorbing about $500,000 in assets of the discontinued Illinois Training School for Nurses. Chicago added few resources to its nursing program, however; 10 years later, there were only four faculty for the school.

By and large, the inauguration of truly collegiate programs lagged. Opposition came from many private physicians who argued that nurses were overtrained, that the service they gave was too costly, and that women with brief training in bedside routines would be just as satisfactory. A number of hospital training schools continued to insist that nursing education meant acquisition of technical skills and manual dexterity only. They believed that intelligence and sound knowledge of theory were unnecessary and might handicap the prospective nurse. Opponents of this view argued that while "dull" young women with proper training could attain skill in technical activities and could carry out certain hospital routines, they were apt to be the same people who would demand the services of a highly competent nurse when some member of their own family became seriously ill. Unfortunately, most of those successful in getting their views into the public press belonged to the reactionary group. They viewed nursing as a form of simple manual work requiring a limited degree of dexterity and a smattering of elementary medical knowledge.

Veteran nurses pointed out that the old-fashioned training of the nurse had been simple and rigorous, stern and even. There had been no great variations in quality. Only women of high moral and physical stamina had survived the hardships of that earlier day. By contrast, students from schools in the 1920s represented every degree of quality. Some of the graduates came from schools that chose their students with care, while others came from "schools" that were only interested in obtaining many strong hands and feet and accepted virtually every young woman who walked in the door.

An editorial in one of the prominent medical journals, entitled "Autocracy of the Sick Room Has Become Vested in the Despotic Realm of the Nurse," had this to say:

The nursing problem is becoming increasingly an example of the frequent paradox that where illness is concerned "the cure is worse than the disease."

As an example of efficiency "hoist by its own petard," the trained nurse situation is one of the most appalling. The medical profession views this Frankenstein of its own manufacture with positive unbelief.

Autocracy of the sick room has become vested in the despotic realm of the nurse who has become a positive czar and who is as luxurious an expense as any Romanoff ever dared to be. Sickness is an expense that no family budget can afford to carry under the best of circumstances, but under the present conditions insisted upon by a trained nurse before she will accept a case, the employment of such assistance in illness becomes enough to actually bankrupt a family.

The registered nurse situation today illustrates perfectly the process of refusing to render service in accordance with hire received. The shift system being forced upon the public makes the patient of less importance than the number of hours a day that a nurse stays under the patient's roof. Yet this discounting of wisdom, skill, and directive science upon the part of the physician is made a weapon of argument by the already overtrained and over-authoritative nurse in her fight for the greatest pay and the least service [11].

Under the weight of such attacks, efforts to improve standards in nurse education lagged in many states. In regard to the educational requirements for nurses' registration of the early 1920s, the laws of no two states were in agreement. In most states registration was permissive rather than mandatory. Of those nurses who wished the R.N. title, little was required. South Dakota overlooked preliminary education entirely, registering all graduates of nurse training schools who had completed a two-year general hospital course. Vermont required a grammar school certificate and training of two years and three months in a general hospital. In Virginia the Board of Health examiners required no preliminary education, simply mandating two years of hospital training. In Ohio the registered nurse was required to have one year in high school along with graduation from a training school approved by the State Medical Board. California demanded a high school education or its equivalent and a three year nurse training course. New York mandated one year of high school and two years of training, with examination by the Board of Nursing Examiners. In Massachusetts nurses were registered after passing the examination of the State Board or upon presentation of registration certificates from other states. Most states placed absolutely no restrictions upon the scope or quality of the training school curriculum.

Perils of Private Duty

By the mid-1920s the private duty nurse was also in serious difficulty. Her counterpart of an earlier day had dealt with a common scope of diseases in patients. Only when people were acutely ill did they call the physician and nurse. Through supportive nursing care, they hoped to help save a life that was close to death. Typhoid fever nursing of six to eight weeks per case was one of the private duty nurse's typical assignments. Influenza, pneumonia, and other contagious diseases were regular events. Surgical emergencies demanding operative procedures under primitive conditions in the home were commonplace.

Medical advances had changed this picture. Typhoid fever and most other contagious diseases had receded into the background, and a major area of private duty nursing had disappeared. Screens, clean milk and water, and assistance from new laboratories and technologic innovations helped close still other areas. Good roads, telephones, and motor cars had moved many medical and surgical patients into general hospitals, where they were cared for by student nurses. For the remaining home cases, shorter units of nursing time were being utilized because less continuous nursing care was needed as a result of therapeutic advances. Consequently, the private duty nurse lost ground in her field.

The slackening demand for private duty nurses was noted in hundreds of nurse registries all over the nation. The early development of nurses' agencies dated from the time when, for the benefit of the graduates of a school of nursing, a list of the names of those wishing to do private duty nursing was kept on file by the superintendent of the training school. The objective was to help supply work to the graduates of a particular school of nursing as well as to

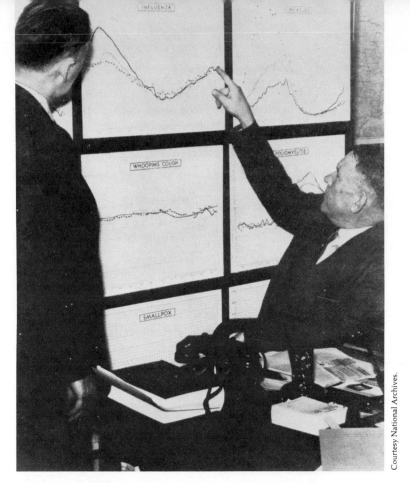

Public health efforts brought significant decline in rates of many communicable diseases—
which vastly altered the demand for private duty nurses.

serve as a convenience to the hospital. The registry functioned only as a center
for the distribution of nurses and the registrar was anyone who happened to be
on duty in the training school office when the call for the nurse was received.
Records were simple and consisted of cards on which the nurse listed the cases
she would not take or was "registered against." No other records were needed,
because the student history of the graduate nurse was on file in the school of
nursing office.

Nurses were sent out on cases in rotation unless the patient or the physician
expressed the wish for a particular nurse. In some instances the alumnae association was privileged to make certain recommendations to the superintendent
of the training school relative to the management of the registry. So-called outside graduates were seldom seen on private duty assignments in the hospital,
as each institution exercised its responsibility to its own graduates. Each registry was an isolated unit and standards were variable.

As schools grew older and the list of graduate nurses increased, the problems
associated with the registry also increased, until it became necessary to take
steps to centralize this important activity. Because many of the hospital regis-

tries had been sponsored by the alumnae associations, the next step was to see what could be done to amalgamate these alumnae activities, and the state nurses' association district organization was the logical unit to approach to assume control of the registry. Soon the proliferation of competing commercial nursing enterprises necessitated the selection by the district registry of a name that would identify it as a functioning unit of the district nurses' association. "Official" was accepted as a term that would so identify the registry, and many registries at once became incorporated as the Nurses' Official Registry. Because of the interest of the American Nurses' Association in the development of these registries, in 1929 the headquarters staff formulated a tentative minimum standard for official registries.

While the demand for private duty nursing was decreasing, schools of nursing were expanding rapidly, in order to staff newly enlarged hospitals. Where the private duty nurse of earlier years had experienced limited competition, the private duty nurse of the mid-1920s was overwhelmed by a fresh deluge of graduates every year. Nurses found themselves waiting longer and longer for cases, and their number of idle days soared alarmingly. It did not seem feasible for the private duty nurse to raise her fees when the majority of the public were living on low or modest incomes and the effect of such a change would simply cause many people to do without nursing, except in crises. Adequate income for the private duty nurse could only come through more work—work that did not exist, because her former patients were going to the hospitals for care.

Hospital Service Improves

The modern hospital of the 1920s contained a large amount of scientific equipment and a degree of specialized service not available in the office of the private practitioner or in the home with a private duty nurse. Of 6830 hospitals surveyed, over 44 percent maintained clinical laboratories and over 41 percent maintained x-ray departments. Used in common by a number of practitioners, equipment and services were available for the diagnosis and treatment of serious illnesses in ambulatory and bed patients, at a cost considerably below that which would be necessary were these provided independently by each practitioner. All told, there were 7370 American hospitals in 1924, with a total bed capacity of 813,926. These included institutions for special groups of disabled persons, such as children, convalescent patients, and maternity cases, and also for special diseases, such as mental disorders, tuberculosis, contagious diseases, disorders of eye, ear, nose, and throat, orthopedic defects, skin diseases, cancer, and the venereal diseases.

Also of importance in bringing patients out of homes and physicians' offices was the growing number of clinics. The clinic was defined as an institution that organized the professional skill of physicians and nurses and provided special equipment for the diagnosis and prevention of disease or for the promotion of health among ambulatory patients. It corresponded to the ward service given to bed patients in hospitals, and, when attached to a hospital, the clinic was

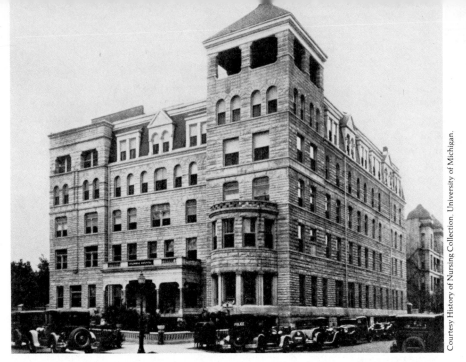

Columbus Hospital in Chicago, one of the 7370 hospitals in the United States in 1924.

frequently called the outpatient department. In a few cases the term *dispensary* was still used because the early clinics had been opened primarily to provide free medicine for physicians' charity patients.

The number of clinics in the United States in June, 1926, was 5726. Of these, 1790 were outpatient departments of hospitals, 2793 were unaffiliated clinics, 923 served special groups only, and 220 were general group clinics. There were at that time 197 clinics attached to hospitals for the treatment of nervous and mental disorders, and 70 of the unaffiliated clinics were for mental cases. Hospitals and sanatoriums for the treatment of tuberculosis had 107 clinics attached to them, and there were 585 unaffiliated clinics for the tubercular. One thousand unaffiliated clinics for baby and child care were reported in addition to the 52 clinics connected with children's hospitals. The 350 clinics for the treatment of venereal diseases were all independent of hospitals.

The growth of health care had resulted in a marked increase in the number of people engaged in it. By 1920 in the United States alone, over one million people were employed on a full-time basis in some phase of the promotion of health.

The Grading Committee Begins Work

Close on the heels of the Goldmark effort came that of the Committee on the Grading of Nursing Schools, which had its origin in two separate movements. One was an attempt by the American Medical Association to study the education and employment of nurses in order to arrive at methods for improving the nursing service available to the members of the medical profession. The other,

Number of Health Workers as Reported by the 1920 Census [12].

Physicians and surgeons	147,000
Attendants of physicians and surgeons	24,000
Retail drug dealers	80,000
Dentists	64,000
Dental hygienists and dentists' assistants	8,700
Trained nurses and student nurses	149,000
Untrained nurses	152,000
Midwives	44,000
Hospital superintendents	2,800
Hospital attendants	330,000
Clinic attendants	5,000
Health department personnel	11,500
	1,018,000

apparently begun earlier, was initiated by the professional nursing associations and contemplated a study of nursing education, especially as it related to the need for qualitative grading of schools. These two approaches to the nursing problem eventually led to an amalgamation of forces and the formation of the Committee on the Grading of Nursing Schools.

The Committee was organized with two representatives each from the American Nurses' Association, the National League of Nursing Education, and the National Organization for Public Health Nursing, and one representative and one alternate each from the American Medical Association, the American College of Surgeons, the American Hospital Association, and the American Public Health Association.

Frances Payne Bolton, who had generously endowed the new school of nursing at Cleveland's Western Reserve University in 1924 and who had been a friend of nurses and nursing since the World War, was asked to serve on the Committee as a representative of hospital trustees and consumers. Her strong committment to the objectives of the Committee was expressed through a gift of $93,000. This sum, combined with the financial contributions of thousands of nurses, allowed the Committee to embark upon the first comprehensive survey of the nation's nursing schools.

The Committee appointed May Ayres Burgess, Ph.D., as director of the study at a meeting in April, 1926. From an academic point of view, Dr. Burgess was a well-trained statistician; from a practical standpoint, she had had many years of statistical work, much of it having been learned from her brother, Colonel Leonard P. Ayres, Chief of the Statistics Branch of the War Department General Staff. Nurses and other hospital workers had a great deal of confidence in her because she had worked in the field of education and with the Committee on Dispensary Development of the United Hospital Fund. Dr. Burgess had also demonstrated her interest in nursing through her studies of private duty nursing in New York.

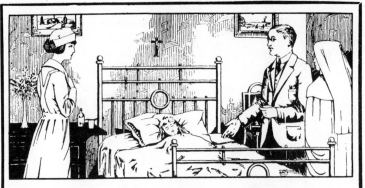

Nurses Training Schools

For the Training of Young Women
In the Noble Profession of Nursing

We believe that many young women would be eager to enter Nurses' Training Schools as pupils, in the state of Wisconsin, if they appreciated the splendid opportunity for service to their fellow-man offered by the greatest profession open to women. There is a large number of such training schools for nurses connected with the many excellent hospitals of this state.

Hence, the subjoined Catholic hospitals of Wisconsin, as members of the Wisconsin Conference of the Catholic Hospital Association of the United States and Canada, present the following facts for the careful consideration and sympathetic appreciation of the young women of Wisconsin who are seriously thinking of what their future life work shall be.

(1) Nursing is a profession whose great purpose is to help the medical profession in the prevention, alleviation and cure of disease in human beings. According to state law each applicant must have finished two years in an accredited high school or the equivalent following the eighth year of the grade schools, and must be of good character and sound health. The nurses' curriculum is of three years' duration and embraces regular courses in the necessary sciences along with daily practice in the technique of service to the sick. It is, therefore, an intellectual profession based on the sciences and arts called for in the highly specialized care of patients.

(2) Nursing is a noble profession because it involves consecrated service based upon the high purpose of caring for fellow human beings in need of watchful and sympathetic regard for all the wants of body and mind and soul.

(3) This deeply human and truly altruistic profession has a serious ethical intent which looks to the securing for the patient of all his God-given rights that affect the life and welfare of life in every contingency of human existence where life and health are involved.

Such a profession can have a strong appeal only to such young women as have an earnest and sympathetic appreciation of the deeper meaning and needs of individual and social welfare, and a strong urge within their own character to render this generous and conscientious service to ailing human beings which is peculiarly distinctive of a woman. The call is an urgent one and our young womanhood will not fail.

The following hospitals offer a course in nursing that is complete in its scientific and technical training, while it embraces with special emphasis the ethical and religious principles and motives which give such depth and satisfaction to one who serves the health needs of her fellowman. The spirit of these schools is beautifully expressed in the words of Florence Nightingale.

"I do entirely believe that the religious motive is essential for the highest kind of nurse. There are such disappointments, such sickenings of the heart, that they can only be borne by the feeling that one is called to the work by God, that it is a part of His work, that one is a fellow worker of God."

Wisconsin Conference, Catholic Hospital Association

ASHLAND	GREEN BAY	MILWAUKEE
St. Joseph's Hospital	St. Mary's Hospital	St. Mary's Hospital
DODGEVILLE	JANESVILLE	Trinity Hospital
St. Joseph's Hospital	Palmer Mercy Hospital	OSHKOSH
EAU CLAIRE	LA CROSSE	St. Mary's Hospital
Sacred Heart Hospital	St. Francis' Hospital	PORTAGE
FOND DU LAC	MANITOWOC	St. Saviour's Hospital
St. Agnes' Hospital	Holy Family Hospital	RACINE
		St. Mary's Hospital

Address, Chairman Publicity Committee, Catholic Hospital Association, 208 Montgomery Bldg., Milwaukee, or Communicate Directly with the Hospital in which you are interested.

In the early 1920s, a cooperative advertisement for 13 Wisconsin hospital schools of nursing mentions two years of high school, good character, and sound health as admission requirements.

In the fall of 1926 the Committee embarked on an ambitious program of three separate studies: (1) an inquiry into the supply of and demand for graduate nurses; (2) a "job analysis" of what nurses did and how they might be taught; and (3) the actual grading of schools of nursing. The supply-and-demand study was carried out virtually as scheduled and resulted in the 1928 publication *Nurses, Patients, and Pocketbooks*. This investigation demonstrated that there was an oversupply of graduate nurses and that this oversupply was increasing much faster than the general population. Unemployment among graduate nurses was serious and chronic. Annual earnings, especially for private duty nurses, were inadequate and educational standards were low. What is more, since nurses congregated in the cities, their geographic distribution was very uneven. While physicians and patients were, in general, pleased with their nurses, and while many nurses were happy with their work, there remained a critical proportion of nurses who were rendering unsatisfactory service and an even larger proportion of nurses who were chronically unhappy because of the inadequacy of their training or because of the conditions under which they were working.

Poorly Prepared Students

In 1925 there were approximately 2100 schools of nursing in the United States. Of the 1500 schools that responded to an American Nurses' Association survey, only 224 revealed a minimum entrance requirement of four years of high school. In half the nursing schools one of every three students had been admitted to training without having finished high school. In some schools none of the students had gone beyond the eighth grade. The minimum educational requirements for entrance lined up as follows [13]:

	Number of Schools	Percentage
Eighth Grade	38	3
1 year high school	813	54
2 years high school	406	27
3 years high school	19	1
4 years high school	224	15
	1500	100

Educational entrance requirements were not the only criteria for good schools. Many schools were so small that they could not provide adequate instruction. Of the 1500 schools responding, there were 104 in which the entire student body numbered nine or fewer and 440 in which the entire student body was composed of 19 or fewer individuals. Students were distributed among those 1500 schools of nursing as follows [14]:

Students	Number of Schools
0–9	104
10–19	336
20–29	334
30–39	210
40–49	128
50–59	86
60–69	86
70–79	60
80–89	39
90–99	26
100+	91

Poor Educational Environment

Not only were many of the schools too small to make adequate instruction feasible, but all too frequently the hospitals themselves were too small to be effective as teaching centers. One hundred and eighty-five schools were connected with hospitals having a daily average of fewer than 25 patients; 562 schools had a daily average of fewer than 50 patients, making one-third of the schools hopelessly below standard. Another 467 schools had a daily average of 50 to 99 patients, which was below the recommended minimum of 100 considered essential for satisfactory clinical instruction. Perhaps the greatest shock came when Dr. Burgess showed the great variation in the hours of duty per week required in the 1500 nursing schools that responded [15]:

Hours of Work Per Week	Number of Schools
25–34	2
35–44	23
45–54	659
55–64	736
65–74	73
75–84	7

The average was 55 hours. When these figures were compared with the 38-hour work week required of most factory workers or with the 42-hour week required of visiting nurses, one could see why young *middle-class* women were thinking twice about pursuing nursing careers.

Defining a teacher in the school of nursing as a person whose main job was instructing, Dr. Burgess compiled the following figures [16]:

Number of Teachers	Number of Schools
None	549
1	639
2	208
3	57
4	21
5	8
6	18

There had been an increase of 102.5 percent in all hospital beds from 1910 to 1927 along with an increase of 138.2 percent in student nurses for the same period. It was significant that the 4322 general hospital nursing staffs in the United States included fewer graduate nurses than the nursing staffs of British or most European hospitals. In this country student nurses carried the greater portion of the general hospital nursing load.

Most schools of nursing had either no full-time teacher or one full-time teacher in the mid-1920s—class at Saint Anthony's Hospital, Rockford, Illinois, 1927.

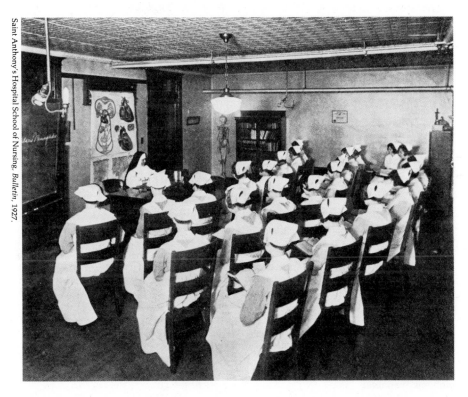

Saint Anthony's Hospital School of Nursing, *Bulletin*, 1927.

It was because the training school had been successful that its growth was extraordinary, reaching a zenith during the late 1920s. The contrast between medical schools and nursing schools was amazing. In 1880 there had been 100 medical schools; in 1890, 133; in 1900, 160. Following publication of the 1910 Flexner report, which attracted nationwide attention to problems of medical education, there had been a widespread campaign by the medical profession aimed at raising the quality of medical education and lowering the number of schools. By 1927 only 79 schools of medicine remained. Nursing schools, on the other hand, showed a totally different picture. In 1880 there had been 15 schools of nursing; in 1890, 34; in 1900, 448; in 1910, 1121; in 1920, 1755; and in 1927, 2286 [17].

Along with the increase in nursing schools came an increase in nurse graduates. Medical schools in 1880 had produced a little over 3000 graduates; by 1900 there were over 5000. Then came the reorganization of medical education, and the number of graduates dropped rapidly until, by 1920, there were barely 3000; by 1926 this number had increased to about 4000. Medical educators were projecting that the numbers of graduates each year through the next 40 or 50 years would probably remain at about 4000. In nursing in 1880 there were 157 graduates for the entire country. In 1890 there were over 500; in 1900, over 3700; in 1910, over 7700; in 1920, about 15,000; in 1927, over 18,000; in 1931, just about 26,000. During the latter year, with over 100,000 students enrolled, the numbers of nursing graduates were expected to continue rising with startling rapidity and at a rate far beyond that of the increase in the general population.

Apprenticeship versus Education

Nurse education of the late 1920s was essentially functioning on an apprenticeship level. In the main, training schools were being conducted primarily to provide student nursing service for the care of patients in hospitals, instead of being operated with the objective of giving the students the best possible nursing education. There was unquestionable value in the apprenticeship method of teaching, and the Committee thought that it should be retained in *any* system of nurse training, because much more depended on repetition and on practice in learning nursing procedures than on didactic instruction. There was, however, no question that hospitals had exploited student nurses in an attempt to avoid the expense required in employing graduate nurses.

Bearing out these findings, Dorothy Dunbar Bromley, in a 1930 article on the nursing crisis published in *Harper's Magazine*, vividly reminded the public:

High school principals, when called upon for vocational advice, have been known to suggest nursing as a possible career for girls unfitted to do anything else. One principal recently wrote the head of a training school saying "Mary Blank's parents are too poor to support her; she is a hopeless failure in her studies, and she is not attractive enough to marry. But I think she would make a good nurse. Won't you take her in?"

That nursing should have so fallen in the esteem of a portion of the community is largely the fault of those training schools which, in their anxiety to get the work of their hospitals done as cheaply as possible, have enrolled whatever young women were at the moment available.

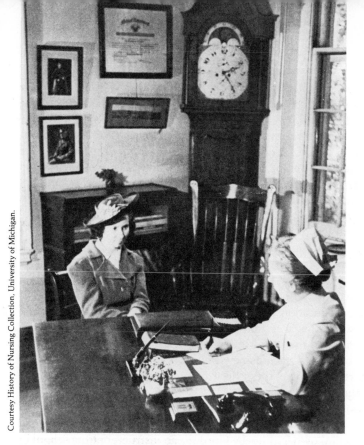

Prospective student being interviewed by a superintendent of nursing.

She concluded that nursing was:

in short, the one line of work open to the uneducated girl which will not only raise her social status and pay her comparatively high wages but will provide her with a living while she is training and perhaps even a monthly allowance. If the standards of nursing are to be salvaged, a good many of the 2200-odd training schools now in existence will have to be discontinued, and this will include most of those conducted by privately owned hospitals. When there are fewer schools and when the requirements for entrance have been raised, there will be fewer graduates and these of a much higher type. [18].

The Grading Committee's findings were published in a series of reports and in a final summary, published in 1934, called *Nursing Schools Today and Tomorrow,* which described weaknesses in nursing education and recommended specific improvements. This report reiterated the belief that providing adequate financial support was the most fundamental problem in placing nursing education on a higher level. In other forms of professional education it was a firmly established principle that funds be supplied to provide teaching personnel and facilities for instruction. The nurse was the only worker whose professional training depended essentially on the service that she rendered in a hospital. This problem and the difficulty of finding faculty with scholastic qualifications for teaching created a serious deficiency in nursing education. Grading Committee statistics showed that 42 percent of teachers in schools of nursing were not even graduates of high school, and that only 16 percent had completed one or more years of college [19].

Dr. Burgess and her associates insisted that it was imperative, if the educational program for a nursing student was to be administered in an effective manner, that an honest attempt be made to correlate classroom instruction and clinical experience. The reason the average hospital training school did not correlate practice with classroom work was that doing so necessitated rotation of a student from one hospital service to another, a program that would provide superior education but interfere with the hospital's freedom to place the student according to ward nursing needs.

Inadequate Financing of Nurse Training

There were few adequately financed hospitals. When the hospital was forced to budget for nursing education, the school of nursing received a minimal allotment. The administrator had a certain amount of money to spend in all departments of the hospital, and the board of directors usually agreed to expenditures that showed tangible assets, such as new buildings and equipment. First consideration was rarely given to the school of nursing by either the hospital administrator or the hospital board.

A central question was: how much did the pupil nurses earn—how much did their employment save the patient, the philanthropic donor, the taxpayer, and the proprietary hospital owner? Phoebe Gordon, an instructor at the school of nursing at the University of Minnesota, studied this matter for the University Hospital and for the Miller and Northern Pacific Hospitals of Saint Paul. The results of Miss Gordon's studies indicated that the then-current system of student staffing was least expensive. For a hypothetical school of 30 graduate nurses and 130 students the total hospital cost was $84,382. Substitution of graduates for students almost doubled the cost of the nursing service, to $167,977.

Against these charges the hospital executives and administrators argued that schools of nursing and nursing care of patients accounted for the high cost of hospitalization. According to Dr. Bert Caldwell, the executive director of the American Hospital Association, part of the cost of hospitalization was the result of expenses incurred by training a nurse over a three-year period. While the three-year training period cost the hospital $2000, by Dr. Caldwell's figuring, the student returned only $1000 in the form of service. Yet each student gave approximately 7000 hours of service to the hospital during her three-year course: if these hours of service were worth only $1000 to the hospital, as Caldwell mentioned, then student nurses were indeed inexpensive labor, for the hospital credited them at the rate of 14 cents an hour.

Students versus Graduates in Hospital Nursing Service

According to progressive nurse educators, graduate nurses were the logical people to provide nursing care in a hospital. A registered nurse could furnish more skillful nursing than could a student, was better prepared to adapt procedures to the individual patient, and had a better basis for judgment because her training and experience made her familiar with the various changing clinical pictures of diseases. A graduate nursing staff assured the patient of competent, safe nursing care. Hospitals might argue that students provided a service that was as good or nearly as good as a graduate service, but if semi-trained students were as well qualified for general duty nursing as graduates, there was little justification for maintaining a three-year course in nursing education.

The conclusions announced in an address given by Dr. Malcolm MacEachern, associate director of the American College of Surgeons, on February 15, 1932, were of interest to many:

Graduate Nurse Service

Advantages:
1. Older nurse—more mature—therefore take responsibility better.
2. The white uniform nurse gains the confidence of the patient more easily.
3. Can work more rapidly because she knows better how to carry out treatment orders.
4. Can do more work on her own initiative—less supervision required.
5. Better health—less lost time.

Disadvantages:
1. Does not like general duty—indifferent to this type of nursing.
2. Objects to discipline.
3. Insists on using her own methods.
4. More extravagant with supplies.
5. Chronic complaints—food, housekeeping, laundry.
6. Uses short-cut methods, thereby becoming careless.
7. Resents criticism.
8. Large salary.
9. Large turnover of help; doesn't stay in one place long.

Student Nurse Service

Advantages:
1. More enthusiastic.
2. More cheerful.
3. More amenable to discipline.
4. More conservative with supplies.
5. More sympathetic.
6. Less turnover.
7. Small salary.
8. Contracts business for hospital with friends and relatives.

Disadvantages:
1. Needs constant supervision.
2. Cost of theoretical education, instructor, etc.
3. Cost of recreational activities.
4. Less experience in handling patients.
5. Wastes time.
6. More mistakes.
7. Does not have as much emotional stability.
8. Less continuity of service [20].

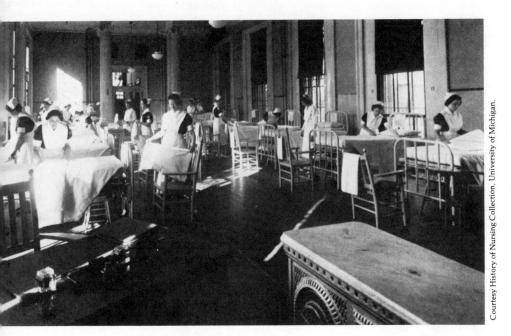

Practice in nursing arts, about 1930.

Resistance to the use of general staff nurses in hospitals had become strongly entrenched. These attitudes were held both by the employer and the employee. The Grading Committee asked 500 superintendents of nurses: "If you had your choice, which would you rather have to take care of your patients—student nurses or graduate nurses?" Seventy-six percent replied emphatically that they would prefer student nurses, and only 24 percent voted for graduate nurses. That this preference was actually put into practice was evident in the disclosure that 73 percent of these same hospitals had no general staff nurses, 5 percent had one general staff nurse, 4 percent had two general staff nurses, 3 percent had three, and 15 percent had four or more.

Grading Committee Conclusions

The findings of the Grading Committee did little to alter what leaders of the nursing profession had long believed although it did furnish data that could be used to strengthen arguments for reform. Such reform, it was decided, should have four basic goals:

To reduce and improve the supply. To make a decisive and immediate reduction in the numbers of students admitted to schools of nursing in the United States, and to raise entrance requirements high enough so that only properly qualified women would be admitted to the profession.

To replace students with graduates. To put the major part of hospital bedside nursing in the hands of the graduate nurses and take it out of the hands of student nurses.

To help hospitals meet costs of graduate services. To assist hospitals in securing funds for the employment of graduate nurses and to improve the quality of graduate nursing so that hospitals would desire to have it.

To get public support for nursing education. To place schools of nursing under the direction of nurse educators instead of hospital administrators and to awaken the public to the fact that if society wants good nursing it must pay the cost of educating nurses. Nursing education is a public and not a private responsibility [21].

The struggle for better nurse education and the debate over its proper role in American health care would focus once again on a question that had recurred elsewhere and would continue to bedevil the hospital for the next half-century. In some ways the central problem of hospital care was nothing less than the question of the true meaning of nursing. Was a good system one that allowed exploitation of students to subsidize the cost of patient care, or was it a system designed to maximize the preparation of quality nurses? Did "quality" imply the kind of quiet, submissive servant that the training schools produced in large numbers, or did it mean much more?

One outstanding attempt to elevate nursing school standards had been the National League of Nursing Education's *A Standard Curriculum for Schools of Nursing*, which had appeared in 1917 under the leadership of Adelaide Nutting and Isabel Stewart. Its purpose had been "to arrive at some general agreement as to a desirable and workable standard whose main features could be accepted by training schools of good standing throughout the country," and it had been hoped that "in this way, we may be able to gradually overcome the wide diversity of standards at present existing in schools of nursing and supply a basis for appraising the value of widely different systems of nurse training."

In 1927, following the general trend to de-emphasize standardization, a revision, entitled *A Curriculum for Schools of Nursing*, was published, introducing "changes needed to keep in line with the newer developments in the field of nursing and the newer ideas in nursing education" [22]. Among the alterations were the inclusion of psychology as a regular course, emphasis on mental health nursing and on public health nursing, and greater stress on a solid scientific background.

The Case of New York State

In 1933 analysis of the curricula in the schools of nursing in New York State showed an amazing lack of agreement on what was essential. The following list gives the range of hours allotted to the various subjects taught. The extremes of variation in the theory component were astonishing [23]:

Subjects	Hours
Anatomy and physiology	48–270
Bacteriology	20–120
Bacteriology and pathology (combined)	32–94
Pathology	0–59
Personal hygiene	8–58
Nutrition and cookery	24–180
Drugs and solutions	15–64
Elementary nursing procedures (including bandaging and hospital housekeeping)	79–325
History and social aspects of nursing	8–34
Chemistry	0–315
Advanced nursing	0–174
Dietotherapy	0–81
Materia medica	16–88
Massage	0–40
Ethics	0–36
Psychology	0–120
General medicine (including skin)	10–130
General surgery and gynecology	15–164
Pediatrics (including infant feeding and orthopedics)	11–116
Communicable (including tuberculosis and venereal)	4–72
Operating room technique	5–62
Obstetric nursing	10–76
Public sanitation	8–42
Diseases of eye	2–18
Diseases of ear, nose, throat	2–22
Hydrotherapy	0–22
Nervous and mental	9–110
Occupational therapy	0–50
Occupational diseases	0–9
Professional problems	0–30
Public health	0–58
Private duty	0–9
Institutional work	0–8
Modern social conditions	0–60
Case study	0–15
Mental hygiene	0–12
Social service	0–43

Examination of school records indicated that students received experience according to what the individual hospital had to offer, and because schools of nursing were located in all sizes and types of hospitals, the clinical experience offered students varied markedly. This list shows the range of experience in the various hospital services [24]:

Service	Days
Surgical	92–453
Operating room	35–145
Pathology laboratory	0–34
Medical	89–475
Tuberculosis	0–130
Communicable	0–114
Pediatric	56–379
Psychiatric	0–483
Physiotherapy	0–56
Occupational therapy	0–41
Obstetrics	62–197
Diet kitchen	24–82
Dispensary	0–103
Pharmacy	0–28
Public health	0–92
Administrative	0–150
Social service	0–58
X-ray	0–36

The range of class hours for a given subject in schools of nursing was astonishing—nutrition laboratory, University of Minnesota School of Nursing, 1932.

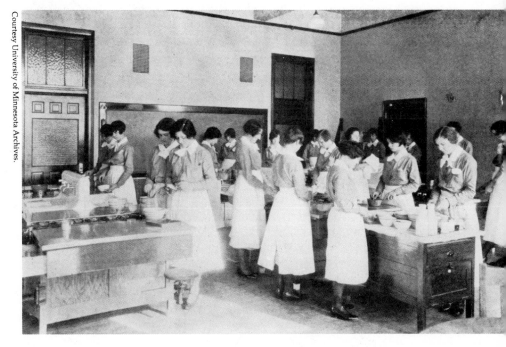

Courtesy University of Minnesota Archives.

The Hospital Association Presents Questions

Lewis A. Sexton, M.D., president of the American Hospital Association, told the 1931 AHA convention that those who were most responsible for both nursing care and the support of the schools had begun to wonder what the nurse of the future would be like and just where her place would be in the scheme of things. Each year saw additions made to nursing school curricula, which were bulging with desirable general education courses but squeezing out, year after year, the essentials upon which the profession had been founded. Dr. Sexton said that he was for education and training that would fit nurses for their greatest sphere of usefulness, but that a feeling had grown among nurse leaders that unless hospitals freed their nursing students from the menial aspects of caring for the sick, their educational duty would not be fulfilled.

He declared that he was old-fashioned enough to believe that one could overeducate people beyond their sphere of usefulness. Some institutions of higher learning seemed to think that unless a nurse had her Ph.D. she was no longer worthy of her place in the profession. Dr. Sexton warned that if, for the next 25 years, all hospitals adhered to the flurry of new recommendations that were being made, there would be no one blessed with a sufficient amount of humility to do the actual nursing necessary for patients' recovery. More than one empire had collapsed under the weight of its own greatness, he noted.

Dr. Sexton pleaded for nurses to enter the profession for the love of the work and the good that they might do; for nurses who were willing to give of themselves to make the long, weary hours of illness less irksome; for nurses the sight of whom was an inspiration and a joy to all who needed their services. Theory in a nurse's training was desirable and essential, he maintained, but the man or woman whose needs called for a gentle, soothing touch cared little whether a nurse knew the solubility of salicylic acid or the atomic weight of sulfur.

Typical Student and Ideal Graduate

Perhaps the best approach to appreciate the situation is to try to understand something of the role of the contemporary student nurse in the social structure and functioning of patient care in hospitals. If you had been a 19-year-old nursing student entering a general hospital in September, 1932, you would have been scheduled to perform 7095 hours of service over the next three years—and in general, you would not have been expected to pay any tuition. In return for your labor you would receive 631 hours of classroom instruction taught by graduate nurses and physician lecturers. Unlike the millions of students in regular colleges and universities, you would not receive a liberal education. The school of nursing was a "total institution," and because you were a first-year student, there would be much you would dislike about the work. Constant fatigue would become your greatest complaint. You were but a cog in a vast authoritarian labor system made up of 100,419 other students in 1844 hospitals all across the nation.

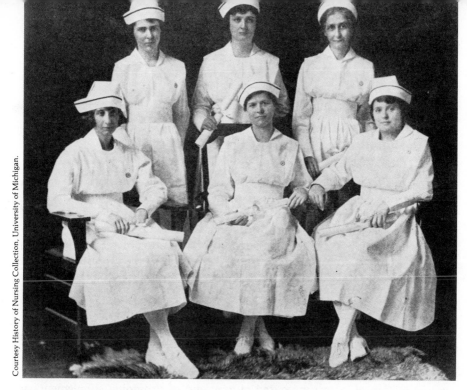

*The old accusations of "overeducated nurses" continued to be raised during the 1920s—
class of 1922 at Saint Joseph's Hospital, Keokuk, Iowa.*

About this time, Clara D. Noyes, former president of the American Nurses'
Association and long-time director of nursing service of the Red Cross, was
asked to depict the ideal nurse. She said that her ideal candidate would be a
young woman about 24 to 26 years of age, of medium height, 130 to 135 pounds.
She would be physically fit and would carry herself well. While a nurse with a
lovely face was good to look at and might be a considerable comfort to a patient—provided that she possessed the other necessary qualifications—this
combination was not often found. Extremes were undesirable. Miss Noyes
went on to say that if she were to paint the portrait of a nurse, it would comprise "a rather low, broad forehead, brownish hair, with a natural wave or
straight, parted in the middle in a more or less Madonna-like fashion." Her
eyes would be "gray or blue, with eyebrows not too heavy, with a nose, mouth,
and chin not necessarily classical, but at least possessing character, well-cared-
for teeth, a skin smooth and free from blemish." Her face would "radiate cheer-
fulness and kindliness." She would also possess dignity and poise. Her voice
would be well modulated and her enunciation clear [25].

As to the ideal nurse's educational background, Miss Noyes reflected that
her preliminary education should be as broad as possible. Whether she was a
high school or college graduate or a product of the private school did not so
much matter as long as her education was sufficient to enable her to meet practical requirements. The broader and sounder the education the better, and a
cultural background of reading, travel, and social experience was essential.
The ideal nurse should possess courage, patience, and willingness to make sac-

rifices. Self-reliance, self-respect, self-control, steadfastness, and honesty were other indispensable qualities.

Failure to Accredit

Many nurses had been eager to have the training schools graded and viewed the publicizing of such information as a way in which hospitals might be stimulated to offer a higher level of education. They also saw listings of accredited schools as a means by which a prospective student could be guided in her choice of nursing school. No schedule of accreditation was attempted by the Grading Committee, however, largely because of "the advice of the representatives of higher education. It was also felt that "the accuracy of a list compiled without personal visits to the schools might be questioned" [26]. It was explained that a firsthand visit to each school, valuable as it would have been, was not financially possible.

Concerned by the lack of accreditation action, in 1931 Isabel Stewart warned that nursing's biggest problems were still those of bringing some order out of the chaos of unregulated and widely differentiated schools, of reducing the overproduction of poorly prepared nurses, and of providing supplementary educational offerings to nurses who had been trained in substandard programs. She insisted that the public had to be made to face this situation and to see that nursing schools needed the same kind of public support that had been given to normal schools and agricultural colleges. Miss Stewart lamented:

In all these years, the public has done very little for nursing education. It has cost the public practically nothing to produce the hundreds of thousands of nurses who have spent their lives in its service. Nurses have paid for their own education, and through their services as students they have contributed in all these years millions of dollars toward the care of the sick in hospitals. They have also put a good deal of money into private pockets. Compare the public cost of training teachers or soldiers or stenographers or workers in agriculture and home economics to the cost which the public has borne for the training of nurses. Without some kind of radical treatment, it is doubtful if the nursing body can ever get back into a healthy condition [27].

Miss Stewart later identified three 20-year stages through which nurse education had passed. The first, from 1873 to 1893, was a pioneering era, in which a few Nightingale schools had been founded in the United States. The second, from 1893 to 1913, was a period of phenomenal expansion, regulated to some degree by legal and professional controls. The third, from 1913 to 1933, was a time of stress and turmoil, of experimentation and painful self-examination.

The facts bore out her analysis. The population of the United States had doubled from 1873 to 1933, but the number of hospitals had increased more than 42 times. In 1873 there were 149 hospitals and allied institutions in the United States; at the close of 1933, 6334 hospitals were able to offer over one million beds. The two factors primarily responsible for this amazing growth were the development of support services and the greater public confidence in

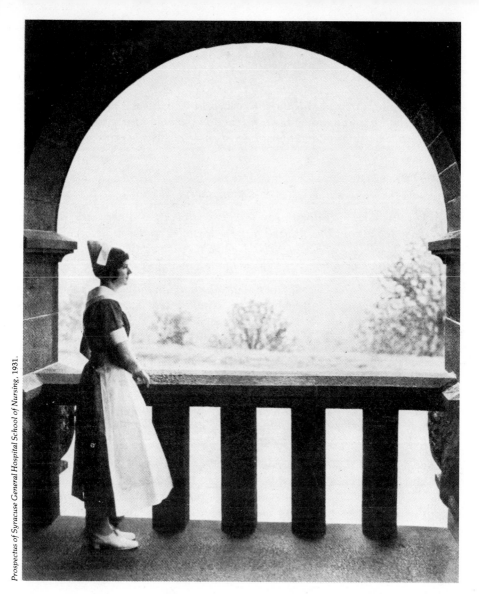

Nurses near the threshold of their careers in 1931 faced the bleak prospects of too many nurses and too few jobs—student at General Hospital, Syracuse, New York.

hospital care. Comparative studies showed that the average per capita period of hospitalization had decreased from 24 days in 1900 to 12 days in 1933.

Meanwhile the confidence essential to prosperous American business had been swept away by the financial panic of October, 1929; soon banks were unable to lend and business began to collapse. Small-business bankruptcies followed bank failures with dismal regularity. Hospitals and public health agencies began to lay off personnel. By the beginning of 1933 the unemployment rate had risen to 25 percent and business was at a near-standstill. During the same time the nation was experiencing crisis, nurses found the integral structure of their profession in chaos.

Summary

The increase of nursing students during World War I was short-lived. Many students who signed up during the war had done so only for its duration. When the Armistice was signed and the influenza epidemic was over, many dropped out.

In 1920 there was a shortage of 55,000 trained nurses. Patient care suffered as a result, and the status and prestige of nursing sharply declined.

Since hospital administrators viewed nursing students as a necessity, and because their labor could be utilized at very low cost under an apprenticeship program, the number of nursing schools rapidly increased. Far too many nurses began to be graduated, many with inadequate training.

In 1920 the Rockefeller Foundation founded a study on the education of nurses which resulted in an exhaustive report by Josephine Goldmark in 1923 entitled Nursing and Nursing Education in the United States.

The Goldmark report pointed out that by establishing independent university schools of nursing, administrative exploitation of the labor of student nurses in hospitals would lessen. It also pointed to the need for recognizing schools of nursing in hospitals as more independent educational departments. As a direct result of the report, Yale University, Western Reserve University, and Vanderbilt University developed collegiate schools of nursing characterized by quality in both theory and clinical experience.

The initial success of the Yale School of Nursing caused the Rockefeller Foundation to assure the permanency of the school, in 1929, with an endowment of $1 million. The 28-month program, the first in the world to be established as a separate university school with an independent budget, initially led to the Bachelor of Nursing degree and included public health and community work as well as hospital service. Yale soon moved to the model of requiring a bachelors degree in arts or sciences for admission and granted the Master of Nursing degree as the first professional degree for the student.

The Yale program remained atypical; the trend in several other universities was to combine a conventional hospital diploma program with two additional years of general education at a neighboring college or university, which led to both the nursing diploma and the B.S. degree. The college counted the diploma school course as the equivalent of two years of higher education.

The private duty nursing field narrowed. Progress in medical science greatly reduced the incidence of typhoid, influenza, pneumonia, yellow fever, malaria, and other diseases that had constituted the bulk of private duty cases. Many more patients went to hospitals instead of being nursed at home, and the per capita time spent in nursing private duty patients declined.

The number of schools of nursing increased to an all-time high in the late 1920s. Very soon the market for graduate nurses became swamped, and competition for jobs intensified.

A study by the Committee on the Grading of Nursing Schools pointed to the oversupply of nurses, inadequate wages, poor training, and a paucity of clinical resources for existing educational programs. The average work week for a student nurse was 55 hours. Most schools had only one nurse, or none, whose major responsibility was teaching.

Compared to England and other Western European nations, American hospital nursing staffs consisted of very few graduate nurses. In 1927, 73 percent of all hospitals with schools of nursing had no graduate nurses on general duty. Hospitals without schools were heavily staffed by attendants.

The Grading Committee's findings, published in 1934 under the title Nursing Schools Today and Tomorrow, *recommended: (1) reduction of the nurse supply and improvement of the quality of training; (2) replacement of students with graduates for routine ward duty; (3) assistance to hospitals to help meet costs of graduate services; and (4) public support for nursing education.*

A Standard Curriculum for Schools of Nursing, *which had been prepared by the National League of Nursing Education in 1917, was revised in 1927 and continued to represent the more ideal educational standards and expectations.*

Isabel Stewart of Teachers College, Columbia University, was particularly concerned about the overproduction of nurses with inadequate preparation. Her view was that, since it had cost the public almost nothing to produce the hundreds of thousands of nurses who had contributed an incalculable amount of service for the care of the sick, the public owed financial assistance to schools of nursing.

The onset of the Great Depression found schools of nursing in the midst of a period of stress and turmoil brought on by overexpansion of the educational plant and continued massive exploitation of student labor in hospitals.

References

1. Isabel M. Stewart, *Developments in Nursing Education Since 1918* (Washington, D.C.:   Government Printing Office, 1921), p. 6.
2. Edwin P. Haworth, "Nursing in the Movies," *Modern Hospital*, vol. 16 (February, 1921): 156.
3. *Ibid.*
4. *Ibid.*
5. Stewart, op. cit., p. 17.
6. *Ibid.*, pp. 17–18.
7. Rockefeller Foundation and Nursing Education, *American Journal of Nursing*, vol. 20 (April, 1920): 525.
8. Josephine Goldmark, *Nursing and Nursing Education in the United States* (New York: Macmillan Co., 1923), pp. 1–36.
9. *Ibid.*, pp. 187–472.
10. *Ibid.*, pp. 310–312.
11. Quoted in "Why Not Be Fair," *Bulletin of the American Hospital Association*, vol. 6 (September, 1932): 6–8.

12. U.S. Department of Commerce, Bureau of the Census, *Fourteenth Census of the United States, 1920* (Washington, D.C.: Government Printing Office, 1923), vol. 4, pp. 42–43.
13. "Some Problems in Grading Our Schools of Nursing," *Trained Nurse and Hospital Review*, vol. 77 (November, 1926): 507–509.
14. *Ibid.*, p. 508.
15. *Ibid.*, pp. 507–508.
16. *Ibid.*, p. 509.
17. Shirley C. Titus, "The Present Position of Nursing in Hospitals in the United States," *Nosokomeion*, vol. 2 (April, 1931): 288–310.
18. Dorothy Dunbar Bromley, "The Crisis in Nursing," *Harper's Magazine*, vol. 161 (July, 1930): 159–160.
19. May Ayres Burgess, "What the Cost Study Showed," *American Journal of Nursing*, vol. 32 (April, 1932): 427–432.
20. Malcolm MacEachern, "Which Shall We Choose—Graduate or Student Service?" *Modern Hospital*, vol. 38 (June, 1932): 97–98, 102–104.
21. May Ayres Burgess, "Nurses, Patients, and Pocketbooks," *Proceedings of the 34th Annual Convention of the National League of Nursing Education*, vol. 34 (June, 1928): 237–256.
22. National League of Nursing Education, Committee on Curriculum, *A Curriculum Guide for Schools of Nursing* (New York: The League, 1927), p. 8.
23. Harlan Hoyt Horner, *Nursing Education and Practice in New York State with Suggested Remedial Measures* (Albany: University of the State of New York Press, 1934), pp. 19–23.
24. *Ibid.*, p. 20.
25. Clara D. Noyes, "How Some Nursing Leaders Visualize the Ideal Student Nurse," *Hospital Management*, vol. 23 (January, 1927): 53.
26. A. C. Bachmeyer, "Systems of Accreditment for Schools of Nursing," *American Journal of Nursing*, vol. 36 (April, 1936): 375–381.
27. Isabel Stewart, "Trends in Nursing Education," *American Journal of Nursing*, vol. 31 (May, 1931): 601–611.

12
Public Health Nursing, 1912–1930

D*espite the rapid growth* of hospitals and other institutions for the care of the sick in the United States, the American public was slow in recognizing the parallel obligation to those who, for whatever reason, were unable to go to hospitals and therefore had to be cared for in their homes. By 1915 no more than 10 percent of the sick received care in institutions. Aside from the small proportion of the unhospitalized sick who could afford to employ private duty graduate nurses at $25 a week, there remained a large majority to be cared for by either untrained practical nurses or well-prepared visiting nurses.

Public Health Nursing Skyrockets

As late as 1891 there had been only 58 associations and 130 nurses throughout the country engaged in visiting or public health nursing. During the next decade a national public health movement took definite form, creating a steadily increasing demand for nurses. Public health nursing surged ahead so that in 1919 nearly 9000 trained nurses were devoting their entire time to this type of work. Some idea of the growth of this movement may be derived from the following table [1]:

Growth of Public Health Nursing in the United States

Year	Organizations	Nurses
1891	58	130
1905	200	400
1914	1922	5152
1919	3094	8770

The first visiting nurses had limited their work almost entirely to bedside care. They soon discovered that the giving of medicine had little effect if there was no food in the house; that to ensure cleanliness required more than just an order from the physician or nurse; that health care and preventive measures required not only technical skill but also a high degree of communicative ability. The nurse soon found that she was making a certain number of visits that were entirely psychosocial in character and that in order to improve the health of a

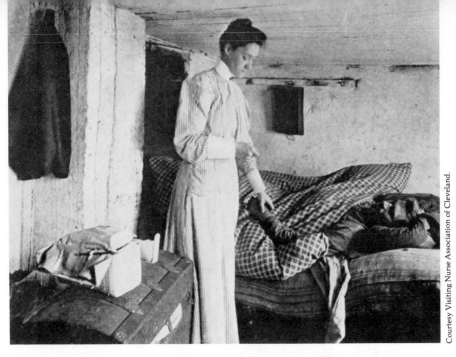

A visiting nurse caring for a poverty-striken man, about 1912.

A wide array of satisfying opportunities were open to the public health nurse.

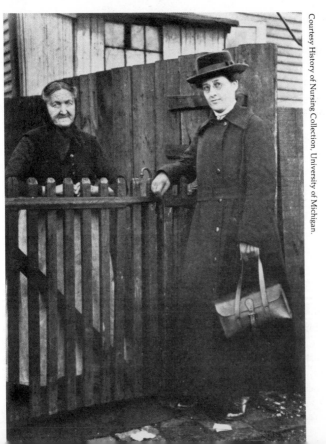

particular patient, her work might require a knowledge of economic, industrial, cultural, or social conditions—knowledge far removed from the therapeutic principles taught in the hospital. Thus the specialty of public health nursing emerged in strength.

While it was essential that the public health nurse first be formally trained in hospital nursing, she also needed preparation in the public health aspects of her field. She could acquire this by special fieldwork in connection with her hospital training, by postgraduate studies in public health at a college, or by on-the-job training with one of the district nursing associations. Some excellent nurses had received their public health training through practical fieldwork under the instruction of a trained supervisor, but in general such education was inferior to the combined theory and practice received in public health nursing courses offered by colleges and schools.

Special courses on the elements of public health nursing soon appeared. By 1916 there were at least eight different colleges, universities, or other institutions offering graduate courses for public health nurses—in Atlanta, Boston, Boulder, Chicago, Cleveland, New York, Philadelphia, and Santa Barbara—along with special courses offered by the state health departments of Kansas and Ohio. The Department of Nursing and Health directed by Professor Adelaide Nutting at Teachers College, Columbia University, was the strongest and most fully developed of these schools. It had a departmental faculty of five professors, with eight special lecturers attached to the staff. It offered one- and two-year programs of study on teaching in schools of nursing, administration of schools of nursing, hospital administration, public health nursing, school nursing and teaching, and supervision in public health nursing. In Boston the District Nursing Association gave both four- and eight-month courses; the public health, household economics, and educational aspects were offered at Simmons College and the sociological aspects at a nearby school for social workers. In Chicago a course given by the School of Civics and Philanthropy covered a period of 16 weeks, including classroom work, visits to social agencies, and fieldwork under the supervision of local public health nursing organizations.

In addition to their usual work, public health nurses were being called to serve as sanitary inspectors, tenement house inspectors, probation officers, hygiene teachers, hospital social service workers, agents of charity organization societies, and welfare workers in large industrial plants. For example, Adelaide Nutting, at the opening of the 1916 fall term, received letters that reveal the type of work that was expected of the public health nurse of that period:

I have just been talking with_____, superintendent of schools at_____. He wants a school nurse . . . . This is a new position, and he is inclined to give the right woman quite a free hand. He says they have 1800 children in the school and practically no foreigners [and] wishes this school nurse to assist the physical education instructor in medical inspection. During the year they conduct some chautauqua work, where the nurse would have an opportunity to deliver lectures to the farmers' wives. They also have a summer school, where they emphasize domestic science, domestic art, and general industrial activities, but this could be arranged later on. Mr._____wants to find a woman who is adaptable and who would be interested in remaining for some time. [He] emphasizes social training, and would like to find a woman of considerable enthusiasm as well as special training.

A letter received from a staff physician at a hospital in one of the large eastern cities stated:

During the past year I have been developing a clinic for the investigation and treatment of diseases of metabolism in one of the large hospitals . . . . Our work thus far has been confined to the treatment of diabetes mellitus and nephritis. The board of managers of the hospital are very much interested in the work, which has been productive of the most gratifying results. Thus far I have been greatly handicapped because of the lack of knowledge on the part of the pupil nurses of the principles of dietetics and the elementary principles of metabolics, and even more handicapped by the fact that we have no teaching nurse who is able to instruct the pupil nurses. It is my plan to secure an educated trained nurse who will come into the hospital, supervise the care of the patients in this ward, and also act as a teacher in the nurses' training school. The position will be one of dignity and will carry with it a reasonable salary. The board of managers of the hospital has instructed me to negotiate for such a teacher. I am appealing to you for assistance in securing such a person. Will you kindly let me know if any of your graduate or present students are or will be available for such work? [2].

In 1916 Mary Sewall Gardner, Director of the Providence, Rhode Island, District Nursing Association and author of the book *Public Health Nursing*, observed the attitude of the medical profession toward public health nursing. The more broad-minded physicians had always recognized the work of public health nurses who helped them produce results that would have been impossible if they had been forced to work alone. The narrow-minded members of the medical profession, however, regarded public health nurses with suspicion and continually feared their interference. There was apt to be a certain amount of antagonism from physicians in any community contemplating the establishment of a public health nursing service. This antagonism could be greatly diminished if the service was started with the cooperation of the medical profession and if the nurses made special efforts to assure everyone that the physician and not the nurse was in charge and that the nurse would not assume the duties and responsibilities of the physician.

Miss Gardner interpreted the rules of professional ethics to mean that the public health nurse "should not diagnose, should not prescribe, should not recommend a particular doctor or a change of doctors, should not suggest a hospital to a patient without the concurrence of the doctor, and should never criticize, by word or unspoken action, any member of the medical profession." These severe rules were sometimes modified so that a nurse would not be compelled to serve under a physician who was professionally incompetent or dangerously careless. In such cases the nurse was to report the problem to her supervisor, who, if she was experienced and resourceful, usually found a way to correct the situation.

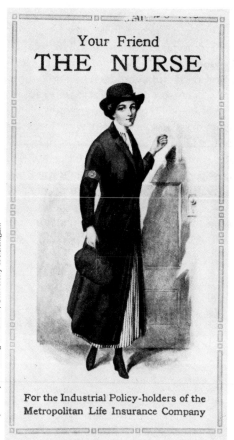

Your Friend
THE NURSE

For the Industrial Policy-holders of the
Metropolitan Life Insurance Company

How to Get the Nurse

1. Post the mailing card,
   or
2. Tell your Agent,
   or
3. Telephone or send some one to the Company's office,
   or
4. Telephone to or send some one for the Nurse.

Things to Remember

Always have a mailing card in your home.

Keep it in your premium receipt book or with your receipts, so that you will know where it is in case of sickness.

If you need more mailing cards, ask the Agent or the Nurse for them.

Have your policy and premium receipt book or receipts ready when the Nurse calls.

Look in *The Metropolitan* for the name and address of the Nurse.

Send for the Nurse When You Need to be Nursed

Form **N.S. 2**— Nov. 1918

Bulletin on the nursing service for Metropolitan Life Insurance policyholders, 1918.

The Metropolitan Life Nurses

By 1920 a program instituted by the Metropolitan Life Insurance Company for its industrial policyholders had gained national attention. It will be recalled that this service, started in 1909 in conjunction with the Henry Street Settlement in New York City, was limited to company policyholders, most of whom were employed in industrial occupations. The service had increased rapidly and was extended to all industrial policyholders who were ill and required bedside treatment. In cities outside the New York City area, visits were made by company nurses, but as a rule Metropolitan Life employed the nurses of the local visiting nurses' association. The total company cost of service during 1918 was more than $810,000, the average cost per visit was 53 cents, and the average number of visits per patient was 4.9. Based upon the entire number of industrial policies, the cost per policy was 4.6 cents.

Metropolitan Life actuaries prepared a table showing the influence of the nursing service and other health and welfare activities upon the mortality rate of their policyholders [3]:

Industrial Policy Holder Experience of the Metropolitan Life Insurance Co., 1911–1917, in Deaths per 1,000

Age Period	1911	1917	Percent Decline
All ages	12.5	11.6	7.2
1 to 4	12.8	10.5	18.0
1	25.2	20.4	19.1
2	16.6	13.5	18.7
3	9.3	7.7	17.2
4	6.6	5.6	15.2
5 to 9	2.7	3.4	3.7
10 to 14	2.7	2.6	3.7
15 to 19	4.7	4.8	*2.1
20 to 24	7.3	6.6	9.6
25 to 34	9.5	8.4	11.6
35 to 44	13.7	12.4	9.5
45 to 54	19.8	19.6	1.0
55 to 64	36.0	35.8	.6
65 to 74	74.5	76.4	*2.6
74 and over	139.3	142.6	*2.4

*Percent increase in seven years.

The above table reveals an average decline in the mortality rate of over 7 percent in seven years. The decline was most marked and most significant during the early years, being over 19 percent in the first year of life. When the rates for the principal causes of death of policyholders were compared with the general death rates for the community at large as obtained from government sources, the results were distinctly in favor of the policyholders. The company thus considered it fair to assume that a significant part of the decline in mortality and

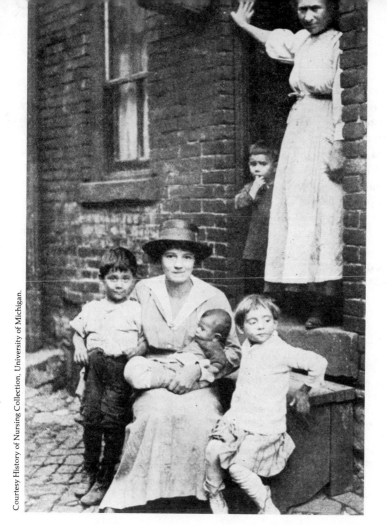

Metropolitan Life attributed a significant part of the decline in policyholder mortality to its public health nursing service.

the accompanying improvement in general health was due to the program of visiting nurses established in 1909.

Activities of Public Health Nurses in the 1920s

Meanwhile, nurses were becoming more and more common in state health departments. Until 1907 no state recognized the public health nurse as a legitimate employee of an official health or education agency. As early as 1898, Los Angeles had employed a few municipal nurses, and in 1902 the New York City Health Department employed several nurses to assist in the control of communicable diseases, but these instances were more or less in the nature of experiments and were not authorized by legislative action. Recognition of public health nursing as a desirable and necessary function of government came gradually in the first 25 years of the twentieth century.

Alabama was the first state to approve the employment of public health nurses by governmental agencies. The County Health Law passed in 1907 specifically mentioned nurses as "employees necessary to accomplish the work of a county health department." The following year New York State passed a law which permitted the employment of nurses to aid in the control of tuberculosis. Ohio was the third state to recognize the public health nurse by specifying her in its school health inspection law which was passed in 1909. Two years later Massachusetts permitted certain cities to employ visiting nurses, and during that same year Pennsylvania authorized the employment of school nurses.

By the early 1920s it was difficult to form any clear picture of the scope of public health nursing. Experts who had carefully studied the public health nursing problem appeared to favor a generalized service combining health instruction and bedside care. The Committee on Nursing of the Rockefeller Foundation concluded:

The question of whether the public health nurse should or should not render bedside care has been hotly debated during the past few years. The arguments for purely instructive service rest mainly on two grounds—the administrative difficulties involved in the conduct of private sick nursing by official health agencies and the danger that the urgent demands of sick nursing may lead to the neglect of preventive educational measures which are of more basic and fundamental significance. Both these objections are real and important ones. Yet the observations made in the course of our survey indicate that both may perhaps ultimately be overcome. Several municipal health departments have definitely undertaken to provide organized nursing service for bedside care combined with health teaching, while in other instances instructive nurses, under public auspices, combine a certain amount of emergency service with their fundamentally educational activities.

Public health nurse teaching by demonstration.

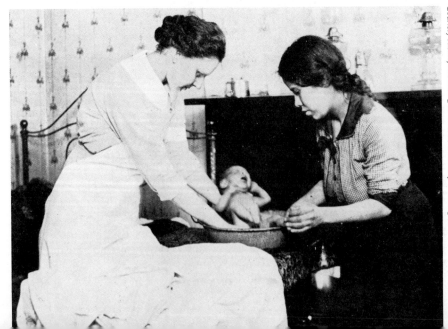

So far as the neglect of instructive work is concerned it results from numerical inadequacy of personnel and can be avoided by a sufficiently large nursing staff.

On the other hand, the plan of instructive nursing divorced from bedside care suffers from defects which if less obvious than those mentioned above are in reality more serious, because they are inherent in the very plan itself and therefore not subject to control. In the first place, the introduction of the instructive but non-nursing field worker creates at once a duplication of effort, since there must be a nurse from some other agency employed in the same district to give bedside care. In the second place, the field worker who attempts health education without giving nursing care is by that very fact cut off from the contact which gives the instructive bedside nurse her most important psychological asset. The nurse who approaches a family where sickness exists and renders direct technical service in mitigating the burden of that sickness has an overwhelming advantage, then and thereafter, in teaching the lessons of hygiene. With a given number of nurses per unit of population, we believe that the combined service of teaching and nursing will yield the largest results [4].

A Census of Public Health Nursing in the United States taken by the National Organization for Public Health Nursing in 1924 found that there were a total of 3629 agencies, with a total of 11,171 full-time graduate nurses. About one-half of these agencies, employing more than one-half of the nurses, were official branches of the federal, state, county, or municipal governments. Among the private agencies listed were 398 public health nursing associations or similar organizations which had 2516 nurses, 473 local clinics and branches of the American Red Cross with 574 nurses, 128 tuberculosis associations which carried 125 nurses; and 424 other non-official agencies employing 1194 nurses. Of the 3045 counties in the United States, 866 had local nursing service available in 1924 for the entire area and 379 for part of the area, leaving 1800 totally unprovided for.

During the 1920s the primary duties of the public health nurse moved more toward advising and instructing—to advise and show others how to care for the sick, to secure adequate care for them, and to instruct people on how to avoid sickness by attention to personal hygiene. Bedside nursing of the sick poor was no longer the primary function of the public health nurse. Among the duties of private public health nursing agency employees were:

casefinding and investigation of cases of communicable disease (tuberculosis, venereal disease, etc.)

sanitary surveys

investigation of home conditions affecting infant mortality

follow-up care of patients with poliomyelitis

facilitating the employment of nurses in industries and cooperating with the work of industrial nurses

inspection and supervision of midwives

instruction in the conduct of infant welfare stations and tuberculosis dispensaries

registration of unreported births

school inspections in cooperation with the school medical inspector

conducting exhibits
educational work, lectures, demonstrations
supervising and instructing local public health nurses

The duies that were usually performed by public health nurses employed by the boards of health of local municipalities were:

casefinding of mild or unrecovered and unreported cases of communicable diseases
investigation and improvement of home conditions which affect infant mortality
conducting of infant welfare stations
securing medical or hospital care for the sick
cooperating with social agencies in promoting public health work, including the control of venereal disease
cooperating with overseers of the poor in improving health conditions among the dependent poor
preventive and follow-up care in poliomyelitis, mental retardation, mental illness, and blindness
antituberculosis work
educational work, such as instruction of Red Cross classes and Little Mothers' Leagues
investigation of food stores, dairies, playgrounds, public toilets
assisting health officers in securing laboratory specimens for diagnostic purposes

The following duties were usually performed by county tuberculosis nurses:

discovery of unreported cases of tuberculosis
promoting the examination and treatment of tuberculosis patients by physicians
studying the morbidity and mortality statistics of the various municipalities with special reference to tuberculosis
arranging for clinic care or admission of tuberculosis patients to hospitals
attending tuberculosis clinics
home visitation and instruction of tuberculosis patients
giving lectures and demonstrations on anti-tuberculosis work

The principal functions of the school nurse were as follows:

casefinding and prevention of communicable diseases among school children
casefinding and treatment of physical handicaps
visiting and instructing parents of school children who had physical handicaps
giving simple routine treatments prescribed by the medical inspector and the family physician

attending school clinics
assisting the medical examiner of the school
instructing special groups of children in "practical hygiene"

The actual work of dealing firsthand with communicable diseases, inspecting milk and other food, maintaining a pure water supply, conducting clinics, providing nursing service, reaching the people with health instruction, and grappling in other ways with the many problems of disease control rested with local health departments. It was important, therefore, that they be provided with adequate staffs and funds for their work. Yet of 818 municipal health departments in cities of 10,000 population and over listed by the United States Public Health Service in 1923, only 41 percent had full-time health officers. Similarly, a 1925 study by the Bureau of the Census of public expenditures in 247 cities having a population of 30,000 or more showed that only 91 cents per capita was used for the conservation of health that year, while over $14 per capita was spent for education and $7.53 for police, fire, and other protection to person and property.

Weighing a baby at an infant health center in the basement of a village church.

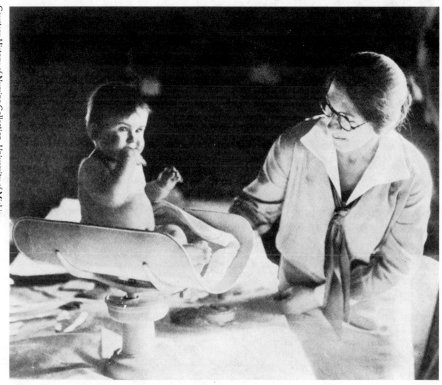

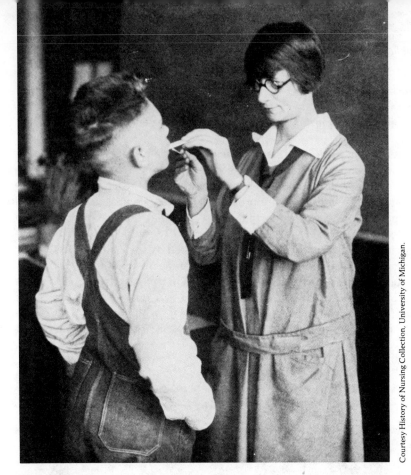

Taking a culture to test for diphtheria infection.

Surveys of Sickness

A most glaring weakness of the nation's total health care system had less to do with individual health professionals than with social and economic realities. A revealing study was made in 1915 by the New York State Charities Aid Association of the modes of health care made in 1600 cases of sickness in Dutchess County, New York. All the illnesses recorded some degree of temporary or permanent disability [5].

Mode of Care	Number	Percent
Medical care provided by a physician at home	11,058	66
Medical care given outside the patient's home, either in a hospital or in other homes	159	10
No medical care rendered	383	24

Another pertinent study, conducted in 1918 by the Public Health Committee of the New York Academy of Medicine, investigated the care secured by families in New York City. It found that among the 8645 people surveyed, 3140 were reported as having suffered from 3536 illnesses during 1918, making an average of over one illness per person. This included partial and complete disabilities. In order to meet the demands of the illnesses, the following forms of treatment were employed by the families [6]:

Form of Treatment	Percent
Private physicians at home	37.7
Lodge physicians at home	4.1
Charity physicians (sent to home from an institution)	0.8
Medical care in hospitals	11.6
Medical care in outpatient clinics	13.2
Midwives at home	10.8
Self-treatment or medication on advice of druggist	21.8

It is significant that the proportion of sick people without direct medical care was about the same as in the Dutchess County survey.

A third survey of providers of health care was carried out from 1921 to 1924 in Hagerstown, Maryland, by the United States Public Health Service. Of 17,217 illnesses for which information was obtained, the following kinds of care were recorded [7]:

Provider of Treatment	Percent
Private physicians	46.00
Medical care in hospital	1.34
Chiropractors and osteopaths	0.41
Self-medication	2.25
No form of care reported	50.00

The Hagerstown cases included a larger proportion of minor illnesses than did the other two studies. But, significantly, 100 percent of the cases of typhoid fever and cancer and 97 percent of the pneumonia patients were treated either in home or in hospital, while almost one-third of the patients with measles reported "no medical care." Of the mass of sore throats, colds, and bronchial conditions comprising over 7000 of the 17,217 total illnesses, fewer than 20 percent received outside medical care.

The Scandal of Self-Medication
Despite its danger, self-treatment through the use of patent medicines was still widespread. Americans consumed more drugs and used more patent medicines than any other country in the civilized world. Self-medication had grown to

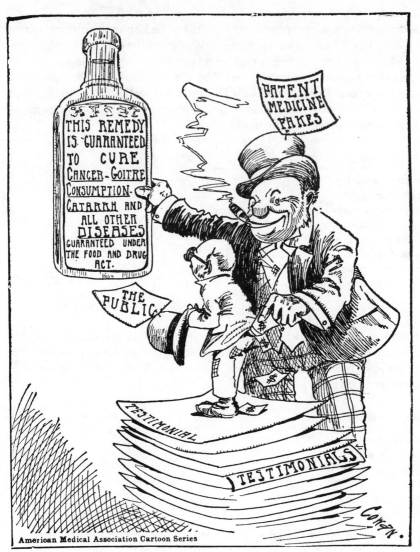

American Medical Association Cartoon Series

Michigan Public Health Magazine, May, 1918.

The patent medicine racket.

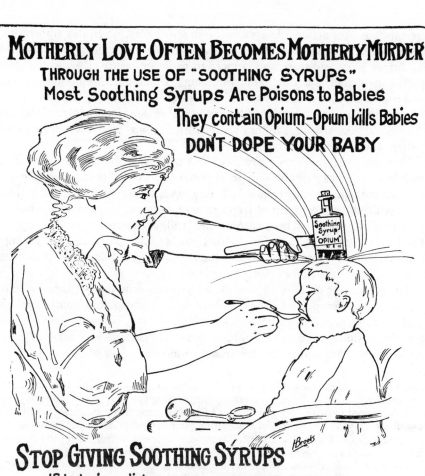

The dangers of soothing syrups for infants and children.

tremendous proportions. Everywhere—in street cars, on trolley transfer tickets, on billboards, in magazines, in newspapers, in the mails—were advertised medicines to cure disease and devices to promote health. Besides the classic patent medicines, such as Lydia Pinkham's Vegetable Compound, castoria, and cod liver oil, came promises of "Colds Cured in One Day" or remedies like "Appendixine" and an array of health foods, massage vibrators, violet rays, "Porosknit" underwear, sanitary tooth washes, soaps, and vitopathic, naturopathic, and assorted faith cures.

New panaceas appeared every day. One product, "Soothing Sirup"—recommended for colicky infants—often permanently doped its small recipients or soothed them into a sleep from which they never awoke. In New York a visiting nurse encountered a group of frenzied women in the hallway of a tenement. Nearby a baby lay on a bed, gasping and "rolling its eyes up into the top of its head." The nurse asked the frightened mother what she had been giving it. "Nothing at all," said the woman—but a telltale "soothing" bottle indicated that the child was dying of morphine poisoning.

The prevalence of ill health and the widespread demand for "cures" also fostered the proliferation of quacks. These were unscrupulous charlatans who, with humbug promises and practices, extorted money from the simple-minded and the credulous. Samuel Hopkins Adams, in his exposé of this sordid business entitled *The Great American Fraud*, observed:

No peril in the whole range of human pathology need have any terrors for the man who can believe the medical advertisements in the newspapers. For every ill there is a "sure cure" provided in print. *Dr. This* is as confident of removing your cancer without the use of the knife as *Dr. That* is of eradicating your consumption by his marvelous new discovery, or *Dr. Otherwise* of rehabilitating your kidneys, which the regular profession has given up as a hopeless job.

The more deadly the disease, the more blatantly certain is the quack that he alone can save you, and in extreme cases, where he has failed to get there earlier, he may even raise you from your coffin and restore you to your astonished and admiring friends. Such things have happened—and pitiful gropers after relief from suffering believe that they may happen again, otherwise charlatanry would cease to spread its daily cure [8].

Through their advertising, quacks spread a pall of fear over the country. "Have you a little pain in your back—look for Bright's Disease! Have you a neglected cough?—look out for consumption!" This artificially created fear drove victims into doctors' offices as well as into the drugstore, and perfectly healthy patients paid needless fees. Elsewhere, quick-cure artists traded on a fundamental human want—the desire to be free from pain and from the fear of pain. Frequently this desire was so urgent that price was no object, and often the sufferer passionately hoped to be cured in the privacy of his bedroom, without friends, family, or even a physician discovering the ailment. Both desires led victims directly to the quacks, sometimes with very serious consequences.

Clare Terwilliger, a public health nurse assigned by the Henry Street Nursing Service to a block on East Thirty-ninth Street, New York, furnished more than

The sad story of
MY FATHER'S GREAT SUFFERING
FROM CANCER
Read the following and be convinced
WE CAN CURE YOU.

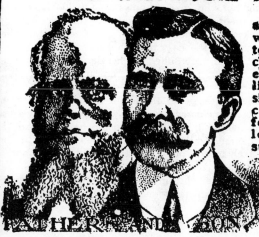

FATHER AND SON

Forty-five years ago my father who was himself a doctor, had a vicious cancer that was eating away his life. The best physicians in America could do nothing for him. After nine long years of awful suffering, and after the cancer had totally eaten away his nose and portions of his face (as shown in his picture here given) his palate was entirely destroyed together with portions of his throat. Father fortunately discovered the great remedy that cured him. This was over forty years ago, and he has never suffered a day since.

This same discovery has now cured thousands who were threatened with operation and death. And to prove that this is the truth we will give their sworn statement if you will write us. Doctors, Lawyers, Mechanics, Ministers, Laboring Men, Bankers and all classes recommend this glorious life-saving discovery, and we want the whole world to benefit by it.

HAVE YOU CANCER, Tumors, Ulcers, Abscesses, Fever Sores, Goitre, Catarrh, Salt-Rheum, Rheumatism, Piles, Eczema, Scald Head or Scrofula in any form.

We positively guarantee our statements true, perfect satisfaction and honest service—or money refunded.

It will cost you nothing to learn the truth about this wonderful home treatment without the knife or caustic. And if you know anyone who is afflicted with any disease above mentioned, you can do them a Christian act of kindness by sending us their addresses so we can write them how easily they can be cured in their own home. This is no idle talk, we mean just what we say. We have cured others, and can cure you. Forty years experience guarantees success. Write us today; delay is dangerous. Illustrated Booklet FREE.

DRS. MIXER, 286 State St., HASTINGS, MICH.

Quack cure for cancer which appeared in newspapers nationwide.

a year's impressions of the segment of life within her jurisdiction, under the title "How Thirty-ninth Street People Secure Care in Sickness." She also showed why they sometimes did not secure care. Miss Terwilliger concluded:

Uncertainty about the nature of the disease which a person seems to have appears to play a greater part than the severity of the illness in determining whether or not to call a doctor. If the disease is recognized, remedies are used which are suggested by some older member of the family or some neighbor who "always knows what to do." If a child with measles, for example, instead of growing better, begins to feel as if it were burning up and breathes very rapidly, that element of uncertainty provides a reason for calling a doctor. If the family belongs to a group of friends or neighbors in which there is one person who has a family doctor, that person is consulted and her doctor is called. The use of a single doctor as the regular family doctor is, however, unusual. If the family does not belong to such a clique the nearest doctor is called.

If the family is Irish and the patient grows better, the doctor's fine qualities are lauded up and down the street for months. If the patient does not grow better in a very short time, another doctor is called. As many as three different doctors have been called in a case of acute illness lasting only four days. If the patient dies, the members of the family and the interested neighbors are likely to state publicly as frequently as the opportunity arises that the doctor killed the patient.

If, on the other hand, the family is Italian and illness is severe, the doctor is requested to bring a "professor" and the money is gathered somehow to pay him before he leaves the house [9].

Health Practices of Immigrants

In a 1921 study by Michael M. Davis, entitled *Immigrant Health and the Community*, a Latvian immigrant was reported to have declared that he did:

not trust hospitals or dispensaries, especially city hospitals, which many of the men from the factory had been to when different accidents happened. One or two of them had died and the family and neighbors looked upon all hospitals as a place where one goes to die.

A statement from the same survey concluded:

Most hospitals give even the sophisticated visitor a sense of being surrounded by very busy, presumably very efficient doctors, nurses, and employees, who are passing rapidly from one duty to another and have no time for him. The attitude towards hospitals revealed in one hundred and fifty interviews with (foreign-born) doctors, and about an equal number with individual immigrants, could be summarized in the following opinions:

A strange place.
A place in which I cannot understand what people say, or be understood.
A place where doctors practice on you, especially young doctors.
A place where people die.
A place where I cannot get the food I like or am used to.
A place where I either have to take charity or pay more than I can afford [10].

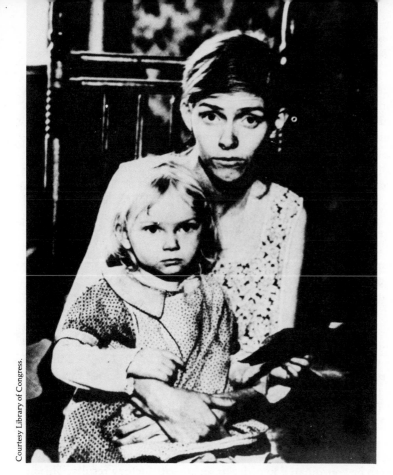

A tubercular New York mother living in the midst of poverty.

A Lithuanian's testimony suggested how the neighborhood drugstore was patronized even without the urge from national advertising, because it was familiar and neighborly, while the hospital was distant and aloof:

All hospitals are the same to Mr. M. "When men are hurt in the factory they are sent there, and if the young doctors do not practice on them they live, but otherwise they die." Mr. M. had no other occasion to use doctors. When he had a cold and sore throat he told the druggist what the trouble was and he gave him some medicine. "Of course the druggist knows what is good for you" [11].

Health Demonstrations

Large-scale health demonstrations were extremely helpful in showing what could be done to improve community health during the 1920s. These intensive programs of health education in carefully defined areas were temporarily supplied with a modern public health service under the direction of trained and experienced personnel. The object of the demonstration was to show the benefits of such services, with the hope that they might become so widely appreciated that they would be permanently adopted by the demonstration community as well as a large number of similar communities. Financial support for health demonstrations came from philanthropic foundations, insurance companies, local contributions, and in some cases state funds.

The first public health demonstration in America was sponsored by the Metropolitan Life Insurance Company. In 1915 that company paid out $4 million in policies for deaths from tuberculosis alone. Such a serious situation warranted an effort to find means of early detection of the disease and of preventing its spread to other members of the community. The task of selecting a typical locality and planning and carrying out the demonstration was entrusted to the National Tuberculosis Association, which selected the town of Framingham, Massachusetts. With the $100,000 contributed by the company, a three-year study was launched. After it became apparent that it would be impossible to fight tuberculosis effectively without carrying on a general health program for the community, the project budget was doubled and the demonstration was extended to seven years. Diagnostic standards were developed, and, for the first time, accurate knowledge of the amount of tuberculosis existing in a given community was determined. As a result of this work the tuberculosis death rate of Framingham fell from 97.5 per 100,000 in 1917 to 38.2 in 1923 and declined to only two-thirds of the rest of the state's tuberculosis rate.

From 1923 to 1929 the Commonwealth Fund conducted demonstrations in Fargo, North Dakota; Clark County, Georgia; Rutherford County, Tennessee; and Marion County, Oregon. From the experience thus gained, Fund directors arrived at the belief that state departments of health needed to give direct aid and guidance to rural health areas and that the efforts of all local health providers needed to be coordinated in order to secure satisfactory results. This included extensive use of local physicians as well as public health officers and public health nurses in programs of mass screening and health assessment.

The Kentucky Frontier Nursing Service

A practical demonstration in uplifting the health status of a remote rural area was also launched, in the form of the Frontier Nursing Service, organized by its director, Mary Breckinridge, In May, 1925. Mrs. Breckinridge had recognized the need for such work and had secured training at the Saint Luke's Hospital School of Nursing in New York and at a nurse-midwifery program in London.

Several years earlier Mrs. Breckinridge had interviewed 53 of the area's midwives and had assembled her data in a manuscript report entitled "Midwifery in the Kentucky Mountains." All but one of the midwives were white and they ranged in age from 30 to 90 years, with the average midwife being 60 years old. Only 12 of the 53 could read or write and none had taken any formal training in midwifery.

As a group these untrained midwives were grossly superstitious and knew nothing of prenatal or postnatal care. Only seven of the 53 carried any equipment with them; the rest "counted on finding at the patient's home the hog grease which is their almost universal requisite." If complications in delivery

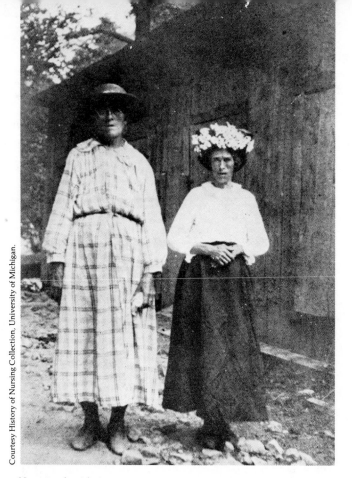

Untrained midwives.

occurred, the midwives would almost never call for a physician, considering such action to be a reflection on their competency. Instead they would attempt to stop hemorrhage by repeating a certain Bible verse or by making tea from black gum bark from the north side of a tree mixed with the bark of sweet apple tree from the south side of the tree. Soot was employed extensively as a medication, some of the midwives preferring chimney soot, others, soot from pots and pans. Generally recommended preventive procedures included placing an axe under the delivery bed with the blade straight up.

Mrs. Breckinridge's field of work was centered in Leslie County and parts of adjacent Clay and Owsley Counties in southeastern Kentucky. Overwhelmingly rural in population, Leslie County's 10,000 inhabitants constituted a density of only 27.1 persons per square mile, the second lowest in the state. The only settlement of any size was Hyden, with 313 inhabitants. The area's poor economy supported only a fragile existence for the population. The absence of highways necessitated travel by horse or mule only. The area was divided into eight districts of about 78 square miles each. In a log cabin in the middle of each district lived two nurses who were responsible for the health of all the people who lived there. They provided midwifery and public health nursing to the

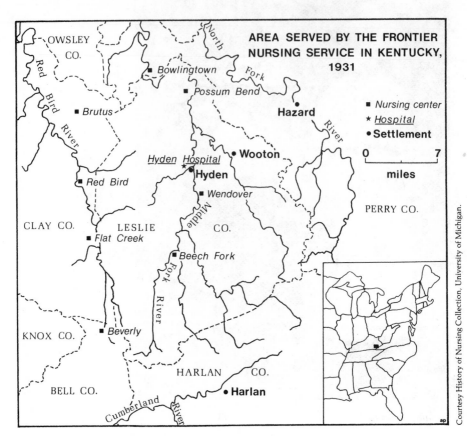

Map of the Frontier Nursing Service area, 1931.

approximately 200 families who lived in the general area.

The work plan was based on one used in the Highlands and islands of Scotland, whose systems had been observed by Mrs. Breckinridge. A generalized service and a decentralized system of organization were the key elements of the plan. A fee of one dollar per year for complete nursing and public health care was charged and, as necessary, an additional five dollars for maternity care—the same fee charged by "granny midwives."

A 12-bed general hospital, the Hyden Hospital and Health Center, was established and operated at near capacity with 375 patient admissions and 31 births in 1935. Assisted by a superintendent and two nurses, the medical director had his headquarters there, taking responsibility for the hospitalized patients and answering calls from the nurses in the various centers.

The bulk of the care offered by the Frontier Nursing Service was delivered by nurses working out of the centers at Wendover, Beech Fork, Possum Bend, Red Bird, Flat Creek, Brutus, Bowlington, and Beverly. All the nurses were required to have had preparation in midwifery in addition to their general nursing

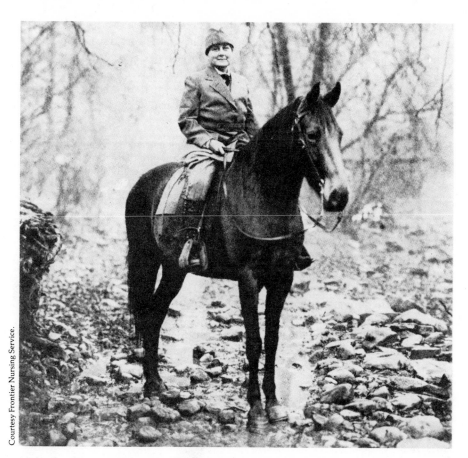

Courtesy Frontier Nursing Service.

Mary Breckinridge, founder of the Frontier Nursing Service.

and public health training. Since there were no quality nurse midwifery programs in the United States until the early 1930s, the early nurses received their
training in England or Scotland. Staff nurses were required to have a certificate
from the Central Midwives' Board in either of those countries. These nurse
midwives gave antepartal, intrapartal, and postpartal care to women in their
districts. They visited their patients at least twice a month until the seventh
month of pregnancy and then every week until the time of delivery. Normal
deliveries were handled by the nurse midwives; for complicated cases, the physician was called. The nurse took care of the patients for 10 days following
delivery.

In 1932 Dr. Louis I. Dublin of the Metropolitan Life Insurance Company
studied the first 1000 cases of the Frontier Nursing Service and summarized the
results. He found that the proportion of complications that occurred during
pregnancy and delivery was lower among the patients cared for by the Frontier
nurses than among the general population. In regard to the mortality among
the 1000 cases analyzed, Dr. Dublin wrote that "not one of the women died as

the direct result of either pregnancy or labor. There were two deaths in the series; but in one the cause of death was a chronic kidney and heart disease, and in the other it was chronic heart disease. Neither of these two cases could properly be ascribed to the maternal state." There were one-third fewer stillbirths and one-third fewer deaths among babies in the first year of life than among the general white population of Kentucky. Dr. Dublin concluded:

The study shows conclusively what has in fact been demonstrated before, that the type of service rendered by the Frontier Nurses safeguards the life of mother and babe. If such a service were available to the women of the country generally, there would be a saving of 10,000 mothers' lives a year in the United States; there would be 30,000 less stillbirths and 30,000 children alive at the end of the first month of life [12].

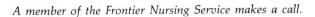

The Frontier Nursing Service also offered care for infants and children. Babies under one year of age were examined twice a month, preschool children from one to six were seen every month, and schoolchildren were examined once every three months. During these visits mothers were taught about diet, cleanliness, health habits, general sanitation, and preventive care. Inoculations against typhoid and diphtheria and vaccinations for smallpox were also given.

The work of Mary Breckinridge and her frontier nurses constituted a vivid demonstration of the greatly expanded role that nurses could play in dispensing

A member of the Frontier Nursing Service makes a call.

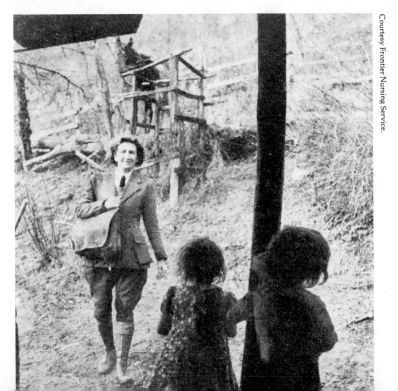

a primary form of health care. While some nurses hoped that this type of service might be emulated elsewhere with the same successful results, the necessary mix of social, economic, and leadership elements failed to materialize, and the Frontier Nursing Service continued as a unique institution.

Trachoma Eradication

Another health demonstration was the trachoma eradication project carried out by nurses of the United States Public Health Service. The cause of trachoma, although it had been intensively sought after by capable bacteriologists, had not been discovered at that time. The disease seemed to be furthered by unusual exposure to wind, dust, and sun and by careless habits of personal cleanliness and the use of the same towel by several or many people—"the common towel." Trachoma first attacked the conjunctiva (the membrane lining the eyelids) causing granulations to form, which thickened the lid and irritated the eyeball. Later these granulations were replaced by scar tissue, which contracted, deforming the lids and bending them inwards so that the eyelashes would rub against the front of the eye. The irritation thus caused was not only very painful but was commonly followed by partial or complete blindness.

In order to combat epidemic trachoma in the Appalachian Mountains, the Public Health Service established special hospitals at Hindman, Hyden, and Jackson, Kentucky, and at Coeburn, Virginia, in 1914 and 1915. Additional hospitals were set up later in the rural areas of West Virginia, Arkansas, and Missouri. Several dozen public health nurses were selected by the Public Health Service Superintendent of Nurses, Lucy Minnigerode, for appointment to the trachoma project. The trachoma eradication project was aimed at the very primitive mountain districts, where roads were impassable for automobiles. Thus one United States Public Health Service nurse making instructive visits and hunting up cases rode 3000 miles on muleback in a single year.

By 1925 United States Public Health Service nurses were working in trachoma hospitals at Rolla, Missouri; Russellville, Arkansas; Knoxville, Tennessee; and Richmond, Kentucky. At Rolla a laboratory had been established so that bacteriological studies could be carried on in connection with the treatment. These temporary hospitals housed about 25 patients. In addition, there were a number of outpatients who also came in for treatment. There were wards for all types of patients, together with treatment rooms, operating rooms, mess halls, kitchens, and bathrooms. The patients were seldom in bed, because they were able to take care of themselves. Generally two nurses were assigned to each hospital.

The treatments alone kept the nurse busy. All eyes were cleansed and irrigated before breakfast. At 9:00 A.M. the physician in charge gave his treatment and orders for the day—atropine for this and silver nitrate for that and so forth. The nurse again, before dinner, irrigated all eyes and carried out the orders. The physician made another call at 2:00 P.M., and the nurse, another round bedtime, making a total of five treatments each day for each patient.

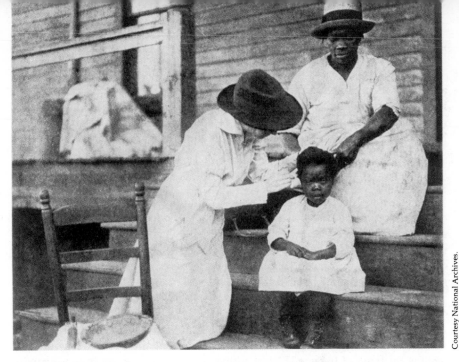

Treating a child with trachoma.

The work was rewarding for the nurse because she knew she was preventing blindness and alleviating much suffering. A weekly report of Blanche Pegg Allen, R.N., special field worker for the United States Public Health Service at Hazard, Kentucky, gives a typical example of this important assignment:

Monday: Left Hazard 8:30 A.M. To Heiner. Got stuck in mud and had to be pulled out. Walked 2½ miles to Heiner and return. To school to see if Mrs. Sarah Combs was home. Gone to her mother's on Troublesome Creek. To home Irvin Smith to see Mrs. Combs, not there. Gone to home of Mrs. J. Erewers. To Brewer home. Mrs. Combs trachoma case, and should go to Hospital. She is Holiness and thinks that her eyes will get well if she has enough faith. Spent a long time trying to get the woman to go to hospital. Said she couldn't make up her mind. Am to return to her home last of week. Walked mile from road to Brewer home and return. To home Mrs. Floyd Engles—former Jackson patient. She is cicatricial trachoma with entropion. Examined six members of family, all trachoma negative. To home Mrs. Green Raleigh, sister Mrs. Combs, trachoma negative. Examined two members of family, trachoma negative. Walked two miles from road to Raleigh and Engle home and return. Returned to Hazard 4:30 P.M. Conference with Miss Connelley, Red Cross Field Representative for this section. Mileage 60.

Tuesday. Left Hazard 6:50 A.M., L.&N. RR. to Wolfcoal. Horseback from Wolfcoal to Turner's Creek. To home Jim Turner's—daughters Margaret and Ida, suspicious trachoma. Examined four members of family, trachoma negative. To home Sam Turner's—four trachoma cases in this home that I have seen before, they are to go to hospital, no one at home. To home Allen Herald, son Patrick trachoma case and to go to hospital. Child doesn't want to go and parents won't send him unless an older person goes along. This child takes to the hills every time I go to this section, and I haven't seen him for six weeks. To home Jesse Herald's, three in this family trachoma cases, and should go to hospital. Mother refuses to let children and husband go. One girl wanted to go and when she isn't around her mother she says she wants to have her eyes treated but when in the presence of her mother she looks at her mother and says no because mother wants her to say this. To home Green Raleigh, trachoma case and should go to hospital. Father says he can't let the boy go to hospital now, has to stay home and do the plowing that they start March 1. Learned from farmers in that section that they will not be able to start plowing before last of March or middle of April. To home John Turner to see if I could stay at their place while on Turner's Creek. Return to home Sam Turner's. Waited over an hour for Mrs. Turner and her children who are to go in to hospital tomorrow, to come home. Didn't come home. Returned to home John Turner's 5:15 P.M. Horseback nine miles.

Wednesday: Left John Turner Home 8:30 A.M. To home Sam Turner. Mrs. Turner said her husband said their children could not go to hospital. Mr. Turner works in Hazard and I have seen him several times about his children going to hospital and he said he wanted them to go and have their eyes treated. He told Postmaster at Wolfcoal Sunday that I didn't need bother going to his place, that his children were not going to hospital. The children had been sent away from home and I did not see them. To home Allen Herald, saw Willie Turner, who has been to hospital. Asked him how he liked it there, said he didn't like it as they kept you in too close. He wanted to get out and run around. To home Elizabeth Turner, trachoma case. Said she couldn't go to hospital on account of her two children. Husband works two days a week and said he couldn't manage with wife gone. To home Mahala Raleigh, cicatricial trachoma with entropion. Examined four members of family, trachoma negative. To home Dora Turner, former Jackson patient. Lids in good condition. To home T. T. Herald to get some one to take me across Middle Fork River. Too high to ford. To home Elliott Turner, following six children suspicious trachoma cases, Bill, age 10; America, age 8; Dullseen, age 5; Johnnie, age 4; Sarah, age 11; Millie, age 16 months. I asked Mother to take part of children now and go to hospital. Said her husband would have to decide. Two older girls said they wanted to go but the boy didn't. To home Wm. Baker, son Alex, former Richmond patient. Lids in good condition. Examined seven members of family—paternal grandfather, age 80; has trachoma, almost blind and aunt cicatricial trachoma, others negative. To home Timothy Herald, have child five years old with bad-looking eyes. Youngster cried and would not let me see her eyes and mother just sat and didn't bother herself about having the child's eyes examined and I naturally couldn't force her if the mother didn't. Examined three members of family, trachoma negative. To home Green Deaton, who is one of the outstanding members of the community. He said, "Oh, these people here are a sight and can't do anything with them." Walked three miles from Middle Fork River to Wm. Baker, Herald and Turner homes and return. Horseback five miles. Returned.

Thursday: Left John Turner's 8 A.M. To home Elizabeth Turner to see if her husband had come home and about her going to hospital. Mr. Turner had gone over on one of other creeks yesterday and they were expecting him home that morning. Not home, waited all morning for him, didn't come and I could see where Mrs. Turner wasn't so anxious about going. Her five-year-old boy was crying and didn't want her to leave, so she wouldn't think of going. To home Allen Herald's, said their youngster could go to hospital if he had an older person to go in with. He had gone back to the hills that morning when he saw me coming and I didn't get to see him. To home Elliott Turner's. Mr. Turner said he didn't want his children to go to hospital now and he wasn't in a position to get them ready to go. The two girls that told me the day before that they wanted to go to hospital said now that they didn't want to go because Mother and Daddy didn't want them to go. At this home I was greeted by two hounds, one of them taking a piece out of back of my coat as I retreated. You don't only get a cold reception from the household but the dogs too. Waited an hour for some one to take me across river as the boat was on one side and I on the other. Walked mile from river to E. Turner home and return. Return to Elizabeth Turner home. Husband had not returned. Left Turner's Creek 2:15 P.M. to Wolfcoal up bed of creek, arrived there 4:20 P.M. Horseback 8½ miles. This creek from Wolfcoal to Turner's Creek is full of large rocks and very hard for horse to travel. Left Wolfcoal 5:17 P.M., L&N. RR.; arrived Hazard 6:46 P.M.

Friday: Left Hazard or Hotel 8:20 A.M. To office Dr. Brown to see if Mrs. Herald from Turner's Creek had reported for treatment as she said she would. She came to Hazard last Sunday. Had not been in to Doctor's office. To office Dr. Carr, County Health Officer, to see about ordering a pass for a patient. To home Mrs. Ann Jones to see if Mrs. Sarah Combs was home. To home Mrs. Combs. Spent the entire morning trying to get the woman to go to hospital. She feels her faith is going to cure her eye and will not go. Walked one mile from car to Combs home and return. To home Sylvester Patrick, old trachoma case. Lids good condition. Examined four members of family, trachoma negative. To home Talbee Williams, cicatricial trachoma. Wife, trachoma negative. To home Fernando Williams, former Richmond patient, some activity in left lid. Referred to County Health Officer's treatment clinic, Hazard. Examined two members of family, trachoma negative. To home Jim Williams, mother Elizabeth Williams, old trachoma case, cicatricial trachoma blind from cataract. Examined five members family, trachoma negative. To home Floyd Jones—daughter Vina, suspicious trachoma, to go to hospital next week. Examined eight members of family, trachoma negative. To home Rose Murrell, examined six members of family, trachoma negative. To home Nellie Engle. Examined two members of family, trachoma negative. To home Jackson Kelley, examined three members of family, trachoma negative. To home Hoey Roberts, suspicious trachoma, right eye. Examined five members of family. Trachoma negative. To home Amy Jones, former Jackson patient, lids in good condition. Examined three members of family, trachoma negative. Walked five miles from car at Ary to all homes beginning with Sylvester Patrick, creek was so deep could not cross in car, returned to car at Ary. Return to Hazard 6:40 P.M. Mileage 51.

Saturday: A.M. worked on reports [13].

Promotion of Maternal and Child Health

Measures to improve maternal and child health as a phase of public health in general did not begin until organized prenatal nursing services and prenatal medical clinics were developed in the first decade of this century, following the more widespread recognition of the tremendous value of prenatal care. The greatest advance in maternal care in the early twentieth century was the recognition of the importance of careful nursing and medical attention throughout the prenatal period. The development of prenatal clinics resulted in a decrease in mortality and morbidity from toxemias of pregnancy and cardiac, renal, metabolic, venereal, and associated complications. Consideration of adequate vitamin, mineral, and caloric content in the diets of pregnant women not only decreased the morbidity but also enhanced the health of all the mothers and children who received competent maternity care.

Effective federal investigation of the special problems of child health dates from the creation of the Children's Bureau in 1912. Investigations of the Children's Bureau fell into three main groups: (1) maternal and infant welfare (including the health and education of the preschool child); (2) the care of special groups of children handicapped by physical or mental problems or through delinquency, dependency, or neglect; and (3) problems relating to the child in industry. Field studies to determine the causes of the existing high rate of infant mortality were carried out in industrial and rural communities, and these investigations, particularly in rural areas, gave special attention to the care provided mothers during pregnancy and at childbirth.

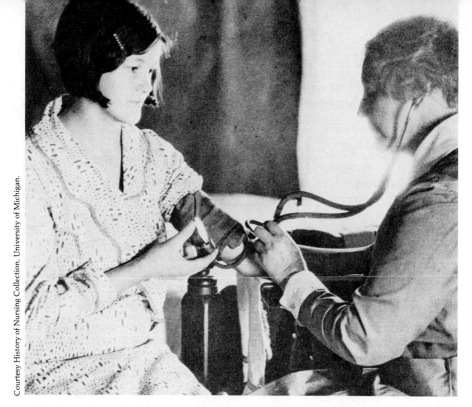

Prenatal visits by the public health nurse were found to be instrumental in promoting the lives of both mothers and infants.

Under the direction of Julia C. Lathrop, the first chief of the Bureau, and Grace Abbott, her successor, nearly 200 studies were carried out during the following 15 years and the results were presented in 195 special bulletins. Besides conducting research in the field, the Bureau compiled, analyzed, and tabulated laws relating to child labor, juvenile courts, illegitimacy, sex offenses against children, mothers' pensions, and interstate placement and adoption of children, and actively cooperated with child welfare and children's code commissions in the revision of state laws.

Early field studies and analyses of statistics indicated that preservation of the lives of both mothers and babies depended upon an expansion of available prenatal care as well as upon improvement in care at the time of delivery. Surveys showed that many births were attended by untrained, unskilled, and none-too-clean midwives. Many other mothers had no trained attendants at childbirth and did not understand the desirability of placing themselves in the hands of a physician or trained nurse for health supervision during pregnancy.

The failure to obtain competent prenatal care was reflected in the number of maternal deaths and also in the neonatal death rate, which peaked during the first month of life, largely due to prenatal conditions or events during delivery. The second most important cause of infant mortality was the gastrointestinal diseases, caused primarily by contaminated milk and water supplies, unhygienic surroundings, and improper feeding methods. Corrective measures included improving milk and water supplies and encouraging breast-feeding, a safer source of milk.

The Sheppard-Towner Act

Increasingly, a massive federal aid program was discussed as an approach to infant and maternal mortality problems. On April 21, 1921, Senator Morris Sheppard of Texas introduced a bill (S. 1039) for the public protection of maternity and infancy and providing a method of cooperation between the Government of the United States and various states. At a hearing before the Senate Committee on Education and Labor, Elizabeth G. Fox, the National Director of the Red Cross Public Health Nursing Service and Vice-President of the National Organization for Public Health Nursing, spoke effectively for the bill:

> I am speaking from a knowledge of public health nursing gained from eight year's experience as a public health nurse and from three years' experience as executive officer in charge of 1,300 public health nurses. As much of the field work provided in the Sheppard-Towner bill will be performed by public health nurses, it is fair to suppose that it will be done according to the high standards and in the thorough manner now prevailing among public health nurses, some of whom are engaged in just the kind of work which is anticipated in this bill. There are now something like 10,000 public health nurses at work in the United States.
>
> It has been said by some of the opponents of this bill that maternal instinct and general intelligence are sufficient to guide a mother safely through pregnancy and in the care of her babies. Those who are familiar with the modern science of medicine and hygiene realize the fallacy of such an argument . . . . The point has also been made by our opponents that agencies would be allowed by this bill to enter private homes. I should like again to describe the practice prevailing among public health nurses. Their work lies entirely in the homes. Sometimes they are called to these homes by members of the family, sometimes by relatives and friends, sometimes by doctors or social workers, and sometimes by other agencies.
>
> When making a first call upon a family, they always explain who they are and why they have come. The family is at liberty to refuse them admittance if it chooses. It has been said that this bill will send large numbers of untrained individuals into private homes. Public health nurses cannot be called untrained individuals. They are not looked upon as nuisances by the people of this country. On the contrary, they are so sought after that they cannot begin to accomplish all the work which they are called upon to do [14].

The bill's proponents pointed to the high infant and maternal death rates in America, especially in rural areas, as compared with other countries. They showed that the latest medical advances were not being extensively used and argued that federal grants would greatly encourage improved care. Senator William S. Kenyon led the fight for the bill, stating: "There are about 250,000 infants who die every year in this country during their first year of life, and approximately 20,000 mothers. The comparison of the infant mortality and maternal mortality of the United States with that of other countries is not pleasing to an American citizen" [15].

Senator Sheppard also spoke strongly in favor of the bill. He noted that it had wide bipartisan support and had been endorsed in 1920 by both presidential candidates. He concluded: "If this Nation declines to take the necessary steps to end the appalling waste of the lives of mothers and children in America, a destruction exceeding every year our total casualties in the most stupendous and terrible war of history, it will invite severest censure" [16].

Opposition to the bill was led by Senator James A. Reed of Missouri. In discussing the leaders of the Children's Bureau who would be administering the program, Reed attacked the "absurdity of putting in charge of a question of maternity and child rearing a band of women who have never had any experience and who have chosen to remain in a condition of single blessedness," since it seemed to him "that they are the last people in the world to whom a position of that kind ought to be consigned." Senator William Borah also opposed the bill because, whatever its merits, he thought it "one of those measures which under the present economic conditions in this country can wait" [17].

After some minor amendments were adopted on the Senate floor, S. 1039 was finally passed by a vote of 63 to 7. Upon passage of this bill, opposing Senator Reed suggested an amendment of the title of the bill to read: "A bill to authorize a board of spinsters to control maternity and teach the mothers of the United States how to rear babies" [18]. The Reed amendment was rejected. The bill was passed by the House of Representatives with only a few amendments. On November 21 the Senate concurred with the House version of the bill, and on November 23, 1921, President Harding signed it into law.

A separate division of the Children's Bureau was organized to administer the Sheppard-Towner Act. Three physicians, two nurses, an auditor, and a few clerks made up the staff of the Division of Maternity and Infancy at its headquarters in Washington. The Board of Maternity and Infancy met three or four times a year to act upon the plans submitted by the states. There were no standards for state guidance, and the states were simply required to use federal and matched funds "in promoting the welfare and hygiene of maternity and infancy" [19]. Usually physicians were in charge of the state programs, but in nine states the work was directed by nurses.

Work of the Sheppard-Towner Nurses

Attempts were made to demonstrate the value of maternity and infancy care to local communities by sending a nurse to a community for a specified period to initiate a maternity and infancy program. It was more common for states to provide funds to communities to employ additional public health nurses as part of a general public health nursing program, which included maternity and infancy work. Under this plan the share of the expense paid by maternity and infancy funds was prorated according to the time given to this phase of the program.

Home visits formed an important part of the work of the child hygiene nurses.

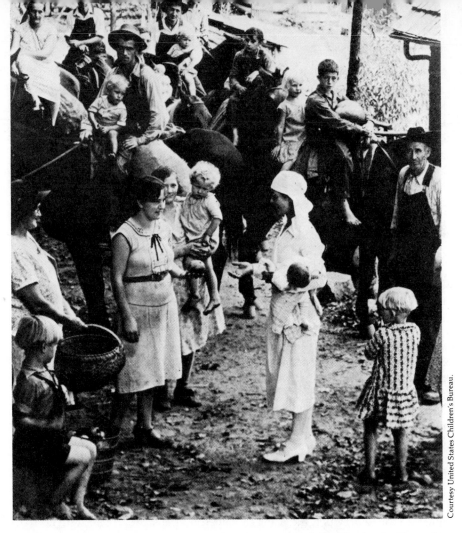

Giving maternal and infant care instruction to a group of families in the Kentucky mountains.

These informal visits provided mothers with excellent opportunities to ask questions and discuss their problems. The nurses used this time to assess the child for possible physical defects and to suggest that the family physician be consulted if problems were evident. The need for medical attention during pregnancy was constantly stressed. Surprisingly large numbers of women had no concept of the value of a physician's care during this critical period and had to be taught that proper prenatal supervision lessened the possibility of complications during pregnancy and promoted the health of mother and child.

One of the problems experienced by the nursing supervisors was difficulty in recruiting trained and experienced nurses for county assignments in maternity and infancy. State directors endeavored to deal with this roadblock in various ways. One method was to teach nurses who had been out of school for some years about the newer methods of maternity and child care, particularly in the areas of nutrition, infant feeding, and the routine to be followed in prenatal care. The directors also drew upon the experiences of nurses who had organized successful clubs, classes, and consultation centers for mothers. Statewide meetings and institutes for maternity and infancy nurses were held in conjunction with state nursing association meetings. Regional and group conferences on local problems were arranged, and newsletters, lending libraries, and other devices were used to maintain the professional standard of rural maternity nursing. Members of the state staffs also gave lectures on maternity and infancy care at training schools and public health nursing classes.

Alleviating the Threat of Incompetent Midwives

Another serious problem that existed in several sections of the country was the supervision and training of lay midwives. An astonishingly large percentage of births were attended by midwives. They were employed extensively throughout the United States, especially by mothers of foreign birth and by those living in isolated communities. It was estimated that in Iowa fewer than 1 percent of births were attended by midwives, while in Louisiana and Mississippi approximately 50 percent were attended by midwives. In the nation as a whole, midwives attended about 30 percent of all deliveries.

The extensive employment of midwives was due in part to objections by the prospective mother or her husband to having a male physician at delivery and also to the family's inability to pay the obstetrician's or general practitioner's fees. "Twenty-five dollars for confinement, if without complications, will be about the average country physician's minimum charge," wrote Samuel Hopkins Adams. "Reasonable though this is, it is still a heavy tax upon a struggling family. A local woman with some little reputation as a 'helper' will come in, more out of kindness than with an expectation of reward, and be quite satisfied

A child health demonstration.

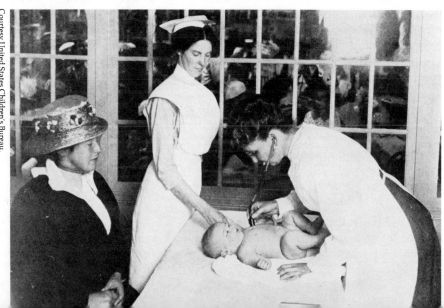

Courtesy United States Children's Bureau.

with a 'present' of two or three or perhaps five dollars" [20].

A study made by Anna E. Rude of the Children's Bureau indicated that in 31 states in 1923 there were 26,627 midwives authorized to practice, and in those and other states over 17,000 were practicing without authorization. These women were for the most part ignorant, often having no knowledge of hygiene. It was useless to prohibit them from practicing. Any woman had the right to call in a neighbor to help her during confinement, and that neighbor became a midwife. Many were illiterate and superstitious and thus were not receptive to training; yet it was imperative to teach them the importance of cleanliness, if nothing else. Thus classes for midwives were held regularly in at least 19 states with the support of Sheppard-Towner funds.

Impact of the Sheppard-Towner Act

Before the introduction of the Shepphard-Towner bill, 12 states had established child hygiene divisions or bureaus. At the expiration of the act in 1929, 45 states and Hawaii had child health agencies. These states reported that, for the period from 1924 to 1929, 144,777 health conferences for expectant mothers and children had been held by nurses and physicians, and 2978 permanent prenatal and child health centers had been established. During the last six years of the Act, public health nurses had made more than three million home visits to mothers and babies, and during the last five years of the Act a total of 19,723 classes for high school girls, mothers, and midwives had been conducted. More than 22 million pieces of literature on infant and maternal care had been distributed, and approximately 700,000 expectant mothers and four million infants and preschool children were reported to have been reached in one way or another.

The effect of the Sheppard-Towner Act and other measures was well documented in the decline in the infant death rate. In 1928 it had fallen from the 1915 rate of 100 for each 1000 births to 69 per 1000 births. The greatest decrease was in the death rate from gastrointestinal disease—a direct result of informing the public about proper methods of infant care and feeding.

Strong efforts were made to renew the Sheppard-Towner Act after Congress allowed it to lapse in 1929, but these were unsuccessful in the face of the reigning political conservatism. The American Medical Association opposed its continuation in the sweeping terms of a resolution of its House of Delegates: "Resolved that the House of Delegates condemns as unsound in policy, wasteful and extravagant, unproductive of results and tending to promote communism, the federal subsidy system established by the Sheppard-Towner Maternity and Infancy Act and protests against a renewal of that system in any form" [21]. Public health nurses supported a renewal and watched the course of debate with deep interest and anxiety, but their concern was of no avail.

Margaret Sanger: Nurse Activist

The attack on maternal and infant mortality was given additional support by the birth control movement. In the United States the birth rate per 1000 women

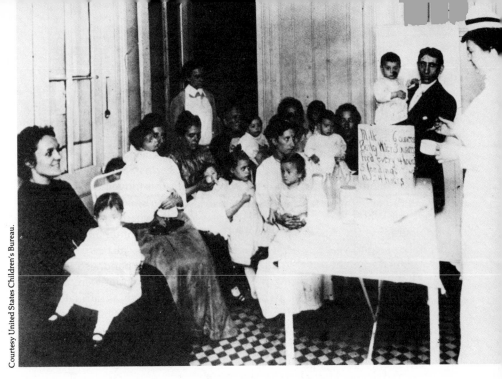

Instruction in the preparation of milk for infants and children.

A group of high school students receiving instruction in infant care.

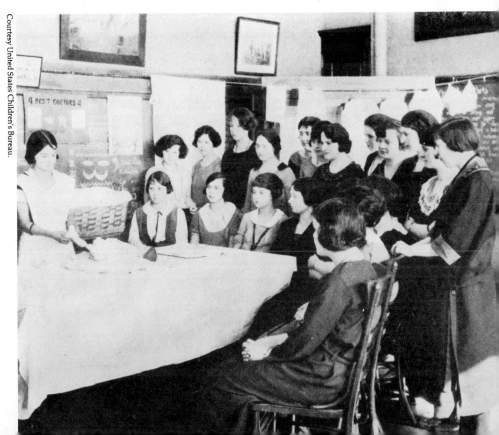

15 to 44 years of age declined precipitously, from 127 in 1910 to 89 in 1930, a decline of 38 percent in a single generation. Despite the unfavorable legal situation for birth control advocates, many Americans considered the declining birth rate a healthy development, asserting that a prime cause of poverty would be removed if birth control were practiced by the poor as well as by the well-to-do. Braving legal opposition, Margaret Higgins Sanger, a determined public health nurse in New York City, spearheaded this movement.

Born on September 14, 1883, in Corning, New York, Margaret Higgins attended the White Plains Hospital, a 25-bed facility where, according to her autobiography, the experience was rigid and sometimes inhumane. She recalls that in her second year she herself underwent surgery and just two weeks later was assigned to night duty. With her right shoulder still bandaged, she could use only her left hand in caring for the patients, all of whom were in serious condition. Margaret received part of her training through an affiliation with the Manhattan Eye and Ear Hospital, where she met William Sanger, an architect and aspiring artist, whom she later married. For the first few years of their married life the Sangers lived in prosperous Westchester County, and her husband commuted to the city to work. During these years she gave birth to three children and devoted herself to homemaking.

Shortly thereafter Margaret began to develop an empathy for the millions of Americans who were living a hand-to-mouth existence. Particularly, she was drawn to the plight of industrial workers, such as those in Lawrence, Massachusetts, where, according to a 1912 United States Labor Commissioner's report, the median family income, with both parents working, was approximately $12 to $14 per week. When only the father worked the median family income was barely $8. In "high-income" families the children always worked.

Doffer girl in New England textile mill, 1912.

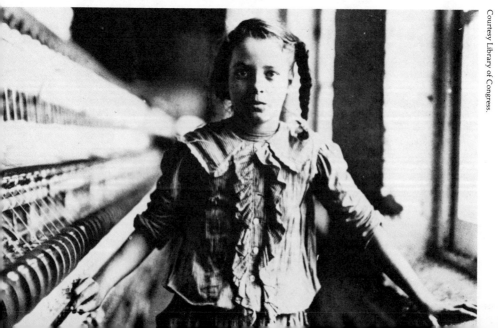

Thus, it was not surprising that a labor strike during January and February of 1912 took 30,000 Lawrence workers away from their jobs in the cotton and woolen mills. Bound to affect the entire textile industry of the United States, the strike was seen as a clash between the radical forces of labor and the reactionary agents of big business. Because the primary reason for the failure of previous walkouts had been the near starvation of the strikers' children, it was decided that the children should be sent to the homes of labor sympathizers in New York until the issue was settled.

Because Margaret's interest in the plight of underpaid workers was well known among militant New York laborers and because she was a trained nurse, she was asked to direct the evacuation of the children from Lawrence. Their condition appalled her:

> We found the boys and girls gathered in a Lawrence public hall, and, before we started, I insisted on physical examinations for contagious diseases. One, though ill with diphtheria, had been working up to the time of the strike. Almost all had adenoids and enlarged tonsils. Each, without exception, was incredibly emaciated.
>
> Our hundred and nineteen charges were of every age, from babies of two or three to older ones of twelve to thirteen. Although the latter had been employed in the textile mills, their garments were simply worn to shreds. Not a child had on any woolen clothing whatsoever, and only four wore overcoats. Never in all my nursing in the slums had I seen children in so ragged and deplorable a condition [22].

By the next week the situation in Lawrence had deteriorated to the point where violence broke out, and some of the parents had been beaten and arrested by the police. In Washington, Representative Victor Berger of Wisconsin was instrumental in securing a congressional investigation of the conditions responsible for the strike. Margaret was called to Washington to testify before the House Committee on Rules on the physical condition of the children:

Rep. Edward E. Pou: Did you talk with those children about their manner of living in Lawrence and about the food they got?

Mrs. Sanger: Yes, sir. I am a trained nurse, and I was especially interested in the condition of the children.

Mr. Pou: Now, as a rule, is it true that the children of the working people in Lawrence— the class we are investigating—now only got meat once a week?

Mrs. Sanger: Those were the assertions of not only the children but of the parents that I interviewed.

Rep. Martin B.: You say you are a trained nurse?

Mrs. Sanger: Yes, sir.

Mr. Foster: And what was the physical appearance of these children that you took to New York? You know something about how they should look; were they properly nourished?

Mrs. Sanger: Well, the condition of those children was the most horrible that I have ever seen.

Mr. Foster: Tell the committee something about how they looked.

Mrs. Sanger: In the first place, there were four little children who had chicken pox that we kept there; we would not allow them to go away; and then one of the children had just gotten over chicken pox, and the father begged us to let the child come; he had one two-year-old and another 3½ years old, I believe, and he begged us to let those children come because he was a widower and had no wife or anyone to take care of these children; he left them with the neighbors during the day. So I took these little children, and we isolated them on the way to New York, and when we got there they were placed under doctor's care. All of these children were walking about there apparently not noticing chicken pox or diphtheria; one child had diphtheria and had been walking around, and no attention paid to it at all, and had been working up to the time of the strike. Out of the 119 children, four of them had underwear on, and it was the most bitter weather, we had to run all the way from the hall to the station in order to keep warm; and only four had underwear.

Rep. Robert L. Henry: Kindly read the letter I now hand you to the committee.

Mrs. Sanger (reading):

New York, February 1, 1912

To whom it may concern:

We, undersigned Italian doctors invited to make a preliminary physical examination of the Lawrence strikers' children, verified that all children were of poor physical build, defective, and underfed. The majority of them had enlarged glands, throat, nose, eyes, defective and affected. All were poorly clad even against the rigor of the season.

(And signed by six physicians.)

Rep. William W. Wilson: Where did those doctors live?

Mrs. Sanger: They were physicians of the Italian Federation of New York City, who volunteered their services to take charge of the children while in New York.

Rep. Irvin W. Lenroot: Have you had an opportunity to become familiar with the condition of the children of other workers in other places?

Mrs. Sanger: Yes, I have.

Mr. Lenroot: Can you give the committee any information as to how the condition of these children compared with that of other children in similar circumstances of life?

Mrs. Sanger: Yes. I have been brought up in a factory town where there are glassblowers and children of glassblowers, and I must say that I have never seen in any place children so ragged and so deplorable as these children were. I have never seen such children in my work in the Italian districts of New York City; in the slum districts, I must say, there are always a few of them who are fat and rugged, but these children were pale and thin [23].

After nearly two months had elapsed and the workers had failed to return, the mills began to offer concessions. The strike committee, seconded by the cheers of an outdoor mass meeting, voted to accept. Within a few days almost everyone was back in the factories, with substantial wage increases all along the line.

After her involvement in labor strife, Margaret, in the spring of 1912, returned to her nursing career, taking work as a public health nurse. She was assigned to care for maternity cases on New York City's crowded Lower East Side, where she found that:

Pregnancy was a chronic condition among the women of this class. Suggestions as to what to do for a girl who was "in trouble" or a married woman who was "caught" passed from mouth to mouth—herb teas, turpentine, steaming, rolling downstairs, inserting slippery elm, knitting needles, shoe hooks. When they had word of a new remedy they hurried to the drugstore, and if the clerk were inclined to be friendly he might say, "Oh,

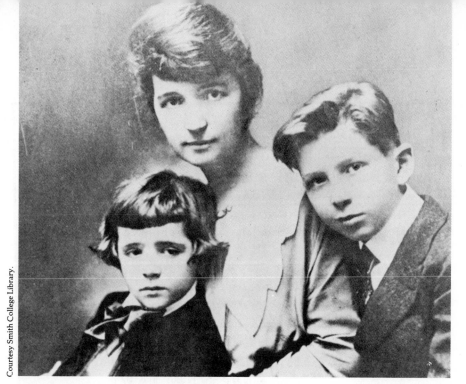

Margaret Sanger pictured with two of her children.

that won't help you, but here's something that may." The younger druggist usually refused to give advice because, if it were to be known, [he] would come under the law;
midwives were even more fearful. The doomed women implored me to reveal the "secret" rich people had, offering to pay me extra to tell them; many really believed I was
holding back information for money. They asked everybody and tried anything, but
nothing did them any good. On Saturday nights I have seen groups of from 50 to 100
with their shawls over their heads waiting outside the office of a five-dollar abortionist
[24].

In mid-1912 Margaret took care of a 28-year-old mother of three who had
attempted to abort herself. After three weeks under Margaret's care the woman
recovered and regained her health. When the physician made his last call, he
admonished: "Any more such capers, young woman, and there'll be no need
to send for me." "I know doctor," the convalescent replied, "but what can I do
to prevent it?" The physician laughed good-naturedly. "You want to have your
cake and eat it too, do you? Well, it can't be done. Tell Jake to sleep on the
roof." She pleaded with Margaret: "Tell me the secret and I'll never breathe it
to a soul, please!" Mrs. Sanger could only remain silent. Three months later,
the husband called Margaret and pleaded with her to come at once. When she
arrived, the wife was in a coma and death followed within minutes. Stunned
and heart-broken, Margaret walked for hours through the New York streets.
In years to come she would cite this experience as a turning point in her life. It
was then that she decided to devote herself to learning about and disseminating
information on contraception [25].

MOTHERS!

Can you afford to have a large family?

Do you want any more children?

If not, why do you have them?

DO NOT KILL, DO NOT TAKE LIFE, BUT PREVENT

Safe, Harmless Information can be obtained of trained

Nurses at

46 AMBOY STREET

NEAR PITKIN AVE. — BROOKLYN.

Tell Your Friends and Neighbors.   All Mothers Welcome

A registration fee of 10 cents entitles any mother to this information.

מומערס!

זײַט איהר פערמעגליך צו האבען א גרויסע פאמיליע?

ווילט איהר האבען נאך קינדער?

אויב ניט, ווארום האט איהר זײ?

מערדערט ניט, נעהמט ניט קײן לעבען, נור פערהיט זיך.

זיכערע, אומשעדליכע אינסקינפמט קענט איהר בעקומען פון ערפארענע נוירסעס אין

46 אמבאי סטריט ניער פיטקין עוועניר ברוקלין

זאגט דאם בעקאנט צו אייערע פריינד און שכנות.   יעדער מוטער איז ווילקאמען

פיר 10 סענט אײנשרײבגעלד דינם איהר בערעכטינט צו ריעזע אינפארמיישאן.

MADRI!

Potete permettervi il lusso d'avere altri bambini?

Ne volete ancora?

Se non ne volete piu', perche' continuate a metterli

al mondo?

NON UCCIDETE MA PREVENITE !

Informazioni sicure ed innocue saranno fornite da infermiere autorizzate a

46 AMBOY STREET   Near Pitkin Ave. Brooklyn

a cominciare dal 12 Ottobre. Avvertite le vostre amiche e vicine.

Tutte le madri sono ben accette. La tassa d'iscrizione di 10 cents da diritto

a qualunque madre di ricevere consigli ed informazioni gratis. 5 5

Multilingual handbill advertising the first birth control clinic in America.

First, she learned everything she could about methods of preventing pregnancy. There was very little such information available to the American public (although contraception was practiced widely in many European countries), largely because the Comstock Act of 1873 had classified contraceptive data with obscene matter and prohibited its passage through the mails. After six months of research at the Boston Public Library, the Library of Congress, and the New York Academy of Medicine, Margaret concluded that there was no practical medical information on contraception available in America. After a visit to France to study methods of birth control, she returned to the United States and published a journal, *The Woman Rebel,* which carried information on contraception and family planning along with a variety of other subjects pertaining to women's rights.

In 1916 Mrs. Sanger opened the first birth control clinic in America, located at 46 Amboy Street in the Brownsville district of Brooklyn, a predominantly Jewish neighborhood. The clinic was operated by Margaret, her sister, Ethel Byrne (also a nurse), and Fania Mindell; and some 150 women sought assistance on the first day alone. For the next week everything went well until a policewoman, disguised as a patient, arrested the sisters and Miss Mindell and took down the names of the angry and frightened clients. In order to publicize the clinic's closure, Margaret refused to ride in the patrol wagon and walked the mile to the courthouse.

When Margaret faced her charges in court several weeks later, the courtroom was filled with friends and supporters, and many reporters were in attendance. It was difficult for the public to believe that the attractive woman seated with her two young sons was either oversexed or mentally ill, as her enemies would have it believed. Margaret did not deny the charge of having distributed birth control information; rather, she challenged the law that forbade such activity. The judge would have been lenient had she agreed to follow the law, but her response was: "I cannot respect the law as it stands today" [26]. She was sentenced to 30 days in the workhouse.

After serving her sentence, Margaret Sanger continued her crusade for many more decades. She allied herself with women of wealth, using those contacts and their financial backing to further her cause. She gave lectures and organized meetings, such as the Birth Control Conference in New York City in 1921. That year she also helped establish the American Birth Control League, serving as its president until 1928, after which she founded the National Committee on Federal Legislation for Birth Control, a forerunner of the Planned Parenthood Federation. Her many books included *What Every Girl Should Know* (1916); *What Every Mother Should Know* (1917); *The Case for Birth Control* (1917); *Women, Morality, and Birth Control* (1922); *Happiness in Marriage* (1926); *Motherhood in Bondage* (1928); and *My Fight for Birth Control* (1931).

The opposition to Margaret Sanger's crusade for the free dissemination of birth control information continued for decades, the most vehement criticism coming from conservatives and various religious groups. Protestant churchmen disagreed on the moral issues involved in birth control. The Committee on

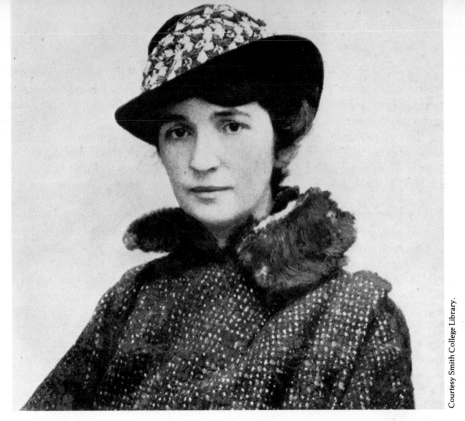

Margaret Sanger.

Marriage and the Home of the Federal Council of Churches recommended in 1930 that the church should not seek to impose its point of view on the use of contraceptives by legislation, or by any other form of force, and should not seek to prohibit physicians from imparting such information to those who in the judgment of the medical profession were entitled to receive birth control information. The General Assembly of the Presbyterian Church, however, criticized this policy statement as morally dangerous. The Roman Catholic Church was uncompromising in its condemnation both of divorce and of birth control. The papal encyclical *Casti Conubii*, issued by Pope Pius XI in 1930, asserted that contraceptive devices were "an offense against the law of God and nature" [27]. But despite strong opposition by many religious denominations, the effort to inform the public about ways of limiting families met a very real social need and flourished. And, along with this crusade, the period from 1912 to 1930 saw a great surge in the number of public health nursing agencies in the United States, and this specialty quickly took its place as one of the most socially relevant occupations for graduate nurses.

Summary

Prior to World War I it was estimated that only 10 percent of the sick received hospital care. Of the remainder, most could not afford to employ graduate private duty nurses. In an effort to help deal with this enormous unmet need, the number of public health nurses had expanded from 136 in 1901 to over 11,000 in 1924.

By 1920 the Metropolitan Life Insurance Company's program of visiting nurses had gained national attention. Company and national statistics showed that the visiting nursing program was responsible for a part of the decline in mortality and for the overall improvement in the general health of policyholders.

The proper mix of health instruction and bedside care in public health nursing was a controversial issue. During the 1920s the primary focus of the public health nurse generally moved away from direct bedside care toward health education, investigation of conditions in homes and public facilities, and preventive work.

A reluctance to utilize physician and hospital care was still common, particularly among immigrants. Frequently there was more trust placed in the neighborhood druggist than in physicians or hospitals.

The use of dangerous or ineffectual patent medicines, including opiates, was still widespread. By using extensive advertising, many charlatans capitalized on public ignorance and superstition.

A series of health demonstrations, largely financed by private foundations, documented the value of intensive health assessment and health education in a given community.

In 1925 the Frontier Nursing Service was organized by Mary Breckinridge to promote the health of a remote rural area through generalized nursing service and a decentralized organization. Nurses in the Kentucky program were required to have training in midwifery, and their service was overwhelmingly successful, as evidenced by a study that showed they were effective in reducing the number of maternal and infant deaths.

A trachoma eradication project, carried out by nurses in the United States Public Health Service, helped to combat widespread blindness in the primitive mountain districts of Appalachia and in the Ozark Mountains region.

Over opposition by conservative forces, including the AMA, the Sheppard-Towner Act was passed in 1921. This program provided funds to 45 cooperating states to develop activities directed at improving maternal and infant welfare. Employing hundreds of nurses, the program emphasized home visits, health education, and health screening of mothers and infants.

Margaret Sanger, a nurse activist, spearheaded the birth control movement and opened the first birth control clinic in the United States. First sensitized to the overwhelming need for family planning as a labor sympathizer and as a public health nurse on New York's Lower East Side, Mrs. Sanger devoted her life to the problem of informing the public about contraceptive methods.

References

1. A. M. Brainard, *The Evolution of Public Health Nursing* (Philadelphia: W. B. Saunders Company, 1922), pp. 429–432.
2. Letters in Nutting Papers, Nursing Archives, Teachers College, Columbia University.
3. Louis Dublin, *The Effect of Life Conservation on the Mortality of the Metropolitan Life Insurance Company* (New York: The Company, 1917), pp. 1–11.
4. Josephine Goldmark, *Nursing and Nursing Education in the United States* (New York: Macmillan Co., 1923), p. 9.
5. New York State Charities Aid Association, *Sickness in Dutchess County, New York, Its Extent, Care, and Prevention* (New York: The Association, 1915), pp. 87–98.
6. New York Academy of Medicine, Public Health Committee, "Problems of Disease," *Modern Medicine*, vol. 2 (March, 1920): 1–23.
7. Edgar Sydenstricker, "Extent of Medical and Hospital Service in a Typical Small City," *Public Health Reports*, vol. 42 (January 14, 1928): 121–131.
8. Samuel Hopkins Adams, *The Great American Fraud* (Chicago: American Medical Association, 1907), p. 70.
9. Clare Terwilliger, unpublished report, Records of the Children's Bureau, National Archives, Washington, D.C., RG 102.
10. Michael M. Davis, *Immigrant Health and the Community* (New York: Harper and Brothers, 1921), pp. 308–309.
11. *Ibid.*, pp. 309–310.
12. Louis I. Dublin, *The First One Thousand Midwifery Cases of the Frontier Nursing Service* (New York: Metropolitan Life Insurance Company, 1932), pp. 1–2.
13. Weekly Report of Blanche Pegg Allen in Records of the United States Public Health Service, National Archives, Washington, D.C.
14. U.S. Congress, Senate, Committee on Education and Labor, *Protection of Maternity. Hearings held April 21, 1921* (Washington, D.C.: Government Printing Office, 1921), pp. 148–149.
15. *Congressional Record*, June 28, 1921.
16. *Ibid.*
17. *Ibid.*, June 30, 1921.
18. *Ibid.*, July 22, 1921.
19. U.S. Department of Labor, Children's Bureau, *Annual Report of Administration of the Maternity and Infancy Act* (Washington, D.C.: Government Printing Office, 1923), p. 23.
20. Samuel Hopkins Adams, "The Vanishing Country Doctor," *Ladies' Home Journal*, vol. 40 (October, 1923): 23.
21. American Medical Association, *Proceedings of the Eighty-first Annual Session of the House of Delegates, June, 1930* (Chicago: The Association, 1930), pp. 35–41.
22. Margaret Sanger, *Margaret Sanger: An Autobiography* (New York: Norton, 1938), p. 81.
23. U.S. Congress, House, Committee on Rules, *The Strike at Lawrence Massachusetts. Hearings before the Committee, March 2–7, 1912* (Washington, D.C.: Government Printing Office, 1912), pp. 226–229.
24. Margaret Sanger, *op. cit.*, pp. 88–89.
25. *Ibid.*, p. 92.
26. *Ibid.*, pp. 93–96.
27. *Ibid.*, p. 237.

13
Depression Doldrums, 1930–1939

Unemployment, increasing rapidly and continuously after the stock market crash of October, 1929, created a major relief problem in the United States. In January, 1930, almost four million people were unemployed. The number rose to about seven million by December of that year, and this figure was doubled by early 1933. It was difficult to exaggerate the utter collapse of national economic life that had occurred before Franklin D. Roosevelt took the oath of office on March 4, 1933. Business had sunk to 60 percent below the normal level. Exports were close to the lowest point in 30 years. Over 1400 banks had failed during 1932, and in the two weeks preceding Roosevelt's inauguration, at least 21 states and the District of Columbia had either declared a banking moratorium or were allowing their banks to operate under special regulations. To a nation waiting with tense expectancy, Roosevelt urged confidence and courage. "The only thing we have to fear," he asserted, "is fear itself." He promised a special session of Congress to deal with the emergency and declared that "our greatest primary task is to put people to work" [1].

Unemployed Nurses
Nurses were a part of the massive unemployment: an estimated 8000 to 10,000 graduates were out of work. Announcements such as the following became commonplace in the *American Journal of Nursing* [2,3]:

Nurses who are contemplating coming to Binghamton, New York, to work, are advised not to do so as there is not enough work for nurses already here.
Secretary, Alumnae Association
Binghamton Training School

District 1 (Birmingham) of the Alabama State Nurses' Association does not wish to be inhospitable but advises nurses planning to come here to do private duty, that unemployment is a serious problem in that branch of nursing here, many local nurses not making enough to live.
Catherine A. Moultis

Will you please publish a warning to nurses contemplating coming to Colorado Springs, Colorado? We do not wish to appear inhospitable, but it might save much time and money to know there is not enough work for nurses who are already here.
M. A. P.

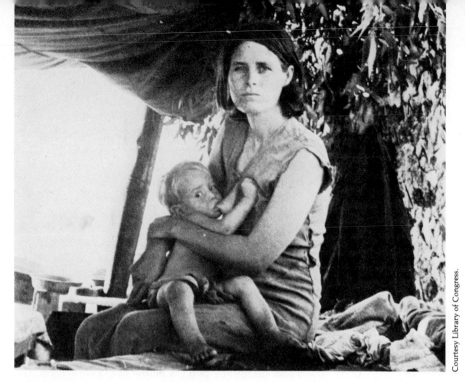

Migrant mother and child during the Great Depression.

To nurses contemplating coming to Miami we wish to present the following facts: There are several hundred nurses out of employment in Miami at the present time. There is less work here now than there has been at any time during the past eleven years. Florida has passed a state law that all nurses practicing their profession in this state pay a tax of $15, this being county and state tax. This, added to the state registration fee, makes a total of $25 that has to be put out in order to nurse in the State of Florida.

Arrie Allen Lambert, Registrar

In 1932 a campaign to promote the hiring of graduate nurses and discontinue training schools, along with provision for an eight-hour day for nurses, was launched by the American Nurses' Association. This move met with considerable resistance. J. A. Diekmann, Superintendent of the Bethesda Hospital in Cincinnati, reported:

There are today 68 Bethesda graduates in this city, victims of unemployment. To remedy this movement the national and state nurse organizations are forcing an issue that looks toward eliminating nurse schools from a large percentage of hospitals, and to employing only graduates for all hospital nursing work.

But what would that mean in point of expense? We have made a careful study of what it would mean to Bethesda. The maintenance of our 112 students costs us $95,036 a year, or $848.53 a student. To do our nursing work through graduate nurses would cost us $132,107, or $37,071 more than student nursing. If we are compelled to give up our nurse school, where would we get that additional $37,071? Hospital rates cannot be raised. There is universal complaint of their being exorbitant now. Will the friends of the hospitals defray that additional large expense by more liberal contributions? The above movement would solve the nurse problem only to create an additional finance problem for the hospitals, most of whom now are in financial desperation [4].

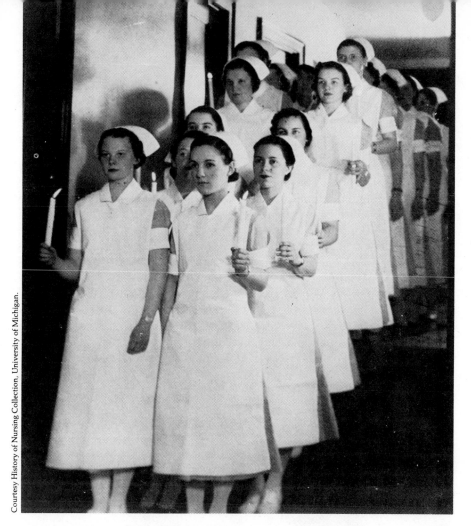

Courtesy History of Nursing Collection, University of Michigan.

Despite an ever-increasing outpouring of unemployed graduates, hospitals still strongly preferred student labor on their wards. Capping ceremony, mid-1930s.

Nurses Working for Room and Board

The suggestion that unemployed graduate nurses be hired by hospitals as graduate floor-duty nurses met with two general arguments. First, graduate floor duty as then organized was not considered respectable by many nurses; second, in the better hospitals, to which graduates would naturally be attracted, there were virtually no positions available. Fifty-nine percent of the beds for sick patients were in hospitals that conducted training schools. The hospitals without schools were heavily staffed by so-called "attendants." Of the hospitals with schools, 73 percent did not have a single graduate nurse on floor duty, and only 15 percent employed four or more.

The few graduates who were employed on floor duty in these hospitals were often looked down upon by students. There was a general feeling among students that graduates on floor duty were unsuccessful private duty nurses who were working in hospitals as a last resort. Floor duty was considered student work, and in some schools floor duty or bedside nursing was not only student work but junior student work, as the seniors who acted as head nurses felt that their function was not bedside nursing but the administration of the ward. Nurses who wanted to do bedside nursing after graduation found little encouragement. Few positions were open to them where they could render quality bedside care and at the same time retain professional standing and dignity.

But amid dismal economic conditions, as 6000 to 8000 nurses found themselves unemployed, dignity became a luxury. Indeed, the question of the month for January, 1933, in *Modern Hospital* was: "Should or should not graduate nurses be allowed to work for their board, room, and laundry?" Many penniless graduate nurses had applied to hospitals for work and were willing to accept room and board for their services. Should hospitals take them in? The nurses were not replacing other graduates but were probably replacing nursing students.

This query was sent to seven eminent hospital administrators, representing various types of hospitals in different sections of the United States. The replies of these authorities were diverse. Dr. Donald C. Smelzer, Director of the Grad-

The question of the month for January, 1933, was: "Should or should not graduate nurses be allowed to work for their board, room, and laundry?"

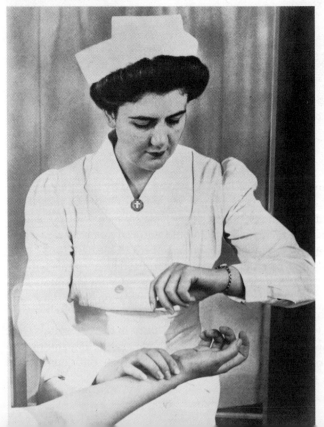

Courtesy History of Nursing Collection, University of Michigan.

uate Hospital of the University of Pennsylvania, thought that this question should be settled primarily by the nurse and secondarily by the hospital. He thought that if the nurse voluntarily applied for work under such conditions, the hospital was justified in accepting her services. In return the hospital should give her the type of work that would be of material benefit to her career. She should be placed on duty in a specific department (such as the operating room or the eye, ear, nose, and throat, medical, or bronchoscopic department) and thus have every opportunity to "brush up." Meanwhile the hospital administration should not reduce either graduate or student nurse staffs to compensate for this additional service.

Dr. Smelzer thought that the hospital should not exploit the misfortune of the graduate nurse. The fact that the nurse was permitted to work in the hospital for her room and board should be looked upon by all concerned as a generous act on the part of the hospital, in that the nurse would be receiving what amounted to postgraduate training. In his view, the room and board would be equivalent to the value of service rendered to the hospital.

Dr. Maurice H. Rees, Director of the Colorado General Hospital in Denver, answered that his hospital did not favor giving board, room, and laundry to unemployed nurses in return for limited amounts of service. His objections were, first, that nurses working only for board, room, and laundry as a rule gave inferior service and often were not even worth their food and lodging, and second, that he was sure no hospital budget could bear the expense of the additional board and laundry that these extra graduate nurses were sure to cause.

Grace Crafts, Superintendent of Madison (Wisconsin) General Hospital, was of the opinion that the period of unemployment was a difficult time for the nursing profession as a whole and for the private duty nurse especially. Economic conditions called for close cooperation between the graduate nurse and the hospital. She felt strongly that hospitals should be helpful and sympathetic and should not take advantage of the unemployed nurse. To accept from her a full day's work in exchange for room, board, and laundry was in her opinion taking most unfair advantage of the graduate nurse's helpless situation.

Nurses Take to the Sky

As the Depression deepened, a new field opened up for a limited number of nurses as airplane travel became common. Back in 1926 there had been about 50 so-called airlines in existence within the United States, but the onset of the Depression had forced widespread consolidation. United Airlines was together by Boeing Aircraft through an amalgamation of smaller carriers. Other corporations molded competitors: American Airlines by Avco, TWA by Curtiss Wright, and Eastern by General Motors. Delta was the outgrowth of a Georgia crop-dusting company. By the early 1930s the airline passenger market was not increasing to any noticeable degree, because of the number of airplane crashes and the attendant publicity. The president of one airline admitted that

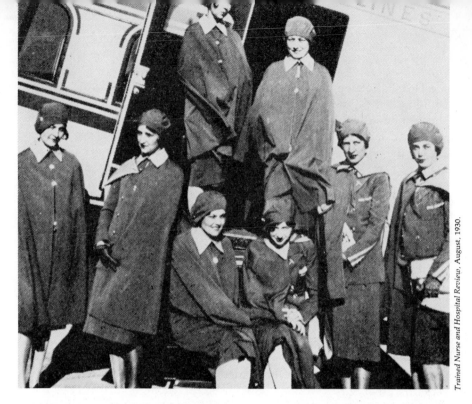

Trained Nurse and Hospital Review, August, 1930.

The tens of thousands of stewardesses who fly present-day world airlines owe their careers to the pioneer work of these original RNs, hired by United Airlines in May, 1930. Shown here are (from left) Margaret Arnott, Jessie Carter, Cornelia Peterman (seated left), Harriet Fly (seated right), Ellen Church, Alva Johnson, Inez Keller, and Ella Crawford.

he never flew in his company's planes whenever he could possibly avoid it and further revealed that his wife refused to fly at all. What is more, the Department of Commerce reported that in 1930 the airlines, on the average, were only filling 5 of 12 available seats per aircraft. The larger carriers realized that in order to survive they must improve their image and counter the widespread fear of flying.

The determination of air transport companies to make their mode of travel appear to be as safe and healthy as possible by having a trained health provider on hand for all emergencies created a new role for the nurse. There were few other lines of work open to the nurse that offered such thrilling experiences as the post of nurse-stewardess on one of the early passenger planes of the major air transport lines. Beginning in mid-1930, the major airlines would employ only graduate nurses of proven ability and although the field was a very new one and positions were relatively few, the work had a strong appeal. This was evidenced by the fact that in the first few months of 1931 there were over 5000 applications from nurses for positions on the transcontinental passenger planes of United Air Lines alone.

The title "stewardess" was used even though it was considered inadequate. "Nurse" was a term too suggestive of the occurrence of illness en route, a contingency that arose much less frequently than was generally supposed. The uniform of the 1930s nurse-stewardess was considered as attractive as that of the Army nurse, which it resembled slightly. It consisted of a dark green wool coat, skirt, and cape, and a beret-like cap. The cape was lined with gray, and gray hose were worn with black oxford shoes. White blouses in summer and white or gray shirts with a tie in winter completed the uniform. On every run the stewardess carried two gray smocks for use on board, designed to cover most of her body and protect her from cabin drafts. There was also a leather coat for cold-weather use.

The transcontinental planes of the early 1930s carried 14 passengers and a crew of three—pilot, co-pilot, and stewardess. With an average speed of 155 miles per hour, the passenger planes never flew in bad weather, and it took two days of good flying conditions to go coast to coast. The cabin looked a little like a small Pullman chair car, but everything was of the lightest material possible. The wicker chairs adjusted to comfortable couches for night runs,

By 1932 graduate nurse Katherine Maye of Virden, Illinois, had traveled more than 250,000 miles as a United Airlines stewardess.

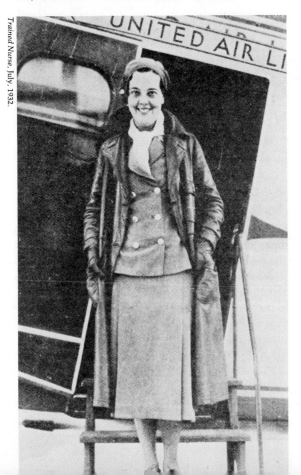

Trained Nurse, July, 1932.

and each had its window with an arrangement for regulating the amount of air admitted, together with a coatrack and an individual electric light. The heating system was run off the engines.

The nurse stewardess was responsible for the passengers' pillows and blankets, pillow slips, seatback covers, towels, napkins, trays, and vacuum bottles, and, most important, the first-aid kit. She also had supplies of stationery and airmail stamps, recent magazines, and in-flight literature issued by the company.

Early passenger planes did not have pressurized cabins, and when the planes climbed over 12,000 feet, many passengers experienced nausea. Airsickness could, in most cases, be prevented by systematic alkalinization before starting on a trip, and when it occurred, the use of an alkaline effervescent was often sufficient to overcome it. If there were signs of faintness, the patient might be entirely relieved by inhalation from a crushed ammonia ampule. The nurse stewardess also carried amobarbital, which helped to induce sleep in nauseated passengers and was also useful in caring for extremely nervous travelers. Individuals who were afraid of high altitudes were assured that fatalities among passengers from that cause were absolutely unknown.

In order to allay the passengers' fears of air travel the nurse stewardess thoroughly informed them about the precautions taken to prevent crashes. She regularly pointed out to the passengers the beacon lights and emergency landing fields that were situated 20 to 30 miles apart along the transcontinental route, explaining that a pilot was never more than a few minutes from a place where he could bring the plane down in case of emergency. The nurse stewardess was instructed to always remain calm and composed, no matter how grave the crisis.

Many pilots looked upon the young women as rank intruders. The hardworking newcomers won their respect before long, however, and came to be regarded as valuable members of the crew. The common belief was that stewardess service was merely a fad, but it soon became evident that this was not true as more and more nurses were employed.

Committee on the Costs of Medical Care

Meanwhile, attempts at health care reform were being pushed. The question of payment was only one of the many complex problems of medical care addressed in 1927 by the Committee on the Costs of Medical Care, a group of representative physicians, public health officers, social scientists, and laymen representing the public. With the financial support of eight foundations, the Committee undertook a five-year study to determine how to provide "adequate, scientific medical care to all the people, rich and poor, at a cost which could be reasonably met by them in their respective stations in life" [5]. Dr. Ray Lyman Wilbur, president of Stanford University and former president of the American Medical Association, was chairman of this distinguished Committee, which included 24 physicians, three dentists, and two nurses.

The Committee revealed the results of its extensive studies in December,

1932. The nation's annual medical bill was found to be approximately $3.5 billion, 30 percent of this amount going to physicians, 24 percent to hospitals, 12 percent to dentists, 19 percent for medicines, 5 percent for private duty nurses, 3 percent for public health work, and 7 percent for all other purposes. For the whole population, payments by private individuals for medical care were found to average $24 a person, or about $108 per family.

A special study of 9000 families over a 12-month period showed that while the need for medical care was approximately the same regardless of economic status, only one-seventh of the well-to-do went without medical attention during the year, whereas the proportion was one-fourth among the middle class and one-half among the poor. Neither rich nor poor were receiving the care they needed. On the other hand, the Committee found that the incomes of medical practitioners—physicians, dentists, and nurses—were not excessive and in many cases were even inadequate. Unrestricted specialization, uncoordinated establishment of facilities, and uneconomical distribution of personnel were declared responsible for extensive waste.

The chief difficulty appeared to be that the individual family could not budget medical costs because of the unpredictability of sickness. To meet this difficulty the Committee pointed to a variety of experiments in organized medical service that had been developing in recent years under the sponsorship of hospitals and public health, industrial, or medical agencies. These included low-rate hospital services, pay clinics, public health nursing, organized service by trained nurse midwives, government hospitals, tax-supported physicians in rural areas, state aid for local medical service, and university medical services. Several plans had been put into operation under commercial sponsorship, such as installment payment for medical care through loan companies and medical benefit corporations operating for profit—practices strongly disapproved by the professional groups in general. These businesses sold insurance services provided through contracts with individual practitioners and hospitals.

The Committee's five basic recommendations were condensed as follows:

That medical care be furnished largely by organized groups of physicians, dentists, nurses, pharmacists, and other associated personnel, centered around a hospital, and rendering home, office, and hospital care.

That all the basic public health services be extended until they are available to the entire population, according to its needs.

That the cost of medical care be placed on a group payment basis through the use of insurance, taxation, or both methods, without precluding the continuation of the individual fee basis for those who prefer it.

That a specific organization be formed in every community or state for the "study, evaluation, and coordination of medical services."

That the professional education of physicians, dentists, pharmacists, and nurses be reoriented to accord more closely with present needs, and that educational facilities be provided to train three new types of workers in the fields of health; namely, nursing attendants, nurse-midwives, and trained hospital and clinical administrators [6].

Attack by the American Medical Association

Few physicians were impressed by these findings. R. G. Leland, M.D., Director of the Bureau of Medical Economics of the American Medical Association, spearheaded the AMA's attack on the group-hospitalization idea. He charged that, to a large extent, such schemes were being suggested as a result of "tactics of desperation" in which hard-pressed hospitals sought "any port in a storm." He warned that all such plans tended to lessen the control of county medical societies over medical practice and thus to decrease the effectiveness of the most important form of professional control of standards and ethics, while at the same time they increased the influence of lay commercial interests.

According to Dr. Leland, group hospital insurance plans tended also to extend hospital care beyond its proper scope: patients who would ordinarily be cared for at home by a family physician would more often insist on going to the hospital, where they felt they had already paid for care. The broad effect of all such plans would be to shift the burden of hospital support from philanthropy and goodwill to taxation of low-paid workers. Dr. Leland asked: "Does the public need at the present time an increased amount of hospital care, or will it benefit more from a greater amount of medical care in the home?" [7].

In December, 1932, the editor of the *Journal of the American Medical Association*, Dr. Morris Fishbein, wrote an emotional denunciation of the report of the Committee on the Costs of Medical Care. Although this committee had been chaired by a former president of the AMA, who had been a member of President Hoover's cabinet, its report was declared to be "socialism and communism—inciting to revolution" [8]. The studies and health demonstrations of several foundations—especially the Milbank Memorial Fund, the Julius Rosenwald Fund, and the Twentieth Century Fund—were criticized in a similar vein. Dr. Fishbein soon began the policy of issuing "research reports" that omitted facts unfavorable to AMA views and personally attacked individuals who disagreed with AMA policy, rather than dealing with the issues they had raised. Dr. Fishbein's innumerable speeches, editorials, and articles were effective in unifying opinion on medical economic questions among the majority of physicians.

Graduate nurses were much less agitated than their brothers in medicine over the dangers of socialized medicine, probably because they had long been accustomed to viewing their work as a service rather than a business. Many nurses were becoming aware of their own need for financial security, and they were beginning to consider health insurance and other plans for illness and retirement more seriously.

Empty Hospital Beds and Sick People

During the early 1930s about one in every 18 people entered hospitals in the course of each year, and the ills of as many more were diagnosed and treated in hospital outpatient departments. There were 6437 registered hospitals in the country in 1933, and hospital bed capacities had mounted steadily. The so-

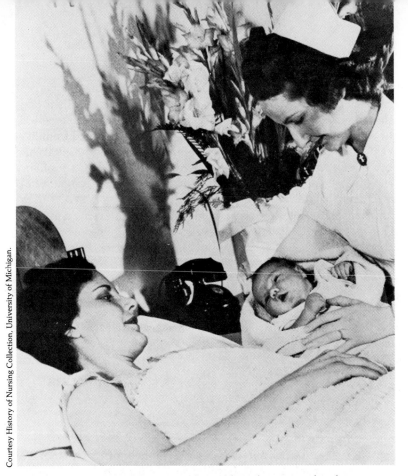

One of every 18 Americans entered hospitals in the course of each year.

called general hospitals—for patients having general or acute diseases—operated mainly under private or nongovernmental auspices. The average government hospital, however, was much larger, containing 162 beds in contrast to the 72 beds in the average nongovernment hospital. In the Pacific Coast states a considerably larger proportion of care was delivered through governmental facilities—43 percent, in terms of bed capacity, compared with 32 percent for the country as a whole.

According to an unpublished study by the Julius Rosenwald Fund, 42 percent of the counties in the United States were without hospitals. These were rural or sparsely settled areas, for the most part, but in certain southern sections they included from 25 to 38 percent of the state populations. In a still larger group of counties, with a population of 44 million, there were plenty of beds in private general hospitals but no government general hospitals at all. In a smaller group, representing 5 percent of the counties and 3 percent of the population, general hospital care was entirely under government auspices.

Low occupancy was perhaps the greatest problem faced by nongovernment hospitals. The average occupancy, which in 1923 was 62.8 percent of all available beds, had fallen by 1933 to 55.3 percent—the lowest being in hospitals owned by individuals or partnerships, which were running at 41.1 percent capacity. Industrial hospitals were operating with 44.4 percent of their beds filled and church hospitals at 54.9 percent capacity. During the same period, however, the rate of occupancy for governmental hospitals advanced from 79.4 to 90.1 percent. The relatively low occupancy of nongovernment hospitals had existed before the Depression and had only been accentuated by it; probably there had already been an oversupply of hospital beds in some communities, while others had no hospitals at all.

Unlike other bills in the family budget, medical bills fell unevenly and unexpectedly. During the 1930s in any given year, about half the people were healthy and had very low medical bills, about one-third had moderate medical bills, and the remaining sixth had very high bills. This unlucky sixth paid half the total medical bills each year. No one could tell in advance whether his family, during the next year, would finish in the lucky half, the moderately fortunate third, or the unlucky sixth. Low income was a major cause of insufficient medical care, but the unpredictable incidence of sickness and the wider range of its costs meant a financial problem even for families far above the poverty level. In proportion, too, as people found it hard or impossible to pay medical bills, the incomes of physicians, dentists, hospitals, and private duty nurses were unstable and often insufficient.

The Hospital Insurance Idea

Hospital insurance plans in the United States had a longer history than many people realized. As far back as 1880, hospital service insurance plans for the benefit of lumbermen had been in operation in northern Minnesota. In other parts of the country, particularly in remote communities such as mining and lumber camps, hospital and medical service plans were common. In 1912 the Rockford Association was organized in Rockford, Illinois. Set up as a nonprofit Illinois corporation with membership open to any community resident over 15 years of age and free from chronic illness, it included six weeks of hospital room and board and all operating room fees. In 1921 a hospital in Grinnell, Iowa, developed a plan covering the costs of room, board, and nursing up to a period of three weeks, exclusive of special services. Six years later the Thompson Benefit Association for hospital service, organized in Brattleboro, Vermont, covered hospitalization expenses up to a maximum of $300, including surgeon's fees.

The plan generally considered to be the nearest prototype of modern hospital insurance systems was organized in 1929 by the schoolteachers of Dallas, Texas. In conjunction with Baylor University Hospital, approximately 1500 teachers were insured for hospital care at the rate of $6.00 per person per year. The plan provided for nursing care in rooms, board, operating room service, anesthesia charges, laboratory fees, routine medicines, surgical dressings, and hypodermics. Full coverage was provided for a period of up to three weeks, with a 33 percent discount for longer periods. Each participant in the plan carried a card that entitled him or her to be admitted to the Baylor hospital.

Under the leadership of Dr. Justin Ford Kimball, vice-president of Baylor University, the program was soon expanded and enrollment was opened to people other than schoolteachers. In 1929 the Baylor plan began with 1400 teachers; by 1933 the plan had 9388 group subscribers and had helped to cover the cost of 1832 patients with 20,500 patient-days. Members continued to be charged 50 cents per month. Various organizations such as schools, businesses, and manufacturing plants, collected the monthly payments and submitted a list of participants along with the dues. The service, which brought in about $60,000 per year, was run at a slight deficit of 6 to 7 percent. This was not nearly as great a deficit as would have been experienced if some of the same patients had been hospitalized as free patients.

In 1933 Dr. Kimball strongly advised other hospitals to undertake insurance plans without waiting for regulatory decisions on specific insurance aspects from state attorneys general: "You do not wait to put a law through the legislature when an Indian is at the point of killing you" [9]. Hospitals, running around 50 percent occupancy, were desperately short of funds, and if they were to keep from going bankrupt, they needed to help devise a system that would not only enable sick people to pay their hospital bills but also to encourage them to come to the hospital for care without fear of personal bankruptcy. Dr. Kimball pointed out that his new approach served the people when they needed hospitalization at a rate that they could pay. It was also beneficial to the physician in that it left funds for patients to meet their bills. Most importantly, it helped the hospital financially, in that it guaranteed the collection of its bills.

The recommendations of the Committee on the Cost of Medical Care gave individual hospital prepayment plans a great impetus for expansion. All these plans constituted a form of social insurance in which individuals or families, usually in employee groups, made equal and regular payments into a common fund used to provide service at a given hospital when required. In some communities more than one local hospital set up its own plan, resulting in competition. By the end of 1934 nonprofit community hospital service plans had begun to be established so rapidly that they were termed a national movement. In that year the multi-hospital Associated Hospital Service Plan of New York (New York City) was organized under a special enabling act. The passage of this unique legislation was a landmark in the development of the movement. The State Superintendent of Insurance had ruled that the proposed hospital service plan was a form of insurance. Previously, in the other states where hospital plans had been set up, their sponsors had assumed that rather than operating insurance plans, they were merely selling hospital service on a prepayment basis. When the attorneys general or insurance departments of those states had been asked for a ruling, they had ruled to that effect, holding that the plans were exempt from the regulations covering stock and mutual insurance companies. This exemption was important in that it meant that subscribers did not have to be liable for assessments and that the plans could start without the large capital required of stock companies.

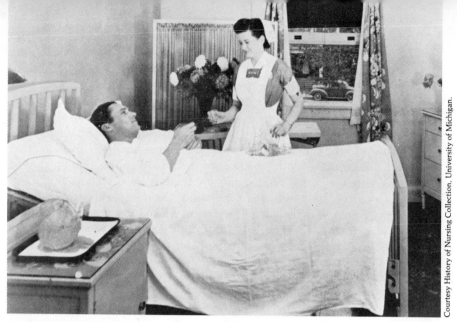

Prepayment plans took much of the fear out of going to the hospital. Patient and student nurse at Bradford Hospital, Bradford, Pennsylvania.

When the New York Superintendent of Insurance ruled that the proposed New York City Plan constituted insurance, local civic leaders, hospital officials, and physicians drafted and sponsored a bill for a special enabling act, which was passed and became law on May 16, 1934. That act stated that any corporation organized for the purpose of operating a nonprofit hospital service plan should be exempt from all other provisions of the insurance law. It also stipulated that rates charged subscribers be subject to review by the insurance department and that the rates of payment to hospitals be subject to the approval of the welfare department. The operatives of such health insurance plans were declared to be charitable and benevolent institutions and exempt from state or local taxes other than taxes on real estate and office equipment. Thenceforth, in virtually all the remaining states, the passage of somewhat similar legislation was a prerequisite for the initiation of such plans.

Blue Cross

The American Hospital Association provided leadership in the development and coordination of hospital insurance plans. Those that were approved were allowed to use the name "Blue Cross." Such plans were sponsored locally by hospitals, the medical profession, and the general public. In most cases the principal initiative in the formation of a plan came from the county or state hospital association. Initial working capital was often provided not only by the hospitals but also by local community chests, business and civic organizations, foundations, and individual civic leaders. A Blue Cross plan was a nonprofit corporation organized under community and professional sponsorship and approved by the American Hospital Association for the purpose of enabling the public to defray the cost of hospital care on a prepayment, group basis. Benefits were paid in terms of hospital service rather than cash indemnity and were guaranteed by the participating hospital through contractual arrangements between the hospitals and the plan. An agreement between the subscriber and the plan listed the benefits to which the subscriber was entitled.

During the late 1930s the annual cost of membership in Blue Cross plans ranged from $5 to $12 per subscriber, depending upon the cost levels of the area, the kind of room accommodation received, the types of sickness covered, and the scope of services offered. A subscriber was admitted to any of the participating hospitals when necessary, but only under the care of a private physician selected by the patient. The typical subscriber paid his own physician's fee, but without charge he received up to 21 days' care in the hospital, including a semiprivate room, nursing service, meals, the operating room, and x-ray and laboratory services.

The growth in enrollment of Blue Cross plans in the United States and Canada proceeded at a rate little short of phenomenal. On July 1, 1938, the total enrollment was 1,949,294; 40 years later it would reach 85 million Americans. Medical insurance, after a slower start due to the conservatism of the AMA, soon expanded at a similar rate, much of it under the medical profession's Blue Shield emblem.

Some of the private life and casualty insurance companies had offered hospital and medical insurance for a number of years, but no widespread demand was built up until the Blue Cross and Blue Shield plans began to achieve national popularity by virtue of their service benefit feature and the low operating cost resulting from nonprofit operation. Moreover, as the American public became more and more conscious of the advantages of medical care insurance, the commercial companies profited by the related publicity and sold their own health and medical policies more extensively than ever before.

Meanwhile, nurses, physicians, and hospital administrators began to note that the health of a large proportion of the population was being affected unfavorably by the Depression. The rate of disabling sickness was found to be 48 percent higher among families having no employed wage earners in 1932 than in families having full-time workers. The group of workers that had dropped from fairly comfortable circumstances to relief roles during the Depression showed a rate of disabling illness 73 percent higher than that of their more fortunate neighbors who had remained in the comfortable class.

In 1934, for the first time in many decades, the annual death rate in large cities was increasing despite the absence of any serious epidemics. Concurrently with these evidences of increased need, local appropriations for public health had decreased 20 percent since 1930. The per capita expenditure from tax funds for public health in 53 cities in 1934 was only 77.5 cents as contrasted with 93.8 cents in 1931.

Federal Health Action under the FERA

Public medical care had been provided by state or local governments to the indigent since colonial days. Nongovernmental agencies, especially local charity hospitals and dispensaries, had also given free care to the needy, but the treatment of the indigent had become more and more a task of government. Over the years, state and local governments had developed varying patterns of administration of public medical care, with a wide range in standards. As the Depression hit bottom in 1931 and 1932, these programs were threatened with disaster because of the great increase in the relief population and the corresponding fall in tax receipts. Accordingly, in 1933 the federal government for the first time entered the picture of medical care for the needy through the famous Regulation 7 of the Federal Emergency Relief Administration.

This administrative regulation stated that health care was a legitimate form of relief and that the regular federal program of grants-in-aid to the states for relief would also cover state programs for medical care in the home. The federal grants were to be confined to severe emergency sicknesses and were not to be used for hospitalization. By September, 1934, 20 states had programs.

Payment for nursing care as well as for medical care of the sick in their homes was increasingly recognized as a legitimate relief expenditure. Under the Federal Emergency Relief Administration (FERA), relief funds were allotted for bedside care to the indigent, and nursing services for patients receiving federal relief was purchased from private agencies with federal funds. The United States Public Health Service was consulted by the FERA in planning this program and was called into vigorous action by many states and communities in

Poverty-stricken family in Hale County, Alabama, summer of 1936.

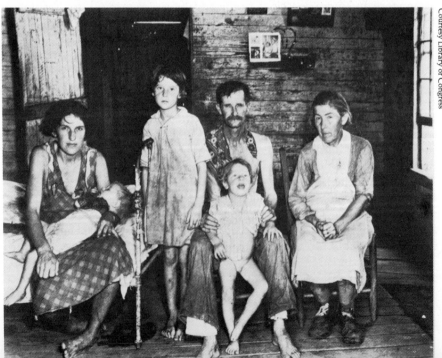

Courtesy Library of Congress

helping to put projects into operation. Provision was made in the rules and regulations for setting up of state advisory committees for the nursing projects. As the federal plan was permissive rather than mandatory, there was much variation state by state, but the principles involved were effectively carried out in many communities.

In West Virginia, for example, the Relief Nursing Service was inaugurated in February, 1933, to meet the need of nurses for employment and the needs of families on relief for nursing care. It was essentially a visiting nurse program. One hundred and sixty-eight full-time registered nurses were employed in 55 counties under the direction of six district supervising nurses.

Most of the counties were covered by two or three nurses, and a few of the most populous counties had organized staffs of from five to 10 nurses. Where two or more nurses were working in one county, one nurse acted as the county supervising nurse. The larger staffs were supervised by nurses trained and experienced in public health work. In counties where there were established visiting nursing services, the relief nurses served as additions to these staffs.

Most of these nurses had had no special training or experience in public health nursing. At the beginning of the program it was necessary to place the nurse at work as rapidly as possible. Typed instructions based on the principles and techniques of the National Organization for Public Health Nursing manual were given to each nurse by the State Director of Relief Nursing. Within two

The Relief Nursing Service in West Virginia was aimed at hiring unemployed nurses and providing nursing care for families on relief.

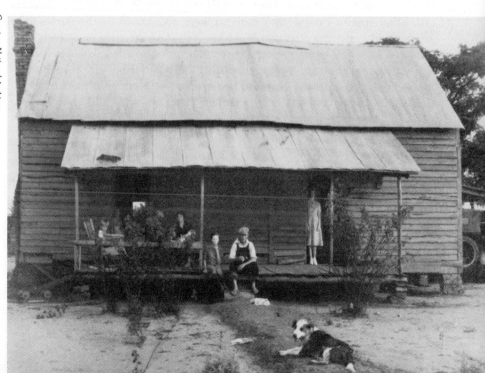

months an advisory committee of physicians was appointed along with six supervising nurses. These supervising nurses were trained and experienced public health nurses. With the advice of the physicians' committee and the State Health Department, the nursing service was organized in the various counties and one day institutes were arranged in each district.

The nurses carried on four fundamental services for families on relief:

Bedside nursing care and health supervision for the family in the home.

Arranging for medical and hospital care for emergency and obstetrical cases.

Supervising the health of the children in emergency relief nursery schools.

Caring for those ill with tuberculosis. A special effort was made to secure physical examination of all contacts in the home and isolation of the actual case was made possible in a great many counties through the construction of portable porches.

Nurses were also responsible for making arrangements for the family physician to attend relief patients needing their care. They saved the physicians many unnecessary calls by making first visits to all patients except in extreme emergency. Immediate report was made to the physician on cases requiring his care, and nursing care was continued under the direction of the physician.

Standing orders based on the National Organization of Public Health Nursing Manual were given to the nurses of each county, to the physicians composing the county medical relief committee, and to the medical association. These orders, as approved, were carried out by the nurses until a physician gave other specific orders. Sick patients were not carried by the nurses unless the case was under the direction of a physician. Special stress was given to the early and complete examination of prenatal cases and adequate provision for delivery and postpartum care of all mothers, no matter how inaccessible their homes might be. In many counties the relief project nurses organized classes for mothers in prenatal and baby care and for adults and children in personal hygiene, home nursing, and first aid.

Nurses under CWA Programs

With the conviction that because of the rapidly increasing volume of relief the winter of 1933 would be one of great hardship, Congress created an additional relief program, the Civil Works Administration (CWA), in November, 1933. Jobs were provided to four million unemployed people on temporary projects submitted by local and state authorities or conducted directly by the federal government.

More than 10,000 unemployed nurses were put to work under the Civil Works Administration. Nurses were employed in numerous settings: in public hospitals, institutions, and clinics; on public health staffs; in bedside nursing; in immunization campaigns and making surveys; and in many other health services. In many instances health and nursing service were carried to remote sections for the first time. In the state of Washington, for example, the public health departments had long been hampered in their work because of the necessity of cutting back expenditures. CWA gave them an opportunity to employ 300 needy nurses. Some of these nurses were so destitute that they had to be given clothing and shoes before they could accept work. With the corps of 300 additional nurses supervised by the public health nurses, from December 8, 1933, to March 15, 1934, thousands of Washington children were immunized against diphtheria and were given smallpox vaccinations. In an area of the state inundated by floods, hundreds were given typhoid vaccine. The impressive results summarized below were amazing, considering that only 300 nurses accomplished all this work in three months' time:

Number having bedside or nursing care	4668
Number of visits to TB patients	1830
Number of maternal case visits	3907
Numbers of pupils inspected in schools	286,193
Number of defects found	40,943
Number of corrections made	6048
Number of pupils excluded	3337
Number of conferences with parents	3447
Number of lectures or talks given	454

CWA nurses were placed in numerous public hospitals.

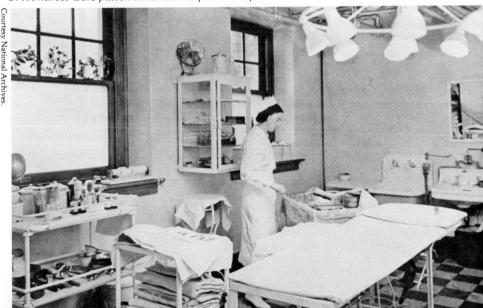

Courtesy National Archives.

Data collected from over 500 CWA nurses in New York about themselves showed the following characteristics:

Ages: ranged from 19 to 64; largest number from 23 to 26 years.

Preliminary education: 47 percent were high school graduates; 3 percent had some college work.

Professional education: out of nurse training for 3 to 38 years; largest number under 5 years.

Postgraduate courses taken by 51 of them, or 9 percent.

Amount of employment in the year preceding FERA service: less than six months, 503; of these 357 had less than three months.

Reasons for unemployment (sometimes a combination): unavailability of work, 476; housewife or other responsibilities, 99; illness, 47.

Average number of months on FERA: 8¼

Duties to which assigned:

General public health	401
School	42
Dispensaries and clinics	36
Hospitals	25
Tuberculosis	23
Nutrition survey	18
Communicable disease	18
Records	8
Social hygiene	6
Camp	3
Preschool cardiac	1
Dental work	1
Swimming pool	1
Social service	1
Laboratory	1
Stockroom	1

Cost of transportation, weekly: city, $1.78; rural district, $5.21; town, $4.41; village, $1.40; county, $5.60. Average, $2.95 per week.

Transportation paid by: self, 236; public funds, 135; VNA, 25; industrial firms, 3; friends, 3.

Reaction to work: very enthusiastic, 425; liked it, 138; no remarks, 20; did not like it, 5.

Employment under the CWA program began on November 16, 1933, and the peak was reached on January 18, 1934, when over 4,260,000 people were at work. It was considerably more costly than anticipated, however. Nearly $1 billion was spent in wages and materials during the four months between November, 1933, and April, 1934, when the program was finally discontinued. Most of the 10,000 nurses it had carried were faced with unemployment again.

The CWA marked the introduction of new principles in the relief of unemployment in the United States. It emphasized the claim that the unemployed wanted work and that the abstract right to a job should be supplemented by a public policy and program which provided a job. Furthermore, the right to a job was extended not only to the destitute unemployed but also to other jobless persons. Weekly wages paid on these projects were not related to family budgets but were based on prevailing rates in the community, and employment was provided for a fixed number of hours per week. The nursing projects were more substantial in character than those that had prevailed under the FERA. The CWA served well in priming the pump while it was operating. It set up standards for work relief projects: all work had to have social and economic value, it could be performed only on public property, and projects could not include work normally performed by the state or localities.

The WPA and Nurses

The Works Program, established by the Emergency Relief Appropriation Act of 1935, was intended to "provide relief, work relief, and to increase employment by providing useful projects." As originally set up, it contemplated that a considerable amount of work would be under the direction of established government agencies whose activities could be expanded through employment of relief workers. But to give direction to the relief employment of these agencies and to provide a large additional number of jobs, the Works Progress Administration (WPA) was established. This soon became the most important single unit in the Works Program. Projects to be approved by the WPA, according to the original plan, had to be useful. They were to be of such a nature that a considerable proportion of the money spent would go into wages. Self-liquidating projects which promised ultimate returns to the federal treasury of a considerable proportion of the costs were to be sought. In all cases, projects had to be of a character to give employment to those on the relief rolls, and they were to be noncompetitive if possible.

All WPA projects were sponsored by tax-supported bodies of states, counties, or towns and represented what the various communities desired and requested. The nursing and public health projects in all cases were sponsored by state or local departments of public health or similar public bodies or agencies. Office space and office and nursing equipment were contributed by the sponsor or by some community agency. The WPA paid the salaries of nurses, technicians, and assistants as were required to render services which the regular staffs of the public health departments, because of their already heavy burdens, were unable to provide.

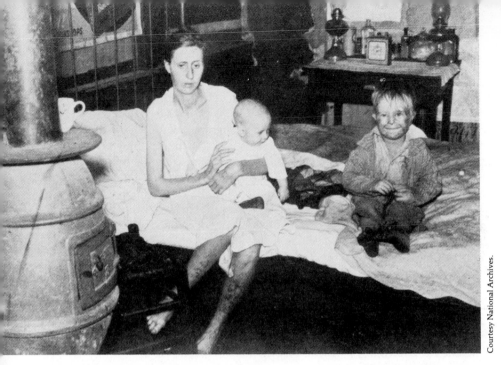

Under WPA projects, hundreds of needy RNs went into underprivileged homes to assist in prenatal care and render nursing service.

Under many of the nursing projects, needy registered nurses, on the recommendation of physicians, went into underprivileged homes to assist with antepartum and postpartum care and also to render nursing service in cases of illness. They performed all types of duties generally listed under the heading of bedside nursing, such as bathing and caring for patients, preparing proper foods for the sick, and providing similar services. WPA nurses were employed on projects to promote physical and oral hygiene. They assisted in a program to examine children for physical and dental defects and in immunization campaigns against whooping cough, typhoid fever, diphtheria, smallpox, and other diseases. On projects in some localities, WPA nurses assisted physicians in administering the Mantoux test.

During fiscal year 1936 approximately 6000 graduate nurses were employed on WPA projects of one type or another. The greatest number of nurses were employed on projects that provided bedside nursing service on a visit basis to families on relief or to families who were unable to provide nursing care for themselves.

Works Progress Administration nursing and public health projects were in operation in 37 states plus the District of Columbia. Up to September 15, 1936, Works Progress Administration nurses had extended services to millions of people through 9,000,000 visits, examinations, or treatments.

A nursing project under way in New Jersey was typical of the WPA projects. In 45 school districts the Works Progress Administration project was supplying public health nurses in public schools where no such service previously existed, and in several other districts the project was supplementing the inadequate regular service. As a result of this activity, 16 school districts had assumed full responsibility for nursing services and 10 of the project nurses had found permanent employment with the schools or with public health nursing organizations. As financial conditions permitted, other school districts proposed to undertake the work as a regular activity.

In Georgia the Works Progress Administration public health nursing program had been taken over by the State Department of Public Health and was now a regular part of the state program. T. F. Abercrombie, State Director of the Department of Public Health, said that the establishment of Georgia's public health nursing division was directly due to the inauguration of the state nursing project operating under the Federal Works Program. During the first year of the new state program all but 46 of the 200 Works Progress Administration nurses had succeeded in getting permanent work, thus removing them from the WPA's rolls. During 1935 WPA nurses had given a half-million immunizations in Georgia. More than 400,000 general home nursing visits had been made, and 30,000 infants and preschool children had benefited by the health supervision of the Works Progress Administration nursing project. Before the government projects were put into operation, there had been no public health nursing programs in the state.

In one county in Wyoming a Works Progress Administration nurse established a tonsil clinic. Any child in the county whose family was unable to employ a private physician was admitted. It had sometimes been necessary to transport cases over 100 miles in order to obtain treatment from physicians who donated their services to the clinic. In the same county the nurse had taken more than 40 persons with eye conditions to one of the leading eye specialists in the state.

In Chicago, 127,540 children in 254 of the city's elementary schools had their eyes tested. Several thousand had treatments resulting in cures or decided improvement in vision. "The value of this work cannot be estimated," said Audrey Haydon, ex-secretary of the Illinois Society for the Prevention of Blindness.

Many other examples could be cited. In New York City the fight against disease was carried on by 6,317 Works Progress Administration physicians, nurses, research and clerical workers, scientists and technicians. Through project clinics, physicians on one project alone treated more than 18,000 victims of venereal disease during the period from December 20, 1936, to January 20, 1937. During the same time, 30,000 schoolchildren were treated in dental clinics. As a result of a drive in Charleston County, South Carolina, made possible by federal assistance, diphtheria had been reduced to a minimum. In a 12-month period, graduate nurses visited 27,408 homes to persuade parents to protect their children from diphtheria by toxoid immunization.

Dr. J. Moss Beeler, County Health Commissioner and Superintendent of the Spartanburg (South Carolina) County Hospital—which consisted of a general hospital, a hospital for blacks, outpatient and social service departments, an isolation unit, a nurses' home, a laboratory and other service units, and a tuberculosis department two miles away—declared, "We would have accomplished about a third of what we have actually accomplished during the past two years if it had not been for the services rendered by WPA nurses," Dr. Beeler was soon able to place 30 WPA nurses on the regular hospital payroll.

Social Security Act of 1935

To deal with the fundamental problems of economic insecurity, Congress passed the Social Security Act of 1935. This was the one New Deal measure clearly inspired by foreign example. Social security measures, first tried in Germany in the 1880s, had spread through western Europe as well as to Australia and New Zealand. They had also been tried out in the United States by state governments and private employers.

The Social Security Act, as approved by the President on August 14, 1935, provided (1) for federal old-age benefits; (2) for grants to the states for old-age assistance, vocational rehabilitation, and unemployment compensation administration; (3) for aid to dependent and/or crippled children, aid to the blind, and maternal and child welfare; (4) for public health work, including the authorization of grants to states for aid in the development and maintenance of state and local health services; and (5) for an annual appropriation to the Public Health Service for additional research and training activities.

It was significant that Title VI of the Social Security Act authorized use of federal funds for the training of public health personnel. When the funds autho-

Two Methodist Hospital of Dallas student nurses make a call on a rural family as part of their public health nursing experience.

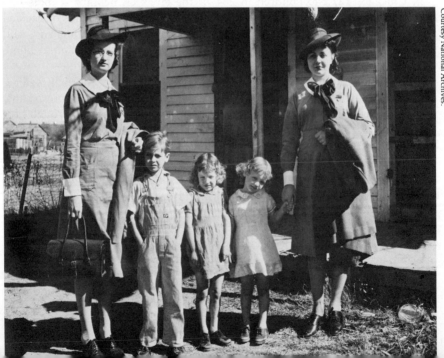

rized by the Act became available early in 1936, about one-third of the states had a functioning public health nursing unit in their state health departments. A considerable number of young nurses who had become involved in public health nursing activities through the work relief projects were eager to acquire formal public health training, and during the first year of the Social Security program about 1000 nurses received scholarship stipends through Social Security funds for study at universities offering public health nursing programs approved by the National Organization for Public Health Nursing. No other professional group in the health care field was able to recruit so many qualified candidates for training in so short a time. Most of the states that had established public health nursing units through work relief retained the same supervisory staff and used grant-in-aid funds provided under the Social Security Act to establish permanent divisions or bureaus of public health nursing.

The success of the training program for public health nurses under the Social Security Act exemplified the soundness of the plan and the effectiveness of the method of cooperation between the states and the federal government. In 1934 only 7 percent of the public health nurses then employed had completed an approved course of study in public health nursing at one of the accredited institutions in the United States, although many of the courses of study at those institutions had been in existence for 10 to 20 years. Within the two years immediately following implementation of the Social Security Act, 2304 nurses (or about 10 percent of all the public health nurses in the United States) received some postgraduate training at approved schools on training stipends. Almost 15 percent of those receiving training stipends attended school for a full academic year or more.

Nursing Education in the Mid-1930s

While nursing education was not experiencing such a dramatic advance, progress had been achieved. A study of the hospital schools of nursing in the late 1930s showed that schools of nursing were conducted in hospitals with a daily average patient census ranging from seven to 6880 and that school of nursing enrollment varied from 6 to 350 students. By 1936 there were 70 so-called collegiate programs in nursing, nearly all of which represented two years of general education either before or after a conventional three-year hospital diploma program. More than half of these had been established between 1930 and 1936. Meanwhile, the number of hospital diploma programs had decreased from over 2286 in 1929 to 1472 state-accredited schools in 1936.

This attrition was attributed to the evaluation studies of the 1920s and the national economic depression. Another major factor in the decrease was the fact that as the Depression had deepened and private patients became scarce, hospitals permitted their graduates to remain at work, often with little more pay than they had received as students. Those without schools of nursing could hire graduate nurses for lower wages than they had been paying their untrained "attendants." By 1937, therefore, the number of graduate nurses in hospitals had risen 700 percent, from 4000 in 1929 to 28,000 in 1937.

Location of the 1472 schools of nursing in 1936.

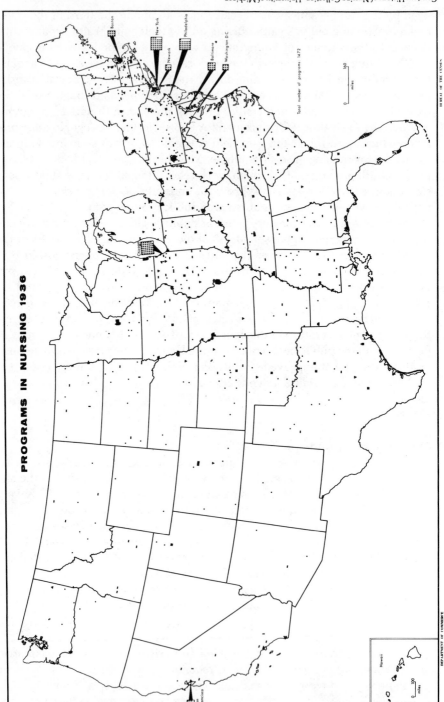

PROGRAMS IN NURSING 1936

The 1937 Curriculum Guide

Toward the end of the 1930s massive unemployment, maldistribution of nursing service, the problems of depression-stricken hospitals, and many other factors called for a change in school of nursing curricula. The third and last revision of the National League for Nursing Education's *Curriculum Guide for Schools of Nursing* appeared in 1937. It was in line with the democratic belief that such a plan could best be put into operation if all concerned contributed to its compilation. Literally thousands of nurses all over the country were involved in the revision, either creatively or critically.

Two innovative assumptions were made in the *Guide*. One of these was that the primary function of the school of nursing should be education of the nurse. This represented a change from the assumption operating during an earlier period, which held that the function of the school was to provide nursing service for hospital patients. This assumption was in no way intended to repudiate the nursing profession's responsibility for the care of the sick, but was meant to remind the community that the preparation of the nurse to care for future patients should not be sacrificed to provision of care in the present. The second assumption underlying revision of the *Guide* was the concept of the nurse serving the total community, rather than just a skewed example of the community—the hospital. Public health nursing, mental health nursing, and understanding of the social setting of health problems and of the economic aspects of health care were all aspects of this concept.

The curriculum covered 2-1/2 to three years. It was set up on a plan of either three terms of 16 weeks or four terms of 12 weeks each, both with four weeks' vacation every year. To hospital administrators the nursing practice time was of special interest. The suggested length of the school week was 5½ days, or 44 to 48 hours, with one or 1½ days off per week. This ideal program included all regularly scheduled classes and nursing practice and provided sufficient time for study, recreation, and rest. In the first four months of the first year, classes and laboratory periods took up 20 to 22 hours per week and did not include any nursing practice. The class hours were decreased to 14 hours in the second term, at which time nursing practice of 18 hours per week was begun. In the third term class hours were held to 14 and practice was increased to 22 hours. In the second and third years classes averaged five or six hours every week; nursing practice, 38 to 42 hours.

The proposed three-year course called for about 1200 to 1300 hours of class and laboratory work and about 4800 hours of nursing practice, as compared to 825 hours of class, 200 hours of ward teaching, and approximately 6000 hours of nursing service in the 1927 version. The courses included in the curriculum fell into three categories. The first included basic courses such as anatomy, physiology, chemistry, microbiology, materia medica, psychology and sociology, and the history and ethics of nursing. These courses supplied a body of principles, facts, methods of study, and laboratory techniques that gave a good background for clinical practice. There was little new or different in this group except that possibly more emphasis was placed upon psychology and sociology.

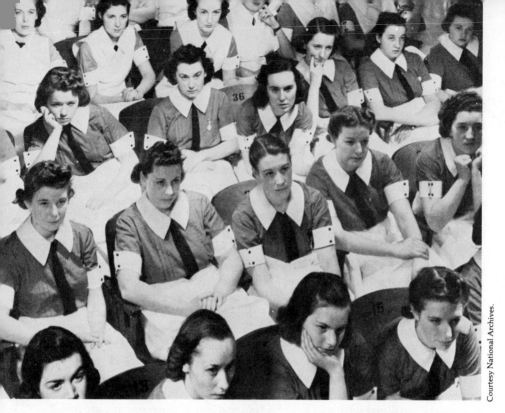

School of nursing class in session, about 1939.

The two other categories of courses contained several new approaches. The major professional and technical courses were concerned with the "art" of nursing and included nursing arts, nutrition and cookery, medical nursing (including nursing in communicable disease), and surgical, pediatric, obstetric, psychiatric, and home nursing. The practical application in actual nursing situations allowed for integration of the basic science courses. A reorientation from sick nursing to a health care focus was proposed. Discussion topics, with content drawn from the nursing content, were a new development and would lead, it was hoped, to a better integration of all the subjects offered to students.

Several other new features were significant. The psychological aspects of nursing were emphasized, and the sequence culminated in a suggested required program in psychiatry in the third year. In the course on pediatrics, the physical and mental development of the well child was stressed as much as the care of the sick child. Public health and health teaching were incorporated throughout the course. Suggested programs of study and practice included applied sociology, social and professional discussion groups, and sessions on the health promotion aspects of nursing in the introduction to the nursing arts course.

Nurses on the Screen

Student nurses of the 1930s—those with the time, energy, and money—began to see Hollywood motion pictures that depicted the nurse in all aspects of her life. The decade started off with *War Nurse* in 1930, moved on to *Night Nurse* in 1931, and *A Farewell to Arms* and *Miss Pinkerton* in 1932, and then bloomed forth in 1934 with *Registered Nurse* and *The White Parade*. In regard to the last film, the review in *Trained Nurse and Hospital Review* expressed whole-hearted enthusiasm:

It is rather fine to discover the ephemeral ideals of youth, which are often crushed into rude shapes by the vicissitudes of life, so sympathetically portrayed in "The White Parade." This interpretation of nursing catches the feeling of altruism so characteristic of youth and gives it wings in a form that is harnessed to practical service. Moreover, it breaks down the thin wall between comedy and tragedy that is so present in reality, until smiles and tears chase across the film and the audience feels itself a part of this life within hospital walls . . . . An underlying spirit of reverence runs through the whole production, yet at times the humor is uproarious—of the boarding school variety—and the audience moves from mood to mood with an appreciation that stamps the sincerity of the production [10].

Loretta Young, as nursing student June Arden, decorates the nurses' Christmas tree in The White Parade. *(Copyright © 1934 Twentieth Century-Fox Film Corporation. All rights reserved.)*

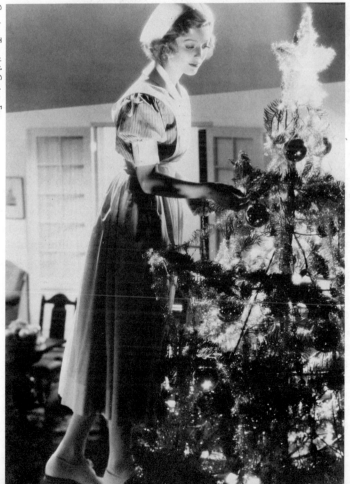

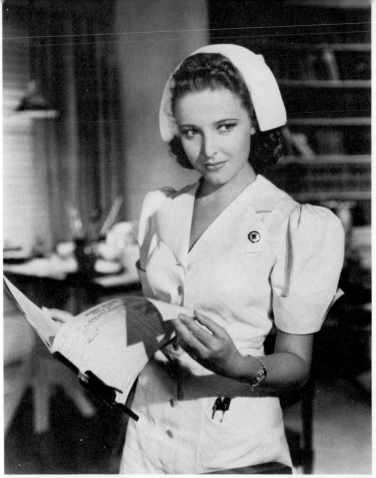

Courtesy MGM.

Nurse Mary Lamont, played by Laraine Day, starred in the highly popular Dr. Kildare *series produced by MGM during the late 1930s and early 1940s. (From the MGM release* The Secret of Dr. Kildare © *1939 Loew's Incorporated. Copyright renewed 1966 by Metro-Goldwyn-Mayer Inc.)*

The remainder of the decade witnessed nurse-dominated films such as *While the Patient Slept; White Angel; The Great Hospital Mystery; Wife, Doctor, and Nurse; Nurse from Brooklyn; Secrets of a Nurse; Four Girls in White; Nurse Edith Cavell;* the *Dr. Kildare* series; and many others. It made little difference that the action in these films, as viewed by more than 85 million people each week, was not totally in tune with reality. What mattered was the enlivening of the public image of the nurse in a relatively positive way.

The PWA Builds Hospitals

Hospitals were also looking better, thanks to massive federal expenditures and low construction costs. The new Public Works Administration, a Depression-inspired "pump-priming" device conceived by President Roosevelt to stimulate heavy industry through construction projects using basic industrial output like steel, cement, and lumber was set up in June, 1933. The PWA received an initial appropriation of $3.3 billion and was placed under the direction of the Secretary of the Interior. It was authorized to start its own construction projects, to support those administered by other federal units, and to make loans and matching grants sponsored by state and local public agencies. The PWA's total achievement between 1933 and 1939 was impressive. During that time it spent $6 billion, created jobs for about four million people in more than 34,000 projects, and helped to build about 70 percent of the new educational buildings and about 35 percent of the new hospitals and public health facilities in the United States. Tremendous skyscraper hospitals in large cities and smaller facilities in rural areas were constructed with the aid of PWA funds.

An Improved Working Environment for the Nurse

During the early part of the twentieth century nearly all hospital equipment had been constructed of cast iron and sheet metal and was generally finished in white enamel or porcelain. In place of crude castings, the new hospitals had streamlined, electrically welded equipment of noncorrosive or corrosion-resistant metal. Such metals were employed in the construction of operating room furniture, laboratory equipment, sterilizing equipment, kitchen and laundry equipment, and elevator cabs, and even in utensils such as basins, jars, and trays. Wood furniture with stain-resistant finishes was also widely used in patients' rooms, waiting rooms, solariums, and offices. Hospitals made extensive use of sound-absorbent materials, and acoustical installations were found in corridors, patients' rooms, preparation and serving kitchens, utility rooms, offices, and other areas.

Improved casters facilitated the introduction of mobile equipment. In the rare instances when it was necessary to move older, stationary beds, a bed conveyor was used. In new hospitals all beds were equipped with casters, and many nurses moved the patient directly to surgery, the x-ray department, the physiotherapy department, or the solarium in his own bed, without first transferring him from bed to wheelchair or stretcher. New mobile equipment included stretcher carts, wheelchairs, food conveyors, linen trucks and linen hampers, and two- and four-wheel trucks for the delivery of supplies. Also equipped with casters were bedside tables, overbed tables, metabolism and oxygen therapy apparatus, therapeutic and examining lamps, and operating room and instrument tables. Stretcher carts and the various types of easily storable folding trucks were also available. Some of the larger hospitals used electrically operated tractors, which made it possible to haul a number of trucks at one time.

The progress in hospital service, made possible in part through the use of modern equipment, could also be seen in the great number of mechanical devices, many of them electrically operated, that had been developed during the 1920s and 1930s. Such equipment was in use in every department, from the operating room and x-ray suites to the offices, kitchens, and laundry. Fever therapy apparatus, respiratory and oxygen therapy machines, iron lungs, electrically heated blankets, stupe and inhalation kettles, incubators, electrically operated breast pumps, suction pressure apparatus, electrically heated ranges, food ma-

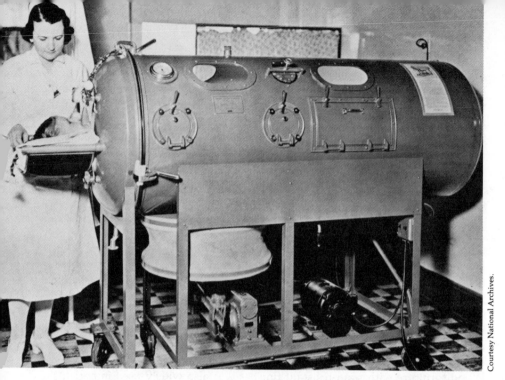

The Iron Lung, a technological innovation in medical care of the late 1930s.

chines and conveyers, electric locks, bedside deodorizers, floor-scrubbing machines, check protectors and check signers, bill machines and photographic equipment: virtually thousands of mechanical devices had been developed for the use of the nurse as well as other hospital workers.

Nurses working in new buildings noted improved illumination. Modern hospitals installed emergency lighting systems, operated by storage batteries or by steam- or gasoline-driven generators, in operating and delivery rooms, corridors, stairwells, and elevator cabs. Operating room fixtures could light the operating field without casting a shadow and were constructed to create a minimum amount of heat, thereby adding to the comfort of the surgical staff. Lighting of patients' rooms had been improved in several ways. Ceiling and wall-bracket fixtures enabled the night nurse to observe the patient without disturbing him, and extensive use was made of illuminated directional signs.

Communication devices had been adopted for hospital use. More and more hospitals were equipped with some type of signaling device that enabled the patient to call the nurse. The type generally used was operated at the patient's bedside by a push button that flashed a light in the corridor, over the doorway to the patient's room, and in other areas where the nurse was likely to be. A few hospitals installed communications equipment between the patient's bedside and the nurses' office, which enabled the patient to speak directly to the nurse. Some hospitals used standard telephone equipment with satisfactory results. The air conditioner was a popular new luxury. Air conditioning was, for the most part, limited to operating room and delivery room suites and nurseries, although a few institutions had installed individual units in a few private rooms, and several hospitals had air-conditioned rooms for the care of premature infants.

In the newer hospitals every effort was being made to make patients' rooms as attractive and homelike as possible. Overbed tables had been installed for the accommodation of food trays, and bedsprings with adjustable, built-in backrests facilitated sitting up in bed and added to the patient's comfort. Many hospitals had replaced the cotton mattress with a comfortable innerspring or sponge-rubber version. Special beds had been designed for cardiac and fracture cases, and many beds featured a special built-in bedpan. Removable side rails, attached to hospital beds in order to protect the semiconscious patient, were newly available. Occasionally, carpeting and attractive window draperies were used in private and semiprivate rooms. Some hospitals used cubicle screening in accommodations for two or more patients in order to assure privacy; this screening consisted of a metal rod, suspended from the ceiling and extending around the patient's bed, on which curtains were fastened.

Despite the Depression and with the assistance of hospital insurance plans and medical advances, by 1939 the hospital had become accepted as a necessary institution in every American community. The 40 million people inhabiting the United States in 1870 had had fewer than 50,000 hospital beds available for their use; the 133 million people in 1939 had 1,200,000 beds. During the 70 years in which the population of the nation had more than tripled, the number of hospital beds had multiplied 24-fold. Health care was increasingly being associated with hospitalization, and graduate nurses were a part of this movement.

A modern hospital of the late 1930s.

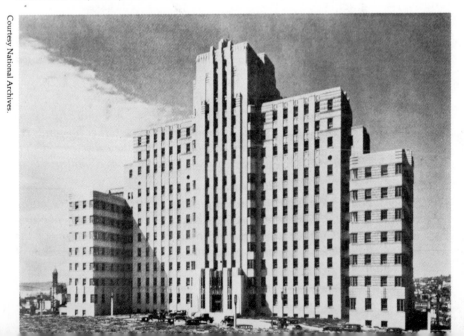

Summary

During the Depression years an estimated 8000 to 10,000 graduate nurses were unemployed. Few families could afford private duty nurses and more than 100,000 student nurses still provided the vast majority of hospital nursing care, leaving little opportunity for graduate nurses to obtain employment. While some hospitals allowed graduate nurses to work for room, board, and laundry, others did not think such concessions were worth the expenses involved.

As air travel became more feasible, nurses were employed as stewardesses.

Attempts at widening access to health care were initiated when the Committee on the Costs of Medical Care, supported by eight philanthropic foundations, conducted a five-year study of ways to provide medical care to all income groups. Among its recommendations was the establishment of group payment for health care through insurance, taxation, or both.

Attacks were launched by the AMA against the prepayment concept on the grounds that it would foster communism and encourage overuse of hospitals at the expense of private physicians. Nevertheless, under the leadership of the AHA, hospital insurance plans rapidly expanded, with many being organized under the Blue Cross emblem. Four decades later, enrollment in Blue Cross plans would reach 85 million Americans.

In 1933 the federal government extended permission for states to use Federal Emergency Relief Administration grants for nursing care of the sick in their homes.

Meeting the needs of both unemployed graduate nurses and destitute families, a series of state- and locally administered nursing programs under the FERA, CWA, and WPA carried community nursing to unparalleled high levels of service.

One of the titles of the Social Security Act of 1935 authorized the use of federal funds for the training of nurses employed by health departments, and many of the formerly unemployed nurses who had worked on relief projects received their public health training with the support of these funds.

The impact of the Depression largely accounted for the decline in the number of schools of nursing—from 2286 in 1927 to 1472 in 1936—as many of the proprietary hospitals with schools were forced out of business. Other hospitals reduced enrollments or terminated their schools because they discovered that they could hire graduate nurses more cheaply than the cost of staffing with students.

During the 1930s nurse educators throughout the country participated in the development of the third revision of A Curriculum Guide for Schools of Nursing. Two new fundamental concepts held that the primary function of the school of nursing was the education of the nurse (as opposed to provision of *student labor for the hospital), and that the nurses' scope of responsibility should include community health as well as hospital service.*

Nurses were widely portrayed in the motion pictures of the 1930s, which were reaching an all-time high of more than 85 million people weekly.

The Public Works Administration, set up from 1933 to 1939 by President Roosevelt to stimulate heavy industry, was responsible for building 35 percent of the new hospitals and public health facilities during the Depression years.

Nurses' working environment in new hospitals was much improved by the utilization of new mechanical devices, many of them electrically operated, which were employed in every department from the operating room to the kitchens.

By 1939 the number of hospital beds had multiplied 24 times from the figure of 70 years earlier, and hospitals had become accepted as a necessary institution in every American community.

References

1. *New York Times*, March 5, 1933.
2. "Binghamton Is Over-Crowded, So Is Birmingham, So Is Colorado Springs," *American Journal of Nursing*, vol. 30 (January, 1930): 97.
3. "Too Many Nurses in These Localities," *op. cit.*, vol. 30 (March, 1930): 344.
4. J. A. Diekmann, "Nursing Schools in Hospitals Under 100 Beds Should Close," *Hospital Management*, vol. 37 (March, 1934): 29–30.
5. Michael M. Davis, "The Committee on Costs of Medical Care Makes Its Report," *Modern Hospital*, vol. 39 (December, 1932): 41–46.
6. Committee on the Costs of Medical Care, *Medical Care for the American People, The Final Report of the Committee on the Costs of Medical Care* (Chicago: University of Chicago Press, 1932), pp. 1–10.
7. R. G. Leland, "Seventeen Defects or Objections to Group Hospitalization," *Hospital Management*, vol. 35 (April, 1933): 25–26.
8. Morris Fishbein, "The Committee on the Costs of Medical Care," *Journal of the American Medical Association*, vol. 99 (December 3, 1932): 1950–1952.
9. "Group Hospitalization Strongly Stressed at Protestant Hospital Convention," *Trained Nurse and Hospital Review*, vol. 91 (October, 1933): 345–352.
10. "The White Parade," *Trained Nurse and Hospital Review*, vol. 93 (December, 1934): 563–565.
11. Frederick A. Washburn, "The Broadened Concept of Hospital Functions Since the Year 1896," *Hospitals*, vol. 14 (November, 1940): 13–17.

14
Nursing in the War for the World

In the spring of 1939 an issue of the *American Journal of Nursing* carried a perceptive editorial entitled "To the Graduates of '39," which alluded to the extraordinary demands looming on the horizon:

We salute you, graduates of '39. We wish you well. The world has need for more nursing.

If such a thing were possible, and all the graduates of '39 could be massed in one great stadium, what a heart-stirring sight it would be.

We don't know what our hypothetical speaker would say to you, you thousands of young and eager American nurses on so great an occasion. Probably he (or she) would begin with some description of the shattering fears of the world we live in, of the undeclared wars, of changing national boundaries, of problems of migration, and of the health problems created by all of them.

Nurses of '39, the world has need of you. If war should come, we have faith to believe that you will fulfill the traditional role of the nurse [1].

A reduction in working hours for undergraduate and graduate staffs had resulted in increased nursing school enrollments from 67,000 students in 1935 to over 82,000 four years later. When enrollment increased by 8000 from 1938 to 1939, many nurse educators began to fear that an overproduction of graduate nurses would lead to a corresponding decline in their quality, as it had in the 1920s. Patients in American hospitals were receiving over 60 million more days of care in 1939 than in 1934; the number of hospital beds had increased by 14 percent.

The Outbreak of War

The 1501 nurses who registered at the Forty-fifth Annual Convention of the National League of Nursing Education in New Orleans in April of 1939 were apparently unaware of the worsening international situation in Europe. Since New Orleans offered a variety of unsurpassed tourist attractions, the delegates explored the quaint streets and fascinating shops of the Vieux Carré, visited the wharves, and dined in exotic restaurants.

Meanwhile international relations in Europe were steadily deteriorating. Ever since the Treaty of Versailles, which had ended World War I, Germany

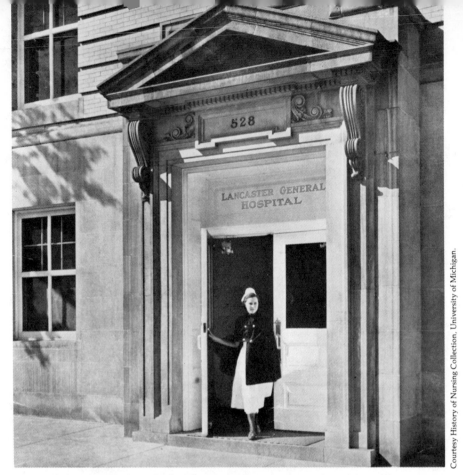

The graduate of 1939 was to be faced with an abruptly changed world.

had been denouncing, among other things, the so-called Polish Corridor, a strip of territory 120 miles long and 60 miles wide separating East Prussia from the rest of Germany. The Treaty of Versailles had awarded this territory to the newly formed state of Poland and had placed the German city of Danzig under the control of the League of Nations. In late August, 1939, the German dictator Adolf Hitler demanded that Danzig be returned to the Reich and that Poland grant him the right to build a road across the Corridor. He also accused Poland of fostering atrocities against its citizens of German ancestry. In order to eliminate the danger of a war on two fronts, Hitler negotiated a 10-year nonaggression pact with the Soviet Union in August, 1939. By demarcating German and Russian spheres of influence in Poland, this pact cleared the way for a joint invasion of the unfortunate country by the new allies. Several days later Hitler delivered an ultimatum to the Polish government, but before it even had time to reply, German troops invaded Poland without making a formal declaration of war.

The Poles expected to offer resistance until at least winter, when bad weather would come to their aid by slowing the progress of the invaders. Long before winter, however, the new German armies won a complete victory. Their rapid, lightning-like movements even caused a new word to be invented—*Blitzkrieg*, or "lightning war." While German armored divisions encircled Polish defenders, the Luftwaffe, which had already destroyed the Polish air force on the ground, ruthlessly bombed cities and fleeing refugees in a deliberate attempt to terrorize the civilian population. Warsaw fell within three weeks, and in little more than a month all Polish resistance to the Germans had collapsed. Meanwhile the Soviet Union, in accordance with the terms of the nonaggression pact, occupied eastern Poland. Two days after Hitler's armies invaded Poland, Great Britain and France declared war on Germany. Their lack of military preparedness, however, prevented them from coming to the aid of the Poles.

The six months following the Russo-German conquest of Poland were quiet, as Hitler paused before assaulting the other European nations. Only Stalin's invasion of Finland excited the American public during this *Sitzkrieg*, or "phony war," which took place during the winter of 1939–1940. This Soviet move to secure the Baltic front against the Germans was fiercely resisted by the Finns and aroused the indignation of most Americans.

Nurses were becoming increasingly aware of the international crisis. In the February, 1940, *American Journal of Nursing* editor Mary Roberts wrote:

Congress, as this is written, has been in session only ten days. The very air is supercharged with tragedy. The wars of other countries are profoundly influencing life in our own, and the Congress is concerned with such matters as neutrality, reciprocal trade agreements, and armaments for defense [2].

Four months later, at the May, 1940, convention of the American Nurses' Association in Philadelphia, Miss Roberts noted that, day by day, the agonies of Europe were growing more acute and that the convention theme, "Nursing in a Democracy," was daily becoming more appropriate in view of the grave war news.

In April, 1940, Hitler's armies suddenly struck in Norway and Denmark. A month later German troops began storming across the Dutch and Belgian borders in the now-familiar blitzkrieg fashion. This lightning thrust caught Great Britain and France unprepared as German dive-bombers wrought havoc behind the Allied lines and massed tanks broke through their defenses. As Belgium neared collapse, German forces penetrated the rugged Ardennes country, avoiding the awesome fortifications of the Maginot Line, and moved across northern France. Veering toward the Channel, the onrushing Germans pinned a half million British and French troops into an ever-narrowing salient around Dunkerque. The near-miraculous escape of the bulk of the British armies from that trap between May 26 and June 3, 1940, could not minimize the catastrophe of the Allied defeat.

Nurses Prepare for the Demands of War

During one session of the 1940 ANA Convention the radio carried President Roosevelt's announcement of national preparedness. Although many delegates immediately asked what preparations were being made for nursing service in case of war, no general plans had yet been formulated. A nurse from Finland spoke at the closing business session. She had come, she said, to express the gratitude of the Finnish people for the material aid and moral support of American nurses. "More than ever I am impressed by our internationalism in the field of nursing," she declared [3]. She vividly described how many of Finland's nurses had lost their lives in their response to the call of duty. Finland, which knew the full meaning of "nursing in a democracy," was painfully recovering from the effects of the Soviet attack. A resolution endorsed by the NLNE and the ANA was passed, offering President Roosevelt "the support and strength of our organizations in any nursing activity in which we can be of service to the country." On that high note, the convention closed [4].

Meanwhile the alumnae of the Army School of Nursing also met. Stimulated by preparations for national defense, this small group discussed reopening the Army School. Although Annie Goodrich was enthusiastic about this suggestion, Julia Stimson, Chief of the Army Nurse Corps and president of the American Nurses' Association, reacted unfavorably. Despite her 11 years as Dean and Administrator of the School and her stout resistance to closing it, she now considered the expense of reopening it unjustifiable if other adequate training schools were available.

After the ANA had failed to support reopening the Army School, Miss Goodrich decided to act on an individual basis. At her suggestion, Frances Payne Bolton, now a member of Congress and still a staunch friend of nursing, appealed directly to Secretary of War Harry B. Woodring. Because of insufficient military appropriations, however, he could not assure her that the school would be reopened.

Nor did Congresswoman Bolton limit her appeals on behalf of the Army School of Nursing to the Secretary of War. Together with Mary Beard, Annie Goodrich, and other alumnae, she called on the Surgeon General of the Army, who told them firmly that the Medical Department had no intention of training personnel for its various technical branches. Mrs. Bolton later recalled that she had kept

... some correspondence with the then Acting Secretary of War to the effect that all of the skeleton framework (for the Army School) would be most carefully kept and if we ever needed it, it would immediately be opened up again. So, in the innocence and naivete, I can't say of youth, when things became embroiled this time, Miss Byrd and Miss Goodrich and Sister Olivia and Miss Hoherty and one other, and myself, called upon the Surgeon General. We thought that all we had to do was to remind him of the skeleton framework that was there and he would immediately start moving. But not Surgeon General Magee! We were told most definitely that the Army was not going to teach all these various branches, he was too busy with the Army, and that it was up to the civilian hospitals to furnish the nurses [5].

Formation of the Nursing Council for National Defense

Five top officials of the nursing profession—Julia C. Stimson, Stella Goostray,

Grace Ross, Mary Beard, and Mary Roberts—gathered for a cheerless meeting in the conference room of the ANA's New York headquarters on July 29, 1940. The main issue was how to prepare nursing for the war that was almost certain to come. Years later, Stella Goostray recalled the events that had precipitated this meeting:

On July 10, 1940, Isabel Stewart, as the newly-elected president of the NLNE, wrote me regarding "the need of some official nursing committee or commission to think through the position that nurses should take with respect to national defense and the many adjustments that may be called for within the next few months . . . . I believe we should have such a commission or board that is representative of the nursing profession as a whole and that it should be at work now, and not wait until Miss Beard calls on us to do something in connection with the American Red Cross." I wrote [to Julia Stimson] on July 9, 1940 . . . . Julia Stimson lost no time, and on July 29, just short of three weeks from the date of Miss Stewart's first letter to me, representatives of five national nursing organizations—ANA, NOPHN, NLNE, NACGN, ACSN, and representatives of several Federal agencies—Army Nurse Corps, Navy Nurse Corps, Children's Bureau, USPHS, Divisions of State Relations and of Hospitals, Nursing Service, Veterans Administration Nursing Service, Department of Indian Affairs, and the ARCNS met in New York. By the end of that day, the Nursing Council on National Defense was on its way [6].

. While the Nursing Council of National Defense was being formed, the news of the war in Europe continued to be bleak. By June 22, 1940, all resistance to Hitler in western Europe had ceased. France had already fallen and Britain stood in mortal danger. Apparently only a miracle could prevent Hitler from winning total victory. Many Americans thought that the fall of France might well be followed by that of England—which would bring Hitler's forces within conceivable striking distance of America.

On September 16, 1940, the President signed the first peacetime conscription measure ever enacted in American history: the Selective Training and Service Act of 1940. This law, which reflected an awareness of imminent danger, was an attempt to satisfy the exigencies of modern warfare, which could no longer be waged on a voluntary basis but required instead the total mobilization and disposition of manpower through a system at once compulsory and selective. The Selective Service System provided for the registration, first of all of men between the ages of 21 and 36, and subsequently of those between 18 and 64.

Six months later, on March 1, 1941, an emergency health and sanitation bill was passed, which provided funds to supplement public health nursing services for the families of workers in major defense industries. The funds for this program, which were administered by the United States Public Health Service, mandated the recruitment of 115 public health nurses. In addition, 90 more were needed at once by the Public Health Service.

Defense Spending Affects Health Facilities and Nursing Education
On June 28, 1941, President Roosevelt signed the Community Facilities Act, which was popularly known as the Lanham Bill. Under the terms of this act,

nonprofit private agencies received grants from the federal government for the equipment and operation of community service facilities in defense areas, including schools, hospitals, and clinics. Within six weeks after the bill's passage, President Roosevelt had approved federal grants from a number of health projects, including hospitals, clinics, and nurses' homes.

In order to insure an adequate supply of well-trained nurses for both military and civilian nursing services, Congress passed the Labor-Federal Security Appropriation Act, which was signed by the President on July 1, 1941. An initial appropriation of $1,800,000 was earmarked for nursing education. Specifically, funds were allocated for refresher courses to prepare retired nurses in modern methods, for supplementary courses in special fields, and for aid to basic schools of nursing to increase the number of students in regular undergraduate classes. Three consultants in nursing education were quickly appointed to draw up requirements for the allocation of funds, which were to be administered by the Public Health Service, and to assist in the implementation of the Act: Margaret G. Arnstein of the New York State Department of Health, Lucile Petry, associate professor of nursing at the University of Minnesota, and Eugenia K. Spalding, associate professor of nursing education at Catholic University in Washington, D.C.

The Subcommittee on Nursing of the Health and Medical Committee of the

The first federal funds ever granted to undergraduate nursing students and schools were appropriated in 1941.

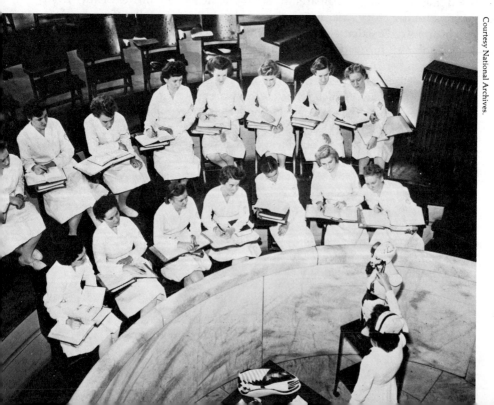

Federal Security Agency, together with three additional consultants to the Subcommittee, served as the Advisory Committee to the Public Health Service for this program. The three consultants to the Subcommittee were Isabel M. Stewart, director of the Division of Nursing Education at Teachers College, Columbia University, Anna D. Wolf, director of the School of Nursing and director of nursing service at Johns Hopkins Hospital, and Elizabeth D. Soule, director of the School of Nursing Education at the University of Washington. Letters specifying the conditions under which funds could be allocated and the procedure to be followed in requesting such funds were sent to all 1400 state accredited schools of nursing and to universities offering programs of study in nursing education. Soon 88 out of the 300 schools of nursing that applied were selected to receive this federal aid to train additional student nurses. Sixty-seven schools in 32 states offered refresher courses to 3000 graduate nurses, and 26 other schools enrolled 500 graduate nurses for postgraduate study.

Crash Program to Train Nurses' Aides

In August, 1941, 800 nursing schools were invited by New York Mayor Fiorello H. LaGuardia, director of civilian defense, to participate in a nationwide program to augment the nursing services of hospitals, clinics, and public health and field nursing agencies. Mayor LaGuardia urged these institutions to cooperate with the American Red Cross and the Office of Civilian Defense in training 100,000 volunteer nurses' aides so that each hospital nurse might have at least one trained aide to help her extend her services to many more patients. "The deficiency in nursing personnel will be overwhelmingly accentuated if this country becomes actively involved in defensive combat," Mayor LaGuardia predicted in extending his invitation to the schools [7].

Five essential requirements for the effective use of volunteer nurses' aides were listed by the Office of Civilian Defense, which urged hospitals and nursing schools to cooperate in training aides: (1) they had to be intensively trained; (2) throughout the period of national emergency they had to continue serving an adequate number of hours in a hospital or clinic, or in field service; (3) they had to be prepared to conform to the discipline of the organization in which they were to work; (4) they were to render service without pay; (5) they were not to replace paid hospital personnel but were to serve specifically as nurses' assistants.

The Drift toward War

As the nation continued to prepare for war, figures indicated that state-accredited schools had admitted 41,397 students for the 1940–1941 academic year, some 5000 short of the estimated need. These figures provided clear evidence of the additional need for federal aid. At the same time on the international scene, two ships carrying nurses of the London-bound Red Cross-Harvard Unit were torpedoed and five nurses and the house mother died. Soon afterwards Presi-

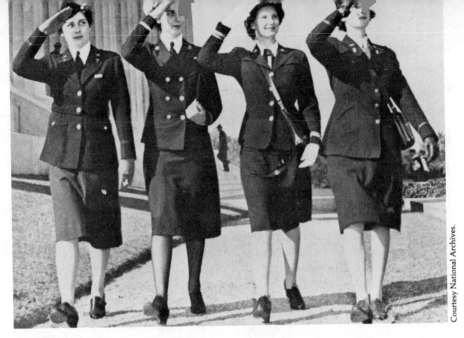

Women of the military services in 1942.

dent Roosevelt decided to furnish naval escorts to merchant ships crossing the North Atlantic.

The incident that finally brought America into conflict with the Axis powers did not occur in Europe, however, but in the Pacific. During the long months when American relations with Germany were growing increasingly tense, Secretary of State Cordell Hull was conducting complicated negotiations with the Japanese. Since the invasion of Manchuria, Americans had observed with growing apprehension the advance of Japanese imperialism in Asia. As December began, hopes for peace were faint.

Although it was known that the Japanese were preparing to mount an offensive, most military experts expected them to attack the British and Dutch possessions in Southeast Asia. Hardly anyone suspected that Hawaii would be the target of a Japanese strike. American commanders had received routine warnings but had taken few precautions. At Pearl Harbor the double row of American war ships, all except for carriers in port for the first time since July 4, presented perfect targets to the first wave of Japanese bombers that burst unexpectedly out of the skies at 7:55 A.M. on December 7, 1941. All in all, the Japanese sank five battleships, severely damaged three others, and hit numerous lesser vessels. Of the 2403 Americans killed during this surprise air raid, nearly half lost their lives when the battleship *Arizona* exploded. Military and civilian nurses at Pearl Harbor rendered heroic service in caring for the many casualties.

Personnel Possibilities of the Military Nurse Services

During the early years of World War II, nurses were in a constant quandry as to whether they should join one of the military nursing services or remain in

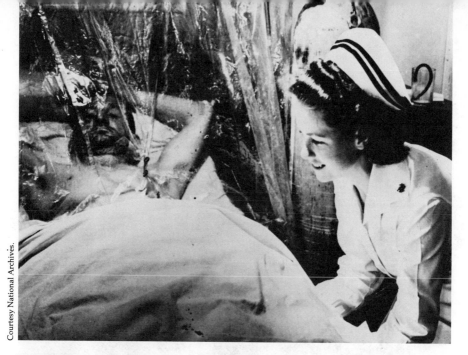

Navy nurse securing oxygen tent for a wounded soldier.

their civilian positions. To help hospitals and other employing agencies as well as individual nurses, the National Nursing Council for War Service established guidelines for two categories of service. These guidelines were approved by the health and medical committee and the nursing subcommittee of the Office of Defense Health and Welfare Service and by the American Red Cross. A nurse should serve with the armed forces, according to the Council, if she was single, under 40, and: (1) doing private duty; (2) on a hospital's general staff; (3) a head nurse not essential for teaching or supervision; (4) a public health nurse not essential for maintaining minimum civilian health service in any given community; (5) in a non-nursing position; or (6) an office nurse.

On the other hand, a nurse should serve at home if she had a position: (1) as an administrator, instructor, supervisor, or head nurse in a hospital having a school of nursing; (2) as an administrator or supervisor in a hospital without a school of nursing; (3) as an administrator, teacher, supervisor, or staff nurse in a public health agency essential for maintaining minimum civilian health services in any given community.

Nurses who joined the military at the beginning of the war received few benefits. The Army offered nurses "relative rank," which amounted to an officer's title and uniform without an officer's commission, retirement privileges, dependents' allowances, or pay. Similarly, the Navy offered only vague "officer's privileges" until this disparity was partially remedied by Congress in July, 1942, when members of the Navy Nurse Corps were also given "relative rank." Even then the injustice of less pay for the same rank prevailed: the nurse ensign received a base pay of $90 a month, compared to $150 for a male ensign.

On December 1, 1943, Frances Payne Bolton introduced in the House of Representatives a bill to remedy this injustice. It would have provided full

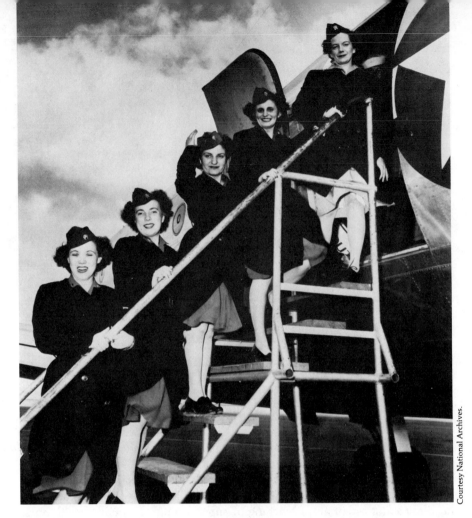

Navy flight nurses on their way to a forward area.

military rank for members of the Army Nurse Corps. After considering this bill for four months, the War Department reported adversely on it, primarily because it authorized permanent officer's rank for nurses. Meanwhile the sad plight of the Army nurse with mere relative rank was highlighted by a reporter in a March, 1944, column in the *Rocky Mountain News*:

Here is the case of Sue—consider it, and reach your own conclusions.

Sue is a college graduate. After an arts degree, she studied nursing and after graduation taught nursing in a university. Early in 1941, believing war was imminent, she volunteered as an Army Nurse. She was at Pearl Harbor when the attack came. She was under fire, and cared for wounded men during long weeks of agony. Exposure, fatigue, the strain of intense and exciting work, shattered her health. She was sent to Fitzsimons Hospital to be treated for tuberculosis. After a year's treatment she was found to be totally and permanently disabled.

Her discharge pay, as an Army nurse, second lieutenant, is $60 a month.

Had she held the same rank as a WAC or a WAVE or a Navy nurse, her pay would be $112.50 a month.

"We are proud to be Army nurses," several young women whose situation is similar to that of Sue told me. "But we don't like to be treated as stepchildren."

At this moment there are more than 100 nurse patients at Fitzsimons Hospital who are facing the same sort of discrimination [8].

After referring to several other cases of blatant injustice to disabled military nurses, the columnist went on to say:

Maybe they will recover, and be able to return to active duty. They hope so, of course. But if they don't—well, they'll be subject to the same sort of discrimination that worked to the detriment of Sue.

Why isn't the Army nurse given a square deal? Because, from some strange quirk—or perhaps from plain neglect—the Army nurse, although she belongs to the oldest service women's corps, holds only what is called "relative rank." A Navy nurse is entitled to the same benefits and privileges of any other officer of her grade; so is an officer of the WACs or WAVES. But, whereas any of the other second lieutenants is allowed under a permanent disability three-fourths of a base pay of $150 a month, the Army nurse is given an allowance on a base pay of $90 a month.

Why? Because the rank of the others is permanent, the rank of the Army Nurse is relative [9].

Finally, on June 22, 1944, Congress enacted a law providing members of the Army Nurse Corps and the Navy Nurse Corps with temporary officer's rank. For the duration of the war and for six months thereafter they were entitled to the same initial pay, allowances, rights, benefits, and privileges as prescribed by law for commissioned officers.

Navy nurses on their way to hospital duty, Naval Air Station, Adak, Alaska, 1943.

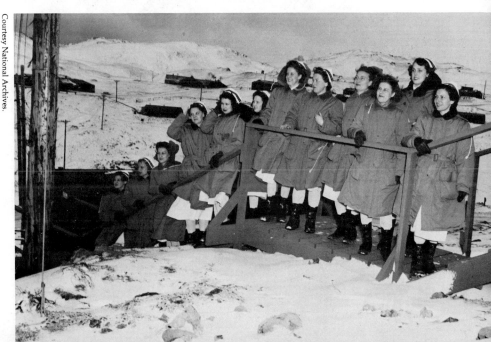

Nurses in North Africa

Meanwhile, after invading North Africa, the Allies waged a seesaw struggle across the desert with the German forces, which were finally defeated at Bizerte in Tunisia in May, 1943. A note written by Lieutenant Charlotte Jean Webber of the Army's Thirty-eighth Evacuation Hospital contained a description of the new African base of operations.

We live in tents somewhere in Northwest Africa and love it. Only we don't take baths, wash our hair, shave, or wash clothes—just one big, dirty, happy family. It's cold at night. I sleep on an Army cot in my sleeping bag with my wool robe on and four Army blankets over me and my fur coat in my little field hospital. Worked like blazes to get it set up these first few trying days—and now we have something to be proud of.

We've named all our little streets in the field—my ward tent is on the corner of Kentucky Ave. and Second St. Our mess tent's called "New York Hotel" and my tent is named "My Old Kentucky Home."

I certainly have a time trying to talk French with these French people. Those two years I had in French in Cynthiana High do come in handy. When I was in town I went to a shop to buy some pins; the French shopkeepers kept jabbering to us and we couldn't understand a thing they said. Finally, I gathered they wanted us to go with them for a drink of wine. Well, they left their shop wide open and took us down to their house, sat us down, and brought out three bottles, and finally FDR's picture, and we all drank a toast to Roosevelt [10].

Army nurses catch some rest between battles in Tunisia during the campaign in North Africa.

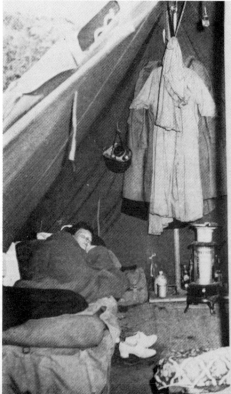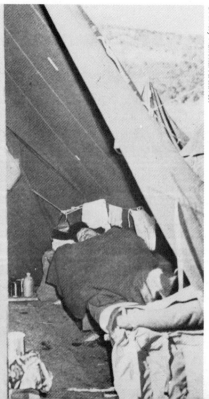

The evacuation hospital was an intermediate link in the medical chain that extended from the battlefield to general hospitals in the United States. Badly wounded men were treated in field hospitals close to the front, but they began actual recovery in the evacuation hospital, located from five to 50 miles farther to the rear. Less serious casualties were sometimes sent directly to the evacuation hospital from front-line medical clearing stations. When patients who needed treatment were strong enough to travel, they were transported to larger, more specialized hospitals far from the battle zone. Those who required more than 30 days to recover were evacuated to hospitals in Sicily and North America, and those who required at least 120 days were returned to the United States. Although evacuation hospitals lacked the tiled neatness of peacetime facilities, they were nonetheless complete and efficient medical units. Many of their patients could be discharged without further treatment. At the evacuation hospital the sick and the wounded enjoyed the luxury of warm baths, clean pajamas, and soft bathrobes for the first time since leaving home. There they also often received medical attention for the first time from nurses.

Ernie Pyle was one of an estimated 1600 American war correspondents, but probably no other combat journalist will be as long remembered. Reporting from the European and Pacific theaters, he captured a devoted following of Americans at home and overseas. His simple style, his directness, and his admiration for the front-line soldier seemed to satisfy the public's appetite for humanized war reporting. Beginning in November, 1942, Pyle followed American fighting men and women from North Africa to Sicily and then to Italy. He made the following comments about the Thirty-eighth Evacuation Hospital's nurses:

The officers and nurses live two in a tent on two sides of a company street—nurses on one side, officers on the other. The street has a neat sign at the end on which is painted "Carolina Avenue." Some Yankee has painted under this "Rebel Street" . . . . The 300 men who do the non-medical work live in their little shelter tents just on beyond. They're mostly from New England. They've built a little wall of whitewashed rocks between the two areas and put up a sign saying "Mason-Dixon Line" . . . . The nurses wear khaki overalls because of the mud and dust. Doctors go around tieless and with knit brown caps on their heads. Pink female panties fly from a line among the brown warlike tents. On the flagpole is a Red Cross flag, made from a bed sheet and a French soldier's red sash [11].

The American nurses—and there were lots of them—turned out just as you would expect: wonderfully. Army doctors, and patients, too, were unanimous in their praise of them. Doctors told me that in the first rush of casualties they were calmer than the men.

The Carolina nurses, too, took it like soldiers. For the first ten days they had to live like animals, even using open ditches for toilets, but they never complained.

One nurse was always on duty in each tentful of 20 men. She had medical orderlies to help her. Most of the time the nurses wore army coveralls, but Colonel Bauchspies [commanding officer] wanted them to put on dresses once in a while, for he said the effect on the men was astounding. The touch of femininity, the knowledge that a woman was around, gave the wounded man courage and confidence and a feeling of security. And the more feminine, the better [12].

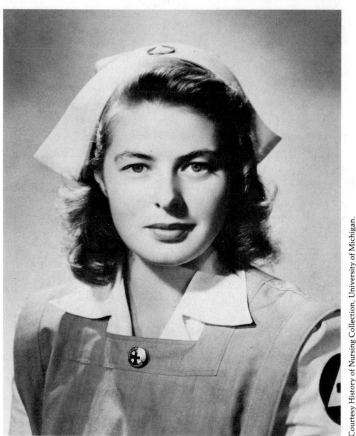

Ingrid Bergman helped popularize the drive to train 100,000 nurses' aides during the early years of the war.

Courtesy History of Nursing Collection, University of Michigan.

Nursing under Fire in Italy

The Allies followed up their victory over the Germans in North Africa by landing first on Sicily and then in Italy. In September, 1943, American troops landed at Salerno and began a long, arduous campaign up the mountainous Italian penninsula. On September 15 the first American Army nurses to set foot on European soil since 1918 landed in the Salerno sector of Italy and immediately went to work in a field hospital. Wearing GI helmets and fatigues with long trousers, these 57 nurses dug in like regular soldiers to take cover during air raids in order to remain with the wounded men.

It was only 100 miles from Naples to Rome, but despite their numerical superiority on land and in the air and their control of the adjacent seas, the Allied troops required eight months to cover this distance. Some of the most mountainous terrain in Europe barred the way to Rome, the objective of the winter campaign of 1943–1944. In an attempt to break the stalemate the Allies made an amphibious landing in the rear of the Germans, at Anzio, 37 miles south of Rome, on January 23, 1944. Even though this landing caught the Germans completely by surprise, they reacted swiftly. Luftwaffe bombers sank a number of Allied transports and warships, and the Allied troops, along with the hospital units, had to dig in on an open plain, where they were subjected to constant air and ground attacks by the enemy. Instead of becoming the spearhead for an Allied military thrust, the Anzio beachhead became a beleaguered fort.

Six nurses, five of them members of the Army Nurse Corps, the other serving as a Red Cross worker, were the first American women killed in the war as a direct result of enemy action. They died of wounds received on the Anzio beachhead on February 7 and February 10, 1944. The nurses were First Lieutenant Blanche F. Sigman, a graduate of Bellevue Hospital; First Lieutenant Marjorie Morrow, a graduate of Iowa Methodist Hospital School of Nursing, Des Moines, Iowa; First Lieutenant Glenda Spelhaug, a graduate of Saint Luke's Hospital School of Nursing, Saint Paul, Minnesota; and Second Lieutenant La Verne Farquhar, graduate of King's Daughters Hospital, Temple, Texas.

Once again military nurses witnessed dreadful suffering. One young University of Minnesota graduate wrote to a relative:

Ensign Jeanne Perriog, Navy Nurse Corps, writes a letter to Mom for Private Odean Sorensen, United States Marine Corps.

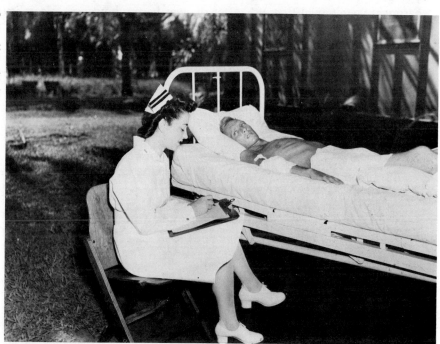

It is now 3 A.M. Most of my patients are asleep so I have a chance to write a few words . . . . Oh, aunt, I feel so tired lately, my stomach feels to be upside down. When I am asleep I wake up constantly and can't get a rest . . . . Recently we are getting very bad casualties. It makes me shiver to just look at them. You can't imagine, aunt, what we see over here. I will never forget it—it is heart-breaking.

One of my patients, only 24, has a piece of shrapnel in his heart, another, 29 and married, has both legs off—his hips are broken, his intestines exposed. Another, 19, was shot through the abdomen, and after the Germans found him lying, they kicked him and shot him into the head, to finish him . . . . He suffers much. His eyes are gone. I have also two patients who were shot through the brain. They lost their eyesight and are crazy. This is just a little part of what we see [13].

The Birth of Flight Nursing

One of the most exciting innovations in military nursing was the development of flight nursing. It appears that Lauretta M. Schimmoler, who as early as 1932 envisioned an "Aerial Nurse Corps of America," deserves credit for the original idea of the flight nurse. By 1940 the Army Nurse Corps and the Red Cross Nursing Service were receiving many requests for information about flight nursing. Answers to these inquiries revealed official opposition to such an organization and a lack of imagination concerning the possibility of using aircraft to evacuate the wounded.

When the war began it was thought that cargo or bomber-type aircraft would be used to transport ill or injured Army personnel. It was not deemed necessary to assign nurses to the Air Corps, inasmuch as enlisted men in the Medical Department were taught first aid. After the war began, however, this policy

Lauretta M. Schimmoler, fourth from the left in this group of auxiliary "Aerial Nurse Corps" flight nurses, originated the idea of the flight nurse.

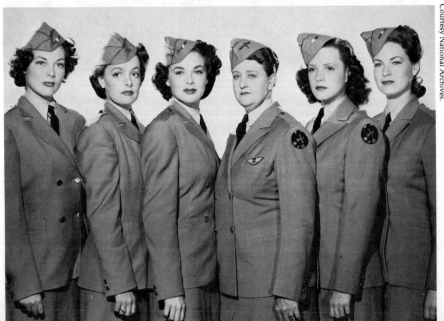

was sharply reversed by the establishment of a Nursing Division in the Air Surgeon's Office in September, 1942.

Nurses clamored for admittance to the new Flight Nursing School organized at Bowman Field, Kentucky. There the flight nurse was trained to perform a variety of duties in connection with air evacuation of the sick, wounded, and injured as well as at ground medical installations. After applying for a commission in the Army Nurse Corps, a graduate nurse had to serve a minimum of six months in an Army Air Force unit hospital before applying for admittance to the Flight Nursing School. In addition, she had to fulfill the following physical qualifications: between 62 and 72 inches in height, between 105 and 135 pounds in weight, and between 21 and 36 years of age.

To a large extent these qualifications limited flight nurse candidates to the young and physically fit who were anxious to fly and practice their profession close to a combat area. They performed most of their duties at flight altitudes of 5000 to 10,000 feet in aircraft without pressurized cabins. Since work under such conditions was extremely strenuous, it was important for the nurses to be in excellent health.

In February, 1943, the first class of flight nurses graduated at the Bowman Field chapel. The 39 members of this group, which included many former airline hostesses, had been poorly housed and had completed a program of instruction still in the experimental stage. The four-week course had included classwork in air evacuation nursing, air evacuation tactics, survival, aeromedical physiology, and flight-related mental hygiene. In addition, the nurses had received training in plane-loading procedures and military indoctrination and had participated in a one-day bivouac.

The School of Air Evacuation, the first of its kind, exerted worldwide influence. In November, 1943, the course of instruction for flight nurses was increased from four weeks to eight weeks. Emphasis was placed on the study of anatomy, physiology, ward management, operating-room technique, nursing, first-aid hygiene, and sanitation. Two weeks of the course were devoted to specialized training at cooperating hospitals in Louisville.

A nurse did not automatically receive the designation of "flight nurse." After completing the course, she had to submit a request to the Commanding General of the Army Air Forces, who had the authority to grant such a designation. Upon certification the nurse was permitted to wear the flight nurse's wings. During the period from December, 1942 to October, 1944, 1079 flight nurses graduated from the AAF School of Air Evacuation.

Adventures of Flight Nurses

The work of the flight nurse was extremely dangerous because the aircraft in which she flew, usually C-46 "Commandos," acted in a dual capacity. After transporting cargo and troops to the battle fronts they were unloaded and rapidly converted into ambulance planes for the return trip. Because of their dual function the C-46s were not marked with the Geneva Red Cross or other

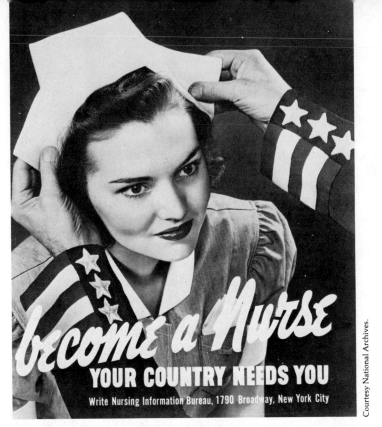

An appeal to the nation's young women to become nurses during World War II.

noncombatant designation and consequently, even though loaded with sick and wounded on return trips, were fair game for enemy fighters. For this reason, all flight nurses were volunteers.

An adventurous life awaited the flight nurse. Second Lieutenant Mary Louise Hawkins of Redwood City, California, had charge of 24 litter patients en route to Guadalcanal when the plane began running low on fuel. As the pilot was passing over a tiny island, he spotted a 150-foot square clearing fringed by tall coconut palms. Rather than ditch the plane at sea, he decided to attempt a crash landing. During the landing a propeller tore a hole in the side of the fuselage, but the patients and crew escaped injury except for one man whose windpipe was severed by a severe cut that fortunately missed the jugular vein. By devising a suction tube from a syringe, a colonic tube, and the inflation tubes from a "Mae West" life jacket, Lieutenant Hawkins was able to keep the man's throat clear of blood until help arrived 19 hours later. After establishing radio contact and receiving supplies of glucose and plasma by parachute, the stranded passengers were picked up by a Navy destroyer and brought to Guadalcanal.

Lucy I. Wilson, one of the nurses who had escaped from Corregidor, later returned to the Philippines as a flight nurse. On its first flight from Leyte, her plane evacuated 15 soldiers. "After watching men suffer and die on Bataan and Corregidor because of lack of medical facilities," she said, "it gave me the greatest satisfaction to realize that these men were being flown to the finest hospital care within a few hours." Elsewhere in the European theater the Distinguished Flying Cross was awarded posthumously to Lieutenant Aleda E. Lutz of Saginaw, Michigan, who was killed after flying more than 190 missions to evacuate wounded personnel from combat areas. Lieutenant Lutz also received the Air Medal with four Oak Leaf Clusters.

Not to be outdone, the Navy instituted a flight nurse training program that included lectures, demonstrations, and practice of skills such as loading patients into planes, the various phases of in-flight nursing care, preparation for emergency abandonment of the plane in flight, and maintenance and use of medical equipment. The nurse was also trained to use oxygen in flight and to administer it to her patients. Survival training prepared her to discharge her responsibilities to preserve life and health in any given situation.

The Navy flight nurse and a pharmacist's mate worked as a team. They evacuated patients from forward naval stations to base hospitals or to larger hospitals where patients received more prolonged treatment. The pharmacist's mates assigned to this service received their training with the nurses in naval air transport squadrons. After completing this training they flew with the nurses aboard hospital planes in the continental United States and thereby gained practical experience on regular hospital flights of the Naval Air Transport Service.

Upon completion of this training the nurse and the pharmacist's mate were ready for assignment to the Navy's new air evacuation service. One of the major goals was to equalize the patient load of naval hospitals in the United States so that those nearest the Pacific combat zones were not overfilled while beds in hospitals farther from the front remained empty. Another objective was to give the sick or wounded men specialized treatment at hospitals that concentrated on certain types of cases. Finally, whenever it was feasible, an attempt was made to place the men in hospitals as near their homes as possible. Two-engine Douglas Skytrains served as flying ambulances for the Navy. Marked with a large Red Cross on each side of the fuselage, the planes could accommodate 24 litter patients or 27 walking wounded. If the plane was not filled, regular passengers could be carried, provided there were no patients aboard with contagious diseases.

The attractive flying uniform of forest green for winter and gray for summer—trousers, shirt, battle jacket-type coat, and a garrison or visored cap—was worn only when the nurses were on actual flight duty. The new flight nurse insignia, a pair of gold embossed wings with a center oval bearing the anchor and oak leaf symbol of the Navy Nurse Corps, was worn on the left breast pocket.

The medical kit for each flight contained equipment similar to that kept in a medicine cabinet on a ward. There were bedpans and urinals for the litter cases, first aid articles, and sterile supplies such as needles, syringes, catheters, Levin tubes, and dressings. Because this medical kit also contained stimulants, narcotics, blood plasma, and intravenous fluids, the flight nurse kept the key in her possession at all times. Thus equipped, an aircraft was ready to carry any type of patient for any distance.

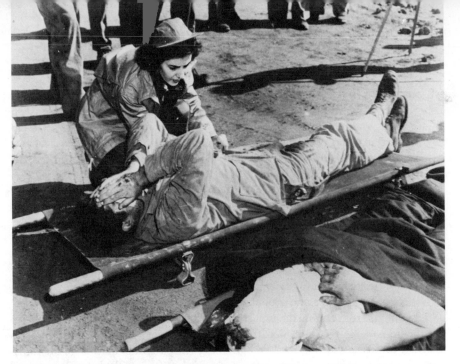

Ensign Jane Kendleigh aids a wounded marine on Iwo Jima.

Ensign Jane Kendleigh, one of the early Navy flight nurses, was the first Navy nurse to fly to Iwo Jima to evacuate casualties. Landing at the airfield under heavy mortar fire, she and the crew took cover in foxholes while planes dispatched by an aircraft carrier wiped out enemy positions north of the field. Later, Ensign Kendleigh became the first Navy nurse to land on Okinawa, where her plane evacuated 20 wounded men on its first flight back to Guam.

Industrial Nursing Booms

Meanwhile, back on the civilian front, nurses were not oblivious to the massive boom in the defense industry that had developed to support the war effort. One of the more striking effects of the war on the nursing profession was a 100 percent increase in employment of public health nurses in industry, from 5512 in 1941 to 11,200 by the end of 1943. The nurse was usually employed by a company to carry out a nursing program of preventive medicine and health education among the employees. Small plants were purchasing increasing amounts of part-time service from visiting nurse associations.

After Pearl Harbor the Committee on Duties of Nurses in Industry recommended that one industrial nurse be provided for up to 300 employees, two or more nurses for up to 600 employees, three or more for up to 1000 employees, one nurse for each additional 1000 employees up to 5000, and one for each additional 2000 employees above that point. The small plant was the most deficient in health care services. Some 26 million workers in the United States were employed in plants having fewer than 500 workers each, and 13 million worked in plants with fewer than 100 workers. Part-time service by a voluntary or

official public health nursing group represented the only feasible way of satisfying the health care needs of these small plants.

In March, 1941, a public health nursing consultant had been assigned to the
staff of the division of industrial hygiene at the National Institute of Health in
Bethesda, Maryland. Her activity did much to stimulate the progress of industrial nursing on a national scale through her many contacts with industrial
nursing on a national scale as well as through the various industrial hygiene
departments. The number of state health departments employing nursing consultants in the field of industrial hygiene grew steadily, and by the end of 1942
there were a total of 18 of these consultants located in the various states.

The nurses were employed in all types of manufacturing plants. As the war
progressed, data issued by the Office of War Information revealed that 65,000
people had been killed in industry in the two years from December 7, 1941, to
December 31, 1943—more than the military casualties for the same period.

*Nurse cleaning a minor cut in the first aid room of the medical department of a large
industrial plant. In addition to first aid and other nursing duties, the industrial nurse engaged in a wide variety of related activities, such as safety education, hygiene, nutrition,
and the improvement of working conditions.*

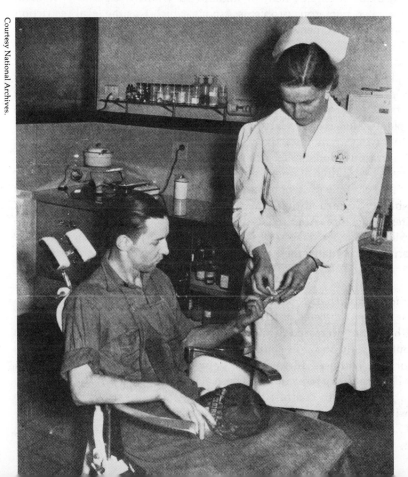

The 210,000 workers injured during the same period exceeded by far the number wounded in battle. According to the same agency, about 50,000 workers were absent every day from industrial jobs because of accidents or injuries. Deaths and injuries on the job resulted in the loss of 270 million work-days per year—equivalent to a loss of 900,000 workers from production lines.

By analyzing the data collected in 1943 from industrial establishments throughout the nation, one investigator concluded that a nurse on eight-hour dispensary duty should be able to attend to and record from 50 to 115 problems per day. These figures were averages for nurses whose full time was spent in the dispensary; the higher number of visits per day per nurse were found in the larger industrial medical units, where nursing service was more specialized. A case load as high as 600 for one nurse in one day was boasted by one company during a successful immunization program. Apparently, all nurses who had an average case load of 75 a day or more were limited to the routine changing of dressings on minor injuries and to the dispensing of medication. On the other hand, it was interesting to note that all industrial medical departments surveyed expected a nurse to see at least 50 cases if she stayed in the dispensary all day.

The war-induced employment of millions of women, especially in small plants, presented numerous problems, among which was the legal restriction on work-hours for women. Another problem was the new Federal Contracts Act, which stipulated that no work should be carried out in surroundings that were unsanitary, hazardous, or dangerous to the health of either women or men. Employers were usually willing to cooperate with these regulations, which nurses helped to enforce. This assistance, however, represented only one aspect of the nurse's usefulness to the tens of thousands of new women workers in industrial plants. Nurses appreciated the special concerns of women, such as rest periods following strenuous activity, facilities to insure cleanliness, the availability of nutritious foods, relief from some of the emotional and physical demands made by children at home, and reactions to the work environment. For example, safe clothing for women presented a problem. Because long hair was fashionable for women at that time, women workers covered their hair with the greatest reluctance. After requesting actress Veronica Lake to pose for photographs illustrating the dangers of wearing long hair while operating machines, the government circulated these pictures widely.

The Nation's Health in 1943

When the nation completed its first year of war in early 1943, concern for civilian health had not decreased. Under wartime conditions, weaknesses in health care would rapidly show in statistics. The general death rate in the United States for 1918 had been 18.1 per 1000 population. For 1942 it was estimated at 10.4. This gratifying reduction had been achieved very slowly.

It was interesting to contrast the 10 leading causes of death in 1918 with those in 1943. In 1918 they were heart disease, pneumonia, tuberculosis, kidney disease, cerebral hemorrhage, birth injuries and other diseases associated with early infancy, cancer, accidents, diarrhea, and diabetes. In the few short years since 1936, the new sulfonamide drugs had revolutionized the treatment of a long list of infections: blood poisoning, puerperal fever, septic sore throat, scarlet fever, and pneumonia. Certain threats to the nation's health had been dealt with in a spectacular fashion and were no longer of great concern; however, others had not been reduced, and still others had actually increased.

The 1918 death rate from typhoid, for example, had been at least 15 times higher than in 1943, and the diphtheria rate for 1918 had been 25 times higher. Despite the disruption of civilian life due to the war, typhoid fever and diphtheria had continued to decline since 1941. Physicians and nurses knew how to prevent these diseases and how to control their spread, at minimum expense to communities and individual families. State and local health departments maintained close supervision of water, milk, and food supplies, vulnerable groups were vaccinated against typhoid, and a higher proportion of children and young people had been protected against diphtheria than at any time in the past.

In 1918 tuberculosis had been the third highest cause of death. By 1943 it had dropped to seventh place, claiming about four lives in every 10,000 of the population. Yet tuberculosis of the lungs still remained the leading cause of death among people 20 to 45 years of age—the young men and women upon whom the nation heavily relied for building the Army and Navy and for producing the weapons of war.

Pneumonia had been the second most frequent cause of death in 1918 and not entirely because of the influenza epidemic. It continued to rank third among the leading causes of death until 1938, when the widespread use of sulfa drugs began to reduce drastically the number of deaths from this disease. The actual number of cases, however, had not substantially decreased, for there still existed no preventive medicine for mass-application.

Although malaria had not been listed among the great killers in the United States during World War I, it was among the 10 highest causes of death in a number of Southern states. It was estimated during the early 1930s that some two million cases occurred each year. No concerted effort was made to eradicate the malaria mosquito in the South until 1935, when federal funds were allotted for work products in 17 states for ditching, draining, dusting, and oiling the breeding waters of *Anopheles quadrimaculatus*, the principal malaria-carrying mosquito.

By 1943 most of the diseases affecting infants no longer ranked among the leading causes of death. On the other hand, diseases associated with old age had become more prevalent since 1918. Cancer, seventh on the 1918 list, had risen to second place in 1943. The mortality rate for heart disease, the number one killer in 1918 and still number one in 1943, had actually increased. Cerebral hemorrhage, kidney disease, and diabetes, which had all moved up a notch or two on the list since 1918, now caused a larger proportion of deaths than they had 25 years earlier.

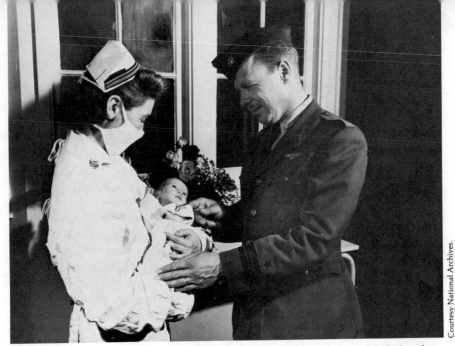

The average newborn baby in 1943 could expect to live 10 years longer than babies born in 1918.

This shift among the leading causes of death occurred primarily because a significant reduction in deaths from childhood diseases had enabled a greater proportion of the population to reach an age at which they were vulnerable to cancer, heart disease, and diabetes. Moreover, medical knowledge about communicable diseases was still inadequate, and methods of preventing and treating adult diseases had not yet been developed. The little knowledge which physicians and nurses had acquired concerning the chronic diseases of middle and late life had not been applied on a wide enough scale to alter the death rates from these diseases.

The first attempts to improve civilian health on a large scale had occurred in the 1920s and thereafter began to yield considerable results. During the period from 1923 to 1943, the average life expectancy in the United States increased from about 55 to 65 years. The average newborn baby in 1943 could expect to live a decade longer than children who had been born during the First World War. This increase was all the more significant when one considers that during the first 20 years of the century the gain had been only five years.

Indicators of Health Problems

Despite these achievements in combating the effects of disease, the results of examinations conducted by local Selective Service boards and military induction centers indicated that the health of the nation's young men was no better at the start of World War II than at the time of the World War I draft. A report of physical examinations from 21 selected states, issued by National Headquarters, Selective Service System, on August 1, 1943, in *Medical Statistics*

Bulletin No. 2, summarized the findings for approximately 121,700 registrants. This publication was a valuable source of information for nurses and other hospital personnel on the incidence of many diseases. The report analyzed the number of draft rejections, which were classified as follows: in a typical group of 1000 registrants examined by local boards, 438 or 43.8 percent were rejected; 90 or 16.0 percent of the remaining 562 were then rejected at induction stations. Thus, of the original 1000 registrants examined, 528 were rejected, representing a combined rejection rate of 52.8 percent.

Rejection rates increased steadily with age. For example, 41.6 percent of the 22-year-old registrants were rejected at either local boards or induction stations, while 80.3 percent of the 36-year-old registrants were rejected.

Tooth defects were the leading cause of rejection, accounting for 16.5 percent of all rejections at local boards and induction stations. Other causes of rejection and the percentages they constituted of all rejections were as follows: eye defects, 11.7 percent; mental and nervous defects, 10.4 percent; cardiovascular defects, 10.0 percent; musculoskeletal defects, 8.9 percent; hernia, 5.9 percent; venereal diseases, 5.9 percent; ear, nose, and throat defects, 5.5 percent; tuberculosis and other lung diseases, 3.8 percent; educational deficiency, 3.8 percent; defects of the feet, 3.0 percent; underweight, 2.9 percent; other causes, 11.7 percent.

Needs on the Home Front

While the emotional appeal of the military service attracted many nurses, the needs of the home front, though less dramatic, were no less real. Dr. William P. Shepard, a public health physician on the West Coast, wrote a letter containing a vivid description of these needs. Health officers in many other parts of the country could recount similar stories:

Increasing pressure for public health nurses to enlist is becoming apparent on the West Coast. It is the public health nurses who are conscious of community needs and, therefore, more prompt in responding to a national appeal.

Knowing what I do of nurses' duties in the Army and Navy, I cannot but feel that this is an unwarranted waste of woman power when public health needs of the civilian population are becoming so urgent and complex. These needs are particularly acute in the many war production areas of this Coast. Out here, industry was less important than mining and agriculture until now.

Almost overnight, great cities of industrial workers have suddenly sprung up where there was little population before. Many small towns have doubled their populations, and I can name 10 or 15 in which the population has been tripled or quadrupled.

Until you see it, you cannot conceive of the serious public health problems this entails. In some of these areas, sewer manholes are overflowing into the streets; rat population, always a serious plague menace on this Coast, has even outstripped human population increases; sanitation of public eating places has broken down; immunization is being neglected. Hospitalization is at a premium in all places and actually unobtainable in many. Remaining physicians are so overworked they must refuse all house calls. One doctor told me the other day a frantic mother phoned that her child had been lying on his head and heels, unconscious, with a high fever, since four that afternoon. He was

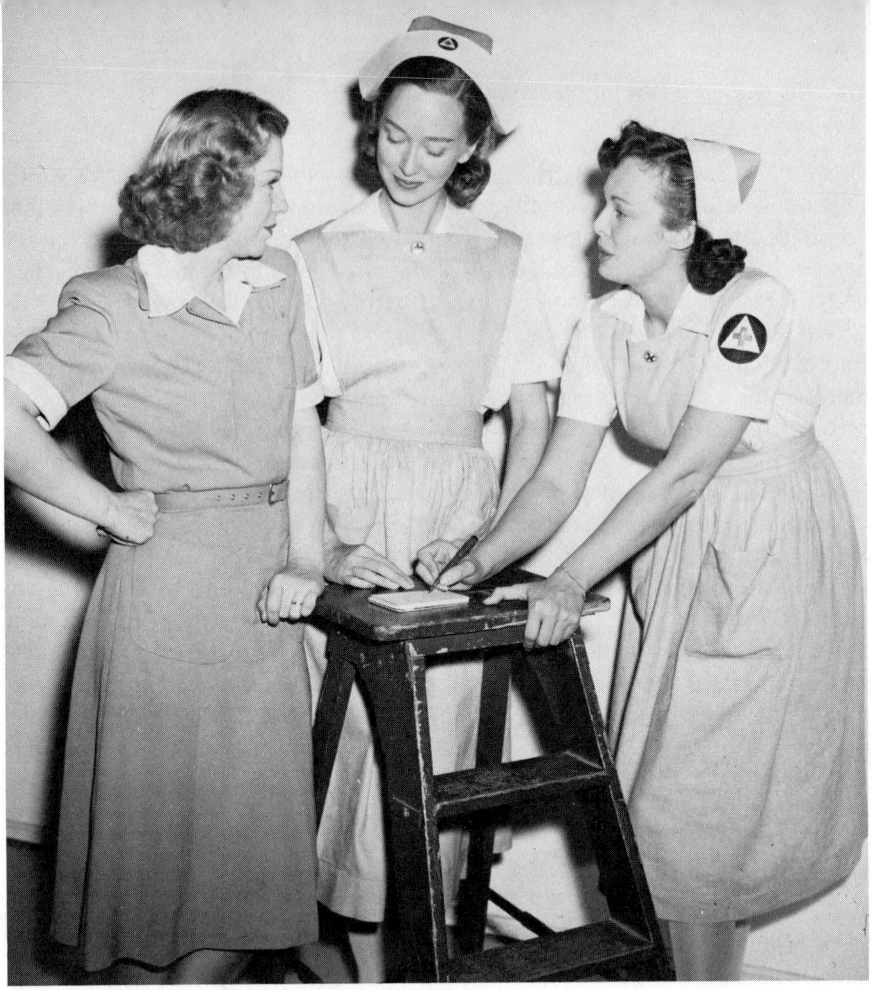

Courtesy National Archives.

As the impact of the withdrawal of more than 75,000 graduate nurses began to be felt, signing up tens of thousands of volunteer nurses' aides was the only recourse.

the fifth doctor she had called and all had been unable to come. He, too, was obliged to decline the call. Deliveries are taking place in homes without even a midwife, let alone a physician, and mothers are being discharged from the hospitals three days postpartum.

For the first time in my memory, organized medical groups, such as county societies and the California Physician's Service, Inc., are appealing for bedside nursing programs. Despite all this, somewhere in the nursing profession there is coercion of public health nurses to join the armed forces. With the winter upon us, which on this Coast means wet clothes and wet feet, and with the overcrowding and migratory problems described above, I am deeply concerned lest this war might be lost on the home front because of lack of wisdom in using trained people where they can do the most good [14].

The quality of service to hospital patients was much poorer in 1943 than in 1938 because patients were receiving fewer hours of care from graduate nurses. Whereas either graduate or student nurses had provided all bedside care in 1938, nonprofessional workers had assumed an appreciable part of this burden by 1943. Full-time personnel had dispensed all bedside care in 1938, while in 1943 part-time personnel were responsible for a significant number of services in some hospitals. In addition, the scarcity of physicians had forced the nursing staff to assume duties formerly performed by doctors. Even worse, the shortage of auxiliary workers—orderlies, ward helpers, and kitchen maids— had compelled the bedside nurses to carry out activities for which these workers had formerly been responsible.

Hospitals in Need of Help

Because of the obvious need of civilian hospitals to bolster their nursing services, they turned to the federal government for help. At the beginning of federal fiscal year 1942–1943, Congress appropriated a sum of $3,500,000 for nursing education, almost double the $1,800,000 that it had voted for the fiscal year 1941–1942. The goals for which these funds had been appropriated, however, were limited. About 3700 inactive graduate nurses had returned to active duty after taking refresher courses. About 4300 graduate nurses had profited from advance study of such specialties as teaching in schools of nursing, nursing in public health, and supervision. Admissions to basic schools of nursing had increased about 12,000 over the first-year enrollments in these same schools during baseline year 1940–1941. Under this program a school could not receive

Although nursing school enrollments had moderately increased, the possibilities for further gains appeared bleak.

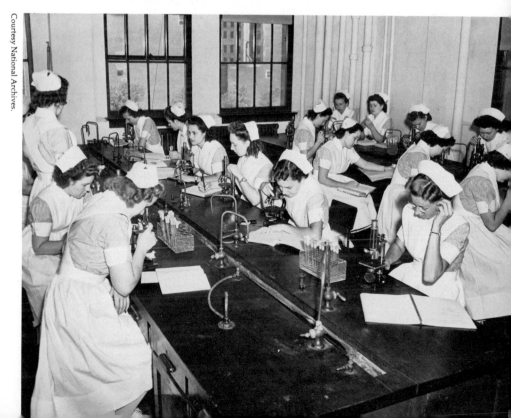

federal aid, except for tuition scholarships, unless it could demonstrate an increase in admissions over the year 1940–1941.

Despite the need for student nurses, federally aided schools achieved only 80 percent of their projected spring 1943 admissions. At the same time, only 67 percent of the expected spring enrollments at all schools materialized. Admission to federally aided schools of nursing declined 10.4 percent in February, 1943, as compared with February, 1942. This difficulty of the nursing schools in attracting an adequate number of student nurses could be explained by the increasingly acute competition for womanpower in 1943. Many young women who would ordinarily have entered schools of nursing were instead joining the women's auxiliaries of the military forces and war industries. Employment statistics for December, 1942, indicated that two to two and one-half million women were needed for war industries, one million for nonwar industries, and 200,000 for the women's armed forces auxiliaries.

Although there were an estimated seven million women in the United States available for full-time work, potential candidates for nurse training were limited largely to young women between 18 and 21 years of age who had graduated from high school and who were physically fit for this strenuous career. It was estimated that 95 percent of all students admitted to schools of nursing were high school graduates. In 1940 the total number of young women graduating from high school was 643,793, of whom a mere 10 percent could be expected to complete a college education.

Employers in other types of war-related work engaged in fierce competition with each other for the services of this tiny group of high school and college graduates. In normal times many young women had been willing to undergo the rigors of nurse training only because of the lack of more attractive employment options. Under the competitive conditions fostered by the war, they could not be expected to limit themselves to nursing when there were opportunities for other types of war service, many of which included paid training. Unless schools of nursing immediately adopted a comprehensive plan for aiding their students, enrollments for 1943 were certain to drop below prewar levels.

Because the armed forces enjoyed the highest priority for receiving nursing care, it was difficult to maintain high standards for nursing services on the home front at the same time. Indeed, the war accentuated the truth of the words of Surgeon General Thomas L. Parran of the United States Public Health Service: "The strength of any nation does not exceed the strength and health of its people." During an all-out war an unchecked epidemic was the ablest ally of the enemy. When for a time armies were being raised faster than ships could be built to transport them, the health of civilian shipbuilders became as important as the health of the Army and Navy. The most obvious solution to this health problem was to educate more nurses. Since a student nurse's potential for service was roughly 60 to 80 percent of that of a graduate nurse, a rapid increase in student nurse enrollments was regarded as the fastest way of enlarging the hospital nurse service force.

The United States Cadet Nurse Corps

To deal with this crisis the Federal Security Agency arranged a series of conferences to explore possible solutions to the acute shortage of nurses. Attended by
representatives from all the major professional nursing and hospital associations, these conferences resulted in a bill introduced into the House of Representatives by Frances Payne Bolton, Congresswoman from Ohio. Widely endorsed by educational groups and professional associations, the bill which
created the United States Cadet Nurse Corps became law on June 15, 1943.

Under the provisions of the Bolton Act the United States Public Health Service subsidized the entire education of nursing students—tuition, fees, books,
uniforms, maintenance, and monthly stipends. In order to obtain the benefits
of the United States Cadet Nurse Corps, a student was not required to prove
actual need of funds, but she did have to promise to engage in essential *military*
or *civilian* nursing for the duration of the war. Candidates were to be between
the ages of 17 and 35 and fulfill minimum admission requirements, which included good health and graduation, with a good scholastic record, from an accredited high school.

The 1944 United States Cadet Nurse Corps recruitment poster.

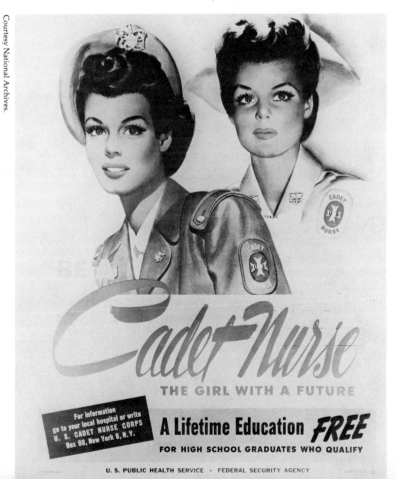

In order to accelerate the period of nurse education, the Bolton Act stipulated that it be reduced from the normal 36 months to 30 months or less. Since state boards of nursing required a three-year program, a compromise establishing three levels of Cadets was worked out: Pre-Cadets, Junior Cadets, and Senior Cadets. Pre-Cadet was the designation given the student during her first nine months in the school, when she was studying the basic sciences and fundamentals of nursing. Junior Cadets were nursing students enrolled for the next 15 to 21 months of their training. Senior Cadets had actually completed their basic educational requirements. The state boards, however, demanded an additional six months' experience. During this period students undertook an important practice assignment either in their home school or in another civilian, military, or government institution.

Immediately after passage of the Bolton Act, the Division of Nurse Education was established within the United States Public Health Service and made directly responsible to the Surgeon General. Lucile Petry, who had been on the nurse education staff of the Public Health Service for two years and had recently been named dean of the Cornell University—New York Hospital School of Nursing, New York City, was appointed as its director. The Federal Security

Lucile Petry, Director of the United States Cadet Nurse Corps.

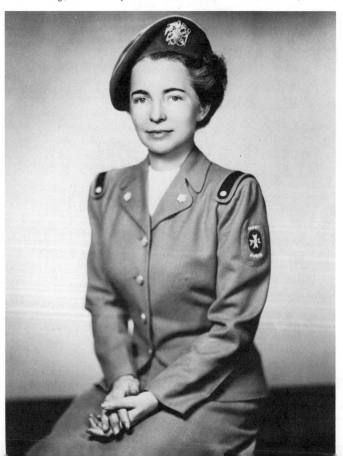

Administrator, Paul V. McNutt, promptly appointed an advisory committee on the training of nurses to assist in implementing the Act.

After a careful consideration of national nursing needs, enrollment quotas were established for the Cadet Nurse Corps: 125,000 for the first two years of the program, 65,000 to be recruited during the first 12 months, and 60,000 the following year, ending June 20, 1945. Under the efficient direction of Miss Petry and her staff, along with major assistance from the War Advertising Council, both quotas were exceeded, a performance that established the nurse recruitment program as the most successful of the war.

Characteristics of Military Nurses

What were some of the characteristics of military nursing during World War II? An examination of the detailed American Red Cross tabulation of the qualifications of the 75,029 nurses in the service—12,239 in the Navy and 62,790 in the Army—reveals several interesting facts. For example, a much larger percentage of younger nurses served with the Navy, as the following table indicates [15]:

Ages of Army and Navy Nurses in 1945 (in Percentages)

Age	Navy	Army	Total
21–25	34.6	26.8	28.1
26–30	40.0	34.6	35.5
31–35	15.6	18.2	17.8
36–40	6.9	11.4	10.6
41–45	1.8	6.3	5.5
46 and over	1.1	2.6	2.4
No record	–	0.1	0.1

As far as educational background was concerned, 97 percent of the Navy nurses were high school graduates, compared to 94 percent of the Army nurses. Of the 75,000 nurses, 20 percent had had some college education, either before or after their nursing education. Almost 90 percent had received their nursing education after 1931, and 72 percent had graduated from hospitals having a daily average of more than 100 patients. Only 16 percent had undergone any undergraduate training in psychiatry, either in their home or through affiliation. The breakdown of postgraduate training was as follows: 1 percent, communicable diseases; 1.3 percent, operating room technique; 0.7 percent, anesthesia; and 4.1 percent, public health. In a sample of 5000 nurses it was found that only 10 percent had done any other type of work, most of it clerical.

Image of the Military Nurse

How did servicemen regard the women military nurses? Male veterans often remarked that the so-called weaker sex was often cooler under fire. Coming

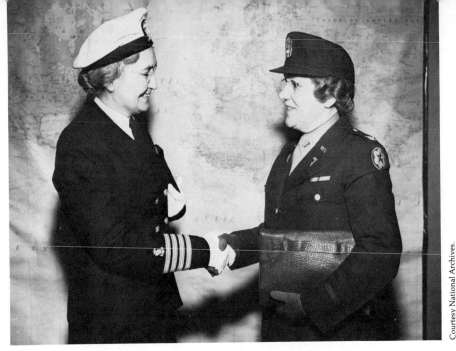

Captain Sue S. Dauser (on left), Superintendent of the Navy Nurse Corps, shaking hands with Colonel Florence A. Blanchfield, Superintendent of the Army Nurse Corps, early 1945.

from wounded men who had recently been in the thick of combat, this was a high compliment. Accustomed to the suffering of patients in peacetime, the nurses tended to take the horrors of war in stride. Death and wounds had been a part of their routine in civilian life. Even so, the kind of death and suffering that the nurses witnessed in war was something new.

An editorial in *America* magazine perceptively analyzed the role of the military nurse:

> Nurses do not receive the publicity of Four Jills and a Jeep. Their pictures do not fill the papers, for there is nothing pictorially pretty about a grimy-faced young girl sponging dirt and blood from the face and body of a wounded soldier. They are not at all glamorous, our nurses, for their profession is not glamorous. There is nothing glamorous in caked blood and torn arms and legs and faces half blown away. There is nothing glamorous in a hospital just behind the lines when the wounded come pouring in, nothing glamorous in the long night's watch at the bedsides of boys in pain, delirious, afraid, crazed, some of them. Nothing glamorous in the washing and the scrubbing and the cleaning. Their days and nights are full of work and sights that strong men could not stand.
>
> Their great glory is that they have offered themselves to service, calmly, almost casually. It is their vocation to tend the sick. Their place is wherever the sick and wounded happen to be. Their task is to be composed in disaster, smiling in the face of suffering, cheerful in the blackest moments, beautiful in the midst of horror.
>
> Their reward is in their giving and in the grateful memory of those to whom they give. Long after the soldiers shall have forgotten the entertainers and come to blush a bit at their silly devotion to pin-up girls, they will remember with a warm, cleansing glow of gratitude the nurse who smiled at their irritable demands, the nurse who helped them to walk again, the nurse who mothered them in the ugliness of their illness [16].

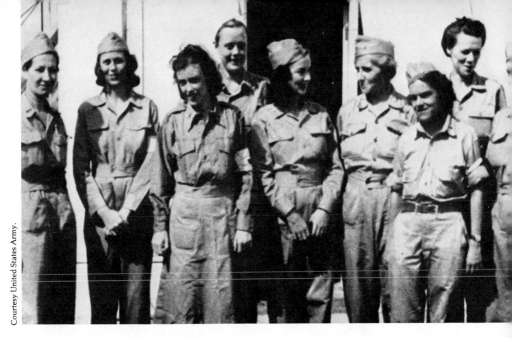

Nine Army nurses who escaped by air from the besieged fortress of Corregidor arrive at Darwin, Australia, on May 2, 1942.

Scores of movies with nurses as leading characters were made during the war. In late 1943 a movie dramatized the heroism of the 100 Army and Navy nurses who served with the embattled American forces in the Philippines during the opening months of the struggle against Japan. Entitled *So Proudly We Hail* and starring Claudette Colbert, Paulette Goddard, Veronica Lake, and Barbara Britton, the film received great acclaim. According to a review in *Life*:

So Proudly We Hail is one of the most terrifying war films to come from Hollywood this year. The reason for this is the authenticity and grim realism of the movie. For 126 minutes audiences see the next best thing to an actual pictorial record of the last bloody days of Bataan and Corregidor. Almost documentary in form, the story tells of the heroic part played by the small band of Army nurses in the Philippines [17].

Photographs of the nurses and their surroundings taken by a war correspondent who had escaped from Corregidor in the last days lent an air of technical authenticity to the film. These pictures were used to reproduce the jungle background and the hospital facilities where the nurses worked.

Another unusual film, *Cry Havoc*, presented a somewhat harsher version of the nurses' story. In this movie, which starred Margaret Sullavan, Ann Southern, Joan Blondell, and Fay Bainter, male roles served only as background cases for the nurses to care for. These two films provided a rare opportunity to display the work of nurses to the public, helped satisfy the public demand for information about the epic battles of Bataan and Corregidor, and improved morale on the home front by depicting the heroism of American nurses in battle.

The Nurse Shortage Becomes Acute
The last Allied offensive in Europe began in early November, 1944, when seven Allied armies pushed forward. It might have been more successful had the weather been better and had the lines of supply been able to keep pace with the advancing troops. On December 16, 1944, the Germans launched a sudden counterattack. For a time it appeared that the enemy, who overran 700 square miles of Belgium and Luxembourg, might actually stem the tide of the Allied advance. As American troops suffered their heaviest casualties of the war, over 1750 per day, the need for nurses quickly became acute. One of the initial reactions to this sudden reversal in the fortunes of war was "Give us nurses—10,000 overnight."

At the same time, a serious shortage of professional and nonprofessional personnel in America's civilian hospitals coincided with an all-time demand for hospital care. According to a survey conducted by the American Hospital Association, certain beds, wards, and operating rooms in 23 percent of the nation's hospitals were not being utilized because of insufficient personnel. This situation, were it allowed to continue, would have an adverse effect on the physical and mental health of the nation.

There were several reasons for the acute shortage of nursing personnel during the winter of 1944–1945. The Army and Navy had enrolled more than 65,000 registered nurses, most of whom had volunteered from civilian hospitals. Some 13,800 nurses were employed in industry—nearly twice as many as before the war—and they proved their worth in maintaining workers' health throughout wartime production. In an attempt to fill this vacuum, student nurses carried about 80 percent of the work of the 1300 hospital-affiliated schools of nursing.

The Nurse Draft Bill
Gradually Washington began to understand how vital nurses were to the war effort. On December 19, 1944, newspapers across the nation carried an article by columnist Walter Lippmann, who charged the Army with gross neglect of wounded soldiers by not having provided an adequate number of nurses to care for them:

The last thing our people will put up with is that sick and wounded American soldiers should suffer because the Army cannot find enough women to nurse them. Yet, I am reporting only the stark truth, which is well known to the Army and to the leaders of the medical profession, when I say that in military hospitals at home and abroad our men are not receiving the nursing care they must have, and that with casualties increasing in number and in seriousness, this will mean for many of the men brought in from the battlefields that their recovery is delayed, and even jeopardized [18].

Lippmann maintained that there were already plenty of trained nurses and nurses' aides in the United States. In addition, there were many women being trained as nurses and more who could be trained as nurses' aides. He further pointed out that, about two months before, some 27,000 nurses had been de-

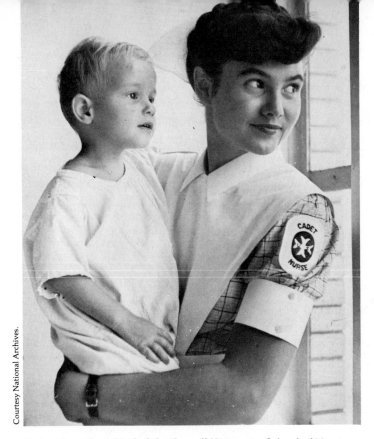

Cadet Nurse Joan Lind of the Cornell University School of Nursing.

clared to be engaged in non-essential nursing in civilian life and were therefore eligible for the Army, pending examination.

In his State of the Union message on January 6, 1945, President Roosevelt startled the nation with the unprecedented request for a draft of women nurses:

Since volunteering has not produced the number of nurses required, I urge that the Selective Service Act be amended to provide for induction of nurses into the armed forces. The need is too pressing to await the outcome of further efforts at recruiting [19].

Many congressmen were also alarmed by the nursing shortage in the Army and Navy as well as by reports of 11 Army units being sent overseas without a single nurse, when each should have had 80 or 90. Considerable debate took place, both in and out of Congress. Since nurses were not volunteering in sufficient numbers, some congressmen supported the President's proposal for conscription as the only practical solution to this problem.

Editor Janet Giester of *Trained Nurse and Hospital Review* wrote that "the story of the 11 hospital units that sailed without nurses had been told to me apprehensively by elevator men, bus drivers, and the cleaning women, all of whom have kin in the services . . . . Another woman told me the nurses' actions in 'letting our boys die' was a national scandal." Congresswoman Clare Booth

Luce, socialite, playwright, and member of the powerful House Committee on Military Affairs, told the press: "Perhaps there is something wrong with our method of training and recruiting nurses, but in this phase American women have not been doing their part as well as the British. American women have done wonderfully, though, in industry."

On February 2, 1945, the Gallup poll posed the following question to a cross section of Americans: Do you approve or disapprove of the proposal to draft nurses to serve with the Army and Navy? The results of this poll showed little appreciation for the nurses' contribution to the war effort thus far, as 73 percent approved, 19 disapproved, and 8 percent had no opinion. Three weeks later another group was polled on a similar question: Do you think that single nurses 20 to 45 years of age should be drafted for service with the armed forces? This time 65 percent answered yes, 28 percent said no, and 7 percent had no opinion.

Reports on conditions in a cross section of civilian hospitals revealed that, far from hoarding nurses, these institutions were serving their communities under extreme hardship and privation. The following examples served to illustrate this problem:

A 475-bed West Virginia tuberculosis hospital. On duty were 20 nurses, 10 of whom had had tuberculosis; five of these served part-time and five full-time on light work only. Two of the 10 healthy nurses were threatening to enter the Army Nurse Corps, lest they be considered slackers.

A New York State hospital of 106 beds. In 1941 it had 32 full-time staff nurses and four part-time on a 48-hour week. In 1945 it had 19 full-time and 22 part-time on a 60-hour week.

A Missouri state mental hospital. For 2600 patients there were nine graduate nurses.

A South Dakota hospital of 125 beds and 30 bassinets. Daily census for 1944 of 150; for early 1945 it had increased to 187. It had already released 50 graduate nurses to the armed services, and 10 others had filed applications. No general duty nurses were employed.

After quickly passing the House of Representatives, the bill to draft nurses into the armed forces became bogged down in the Senate. Because of the military successes of the Allied armies on both the eastern and western fronts of Europe, Congress began to question the need for additional manpower legislation. On March 24, 1945, the Allied armies succeeded in crossing the Rhine, and five days later General Patton captured Frankfurt. Just as VE Day was approaching, all the drastic attempts short of conscription to recruit nurses became embarrassingly successful. Stimulated by the threat of the draft, the nursing profession had responded with an overwhelming mass of applications for commissions, 10,000 of which were filed between January 8 and January 29, 1945, alone. Similarly, the pressure of possible conscription had induced 60 percent of the Senior Cadets to choose the Army instead of civilian employment.

Despite charges to the contrary, most hospitals had turned over the best of their nursing staffs to the military.

Courtesy National Archives.

When Colonel Florence Blanchfield, Superintendent of the Army Nurse Corps, returned from Europe, she found that there were actually too many nurses. By late April, 1945, the Medical Department was in an embarrassing position. Too many of its 54,000 graduate nurses were idle, while the number of Senior Cadet nurses in military hospitals had more than doubled, to a total of 6000. This excess of nurses posed a serious problem, for the overstaffing of hospitals had caused a plunge in morale. In view of this overabundance, Colonel Blanchfield recommended that 2000 civilian nurses be released and that Congress cease efforts to pass the proposed draft legislation.

The War Ends

The last days of the Third Reich were a nightmare. As the Allies overran Germany, they encountered indescribable examples of Nazi barbarism in the concentration camps of Belsen, Buchenwald, Gotha, Auschwitz, and Dachau, where more than 10 million civilians had been executed in gas chambers and in "scientific experiments." About six million of these victims were Jews, including children; most of the others were eastern Europeans and political prisoners. Army nurses in Germany had a rare opportunity to observe the effects of starvation upon the human body and to learn how survivors recovered from such a grim ordeal. The physical abuse suffered by prisoners in German concentration camps was worse than anything that they had ever seen.

The invasion of Japan, scheduled for the autumn of 1945, was expected to encounter stubborn resistance and to exact a heavy toll on American and British lives, for the Imperial Japanese Army, unlike the navy and air force, was still relatively intact. Its strength was estimated at five million—two million on the islands of Japan and an additional three million in Manchuria, China, and Formosa. In view of such a formidable military obstacle, it had been calculated that the war could drag on until late 1946 and that the assault on Japan would cost between 500,000 and one million American casualties.

The atomic bomb brought the war to a sudden and dramatic end. On August 6, 1945, an American B-29 flew over Hiroshima and at 9:15 A.M. dropped an atomic bomb over the center of the city. Hiroshima had been selected as the target because it was the headquarters of the Japanese army in southern Japan and a key military assembly and supply point. This atomic bomb, the first ever used for military purposes, plummeted five miles before exploding with a destructive force equal to 20,000 tons of TNT. The explosion blotted out the sky in a blinding flash. In that instant thousands died. A mushroom-shaped cloud of dust and smoke swiftly rose to a height of 40,000 feet. More than 78,000 people perished in this holocaust, 37,000 were injured, and about 13,900 more were reported missing. Japanese nurses played a heroic role in the terrifying chaos that followed.

Despite the horrible destruction of Hiroshima, Japanese militarists obstinately refused to surrender. On August 8 the Soviet Union declared war on Japan, and on August 9 a second atomic bomb leveled Nagasaki, another major railroad junction, supply depot, and industrial center in southern Japan. After this second blow Japan could endure no more and sued for peace on August 10, 1945. On August 14 President Truman announced that Japan had accepted the Allied terms of surrender. The formal end of World War II came on September 2, 1945, when General MacArthur conducted the official ceremonies of surrender on the Battleship Missouri in Tokyo Bay.

The Contribution of Nurses

"There has been a larger number of war-service volunteers from nursing than from any other American profession," stated the American Journal of Nursing in evaluating the performance of nurses in the war. Almost half of the 240,000 active registered nurses in the United States, many of whom could not meet the physical requirements, had volunteered for military service. As of June 30, 1945, about 29 percent of all active nurses (65,377) were on duty with the armed services.

In the nation's schools of nursing the total student nurse enrollment had increased 30 percent since 1943, thanks largely to the 179,000 young women who joined the Cadet Nurse Corps and pledged to engage in essential civilian or military nursing for the duration of the war. To comply with President Truman's request for an orderly termination of this massive educational program, the United States Public Health Service established October 15, 1945, as the final date for new admissions to the Corps. By permitting students admitted before this date to graduate, the federal government temporarily cushioned the impact of the withdrawal of its funds from the schools.

When the Cadet Nurse Corps program finally terminated in 1948, it had received over $160 million in federal appropriations and had graduated 125,000 students. In addition, approximately 15,000 graduate nurses had received federal funds for advanced study before the grants were discontinued on October 15, 1945. Of this group, about 5000 took intensive courses designed for nurses who could not leave their jobs. The importance of nursing within the United States Public Health Service reached an all-time high in fiscal year 1945, when the appropriation for the Cadet Nurse Corps amounted to $62,140,760, over one-half the total PHS budget of $120 million.

Cadet Nurses at Freedmen's Hospital School of Nursing, Washington, D.C.

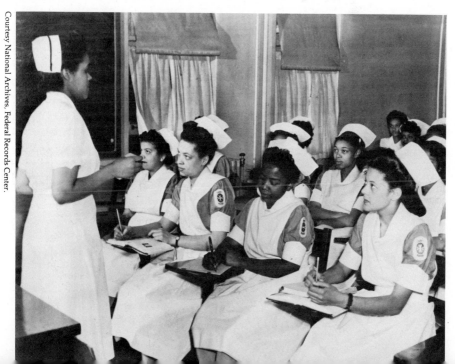

Registered Nurses Serving in the Military Nurse Corps, as of June 30, 1898–1977.

Year	Army	Navy	Air Force	Total
1898*	1,158			1,158
1899	202	Contract nurses		202
1900	210			210
1901	176			176
1902	170			170
1903	152			152
1904	126			126
1905	120			120
1906	118			118
1907	108			108
1908	95			95
1909	80	20		100
1910	100	52		152
1911	125	70		195
1912	125	101		226
1913	125	130		255
1914	150	135		285
1915	150	148		298
1916	276	145		421
1917	403	550		953
1918	21,480†	1,613		23,093
1919	9,616	533		10,419
1920	1,551	535		2,086
1921	851	492		1,343
1922	828	495		1,323
1923	705	486		1,191
1924	675	488		1,163
1925	725	484		1,209
1926	673	474		1,147
1927	681	484		1,165
1928	699	487		1,186
1929	734	495		1,229
1930	807	503		1,310
1931	809	501		1,310
1932	824	504		1,328
1933	669	455		1,124
1934	609	355		964
1935	603	336		939
1936	603	366		969
1937	625	398		1,023
1938	671	425		1,096
1939	672	438		1,110

Year	Army	Navy	Air Force	Total
1940	946	488		1,434
1941	5,433	823		6,256
1942	17,247	1,778		19,025
1943	30,316	5,431		35,747
1944	40,018	8,399		48,417
1945	54,291	11,086		65,377
1946	13,617	5,580		19,197
1947	5,979	2,100		8,079
1948	4,317	1,956		6,273
1949	4,662	2,010	1,199	7,871
1950	3,401	1,950	1,158	6,509
1951	5,361	3,238	2,365	10,964
1952	5,323	3,117	2,816	11,256
1953	4,692	2,600	2,991	10,283
1954	4,189	2,345	2,609	9,143
1955	3,757	2,165	2,289	8,211
1956	3,556	2,146	2,609	8,311
1957	3,384	2,122	2,949	8,455
1958	3,359	2,088	2,833	8,280
1959	3,364	2,168	2,880	8,412
1960	3,310	2,198	2,977	8,485
1961	3,283	2,200	3,113	8,596
1962	3,402	2,145	3,438	8,985
1963	2,981	2,038	3,409	8,428
1964	2,969	1,968	3,412	8,349
1965	3,121	1,874	3,488	8,483
1966	3,704	2,038	3,757	9,499
1967	4,545	2,322	4,102	10,969
1968	4,734	2,374	3,928	11,036
1969	4,829	2,382	3,961	11,172
1970	4,825	2,242	3,818	10,885
1971	4,752	2,231	3,811	10,794
1972	4,172	2,336	3,817	10,326
1973	3,769	2,436	3,785	9,990
1974	3,731	2,646	3,750	10,127
1975	3,706	2,562	3,883	10,151
1976	3,555	2,542	3,776	9,873
1977	3,646	2,566	3,736	9,948

*Strength for September 15, 1898.
†Strength for November 15, 1918.

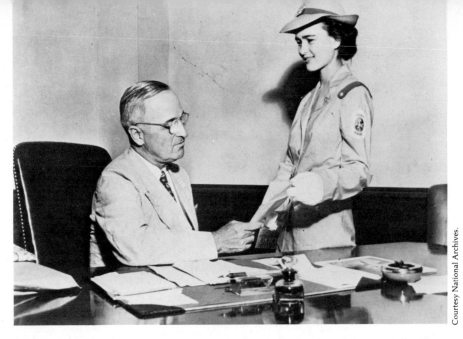

President Truman authorized a gradual phase-out of the United States Cadet Nurse Corps from 1945 to 1948.

As a result of these federal aid programs, hospital schools of nursing obtained more students and better qualified instructors and head nurses. In addition, over $17 million worth of Lanham Act building funds were allotted to schools in the Cadet Nurse program for the construction of nurses' residences and instructional facilities. During the Senior Cadet period of instruction, 73 percent of the Senior Cadets remained in their home hospitals, while the other 27 percent served in the Army, Navy, Veterans Administration, Public Health Service, Indian Service, or other civilian hospitals or public health agencies.

The price of America's victory in World War II had been high. Some 16,300,000 Americans had served in the armed forces, of whom 292,131 were killed and 671,000 were wounded. The excellent record of lives saved—96 of each 100 wounded—had been achieved because of nursing care, effective first aid treatment, front-line surgery, the availability of blood plasma, chemotherapy, and early evacuation from battle areas. Had it not been for these essential factors, the number of deaths would have been far greater.

Summary

In 1940 the ANA offered President Roosevelt the support of nursing organizations in the nation's defense effort. The Nursing Council of National Defense, an umbrella organization of all the professional nursing associations, was formed to assist in the war effort.

As huge defense expenditures impacted on industrial communities throughout the United States and health facilities became overtaxed, the United States Public Health Service implemented an emergency health and sanitation program that provided extra services in defense areas. In 1941 a federal appropriation for basic nursing education was enacted for the first time in order to secure an adequate supply of nurses for heightened military and civilian needs.

In 1941 New York's Mayor LaGuardia, Director of the Office of Civilian Defense, initiated a massive training program to secure 100,000 volunteer nurses' aides.

The National Nursing Council for War Service established guidelines to help nurses determine whether they should remain in their civilian positions or join the military nursing services. It was recommended that a nurse join the military if she was single, under 40, and working in a position not essential for teaching or providing minimum health service in a community.

Since 1920 Army nurses had been authorized only "relative rank" and were thus not entitled to regular military benefits such as retirement privileges and dependents' allowances. Nurses also received substantially less pay than male officers of the same rank. In 1944 Congress legislated a more equitable ranking system and benefit package for nurses that was to last for the duration of the war. Military nurses would receive actual permanent rank two years after the war ended.

As the United States took the offensive, Army nurses served in the successful North African campaign and landed in Italy in late 1943. War correspondents described them as flexible and willing to live under primitive conditions.

After the value of flight nurses was recognized by the military, a flight nursing school was established at Bowman Field, Kentucky. The flight nurse was responsible for specific duties in air evacuation such as loading patients, performing emergency first aid, and administering medications.

The number of public health nurses employed in industry nearly doubled from 1941 to 1943. In addition to her traditional duties, the industrial nurse was able to appreciate the needs of the tens of thousands of new women industrial workers and help improve health and safety standards.

During the period between the world wars, diseases associated with old age, such as cancer, heart disease, and diabetes, had replaced communicable, infant, and childhood diseases as the leading causes of civilian deaths. Nevertheless, Selective Service records revealed large-scale rejections of young adult males for physical reasons as more than half of a selected sample of male registrants were rejected by local boards and induction centers.

By 1943 the rapidly growing industrial centers were in urgent need of expanded health facilities. Nursing services in hospitals in many parts of the country were severely understaffed.

Fierce competition for womanpower was causing a lag in enrollments at nursing schools at a time when larger classes of students were desperately needed to bolster hospital nursing services.

In 1943 Congress passed the Bolton Act, which created the United States Cadet Nurse Corps. Under the provisions of this act the United States Public Health Service subsidized the education of nursing students who would agree to engage in essential military or civilian service for the duration of the war.

Under the efficient leadership of Lucile Petry, annual admission quotas for the Cadet Nurse program were exceeded and the acute shortage of student nurses was thereby alleviated.

Numerous motion pictures produced during the war presented the popular image of the military nurse as a cool, resourceful, and efficient worker during her repeated confrontations with death and injury.

Large numbers of additional military nurses were urgently needed when, in late 1944, the Army suffered its heaviest casualties of the war. On the home front a serious scarcity of graduate nurses already existed in civilian hospitals, where record numbers of patients were being treated. Because of a severe labor shortage, many nurses were performing functions previously carried out by physicians and nonprofessional staff members.

In January, 1945, President Roosevelt made an unprecedented request for the conscription of women nurses. After a bill had been passed by the House of Representatives, Allied successes in Germany caused many Congressmen to question its value, and it subsequently became bogged down in the Senate.

Even though nearly 30 percent of the nation's graduate nurses had already entered the military service, fear of conscription prompted over 10,000 additional applications for nurse commissions during three weeks in January, 1945. By April of that same year the Medical Department found itself in the embarrassing position of having too many nurses serving in European hospitals.

By the end of the war, in August, 1945, almost half of the 240,000 active registered nurses in the United States had volunteered for military service and some 76,000 had served. Nationwide student enrollment had increased by 30 percent since 1943.

By the time the United States Cadet Nurse Corps program was phased out in 1948, 125,000 students had graduated under its auspices. The appropriation for the Cadet Nurse Corps in fiscal year 1945 represented over one-half of the total Public Health Service budget, a fact that emphasizes the tremendous importance of nurses in the war effort.

References

1. "To the Graduate of '39," *American Journal of Nursing*, vol. 39 (May, 1939): 529–530.
2. "Federal Legislation—and the World We Live In," *American Journal of Nursing*, vol. 40 (June, 1940):176.
3. "The Philadelphia Biennial: · Nursing in a Democracy," *American Journal of Nursing*, vol. 40 (June, 1940):673.

4. *Ibid.*
5. U.S. Public Health Service, *Minutes, First Meeting of the Advisory Committee on Rules and Regulations of the Surgeon General.* Federal Record Center, Suitland, Maryland, RG 90, p. 8.
6. Stella Goostray, *Memoirs: Half a Century in Nursing* (Boston Nursing Archive, Boston University Mugar Memorial Library, 1969), pp. 116–117.
7. "Training Program Announced for 100,000 Nurses' Aides," *Hospital Management* vol. 52 (September, 1941): 44–45.
8. Quoted in the U.S. Congress. House. Committee on Military Affairs. Seventy-eighth Congress, Second Session, *Army Nurse Corps, Hearings on H.R. 3718* (Washington, D.C.: Government Printing Office, 1944), pp. 28–30.
9. *Ibid.*, p. 30.
10. Legette Blythe, *38th Evac: The Story of the Men and Women Who Served with the 38th Evacuation Hospital in North Africa and Italy* (Charlotte, North Carolina: Heritage Printers, Inc., 1966), pp. 43–45.
11. Ernie Pyle, *Here is Your War: The Story of G.I. Joe* (Cleveland: World Publishing Co., 1944), pp. 71–84.
12. *Ibid.*, pp. 82–83.
13. Personal letter, copy in Katherine Densford papers, University of Minnesota Archives, Minneapolis.
14. "When Does the Home Front Have Priority?" *Public Health Nursing*, vol. 35 (February, 1943):77–78.
15. Unpublished document, Records of the War Manpower Commission, National Archives.
16. "The Nurse," *America*, vol. 41 (January 15, 1944):407.
17. "So Proudly We Hail: Realistic Story of Nurses in the Philippines," *Life*, vol. 15 (October 4, 1943):69.
18. "American Women and Our Wounded Men," *Washington Post*, December 19, 1944 (reprinted in *Congressional Record* as an extension of the remarks of Hon. Edith Nourse Rogers, December 19, 1944).
19. U.S. Congress. House. Seventy-ninth Congress, First Session, *Message from the President of the United States Transmitting a Message on the State of the Union* (Washington, D.C.: Government Printing Office, 1945), Document No. 1, p. 7.

15
Postwar Reappraisal, 1945–1950

The end of World War II did not ease the demand for nurses. The greatest turnover ever known among American nurses began with the war and received new impetus with V-J Day. The coming of peace affected not only the 76,000 graduate nurses who had served at some time with the armed forces but also the more than 164,000 who had both carried on their own jobs and also filled in for those away in the armed services. All through the war, nursing staffs at home had been weakened in order to supply the imperative needs of military service hospitals. Under these conditions, hospitals welcomed any help that could be obtained, and practical nurses, volunteer aides, and orderlies had played an important part in the nursing of patients. In such an atmosphere it was understandable that the home-front nurse eagerly anticipated the return of the military nurse.

The Case of the Missing RNs

Although the war had ended, the surrender of the Axis powers did not bring the civilian hospitals relief. Instead, it shattered illusions about the supply of nurses. While millions of men and women returned to civilian life, the anxiously awaited nurse reinforcements failed to reach overburdened hospitals. Questionnaires returned by 31,000 members of the Army Nurse Corps and tabulated by the American Red Cross revealed that only one Army nurse in six expected to return to her prewar position. Although 69 percent planned to remain active in nursing, their interests covered a wide range. More specifically, when one realized that 64 percent of Army nurses had come from posts in hospital nursing, the finding that only 26 percent planned to return to civilian hospital nursing and 4 percent to teaching in hospital schools of nursing portended disastrous consequences for hospitals. Many military nurses claimed that the reason they did not wish to return to general duty hospital positions was that they had carried considerable responsibility in the Army or Navy and had found real satisfaction in more flexible, autonomous roles.

The extent to which civilian hospitals were short of both nursing and non-nursing personnel was evident in the 1060 responses to a questionnaire sent to institutional members of the American Hospital Association by the Council on

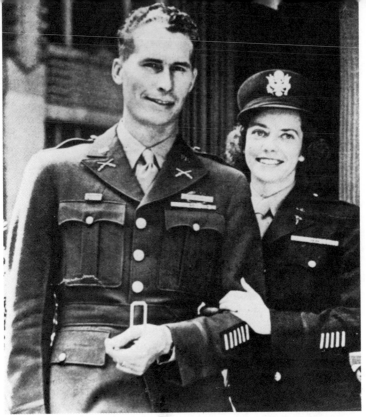

Trained Nurse, June, 1945.

Marriage was an almost inevitable correlate with military nursing service during and after World War II.

While the birth rate soared, the supply of registered nurses plummeted.

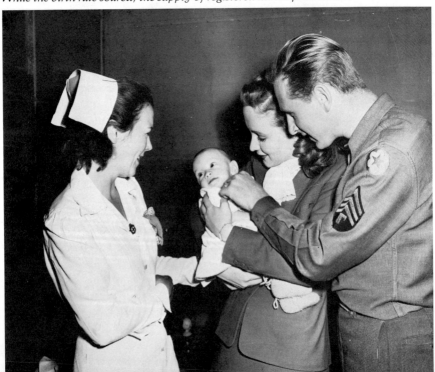

Courtesy History of Nursing Collection, University of Michigan.

Professional Practice. Administrators of member hospitals were asked to estimate the number of employees needed in the different categories. Their replies produced the following figures on unfilled positions in late 1945:

Registered nurses	65,000
Nurses' aides	90,000
Nonnursing personnel	90,000
Untrained volunteers	45,000

In brief, 65 percent of the hospitals reported that they were acutely short of nursing personnel. These hospitals had an average census of 220 patients per day, whereas the group not acutely short had an average census of 125 patients per day. The hospitals acutely short reported a 379 percent increase in part-time employment of nurses, and the others reported a 150 percent increase.

Nearly 6000 vacancies on the nursing staffs of hospitals and health agencies in New York City made it necessary to close 1200 beds during a time of unprecedented demand for hospital facilities. No solution was in sight, and nursing and hospital officials predicted that the situation would worsen with the increasing incidence of illness in fall and winter. Factors contributing to the shortage of nurses were, according to a *New York Times* survey, the poor pay for hospital nurses compared with the pay for nurses in industry, in physicians' offices, and in nonnursing jobs; the shorter hours in nonhospital jobs; the increase in retirement and marriage of nurses; the opportunities for advanced education under the GI Bill; and the housing shortage. The report said that volunteer help in New York hospitals had also declined since the end of the war, which contributed to the difficulty.

Poor Wages and Bad Working Conditions

In a 1946 national salary survey, the American Hospital Association found that the average starting salary for a staff nurse was $35.75 a week. The average work week was 48 hours, yielding a pay rate of 74 cents per hour. Most nurses wanted the work week cut to 40 hours and the pay increased to at least $40. In sharp contrast, typists were averaging 97 cents an hour, bookkeepers $1.11, and seamstresses $1.33. Sue Z. McCracken, general secretary of District No. 4 of the Ohio State Nurses' Association, told of hospitals in her area that paid their regular nurses $30 per week and hired "extras" at $60 weekly to tide them over acute nurse-shortage periods. Two nurses might be working side by side, one knowing that the other was getting twice as much pay for doing exactly the same work. As one superintendent explained, "When the Depression comes, we'll just fire the $60 ones" [1].

Practices such as this were not uncommon in hospitals across the nation. Because of the shortage, at one major hospital in New York a head nurse was paid $35 a week while the staff nurses who worked under her were hired at $40. In this case, as at many other hospitals, salaries had to be kept secret or dismissal was risked. But the facts leaked out and the head nurse went in to ask a few questions. "We'll raise you to $45 if you promise not to say a word to the others," she was told. Nurses wanted to see the end of such outmoded personnel arrangements and, in their place, the establishment of uniform, aboveboard salary scales [2].

The RN had achieved a status of "professional" in the nomenclature but often was not treated accordingly by physicians, administrators, or the public. Few nurses thought of hospital nursing service in terms of professional career work. In one postwar study of 500 registered nurses, only 12.2 percent reported that they looked forward to making a career out of hospital nursing. About 5.2 percent planned on careers in nursing education, and 6.2 percent were planning careers in nursing administration. The remaining 76.4 percent planned either to use nursing as a desirable "pin-money" job supplementing the husband's income or to stop nursing altogether upon marriage. Nearly 20 percent of the hospital nurses sampled reported that they planned to switch to another line of work or study. Such data generally reflected the low level of job satisfaction and a lower esteem for hospital nursing.

Hospital nurses saw themselves as working under more rigid discipline than women in other occupations. They felt that there was less opportunity for social activities and that they had to follow more rules and orders than women in other occupations. Moreover, there was a preponderant feeling among nurses that their work required greater precision than was required of women in other lines of work. According to most nurses' appraisals of their work, satisfaction in a profession was associated with independence of action and self-direction, along with opportunity for social activity and recreation. Nurses sought recognition as professionals worthy of trust and responsibility. They were unhappy at being held to a student-like status entailing blind obedience and uncomplaining acceptance of criticism rather than being accorded a status involving cooperative effort and participation in planning and decision-making.

In 1941 the hospital nurse had generally worked a 48-hour week; in 1946 she worked 46 hours. These figures did not tell the entire story. In 1940 approximately 70 percent of all hospitals had required their nurses to work "split shifts," which meant that the nurse's working day consisted of two segments of duty hours with an intervening period of time off without pay. Since it was difficult to make effective use of three to four hours of leisure time between assignments, the split shift was exceptionally burdensome. By 1946 one of every four hospital nurses was still working a split shift. Without the split shift, it took three or more nurses working a seven- or eight-hour day to do the work that formerly required two persons, each paid for nine or 10 hours a day.

Another 1946 survey reported that one of five hospital nurses was critical of her job as a whole. In addition to the conditions that were major grievances in almost all branches of nursing, hospital nurses frequently objected to the unevenness of their workload, the number and arduousness of their duties, the proportion of time spent on nonprofessional work, the quality of supervision, the lack of educational opportunities, and the long hours of work. Half of all

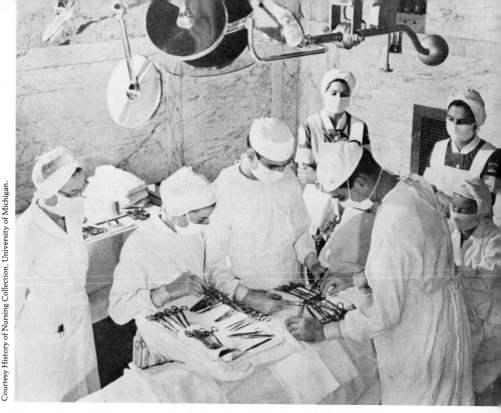

During the postwar period numerous complaints were expressed about the arduous work and physical strain associated with nursing.

hospital nurses who expressed opinions on any aspect of their job were dissatisfied with the quality and quantity of nonprofessional help, provision for retirement, and employment security.

The complaints regarding the arduousness of the work referred both to heavy workloads and to the general physical strain associated with nursing assignments. Examples were numerous:

At times it requires a strong, large nurse to lift the heavy patients—and the transporting of heavy equipment and oxygen tanks. It is hard work and there are never people available to lift these things. It is much easier to turn to a different position than to suffer these strains.

Work is very heavy everywhere. Everyone leaves the floor with the feeling that his work is incomplete—if one stayed two hours longer the feeling would still be the same.

You work like a demon, wondering why you couldn't be an octopus and a centipede at the same time. You stay on duty until everything is completed, and if you punch the clock an hour or more late, it apparently is your own fault for not being able to plan your work better. Our time clock seemed to be installed as a means of checking on the time we reported for duty, but the payroll department blindfolded their eyes and their conscience to any overtime.

I feel a little more understanding and a little more kindness and consideration from doctors, hospital executives, and also from private individuals would have prevented the present shortage of nurses. Don't get me wrong, in my quarter of a century of nursing I have had more good than bad but surely hope [that the nurse of the future has] a life with more time for fun and play and normal living, that she won't be considered a queer duck because she works nights, etc.

The daily load carried by each nurse is so heavy that of necessity minor details are neglected that the important things might be done for the patient. Instead of receiving the slightest bit of encouragement from the people that sit in the office and make rounds very infrequently, these small things are criticized, and the nurse, who is overworked physically [and] as a result, tense mentally, is made to feel that she is doing nothing.

People expect nurses to be more or less like a high-class servant, instead of giving them the status of an actual professional [3].

ANA Becomes Aggressive

With the theme "Nursing in the Nation's Plans for Health," 12,000 nurses from all parts of the United States gathered in Atlantic City during the last week of September, 1946, as the American Nurses' Association, the National League for Nursing Education, and the National Organization for Public Health Nursing met for the fourteenth time in a joint biennial session. The convention also marked the golden anniversary of the ANA.

The convention concerned itself primarily with the adoption of a series of resolutions, known as the platform of the American Nurses' Association. The 1946 platform contained the following 10 points:

1. Improvement in hours and living conditions for nurses so that they may live a normal personal and professional life. Specifically, action toward: (a) wider acceptance of the 40-hour week with no decrease in salary, thus applying to post-war conditions the principle of the eight-hour day adopted by the American Nurses' Association in 1934; (b) minimum salaries adequate to attract nurses of quality and to enable them to maintain standards of living comparable with other professions.

2. Provision for optimal nursing care for all, and the furtherance of a positive health program in all communities.

3. Increased participation by nurses in the actual planning and in the administration of nursing service in hospitals and other types of employment.

4. Greater development of nurses' professional associations as exclusive spokesmen for nurses in all questions affecting their employment and economic security. Such a development should be based on past successful experience of professional nurses' organizations in collective bargaining and negotiation.

5. Removal, as rapidly as possible, of barriers that prevent the full employment and professional development of nurses belonging to minority racial groups.

6. Employment of well-qualified practical nurses and other auxiliary workers under state licensure, thus protecting both the patient and the worker.

7. Continuing improvement in the placement and counseling of nurses, to give greater stability and job satisfaction to the profession and to facilitate a better distribution of nursing service to the public.

8. Further development of nursing in prepayment health and medical care plans, in order to spread the cost of nursing service to the public.

9. Maintenance of educational standards, and development of educational resources, that nursing may keep abreast of the rapid advances in medicine and other sciences. Such a development may well require federal subsidies and contribution from foundations and other educational philanthropies.

10. Appraisals of our own national organizations through the report of the Structure Study and fearless action based upon such appraisal to make sure that the nursing profession will be organized and equipped to deal most effectively with its problems and its opportunities [4].

In an obvious step to counter union organizers who had begun efforts to unionize nurses, the ANA adopted a carefully worded resolution in which it went on record as endorsing the qualifications of the several state and district associations to act as the exclusive agents of their respective memberships in the field of economic security and collective bargaining. The resolution continued:

The association commends the excellent progress already made and urges all state and district associations to push such a program vigorously and expeditiously. Since it is the established policy of other groups, including unions, to permit membership in only one collective bargaining group, the association believes such policy to be sound for the state and district nurses' associations [5].

It was emphasized that adoption of this policy by any state association would be optional and that the individual nurse had free choice whether she wished to join her professional organization or a union.

Under the sponsorship of the NLNE, the convention delegates held a panel discussion on the general subject "Who shall pay for nursing education?" The panel concerned itself with whether student nurses were serving primarily as manpower in caring for patients or as students acquiring a professional education. The group argued whether or not the prevailing system of nursing education—carried on largely by hospitals, which were primarily service institutions and only secondarily educational institutions—was adequate to meet national nursing needs.

The panel generally agreed that it would be wise to foster the establishment of schools of nursing in universities and colleges, since 91 percent of the nursing schools were being operated by hospitals. Senator Claude Pepper of Florida, one of the participants in this discussion, abhorred the fact that, under the current hospital nursing system, the patient was paying for what Senator Pepper called a "deterioration in nursing service" by reason of increased fees for medical care accompanied by a nursing shortage and a relative decline of enrollments in nursing schools. He stated that adequate nursing care for all could come about only when conditions in the nursing field were such as to attract sufficient numbers of high-quality personnel. According to the Senator, nursing education, like other forms of professional education, should be directly financed by the individual or the student's family, and by tuition grants, loans, scholarships, and fellowships paid from private and government sources.

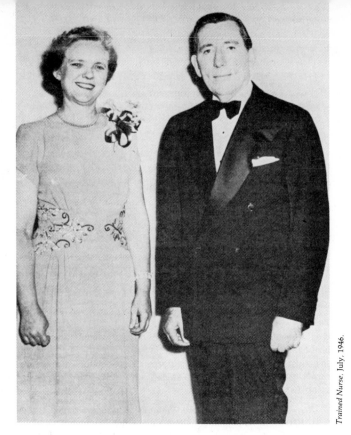

Ruth Sleeper, president of the NLNE, with Senator Claude Pepper of Florida, exponent of a comprehensive national health insurance program during the 1940s.

Continued Peacetime Nurse Shortages

The postwar shortage of registered professional nurses in the United States was due primarily to a decline in enrollment of nursing students at a time of rising demand for nursing care and heavy losses of graduate nurses through marriage. The lag in student enrollment seemed related to problems of student training and to competition from fields of employment that required less specialized education and thus provided almost immediate earnings. Workers in industry generally had shorter hours and fared better with respect to overtime pay and retirement pensions, although nurses typically received more liberal vacations and sick-leave benefits.

By midsummer 1948 there were 380,500 active registered nurses in the United States. They were distributed among the major fields of nursing as follows: 167,400 in institutions, including 4400 full-time instructors in schools of nursing; 22,100 in public health; 52,800 in private duty; 12,700 in industry; and 25,500 in other areas, including physicians' offices. The better hospitals were slowly learning that efficiency and productivity in the nursing service was far less a matter of the amount of hard work done by each individual than of the engineering of the job, the kind of mechanical equipment used by the nurse, the size and flexibility of the institution, the layout of work space, and the relationship of jobs to one another.

In 1948, in a report from the Bureau of Employment Security of the Social Security Administration to Federal Security Administrator Oscar R. Ewing, the national nurse shortage was estimated at approximately 40,000. This report examined nursing needs in hospitals, physicians' offices, schools, industry, and public health agencies. It was estimated that there was also a "potential demand" for an additional 40,000 nurses to staff new hospital facilities and to meet other nursing requirements during the next three to five years.

The report said the nursing shortage was still acute, with thousands of vacant beds in hospitals attributable to lack of nursing personnel. The estimated shortage of 40,000 was broken down as follows: hospitals and clinics, 20,000; public health, 6000; private duty, 4000; nursing schools, 3000; physicians' offices, 3000; industry, 2000; and miscellaneous, 2000. The report revealed that institutional nurses received the lowest pay and industrial nurses the highest. The average work day for nurses was eight hours, and weekly schedules ranged from 40 to 48 hours, with the longest schedules prevailing in institutions. Also noted was a tendency toward shorter hours in large communities.

The Cadet Nurse Corps Program had exerted a marked effect upon the num-

New student nurses were increasingly hard to recruit during the postwar years.

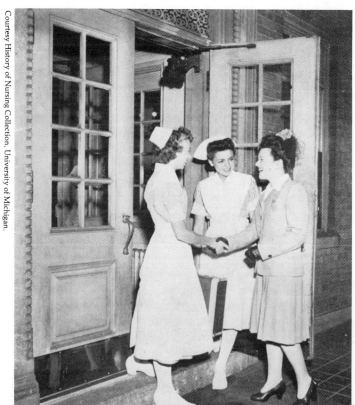

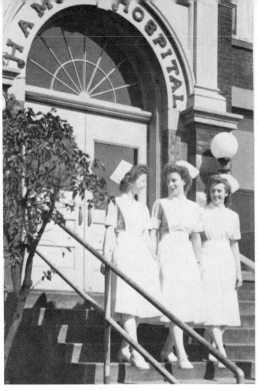

Hamot Hospital School of Nursing Bulletin. 1946.

Hospital schools of nursing accounted for 96 percent of 1947 graduates.

A big question during the postwar years was whether or not a young lady could stand up to the rigorous training given to student nurses.

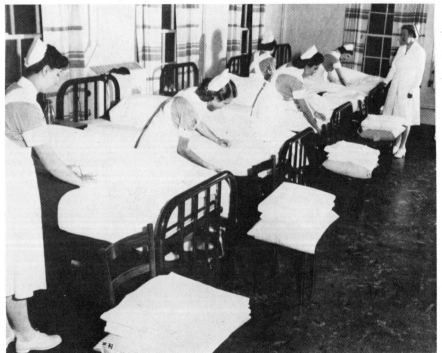

Courtesy National Archives.

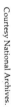

ber of young women applying for admission to nursing schools. During the war years these classes gradually increased, not only because of the patriotic urge that prompted applications but also because of the financial program inaugurated and carried out by the government. Following graduation of large Cadet Nurse classes came a dearth of student nurses in many schools. In 1941 there had been 93,977 students enrolled in accredited schools of nursing. In 1945 there were 130,909. In 1947 there was a marked decrease in enrollment; these schools had 94,133 students.

Falling Popularity of Nursing as a Profession

Fewer young women were choosing a nursing education. In 1910 the number of American women who entered nursing approximated 1.5 percent of those eligible. This proportion had passed 3 percent by 1940, and wartime enrollment rates averaged almost 5 percent. The first few postwar years brought a sharp drop. An all-time-high withdrawal rate of student nurses, 30 percent, was reported during 1947 in a statistical survey of graduating classes from state-accredited schools of nursing. The national graduating class total reached a new high of 40,744, but this reflected the war-swollen admission figures of 1944. Only 1779 students, or 4 percent of the total graduated, received university degrees. A mere 42 nursing graduates of 1947 were men. The 582 black graduates constituted an increase of 50 over the previous year.

Schools of nursing were having great difficulty in filling their classes. There was no telling, of course, how many prospective nurses were scared away from nursing by Clarence Woodbury's critical article entitled "Student Nurse— Could You Take It?" in the June, 1949, *Woman's Home Companion* [6]. Commenting on the piece, administrator John F. Latcham of Trumbull Memorial Hospital in Warren, Ohio, felt that the article was a "pincer movement" in the government's plan to socialize medicine. Latcham noted that "at the Trumbull Memorial Hospital we know that our students are properly housed and fed. The Nurses' Home is a modern building, with attractive rooms, a parlor, a good library, adequate classrooms and excellent bath facilities." He noted that "some religious schools of nursing were noted for harsh discipline, but, as far as the majority of schools go, I would believe that lack of discipline would be the more proper charge." He emphasized that "no apprentice ever learned a trade from theory. Our nurses work a 44-hour week, with classroom time included" [7].

Another hospital executive felt that "nurses should either get off their high horses and do the physical work they started out to do or move over and let others do it. There is too much talk about 'high professional standards' and not enough about taking care of the sick." A third hospital administrator did not think that there was any use in castigating the *Woman's Home Companion* over the article. He thought the real fault for declining interest in nursing was the small but highly vocal lunatic fringe, the current vogue group in high nursing circles [8]

The Anticollegiate Nursing Faction

The big controversy was whether nursing education should go the collegiate route. Dr. Frank Lahey, former president of the American Medical Association, charged that nurses were "legislating and educating themselves out of jobs." On the other hand, nurses like Eunice D. Johnson, director of the nursing school of Saint Luke's Hospital, New Bedford, maintained that "you can never overeducate a nurse" [9]. The editors of *Hospital Management* submitted this dispute to a panel of hospital administrators. Hundreds of different views were expressed, making it very difficult to tabulate the results accurately. Still, an attempt was made to set down some figures in response to the question of whether nurses were pushing for too much education. Forty-eight percent said no, 30 percent said yes, and 22 percent were undecided.

Edith W. Bailey, administrator of the Canonsburg General Hospital in Canonsburg, Pennsylvania, commented:

The nurses attending universities and colleges insist only on supervising—no physical work . . . Not everyone is fitted for supervising—and strangely enough, a sick person doesn't give a hang whether his nurse possesses a B.A. or B.S. The root question is "Can she make him comfortable?" [10].

Another comment along this line came from A. M. Frank, M.D., chairman of the staff at Lutheran Hospital, St. Louis. He predicted that practical nurses would be in greater demand than those with degrees and added that "one definitely does not need a Ph.D. degree to carry a bedpan. The patients are only interested in whether it is hot or cold. Student nurses are spending too much time in the lecture halls and too little time on the floor so that we are getting too many desk models and insufficient floor models" [11].

According to a postwar survey made by the American College of Surgeons, less expensive nursing care was needed. The survey revealed that the quantity of nursing was 50 percent of the total need and that the quality had deteriorated about equally. Eighty-four percent of the replies stated that, with few exceptions, the needs of the sick could be met by auxiliary help.

The ACS held that such requirements were incompatible with the expensive developments in nursing education over the years. The professional nursing associations had been concerned with elevating their professional status and advocating more years of education. Actual nurse training had been relegated to a place of secondary importance behind general educational aspects. It was agreed that, as nurses, such graduates had been less well prepared. The immediate need to initiate action independent of the control of nursing organizations was apparent and urgent. The Board of Regents of the American College of Surgeons adopted the following resolution on December 20, 1946, during its annual meeting at the time of the Clinical Congress in Cleveland: "The American College of Surgeons advises hospitals to admit and utilize the assistance of auxiliary nursing aides. In addition, approved hospitals should provide training for such vocational nurses by means of short courses" [12].

Staffing Dilemmas

During the war four types of nurse staffing were common: (1) graduate registered nurses only; (2) graduate registered nurses and paid auxiliary workers; (3) graduate registered nurses and student nurses; and (4) graduate registered nurses, student nurses, and paid auxiliary workers. In 1943 the most important facts established about the variation in hours of care per patient per day by different types of personnel were:

Students gave almost two-thirds of the hours of care in the hospitals with schools of nursing.

The total hours of care per patient per day decreased consistently as the size of the hospital increased.

The hours of care per patient per day given by general staff nurses in hospitals without schools decreased as the size of the hospital increased.

The hours of care given by students decreased as the size of the hospital increased.

The hours of care given by paid auxiliary workers in hospitals without schools decreased as the size of the hospital increased; by contrast, in hospitals with schools, such hours of care increased as the size of the hospital increased.

The hours of care given by general staff nurses ranged from an average of 2.1 hours of care per patient per day in hospitals without schools of nursing and without paid auxiliaries to only 0.6 hour in the hospitals with schools and without paid auxiliaries.

During World War II, in the average hospital, the proportion of direct nursing care supplied by RNs dropped drastically; an estimated 3100 of the total 4200 general and related special hospitals throughout the United States employed paid auxiliary nursing workers in 1944. The practice of employing paid auxiliary nursing workers was considerably more prevalent among hospitals without schools of nursing than among hospitals with schools of nursing—81 percent and 58 percent, respectively. In the hospitals without schools of nursing, 42 percent of the total nursing care was given by paid auxiliaries. The remainder of the care was provided by the only other group of workers giving nursing care or by the general staff nurses. In the hospitals with schools of nursing, only 17 percent of the care was given by the paid auxiliaries. The remainder of the care in these hospitals was provided by the general staff nurses and the students.

Widespread Introduction of Nurses' Aides and Practical Nurses

It was widely felt that the registered nurse represented too large an investment in education for some of the tasks she was given to perform. One study showed that of 150 practices and procedures involved in nursing care, only 35 percent needed to be done by a registered nurse, while 65 percent could be performed by a practical nurse. During the war approximately 150,000 volunteer nurses' aides had been trained and had served in wartime hospitals. They had literally "saved the day" in many hospitals. Additionally, they had been prepared to

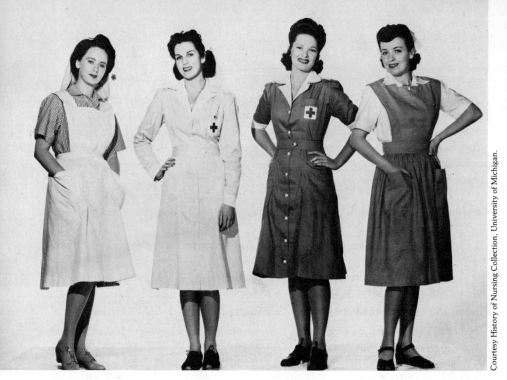

Women who helped ease hospital nursing shortages.

care for family members with mild illnesses in their own homes. Another group of volunteers, the more than 500,000 certificate holders from the Red Cross home nursing classes, were also urged to offer their services to hospitals in nonprofessional capacities. Many members of these two groups gave voluntary service of not less than 150 hours a year in more than 100 Army hospitals, more than 25 veterans' hospitals, and over 2000 civilian hospitals. Others undertook this work at a rate of pay approaching that of the graduate nurse.

Those who received this training had at first been asked not to use their preparation in any paid capacity. Later, to relieve a serious personnel shortage in Army hospitals, the Civil Service Commission, through its regional offices, recruited nurses' aides who had taken the Red Cross course for paid jobs at $1440 a year, with overtime. This was close to the professional nurse's salary and was considered to infringe on the professional nurses who had helped to train the aides.

Due to the recruitment of nurses by the armed services, the limited number of student nurses, and the increased patient-load of civilian hospitals, it became increasingly necessary to pay auxiliary nursing workers to carry out many of the more routine and less technical nursing duties previously performed by graduate registered nurses. An auxiliary worker was defined by the three major national nursing organizations to include "all persons other than graduate registered nurses, attendants, trained attendants, licensed attendants, licensed undergraduate nurses, licensed practical nurses, ward helpers and orderlies, nurses' aides, nursing aides, etc." [13].

Schools of Practical Nursing Proliferate

The term *practical nurse* had been approved by the Joint Board of Directors of the American Nurses' Association, the National League of Nursing Education, and the National Organization for Public Health Nursing. A practical nurse was defined as a person trained to care for subacute, convalescent, and chronic patients requiring nursing services at home or in institutions. She worked under the direction of a licensed physician or a registered professional nurse and gave household assistance when necessary. A practical nurse might be employed by physicians, hospitals, custodial homes, public health agencies, industries, or by the public. This definition suggested specific controls and limitations on practical nurse activities as well as a specified relationship with physicians and professional nurses.

If the above functions of the practical nurse were used as a criterion, during the 1940s thousands of self-styled practical nurses lacked the range of training and the supervised experience necessary to qualify them to use the title. In many states, anyone who assisted in homes or institutions where illness prevailed might designate herself a practical nurse, although her qualifying experience might have consisted only of raising a family in her own home or serving in a limited capacity as a hospital aide.

There were comparatively few standards governing the practice of practical nursing. As of December, 1945, only 19 states and one territory had any legislation dealing with practical nurses, and licensure of practical nurses was mandatory in only one state. Many titles were used to describe workers in the field of practical nursing. There was also considerable variation in the interpretation of the range of duties of the practical nurse and her requisite training.

The first school for training practical nurses had been organized in 1897. By 1930 only 11 schools had been established, but between 1930 and 1947, 25 more were opened. In contrast to the 36 schools established over a half-century, there was an increase of 260 between 1948 and 1954. Most of the early practical nurse schools were attached to hospitals and to institutions for chronic, crippled, aged, or mental patients. Some training programs had been organized under the auspices of YWCAs and other private institutions and agencies. In a few states, practical nurse training was offered in publicly supported vocational education programs.

Under the provisions of the federal vocational education acts, funds to support the training of practical nurses could be provided only as part of a program of trade and industrial education. The federally aided classes, conducted by local public schools, included practical experience in cooperating hospitals. In 1949 federal money went to 50 classes operating in 22 states and graduating approximately 1100 practical nurses per year. The classes averaged about 20 students each, and the courses ran in length from nine months to a year. The greater proportion of time spent in the first part of the course was given over to classwork. The latter part was devoted largely to practical hospital experience gained under immediate medical and nursing supervision. Graduate nurses were used as instructors and supervisors.

Practical nurse programs in the public schools generally did not charge tuition unless the student resided outside the school district. Elsewhere, however, a fee might be charged, and in some schools it was as much as $200. Without any strong professional association to police the programs, some schools resembled exploitative trade schools. In some there were no provisions for a maintenance allowance, but a few cooperating hospitals paid the students as much as $1820 for the service portion of their training.

Duties of the LPN

At mid-century there were more than 144,000 practical nurses, 95 percent of them women. This was a 35 percent increase over 1940. Many hospitals gradually expanded the range of duties assigned to practical nurses; for example, they were increasingly being trained for service in the operating room. In effect the practical nurse was repeating the history of the registered nurse, who had inherited tasks from the physician. She was broadening her work spectrum by piecemeal accumulation of activities that the registered nurse lacked time to complete. Once the LPN had begun to undertake a certain task she was likely to think of it as being within her domain. Some professional nurses worried that, as the salary of the diploma-holding nurse was raised higher, every purchaser—hospital administrator, clinic administrator, nursing home administrator—would seek protection through substitution. Each would try to get his job done by using less expensive personnel.

By 1952 the nonprofessional group employed in nursing service accounted for 56 percent of professional and nonprofessional personnel combined. Although it was apparent that acceptable nursing care could be provided by people with less training, refusal to acknowledge that in the future most nursing personnel would be other than RNs created some bitterness among registered nurses. In addition to the general criticism of the quality and quantity of nonprofessional help, there was a good deal of resentment about the status, privileges, and responsibilities granted to practical nurses. Objection was also voiced that uniforms of practical nurses did not adequately distinguish them from professional nurses. Comment elicited in one study included the following:

Nonprofessional help are literally treated with kid gloves at the expense of the nurses. They refuse to do their work, do it slovenly, are openly abusive, and when such situations are reported, the nurse is invariably held at fault.

The once "thrill" of being "capped" is gone. We find a few months' course and we can become a "trained" nurse, cap and all, and practically receive the same salary as an RN. Many of our public do not know the difference. We once had something to look forward to at the end of our three- or five-year course, a cap and that wonderful distinction of being an R.N., an honor we wanted the whole world to know; we were a little different than others. Now we even take orders from nonprofessionals, instead of doing what we know is best, and like it.

I believe that where there is a shortage of registered nurses, there is a need for nurses' aides. There are many things which nurses' aides can be trained to do, but I feel that the

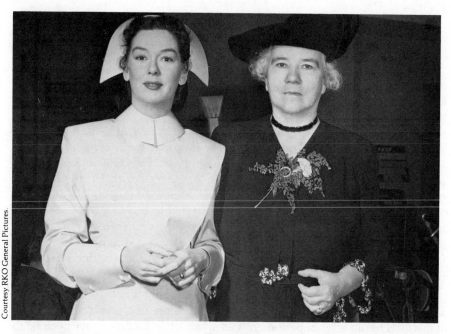

Amidst unsettled postwar nurse-physician relations, Sister Elizabeth Kenny (right), a tough-minded Australian nurse, battled physicians over the proper treatment of infantile paralysis, and was identified by Life *magazine as "the most publicly controversial figure in the medical world today." On the left is Rosalind Russell, who portrayed the nurse in the 1946 RKO film* Sister Kenny.

administration of medicines and assisting with operations, etc., should be done only by those trained professional nurses who are fit for the responsibility involved.

This hospital allows these practical nurses to do medications, intravenous, and all procedures in general; however, you hear complaints from patients continuously about poor treatment. This hospital also calls practical nurses to do private duty when there are registered nurses available.

I really don't blame girls for not taking up nurses' training when they can get positions in the profession without a moment's training of any sort, right out of high school, are requested to wear white caps, white uniforms . . . and receive a higher wage than RNs working in an MD's office. The nurses' white uniform is worn by anyone who wishes to don it and it certainly burns [us] up [14].

The Brown Report

About this time, far-reaching changes in nursing practice and nursing education were recommended in a 1948 report, *Nursing for the Future*, by Esther Lucille Brown, Ph.D., of the research staff of the Russell Sage Foundation. "Today the nurse probably ranks close to the teacher as a social necessity," observed Dr. Brown. Nevertheless, society did not assist nursing education as it did teacher training, and other conditions within and outside the profession had alarmingly reduced the number of applicants available for training. Nursing was fighting a losing battle in attracting the needed numbers of young women.

"Many thoughtful persons," remarked Dr. Brown, "are beginning to wonder why young women in any large numbers would want to enter nursing as practiced, or schools of nursing as operated today." The report also pointed to "authoritarianism" in the hospitals, where the nurse was caught between the dictates of the medical administration and those of the hospital administration; it pleaded for more freedom for nurses and a larger share in policy determination [15].

Conditions in nursing education were regarded as central to the whole problem of the profession. "By no stretch of the imagination," the report charged, "can the education provided in the vast majority of some 1250 schools be conceived of as professional education." Dr. Brown perceived that many hundreds of hospitals still operated schools to avail themselves of the services of student nurses. She recommended "that effort be directed to building basic schools of nursing in universities and colleges, comparable in number to existing medical schools, that are sound in organizational and financial structure, adequate in facilities and faculty, and well-distributed to serve the needs of the entire country" [16].

Without giving approval even to the best hospital schools for the indefinite future, the report stated that "the continued existence of a considerable number is essential for an interim period until adequate other facilities have been established and are sufficiently patronized to guarantee a steady flow of personnel into nursing." But the report added that there had long been "consensus that an undetermined number of weak schools—running certainly into several hundreds—should be closed." The smaller schools, in particular, had rendered a poor performance record. Dr. Brown pointed to a 1945 evaluation by the Division of Nursing of the United States Public Health Service of 602 schools of fewer than 100 students that rated only 4 percent as excellent or good, 50 percent as fair, and 46 percent as poor or very poor. Dr. Brown's report recommended:

That nursing make one of its first matters of important business the long overdue official examination of every school.

That lists of accredited schools be published and distributed, with a statement to the effect that any school not named had failed to meet minimum requirements for accreditation or had refused to permit examination.

That a nationwide educational campaign be conducted for the purpose of rallying broad public support for accredited schools and for subjecting slow-moving state boards and nonaccredited schools to strong social pressure.

That provision be made for periodic re-examination of all schools listed or others requesting it, as well as for first examination of new schools, and for publication and distribution of the revised list.

That, if organized nursing committed itself to this undertaking of major social significance, the public assume responsibility for a substantial part of the financial burden [17].

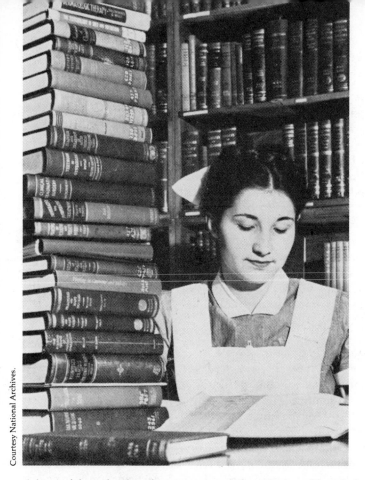

A bitter debate developed among nurses, physicians, and hospital administrators over the desirability of increased amounts of theory in nursing curricula.

The Brown report was predicated on the assumption that a solid basic education is an essential for every citizen of a free and self-governing nation, and particularly for every nurse, regardless of her work. Formerly a system of apprenticeship, nursing education was slowly becoming a well-planned program of preparation for a calling that could rank as the equal of other professions. In making this transition, nursing education was moving unmistakably into colleges and universities. Like other professions, it was finding in colleges the proper intellectual climate for the preparation of the professional worker. Nurse educators with vision were strongly impressed with the need for better teaching and for better resources in libraries, laboratories, and other physical facilities for education available in colleges and universities. They were beginning to realize the need for developing research in nursing and for professional writing and publication if nursing were to be brought abreast of its associated professions. Alert nurses, because of new insights into the advantages of higher education, were also anxious to associate with stimulating persons in other fields within higher education.

Reactionary Attack on the Brown Report

Many physicians and hospital administrators were hostile to these aspirations. In his final appearance as president of the American Hospital Association, Graham Davis of Battle Creek, Michigan, told the 1948 AMA convention in Atlantic City that Dr. Esther Lucille Brown's report ignored the facts of life. "Nurses 20 years from now will not look back with pride on this period in their history," Davis said, referring to what he termed the "trade unionism element" in nursing. "There is a better way to seek economic security," he declared. Davis pointed out that Dr. Brown was not a nurse and that the survey on which the report was based covered a comparatively small number of nursing schools. He was especially critical of her characterization of many small hospital schools of nursing as "socially undesirable." He defended these schools, pointing out that they had made it possible for hospitals to deliver nursing service throughout the wartime and postwar shortages [18].

Accreditation Finally Becomes a Reality

To strengthen schools to meet the new needs for better prepared nurses, the nursing organizations began to establish their long-discussed accreditation program, through the Committee to Implement the Brown Report, soon renamed the National Committee for the Improvement of Nursing Services. It was recognized that some classification method was necessary to focus attention on the need for more rapid improvement in basic nursing programs. Accordingly, the Subcommittee on School Data Analysis was appointed to make a study of all schools of nursing in the United States. Although participation was voluntary, 96 percent of the schools returned the Subcommittee questionnaire.

Statistical procedures were utilized in analyzing information submitted on the questionnaires, and each school was evaluated in terms of long-accepted criteria by the profession. Schools were classified according to their total score, on a 100-point scale based on standards of nursing recommended by the professional organizations. The weight given to various criteria and the maximum scores assigned to them were as follows [19]:

Administrative policies	3
Financial organization	3
Faculty	22
Curriculum	16
Clinical field	22
Library	6
Student selection and provisions for student welfare	13
Student performance on state board examinations	15
Total score	100

When ranked according to general, overall excellence, schools in the upper 25 percent were classified as Group I, those in the middle 50 percent as Group II, and those in the lowest 25 percent as Group III. The schools reporting to the

Subcommittee (1150 out of 1190 state-accredited schools) were classified as follows [20]:

	Number of Schools	Number of Students
Group I	301	36,436
Group II	567	46,483
Group III	282	13,779

All of the 114 college-controlled schools participated and were classified in Group I or Group II. The findings were published in a report, *Nursing Schools at the Mid-century*.

The NOHSN Fights Back

As a reaction to the classification project, as well as to the general thrust toward nursing in higher education, the National Organization of Hospital Schools of Nursing, with headquarters in Atlanta, was formed for the avowed purpose of aiding hospital schools of nursing in what was termed a "struggle for existence." The new association protested that approximately 240 schools of nursing had been omitted from the list "accredited" by the National Committee for the Improvement of Nursing Service. The NOHSN believed that too many "good schools of nursing which have served their communities well do not appear on this list" and that all "present schools are needed and should continue." It was claimed that accreditation had been arbitrary, since the classification had been based on a survey questionnaire that the schools had not known would be used for this purpose and no visits to the unaccredited schools had been made [21].

Because the Brown Report had advocated the movement of nursing education into a collegiate setting and the National League of Nursing Education had urged that hospital schools "give early consideration to the transfer of control and administration to educational institutions," the NOHSN felt that a new organization was justified in order to aid existing hospital schools of nursing. According to Lucy I. Mace, secretary-treasurer, "the incorporators believe that all hospital schools of nursing approved by State Boards of Nurse Examiners should be accepted for membership. We will publish our own list of approved schools and conduct a general public relations program which will be favorable to the hospital schools" [22].

"Confusion, discouragement, and even despair exist among nurses, physicians, and hospital administrators today," said one NOHSN release. It also mentioned that "it is well known that the described conditions furnish fertile fields for the seeds of ideologies contrary to Americanism." It was also charged that the accreditation and collegiate nursing movements were "contingent upon use of federal subsidy and therefore inevitable federal control." To accept such programs knowingly was characterized as a step "to aid and abet the enemies of free enterprise and freedom" [23].

Controversy over National Health Insurance

The postwar crusade to upgrade nursing education carried over into the emotionalism and controversy about national health insurance. On November 19, 1945, President Truman submitted to Congress his recommendation for a comprehensive, modern national health program. It consisted of five parts:

Federal grants for construction of hospitals and related facilities.

Expansion of public health, maternity, and child health services.

Federal grants for medical education, nursing education, and research.

Establishment of a national social insurance system for the prepayment of medical costs.

Expansion of present social insurance systems to furnish protection against loss of wages from sickness and disability.

The same day, Senator Robert F. Wagner of New York introduced, with Senator James E. Murray of Montana, a bill to establish such a plan. Representative John Dingell of Michigan introduced a companion bill in the House. The Wagner-Murray bill, S. 1606, was the subject of extensive hearings between April and July of 1946. Chances of passage looked poor at the outset when Senator Robert A. Taft of Ohio got involved in a heated argument with Committee Chairman Murray after declaring that the bill was, to his mind, "the most socialistic measure that this Congress has ever had before it, seriously" [24].

The medical provisions were the most controversial part of the bill, which provided for a single payroll deduction of 6 percent on annual incomes up to $3000, with employers paying a like amount. Self-employed persons such as grocers, farmers, and physicians would pay 7 percent. One-quarter of the total funds would be applied to medical care costs, the balance going to insurance against old age, unemployment, maternity, temporary illness, and permanent disability. For the employed person, complete medical care for himself and his dependents would cost 1.5 percent of his income, up to $3000, or not more than $3.75 a month. An average, middle-income family in 1946 paid 4 percent of their income on medical bills alone, or about $120 annually on $3000. Of course, most families would not pay the maximum $3.75 monthly, or $45 annually, for medical and hospital care, because three-fourths of them made less than $3000 a year.

Opponents charged that the bill was "communistic," "un-American," "a stab at free enterprise," and a scheme to provide an inferior kind of "political medicine" to the people. Led by the American Medical Association, the opposition included several large national drug chains, some private insurance companies, a group of patent medicine and drug manufacturers, the American Bar Association, and the American Hospital Association.

Those in favor of the bill argued that tax-supported medicine was no more un-American than tax-supported education. They were led by sponsoring

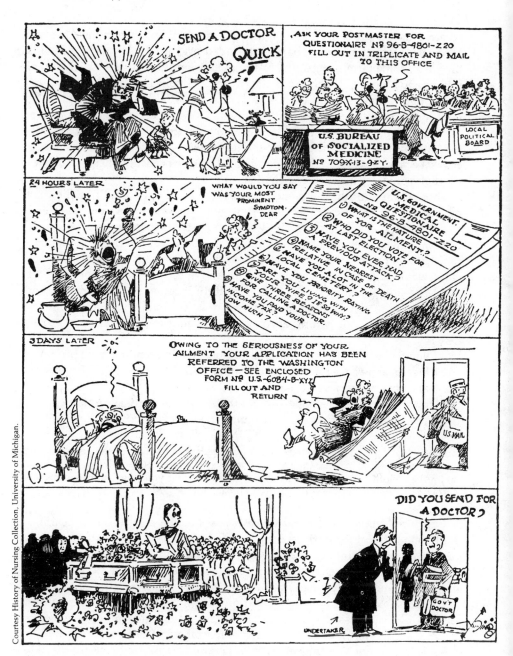

Anti-National Health Insurance cartoon.

senators and congressmen and by a minority of physicians within the American Medical Association. Other backers included organized labor (The AFL and the CIO), some farm groups, the National Lawyers' Guild, the Association of Interns and Medical Students, and the American Public Health Association.

The opposition forces insisted that: (1) the bill would rob the patient of his right to choose his own physician; (2) it would lower standards of medical care; (3) it would make physicians "slaves" to bureaucrats; (4) it would cut the doctors' incomes by ending the fee-for-service system; and (5) the bill was unnecessary because anyone could get the medical care he needed, either privately or through voluntary insurance or charity.

Those in favor of the bill replied that: (1) the bill did not limit free choice of physicians; rather, it extended the privilege to those who had not had much choice before; (2) standards of care would be raised, because a physician would be able to make free use of costly equipment, specialists' services, and laboratory tests that were often beyond the financial means of his patients; (3) physicians would still be independent, and under National Health Insurance they would be sure of getting paid; (4) most doctors' incomes would be raised, and those who wished to keep on with private practice could do so; and (5) many people who were not getting adequate care would at last gain access to its benefits.

Although results differed from poll to poll, public opinion seemed to favor some federal assistance for medical care payments. One poll, commissioned by the California Medical Association to determine how physicians could meet the "threat of federal medicine," found that 50 percent of California's citizens definitely favored federally supported medicine. They noted:

Among upper-income groups, federal medicine is desired because of the poor. Among the poor it is desired because they want proper care themselves . . . . If it were to come up on the ballot today . . . it seems abundantly clear that you [the California Medical Association] would lose the issue—perhaps by a landslide [25].

Organized nursing produced two witnesses at the congressional hearings. Katherine J. Densford testified for the American Nurses' Association before a Senate Committee on April 24, 1946, but could only state that the 181,000-member ANA had taken no action regarding S. 1606, since the House of Delegates would not be meeting until September 1946. Ruth Sleeper, president of the National League of Nursing Education, submitted a statement that favored the bill. She emphasized that in order to meet current and future demands of the health care system it was essential that federal grants be provided to nursing schools to improve clinical courses in undergraduate nursing education and to improve, expand, and develop new programs for graduate nurses preparing to become teachers or administrators in schools of nursing and administrators or supervisors in all types of nursing services. According to Miss Sleeper, the NLNE favored federal aid to nursing education on a direct basis, from Washington, rather than through individual state health departments.

Because congressional support for National Health Insurance was insufficient to bring about passage of the program, President Truman convened in May, 1948, a National Health Assembly, attended by 800 professional and community leaders, including several prominent nurses. Using this assembly as a publicity springboard, Federal Security Administrator Oscar Ewing prepared a report to the President entitled *The Nation's Health: A Ten Year Program*, outlining a plan for comprehensive, federally sponsored, compulsory health insurance. This report was regarded as a danger signal by the leaders of the American Medical Association. They were frightened by its attractive format almost as much as by its content. They decided that a grave danger had arrived, to be forcefully attacked if Truman won his second term.

The AMA "Educates" the Public

In December, 1948, shortly after the election, the AMA assessed its members $25 each for a nationwide plan of "education," and during the next 3½ years it spent over $4.5 million in informing the American people about the hazards of "socialized medicine." A public relations firm managed the campaign, which on the whole allied organized medicine with the Republican Party and with Senator Robert A. Taft of Ohio.

Rhetorically, they asked, "Does the report on the nation's health give a factual picture of the people's health in America?" They answered: "No. This widely publicized report is a hoax. It is a propagandist treatment of a subject far too important for such loose handling by political experimenters." They asked, "Who is for Compulsory Health Insurance?" and answered, "The Federal Security Administration. The President. All who seriously believe in a Socialistic State. Every left-wing organization in America . . . the Communist Party." The plan to improve the nation's health was dismissed as part of a trend toward complete socialization of American life: "The Government proposes to assume control not only of the medical profession, but of hospitals—both public and private—and drug and appliance industries, dentistry, pharmacy, nursing and allied professions" [26].

In terms of money spent, the heart of the AMA's National Education Campaign was the production and distribution of pamphlets. Literature was produced by the national office and distributed by physicians, through cooperating organizations, and by direct mail. In the first year of the campaign alone the total distribution of literature ran to more than 54 million pieces, at a cost of over $1 million. Although the principal distribution agents were physicians and organizations of physicians, dentists, druggists, the insurance industry, and other groups made substantial contributions.

Clem Whitaker and Leone Baxter, directors of the campaign, addressed the Conference of State Medical Societies in Chicago on February 12, 1949:

Mr. Chairman and ladies and gentleman; every minister preaches from a text—and every campaign, if it is a successful campaign, has to have a theme!

The theme, if it is geared to reach more than 100 million people, as we must in this campaign, should have simplicity and clarity. Most of all, it must high-point the major issues of the campaign with great brevity—in language that paints a picture understandable to people in all circumstances.

That's one of the reasons we have a large blown-up color reproduction of the famous Fildes painting, *The Doctor*, on exhibit here today, with the simple caption under it: "Keep politics out of this picture!"

The picture and the caption, even without elaboration, focus attention on one of the most important arguments against government-controlled medicine.

Smaller color reproductions of this famous painting soon will go up in doctor's offices all over America as one of the first steps in dramatizing our case to the American people—and more important—as the first step in making doctors campaigners in their own behalf. For this purpose we have added a hundred words of text which help to establish the theme of this campaign.

The public relations experts then read the 100-word text that accompanied the painting:

"Keep Politics out of this Picture!"

When the life—or health—of a loved one is at stake, hope lies in the devoted service of your doctor.

Would you change this picture?

Compulsory health insurance is political medicine.

It would bring a third party—a politician—between you and your doctor. It would bind up your family's health in red tape. It would result in heavy payroll taxes—and inferior medical care for you and your family. Don't let that happen here.

You have a right to prepaid medical care—of your own choice. Ask your doctor, or your insurance man, about budget-basis health protection.

This is signed: American Medical Association [27].

Physicians at the state and local level nearly abandoned their professional ethics to political arm-twisting. One letter to the patients of a number of New York physicians appealed frankly to the patients' sense of gratitude for services rendered. "You and I have been friends for some time," it said. "I believe I have served you faithfully and well with sympathy and understanding in your hours of need. There are evil forces creeping into this country which would destroy this personal relationship. They would deny you my services and would deny me the freedom of exercising my skill in serving you." The letter went on at length and closed with the request, "as a service to yourself and to me and to America, that you, your family, and your friends vote in this coming election"—for John Foster Dulles, described earlier in the same letter as "thoroughly opposed to socialized medicine and all other European 'isms'" [28].

Federal Aid to Nursing Stymied
Aware that the controversial national health legislation package was effectively

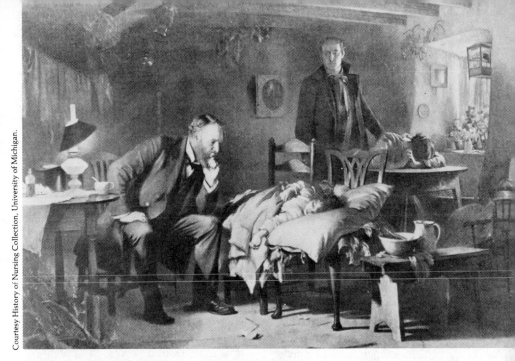

The nineteenth century artist Luke Fildes' The Doctor was effectively used in the AMA campaign with the slogan: "Keep Politics Out of this Picture!"

blocked by a coalition of conservative Republicans and Southern Democrats, Senator Elbert D. Thomas of Utah in June, 1949, extracted the Title I health manpower provisions out of a pending national health insurance measure and introduced them as a separate bill. This proposal envisioned a five-year program of aid for nursing education ranging from $13 million in fiscal year 1950 to $20 million in fiscal year 1954. Eligibility for federal aid for schools of nursing was to be determined by an agency designated by the Surgeon General of the Public Health Service.

Under the management of Senator Claude Pepper of Florida, the Emergency Professional Health Training Act of 1949 passed the Senate unanimously on September 23. Hopes for passage were high as the House Committee on Interstate and Foreign Commerce reported favorably on the accompanying House version of the bill, sponsored by Representative Andrew Biemiller, on October 11, 1949, but now the new National Organization of Hospital Schools of Nursing flexed its muscles. According to the NOHSN, the bill was aimed at "regimentation or nationalization of the medical, dental, and nursing professions." It would enable the Surgeon General of the United States Public Health Service to control hospital schools of nursing, since it would give him the power to select the body or bodies approving schools eligible to receive federal funds.

The bill bogged down in the House Rules Committee, as a result of the efforts of some Georgia and North Carolina nurses:

A small group of insurgent members of the nurses' organization in Georgia and North Carolina, and the owner of a private hospital in the latter state, got the impression that the measure would somehow set up the American Nurses' Association as an accrediting body for all nursing schools—and thus force the closing down, for lack of accreditation, of some of the less qualified schools in the Southern States.

On behalf of this group, Representative Robert L. (Muley) Doughton of North Carolina protested to the Rules Committee. The sponsors of the Bill offered to amend the measure to overcome the objection. This satisfied Doughton and he withdrew his protest.

But the Biemiller bill had, by then, become "controversial." The Rules Committee, fearful of setting a precedent that would throw a host of other controversial measures on the House Floor in the last two weeks of the session, withheld its approval. The bill was held up until Congress could meet again [29].

Although reintroduced in the next Congress, the bill failed even to pass the Senate, because supporters such as Claude Pepper, Elbert Thomas, and Frank Graham of North Carolina had met with defeat in the 1950 congressional elections, a defeat due partly to the efforts of the AMA lobby.

The postwar phenomena of an acute shortage of graduate nurses brought entirely new demands upon a profession formerly faced with perennial oversupply. As preparation for nursing began shifting from a process of apprenticeship and training to one of education, the student labor component was accordingly diminished at the same time general hospitals were expanding. Many nursing leaders looked to the federal government for a solution to the nurse shortage, but the mood of the country was growing conservative and plans for federal assistance were successfully blocked.

Summary

As the war came to a close, it was anticipated that military nurses would return to civilian nursing positions and that the acute shortage of graduate nurses would be eased. Unfortunately, however, great numbers of nurses left the profession for marriage or because they were dissatisfied with the working conditions, pay, and small degree of autonomy. Moreover, thousands of students dropped out of nursing programs as the patriotic urge diminished. Concommitantly, recruitment of students was hampered by the phase out of the Cadet Nurse Corps.

In September, 1946, at the joint convention of the ANA, NLNE, and NOPHN in Atlantic City, a platform was adopted that called for reforms aimed at making nursing an economically viable and professionally satisfying occupation.

According to a national survey in 1946, nurses worked an average of 48 hours per week and were paid less than women in other similar occupations. Another postwar study found that 76.4 percent of nurses planned to leave the field for one reason or another. Job satisfaction among hospital nurses was low and fewer young women were choosing nursing as a career.

Amid continuing nurse shortages and controversy over the so-called high costs of nursing service, nurses' aides, and practical nurses, who had gained a foot-

*hold during the war, skyrocketed in numbers. Although these auxiliaries gen-
erally performed the less technical, more routine tasks, some hospitals turned
over much greater responsibilities to them, and confusion ensued as to the
proper range of their duties and responsibilities. The great variance in practical
nurse training programs was also of concern.*

*As nonprofessional groups rapidly entered the hospital field, the ratio of pro-
fessional to nonprofessional workers within hospitals changed. By 1952, 56
percent of the workers were of nonprofessional status.*

*Meanwhile, far-reaching changes in nursing practice and nursing education
were recommended in 1948 in Dr. Esther Lucille Brown's* Nursing *for the Future.
Among her recommendations were that schools of nursing be moved into collegiate settings and that the profession undertake a program of accreditation of
all nursing education programs.*

*Although most physicians and hospital administrators were hostile to the ideas
put forth in the Brown report, the professional nursing organizations formed
the Committee to Implement the Brown Report to work on the development of
an accreditation program.*

*A subcommittee on School Data Analysis was established to survey and analyze
information about the country's schools of nursing. Based on questionnaire
results, a classification system was created, and participating schools were
ranked according to level of excellence.*

*The National Organization of Hospital Schools of Nursing objected to the
classification scheme and claimed that many good schools were omitted from
the "accredited" list. Its members felt that the results of the survey were arbitrary, and they attempted to counter this with their own accreditation program.*

*In 1945 President Truman recommended a comprehensive, progressive national
health program that included national health insurance. Opponents, rallying
behind the AMA, the American Bar Association, the AHA, and other groups,
charged that the measure was "un-American and "communistic."*

*Advocates of national health insurance included socially-minded legislators, a
minority of physicians, organized labor, the National Lawyers' Guild, the Association of Interns and Medical Students, and the American Public Health
Association. Public opinion polls indicated that a majority of Americans favored the bill.*

*After President Truman had been reelected in 1948, the AMA staged a nation-
wide plan of public "education." During the next 3½ years the AMA spent
over $4.5 million in propaganda literature to inform the American people
about the hazards of "socialized medicine."*

After a coalition of conservative Republicans and Southern Democrats had effectively blocked the comprehensive national health insurance bill, Senator Elbert D. Thomas of Utah extracted the Title I health manpower provisions out of the legislation and introduced them separately. This new bill, proposing a five-year program of federal aid for nursing education, was passed by the Senate but it failed in the House.

References

1. Howard Whitman and Douglas J. Ingalls, "Don't Curse the Nurse," *Colliers*, May 31, 1947, pp. 26, 67–69.
2. *Ibid.*, p. 67.
3. U.S. Department of Labor, Bureau of Labor Statistics, *The Economic Status of Registered Professional Nurses, 1946–1947* (Washington, D.C.: Government Printing Office, 1948), pp. 42–43.
4. "The Biennial," *American Journal of Nursing*, vol. 46 (November, 1946): 728–783.
5. *Ibid.*, pp. 728–729.
6. Clarence Woodbury, "Student Nurse–Could You Take It?" *Woman's Home Companion*, vol. 76 (June, 1949): 36.
7. "What's All This About the Deplorable State of Nursing Schools?" *Hospital Management*, vol. 67 (June, 1949): 31.
8. *Ibid.*, pp. 31–32.
9. Kenneth A. Brent, "Are Nurses Getting Too Much Education?" *Hospital Management*, vol. 67 (April, 1949): 68.
10. *Ibid.*, pp. 68–70.
11. *Ibid.*, p. 70.
12. "College of Surgeons Surveys the Nursing Situation," *Modern Hospital*, vol. 69 (August, 1947): 59.
13. Joint Committee on Auxiliary Nursing Service, "Annual Report to the NLNE," *Proceedings of the 50th Annual Convention of the National League of Nursing Education*, vol. 50 (September, 1946): 239–250.
14. U.S. Department of Labor, Bureau of Labor Statistics, *The Economic Status of Registered Professional Nurses, 1946–1947* (Washington, D.C.: Government Printing Office, 1948), p. 46.
15. Esther Lucile Brown, *Nursing for the Future* (New York: Russell Sage Foundation, 1948), pp. 45–46, 165–166.
16. *Ibid.*, pp. 48, 178.
17. *Ibid.*, pp. 132–170.
18. "Graham Davis Attacks Brown Report on 'Nursing for the Future,' " *Modern Hospital*, vol. 71 (October, 1948): 138.
19. M. West and C. Hawkins, *Nursing Schools at the Mid-century* (New York: National Committee for the Improvement of Nursing Services, 1950), p. 56.
20. *Ibid.*, pp. 81–85.
21. "New Group Will Combat Legislation Unfavorable to Unclassified Nursing Schools," *Modern Hospital*, vol. 74 (February, 1950): 128.
22. "Survival of Hospital Schools Called Matter of Utmost Urgency," *Hospital Management*, vol. 69 (January, 1950): 30.
23. *Ibid.*
24. U.S. Congress, Senate, Committee on Education and Labor, *National Health Program*. Hearing, Seventy-ninth Congress, Second Session on S. 1606, a bill to provide for a national health program. Part 2. (Washington, D.C.: Government Printing Office, 1946), pp. 46–47.

25. N. Adams, "Why Opinion Polls on Socialized Medicine Don't Agree." *Medical Economics*, vol. 24 (February, 1947): 72–74.
26. James G. Burrow, *AMA: Voice of American Medicine* (Baltimore: Johns Hopkins Press, 1963), pp. 368–369.
27. U.S. Congress, House, Committee on Interstate and Foreign Commerce, *National Health Plan*. Hearings, Eighty-first Congress, First Session. H.R. 4312 and H.R. 4313 and H.R. 4918 and other identical bills (Washington, D.C.: Government Printing Office, 1949), pp. 28–31.
28. R. M. Cunningham, "Can Political Means Gain Professional Ends?" *Modern Hospital*, vol. 77 (December, 1951): 51–56.
29. *Congressional Record*, October 3, 1951.

16
Nursing at Midcentury

Close to 390,000 professional registered nurses were employed in 1950 in the United States and its territories. About half of the active professional nurses were now working in hospitals and other health institutions, whereas in 1928 less than one-fourth of the active RNs had been so employed. In the period following World War II, it had been feared by some that the release of nurses from military service would create a civilian oversupply, but the exact opposite occurred.

Persistence of an Acute Shortage of Nurses

In 1950 the American Hospital Association stated that 22,486 vacancies for graduate nurses existed in 2677 of the 4830 hospitals which reported on the nurse shortage. More registered nurses were working than ever before in the nation's history, yet a critical shortage of nursing service existed in almost every city and rural area. Reports from all over the country described the shortage as "critical," "severe," "serious," "acute," and "pressing." What was meant was that hospitals had been forced to shut wards, new units could not be opened, and new programs for health services could not be started.

In Birmingham many hospitals were working nurses on 12-hour shifts instead of on the normal eight, with some nurses performing double-shift duty. Many hospitals were using practical nurses to cover situations where professional nurses were needed. The Alabama Nurses' Association and the Alabama Hospital Association pooled $5000 and appointed a full-time nurse recruiter for the state. While many young women were recruited during the year that this drive took place, the funds were exhausted and the drive had to be closed.

In Boston the Massachusetts General Hospital affiliated with a school of practical nursing, giving students from that institution 13 months of bedside training out of a 15-month program. The practical nursing students helped to free professional nurses for other duties as did the aides the hospital hired who were trained in a short, six-week course. These persons were replacing the volunteers of the war years. The hospitals operated on a team plan whereby a graduate nurse served as team leader and was assisted by aides and practical nurses to care for a group of patients. The auxiliary workers took the morning temperatures, got breakfast trays passed, and then received instructions for the day's assignments from the team leader. Nursing students and occasionally other graduate nurses were also assigned to these teams and carried out selected aspects of patient care. The team leader received her instructions from the head nurse.

In Chicago the Illinois Hospital Association and the Blue Cross Plan for hospital care were entering the third year of a joint drive to increase enrollment in schools of nursing and reduce the nursing student withdrawal rate. The group's goal was 3500 admissions each year and 2250 graduations. Cooperating in the drive were the Illinois State Nurses' Association, the Illinois League of Nursing Education, and the Illinois Medical Society. A feature of the campaign was student nurses' week, which was to be proclaimed annually by the governor. Prior to the week's opening, sponsors of the drive got their message to the public through the newspapers, television, radio, church sermons, hospital-sponsored poster contests in schools (with scholarships awarded to the winner), hospital equipment exhibits in department stores, open houses at hospitals for high school students, and teas for prospective nurses. Also supporting the drive were civic and fraternity organizations and women's groups. Meanwhile, the Chicago Council on Community Nurses had assumed leadership in educating practical nurses as one approach to easing the shortage. Working with the Board of Education and aided by several grants, the Council had training branches in two Chicago schools.

Cleveland hospitals, in a desperate attempt to obtain qualified nurses, had adopted a general, 40-hour work week, increased wages, and improved working conditions. One hospital opened an adjacent nursery in an effort to attract nurses who had married and left the work force. Ten nurses with young children took advantage of the project and returned to active nursing. Several hospitals experimented briefly with nurseries for the children of hospital personnel but abandoned the plan for fear of an epidemic of childhood diseases. Other hospitals did not initiate nurseries because of the high cost of operations. In the emergency shortage of registered nurses, hospitals had been employing students as nursing assistants, and many interns were also picking up spending money by working extra hours as nurses.

In Los Angeles the nurse shortage had caused a mushrooming of hit-and-run commercial schools which advertised that, for less than $200 tuition and in as little as 24 hours of instruction, they could prepare practical nurses who could earn "big money." Such schools actually did not even have nurse-aide training, much less a practical nurse course, but they gave graduates a cap and a pin and turned them loose. Several such schools were transplanted Eastern enterprises, one of them having taught air conditioning and television repair in Baltimore.

In Philadelphia the Community Nursing Bureau of Metropolitan Philadelphia, organized by professional and lay people who contributed funds and material, opened in February to register nurses to supply hospitals, physicians, and the general public. Nurses were able to register for full-time, part-time, or hourly work. The Careers in Nursing Committee of the Nursing Council of Metropolitan Philadelphia had been conducting a vigorous enlistment campaign. It held career forums in various sections to stimulate interest in nursing.

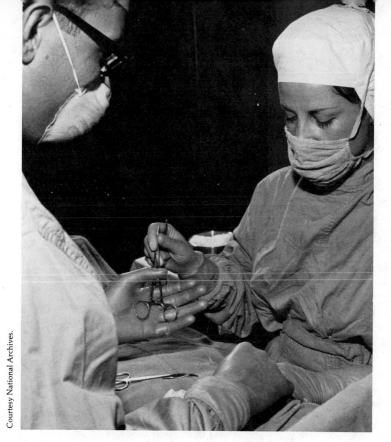

An acute nurse shortage endangered standards of nursing care.

Since the program started four years prior to that time, schools of nursing and hospitals had held open house each spring so that parents and prospective students could see nurses in action. The Nursing Council also was encouraging the training of practical nurses. The Philadelphia Public School System had a program for educating practical nurses with students receiving three months of classroom work and nine months in hospitals.

In Seattle the legislature had passed a law providing for the licensing of practical nurses with only 450 hours of special preparation and five months of on-the-job training. The University of Washington School of Nursing planned to announce a working agreement with the Virginia Mason Hospital, Seattle, to conduct a training program tied-in with the nursing school. Hospitals in Seattle were using more practical nurses and nurses aides than ever before. Practical nurses were assigned by the Professional Nurses Registry, for duty both in private homes and in hospitals under supervision. The King County Nurses' Association voted against the use of practical nurses for private duty in hospitals, feeling that enough responsibility had been delegated to practical nurses already.

The nationwide shortage of nurses hit New York harder than any other large city in the country. Nurses were leaving the city hospitals faster than replacements could be found. Those remaining could not give adequate care to patients because of their increased work load in already overcrowded facilities. As a result, the department of hospitals was operating with only 53 percent of the registered nurses it needed. The shortage in the hospitals was paralleled in the department of health. To maintain its public health services, it needed at least 1600 nurses; the department, however, had an authorization for 1071 but employed only 795.

Why was the shortage so great if there were more nurses than ever? There was general agreement among nursing and other health groups that, while there was a need for more nursing service because of the tremendous expansion of health and medical services emphasized by the mobilization program, the following factors had changed the pattern of medical and nursing care: the rising average age of the population; the growth of population and its urbanization; the growth of hospitalization and group health insurance plans; the change in the techniques of medicine such as the use of "miracle" drugs that kept patients alive who formerly would have died; the spread of nurses out of hospitals into industry and public health services; and the large increase in the number of mothers who had their babies in hospitals.

Characteristics of the Labor Force Pertaining to Nursing

In 1940 the number of women 15- to 19-years-old in the population was 6,153,370, but in 1950 the number was only 5,431,000. According to decennial census figures, in 1950 there were about 300,000 fewer women 18 and 19 years of age than in 1940. Not until 1960 would the declining trend in the number of young women in the population be reversed. Meanwhile the general population increased in the decade 1940–1950 among the youngest and the oldest age groups. The lowest point in the nation's recorded national birth rate had been in 1933. From 1933 to 1940 the birth rate had increased only 8 percent, whereas from 1940 to 1947 it rose 45 percent. The number of young women available to enter a nurse preparation program was less than in former years because the high school graduates of the 1950s were born in the depression period, when the nation's birth rate was at its lowest ebb.

Also of importance was that in 1950, 54 percent of all women 18 to 24 years of age were married (with husbands present), compared with 39.8 percent in 1940. The birth rate per 1000 female population aged 15 to 19 increased from 48.9 to 79.7 by 1950, and the number of children under five years of age increased by 54.7 percent from 1940 to 1950. The increase in the number of marriages among young women was reflected in the accelerated withdrawal rate of nurses from the work force, which was estimated at 6.5 percent per year.

In the 1950s the birth rate astonished all the experts by maintaining the rise it had shown just after World War II. Despite the insecurities of the postwar world and the apparent degree of relaxation in the family structure, it was obvious that most young American married couples wanted several children. Another shift in family patterns was the marked tendency toward earlier marriages and the consequent necessity that many wives support their husbands until they had finished preparing for professional careers.

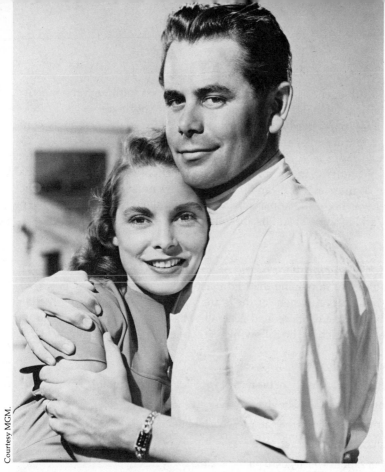

Marriage and children assumed a postwar high about 1950—a fact emphasized in the entertainment of the year as Dr. Michael Corday (Glenn Ford) married Evelyn Heldon (Janet Leigh), who became his office nurse in The Doctor and the Girl. *(From the MGM release* The Doctor and the Girl © *1949 Loew's Incorporated. Copyright renewed 1976 by Metro-Goldwyn-Mayer Inc.)*

In most professions, the majority of new graduates immediately became active and in many cases remained active until death or retirement. This was not the case with nurses. Although most new graduates were active immediately following graduation, a substantial proportion dropped out of their profession within the first three years after graduation and did not reenter the labor force until they were 45 or older, if indeed they ever returned. In other words, nurses tended to withdraw from the labor force in order to marry and raise families.

For young single women, possibilities for marriage and for pregnancy were the most important factors in determining work-life expectancy. The overriding effect of marriage and childbearing upon women's work patterns was obvious. While a nursing education supposedly provided excellent preparation for homemaking, marriage, except in restricted instances, was not compatible with the practice of nursing. Married women generally were not accepted as students by most schools of nursing due to the conflict between living in the hospital and maintaining an outside home. Most hospitals and institutions and some public health agencies also preferred single nurses (although the married nurse had briefly become popular during the wartime shortage).

Married nurses, particularly those with children, tended to be strongly committed to their families. For most student and graduate nurses, marriage and children seemed more important than nursing, and although the motivation for nursing was higher than for any alternative occupation, it could not equal the attraction of marriage and family. Even among nurses who remained active, turnover was high: the nurse shortage was conducive to a high degree of job mobility, and in some hospitals annual turnover exceeded 66 percent.

The Origin and Development of the State Board Test Pool

A postwar movement in nursing that did much to improve standards in schools of nursing was the development of the State Board Test Pool. During the late 1930s, state board examinations had generally been poorly constructed and unreliable. Questions such as the following were asked in a test on hygiene [1]:

Name the six essentials for personal hygiene.

What is the peculiar opportunity of the nurse in public health education?

How often should a schoolchild be given a physical examination?

Lacking an instrument, what is the natural guide for humidity of a room?

Name two health essentials for a student nurse.

Name two organizations which guard public health.

For the test on anatomy, students were asked the following questions:

Designate on or in which bone each of the following is found:
a. foramen magnum
b. olecranon process
c. greater trochanter
d. antrum of Highmore
e. spinuous process

Locate:
a. the visceral pleura
b. the parietal pleura

Name five classes of tissue.

Give an example of each.

By what means are muscles attached to bones?
a. Name and locate the longest nerve in the body.
b. Which nerve has the greatest diameter?

To what system do the following belong?
a. lungs
b. skin
c. urinary organs
d. bones

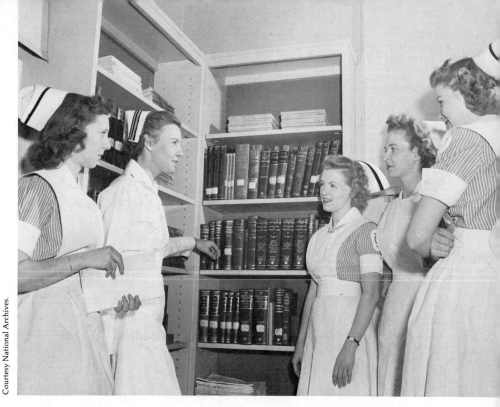

As senior cadets from a number of schools served in military hospitals, variations in state licensing examinations became more apparent.

The outbreak of World War II had increased the pressure on licensing authorities to license eligible candidates as quickly as possible after they had completed their basic programs. Schools quickly found that preparing students to meet the minimum standards for their own state board licensing examinations was no longer adequate; the national norms of competence in nursing had to be taken into consideration. As graduates joined the Army or Navy Nurse Corps and many senior cadets served in federal hospitals, individual schools were compared informally with other schools of nursing in other states.

In December, 1942, at an emergency conference of state boards, the Subcommittee on Tests of the Committee on State Board Problems of the National League of Nursing Education had met and recommended that the League assist states in adopting machine-scored examination questions and implement the proposed plan of developing prepared state board examinations "for the use of all states in order to have more valid and reliable sets of examination questions and to have these available for more frequent examinations."

The objectives which the Committee set up and which the state boards of nurse examiners approved for the State Board Test Pool were as follows:

To provide objective tests of nursing competency which will enable each state board of nurse examiners to discover the level of ability of each candidate and the average for each school in the state, and for the state as a whole, in comparison with the level of all other candidates tested, and the average for each other school and state.

To develop improved tests of nursing ability and work towards a comprehensive test battery of high validity and reliability.

To study nursing ability, as revealed in the examinations, in order to arrive at a clearer concept of the minimum level of competency as well as the average level of expectancy of professional nurses.

To secure data which will be of help to the state boards of nurse examiners and the schools of nursing in improving the level of nursing preparation.

To lighten the burden of busy state boards of nurse examiners by serving as their agent in preparing and scoring the licensing examinations [2].

State boards were asked to submit sample questions to the Committee on Nursing Tests, which selected those judged most suitable. The examinations were then set up for machine scoring. Within one year, by January, 1944, the pool was in operation and six states had agreed to use the examinations.

During the first complete year of operation, 15 states administered these examinations. Licensing authorities in other states were quick to recognize the values to be derived through such a cooperative effort, and within a very short

The State Board Test Pool in 1944 included an examination in surgical nursing. Students observing surgery through binoculars into an amphitheater below.

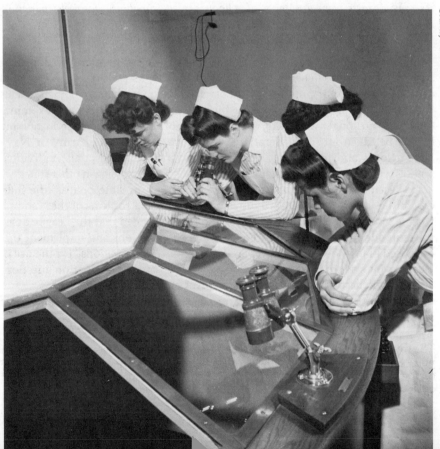

time the State Board Test Pool had become well established. It was operated by the Committee on Measurements and Educational Guidance of the National League of Nursing Education and by the State Board Test Committee—a subcommittee of the Committee on State Board Problems of the League.

The pool simplified the administration of state licensing examinations for nurses and provided participating members with a comparable system of measures for evaluating nursing ability. Participation in the Test Pool program saved time for busy state boards of nurse examiners in correcting papers, speeded up the issuance of licenses to newly graduated nurses, and simplified registration of nurses who moved from one state to another in which the same tests were used.

When the pool was initiated in 1944, the licensing examination had included 13 tests: anatomy and physiology, chemistry, microbiology, nutrition and diet therapy, pharmacology and therapeutics, nursing arts, communicable disease nursing, medical nursing, nursing of children, obstetric and gynecologic nursing, psychiatric nursing, surgical nursing, and social foundations of nursing. The number of tests used varied from state to state: some used all of them, while others used only one. By 1949 the number of tests had been reduced to six: medical nursing, surgical nursing, obstetric nursing, nursing of children, communicable disease nursing, and psychiatric nursing.

Each test included questions designed to evaluate the candidate's understanding of the principles of physical, biological, and social sciences considered important for the learning experiences in the various clinical areas as well as questions designed to test the candidate's nursing skills and abilities in a given clinical area. A concerted effort was made to center most of the test questions around nursing care in given situations. The questions were also designed to test candidates' ability to apply knowledge gained through classroom and clinical experience. Some faculty members had long criticized the mechanical acquisition of factual data required by state board examinations. Because the pool tests emphasized principles rather than facts, instructors could now concentrate on the mastery of working theories and thus better prepare their graduates for nursing.

Since the tests had been devised to challenge even the most able students, the average candidate was able to answer only about half of the total number of questions asked. Nurses who failed to understand that the new tests were based on the principle of "achievement" tended to regard them as too difficult, for they still thought that a successful candidate had to answer 70 to 75 percent of the questions correctly in order to "pass."

Although each state determined its own passing score, the basic fund of knowledge required for licensure as a registered nurse was the same nationally. Only the degree of knowledge required for licensure varied. From time to time the members of the conference of state boards of nurse examiners considered the feasibility of establishing a common score on each test, which they would accept as the minimum level of performance for licensure of professional nurses. In 1951 the conference recommended that a standard score of 350 be used as the passing score in as many states as possible for purposes of interstate registration or for registration by reciprocal agreement. As a result of this action, state boards of nurse examiners in many states accepted this standard for each test as the minimum level of performance acceptable for licensure.

The growth of and the participation in the State Board Test Pool was rapid. Within a five-year period, from January, 1944, to March 1, 1949, this service expanded from the original six states to 41 states. During 1950 the last of the 48 states joined the State Board Test Pool, and nursing became the first profession for which the same licensing examination was used throughout the nation, the District of Columbia, 'and Hawaii. In addition, the Canadian provinces of British Columbia and Alberta were members of the Test Pool. The development of the State Board Test Pool further broadened each school's concept of its goals.

Psychiatric Hospitals

A significant postwar social phenomenon was the increase in psychiatric disorders in society as a whole. By 1948 there were 540,000 inmates in American mental institutions, representing a ratio of 3.7 for every 1000 people, in contrast to only 1.1 per 1000 in 1910. Among young men of draft age during World War II, 1,825,000 were rejected and 600,000 were discharged because of psychoneurotic disturbances. This high figure was widely interpreted as an indication that the pressures of modern living caused increases in anxiety and insecurity. But this increase was perhaps more apparent than real, inasmuch as people had now acquired a better understanding of what constituted emotional and mental disorders. Many people who in the nineteenth century would have been considered a little strange but in no need of medical attention were now diagnosed as having neurotic tendencies. The emergence of psychiatry was one of the major scientific developments of the twentieth century, and most educated Americans acquired some understanding of its basic concepts.

Karl Menninger defined mental health at midcentury as "the adjustment of human beings to the world and to each other with a maximum of effectiveness and happiness" [3]. He added that this definition did not mean only the attainment of contentment or the grace of obeying the rules of the game cheerfully; rather, it was a combination of both these states—the ability to maintain an even temper, an alert intelligence, socially considerate behavior, and a happy disposition. Mental health, like physical health, varied greatly in form and degree from individual to individual.

Government agencies spent $250 million a year on institutions for the mentally ill, as compared with less than $1 million allocated annually for research into mental and nervous diseases. Even though such disorders caused the major share of chronic disability in the United States, they represented one of the least explored fields of investigation. The problem of mental disease, in fact, illustrated the nation's deficiencies both in medical knowledge and in the application of knowldge already acquired. Since the founding of the first psychiatric hospitals in the United States in the eighteenth century, mental illness had gradually come to be accepted as a public responsibility. Unfortunately this concept of public responsibility for the mentally ill had not expanded beyond the original idea that persons whose abnormal behavior could no longer be tolerated should be placed in institutions.

The quality of care given to patients in public mental institutions varied in different parts of the country. A few state institutions provided a reasonably high standard of care, including specialized treatment and medical and hospital care for physical illness. Surveys made by the Public Health Service revealed deficiencies in the care of patients, however, that could not be attributed solely to lack of funds, personnel, beds, and facilities. The average public mental health institution did not deserve the name *hospital*; rather, it was a storehouse for human wreckage that had to be removed from the sight of the more fortunate members of society. States and communities, and indeed the nation as a whole, needed to reappraise their services for the growing numbers of mental patients.

Psychiatric Nursing

In 1940 there had been only 4252 graduate nurses employed in state mental hospitals. In one of the West Coast states, for example, there were seven state hospitals, with a patient population of approximately 27,000; yet a total of only 18 graduate nurses were employed. In January, 1944, there were 14 states in which no psychiatric nursing courses had ever been given; yet each of these states had hospitals for the care of psychiatric patients as well as general hospital schools of nursing. Often nursing schools operated by psychiatric hospitals did not deserve their official status: one school visited had been in operation for many years, yet never in its history had an instructor been employed on the staff.

Graduate nurses in psychiatric hospitals represented several different types of preparation. Some were graduates of general hospital schools who had moved into psychiatric nursing either by taking a postgraduate course in it or by learning through experience in a psychiatric hospital. Others, graduates of psychiatric hospital schools of nursing, had acquired in their three years of preparation some degree of knowledge of general nursing and a special knowledge of psychiatric nursing. Still others were older graduates of two-year courses who, for various reasons, had not pursued work in other schools to qualify themselves for registration under the requirements of state boards of licensure.

The duties of psychiatric hospital nursing personnel included much more than the care and treatment of the physically ill; such patients were a minority in the hospital population. Many more psychiatric patients were ambulatory rather than bedfast. Olga Weiss, in the March, 1947 issue of the *American Journal of Nursing*, effectively described the psychiatric nurse's role:

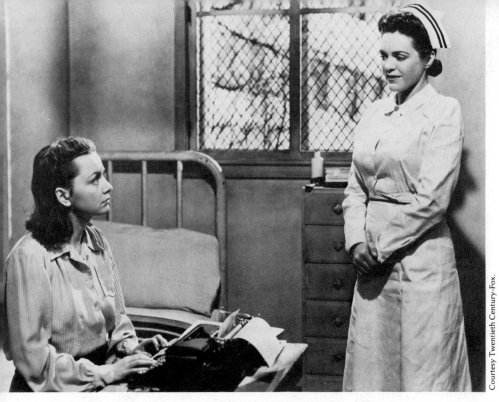

The motion picture The Snake Pit *helped generate a vigorous effort to improve mental health facilities in the late 1940s. (Copyright © 1948 Twentieth Century-Fox Film Corporation. All rights reserved.)*

She must learn to respect her patients as fellow human beings. The person who develops a wholesome respect for other persons as individuals with the same rights and privileges as himself has taken great strides toward reaching understanding.

This is perhaps the most difficult lesson for the nurse to learn, as it means giving up some of the "privileges" of being a nurse, an authoritative creature in a white uniform whose word is law. Because nurses are trained so rigidly, they tend to become rigid, and it is not easy for them to give up some of the precepts learned so painfully. It is difficult to substitute skillful conversation for manual dexterity; the former actually demands more of the nurse. The psychiatric nurse must learn to give much of herself to the patient: her time, patience, and understanding. By understanding we do not mean the useless, sweet, blanket understanding of the willing, but untrained volunteer who pats the head of a withdrawn schizophrenic and speaks condescendingly to him. The nurse working with such patients must have a true scientific knowledge of the illness and its symptoms and must recognize that these people, no matter how withdrawn they seem, are acutely aware of what goes on around them and that condescension is as infuriating to them as to any well person [4].

Although over 50 percent of all patients in the United States in the early 1950s were mentally ill, nurses were taught primarily to care for the other 50 percent, and the nurses' educations usually did not cover psychiatric nursing. Progressives of the era pointed out that a psychiatric nurse should have all the education and ability of a general hospital nurse and much additional experience in the psychological aspects of mental illness. It was not generally recognized at this time that psychiatric nursing content was helpful for all aspects of nursing practice.

The National Mental Health Act

The federal government launched an attack on the deficiencies in the care and treatment of the mentally ill in July, 1946, with the passage of the National Mental Health Act. The purpose of the Act was to provide a method for financing research and training programs and to assist the states in establishing community mental health services. The National Institute of Mental Health (NIMH) of the United States Public Health Service had responsibility for administration of the program. The Act provided for the establishment of a National Advisory Mental Health Council composed of six outstanding civilian mental health authorities. This Council made recommendations to the Public Health Service on all matters relating to mental health and formed committees on community services, research, and training. The training committee consisted of four subcommittees set up to evaluate training projects in psychiatry, psychiatric social work, psychology, and psychiatric nursing. The approval of the Council was necessary to obtain a grant for research or training.

Soon research grants were awarded for the investigation of child personality and development, psychosomatic disorders, neurosurgery, epilepsy, schizophrenia, marital counseling, social factors in mental illnesses, and a number of other related areas. Research fellowships were granted to psychiatrists, psychologists, neurophysiologists, neurologists, anatomists, pediatricians, sociologists, and biologists.

In 1949 graduate-training grants totaling about $2.5 million were made to 28 schools of psychiatric social work, 18 collegiate schools of nursing, 46 clinical psychology training institutions, and 56 psychiatric centers. Training stipends were awarded to 471 people through these graduate training centers. The NIMH traineeship program, which began in 1948 (at the same time the United States Cadet Corps program was in final phase-out), kept alive the principle of federal aid to nursing education.

Several other NIMH activities pertained to nursing. During 1949 the National Institute of Mental Health awarded grants to support training institutes that brought together individuals engaged in the education of psychologists, psychiatric social workers, and nurses. A conference was held in Pittsburgh in January, 1950, to discuss the program of preparing mental health nurse consultants in the field of public health nursing. The conference was regarded by the participants as a unique opportunity to exchange concepts and methods and to allow the individual educator to become aware, through contact with clinicians, of the needs in the field.

In 1949, $3.5 million was made available for state grants-in-aid to community services programs. The amount granted to each state depended on its population, its financial need, and the extent of its administrative problem. Annual grants varied from $20,000 to $283,000. Each state designated a particular agency as its state mental health authority empowered to administer the federal funds that became available. These designated agencies had to prepare both a plan and a budget for approval by the Public Health Service in which one dollar of state or local public funds was to be matched by two dollars in federal funds. The federal funds could be used to finance mental health activities other than those pertaining strictly to the care and treatment of hospital patients. By 1950 all but one of the states and territories had initiated or expanded their mental hygiene program by utilizing the grant-in-aid funds made available under the National Mental Health Act along with new or increased state appropriations.

The Hill-Burton Act and Hospital-building Programs

On another front, passage of the Hospital Survey and Construction Act of 1946 laid the foundation for development of an integrated, balanced system of hospitals throughout the country, for coordination of hospitals and public health centers, for ultimate organization of all personal health services to the states, and for construction of additional facilities. This act applied to all types of nonprofit (voluntary as well as public) hospitals and established quantitative and qualitative standards for facilities eligible for aid. General tax funds were allotted to the states on the basis of a special schedule. The total costs of approved projects was borne jointly by federal and state governments, the federal share ranging from one-third to two-thirds. During its first six years, the program, which allocated funds mainly to general hospitals in rural areas, resulted in the total addition of some 88,000 beds.

Although priority had been given to the construction of hospitals and public health centers in badly undersupplied areas, the few states with high per-capita incomes continued to have much larger proportionate numbers of hospital beds and more public health centers than did many states with comparatively low per-capita income. Most of the hospitals meeting high standards were in large cities, and the new-hospital movement was slow to reach sparsely settled rural areas. Because rural people had been unable to establish tax-supported hospitals in their communities, the burden of initiating building programs fell upon local physicians as personal ventures, undertaken chiefly to provide places where surgery might be performed. Thus, rural hospitals were frequently proprietary institutions.

The rural proprietary hospital was fast proving to be an economic impossibility. Rural populations were constantly declining, and the relatively low earnings of the physicians who owned rural hospitals did not allow for institutional operation in accordance with acceptable standards. Improved roads enabled rural people to go to larger towns for better hospital care. Nevertheless, an estimated 20 million people still lived in sparsely settled areas beyond the range of satisfactory hospital care. Rural people were also losing their physicians and nurses to the cities. Authoritative studies of this trend revealed a declining ratio of nurses and physicians to population, an increasng average age of nurses and physicians, and a negligible number of new graduates settling in rural communities.

The Rise in Nursing Homes

The early 1950s saw many changes in non-hospital institutions for the chronically ill. The Social Security Act of 1935 and its amendments of 1950 led to the closing of public homes for the aged and resulted in a tremendous growth in the number of proprietary nursing homes. The number of public homes had declined from 2350 in 1929 to 1260 in 1949. The number of private nonprofit homes had increased from 1270 to 1500, and the commercial nursing homes had shot up from a negligible number to a total of about 8500. The population of the proprietary homes had increased to an estimated 111,000.

The greatly increased number of private nursing homes made it difficult to enforce acceptable standards through inspection and licensure. The 1950 amendments to the Social Security Act required that states claiming matching funds for the costs of care of individuals residing in medical institutions establish and maintain adequate standards for them, and by mid-1953 only four states—Arizona, Florida, Mississippi, and Wyoming—had no statutes regarding such standards. Few public assistance programs provided sufficient funds to help pay for adequate private nursing home care, and the great majority of the homes lacked organized affiliation with other medical-care facilities. Despite these serious deficiencies the demand for beds was so urgent that substandard care was sometimes tolerated. Many state and local groups recommended that religious, fraternal, and government organizations undertake more construction and operation of non-profit nursing homes.

Restructuring the Professional Organizations

Meanwhile, as far as a revision of the organizational structure of the nursing was concerned, the initial move was taken at the biennial convention of the American Nurses' Association in 1950, when delegates approved the division of the profession into two large organizations to replace existing operating associations. Under the reorganization plan the American Nurses' Association and the National Association of Colored Graduate Nurses merged, while the National League of Nursing Education, the National Organization of Public Health Nurses, and the Association of Collegiate Schools of Nursing formed another group, the National League for Nursing.

The convention also tabled a resolution opposing compulsory health insurance. In tabling the resolution the convention ignored a telegraphed appeal from the American Medical Association to join the "fight against socialization of medicine." During a discussion of a resolution that the association formally declare its opposition to compulsory health insurance, representatives of the New York, Florida, and Georgia associations spoke in favor of the resolution, claiming that compulsory health insurance had caused a decline in national health and a deterioration of medical standards and facilities wherever it had been introduced. Speakers opposing the resolution urged the nurses to avoid becoming a "pressure group" and maintained that the ANA had not studied the problem of health insurance sufficiently to take any position.

In reaffirming the "principles relating to organization, control, and administration of nursing education" adopted in 1947, the ANA again asserted that nursing education, "in common with other types of education, should be the charge of the educational institutions of the country." The ANA further declared that the education of professional nurses should be an integral part of an institution of higher education, managed according to approved principles, and the basic professional nursing program" should include or be built upon at least two years of general collegiate education" [5].

War Again

The peacetime complacency of nurses was suddenly shattered on June 25, 1950, when the Korean War broke out. At the beginning of the action the total strength of the Army Nurse Corps was below 3500 and that of the Navy Nurse Corps, below 2000. The Army Nurse Corps could draw from only 6300 inactive reservists. Many nurse leaders, anticipating a major war, had predicted dire consequences for nursing service in civilian hospitals. Alice Clarke, editor of *R.N.*

The outbreak of the Korean War shattered the peacetime complacency of nurses.

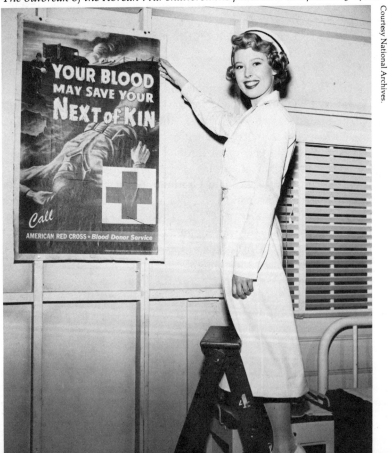

magazine, thought it a foregone conclusion that, in case of full-scale war, there would be "a general exodus from these hospitals—for nurses in large numbers will always volunteer for military service when they are needed" [6].

Aware that the civilian and military needs for nurses required cooperative planning, the special Joint Committee on Nursing in National Security recommended that the mobilization of nurses be guided by several basic assumptions. First of all, it was thought that military needs for nurses should receive highest priority, provided that the military set reasonable quotas, recruit personnel according to functional category and field of nursing, and make full use of male nurses and auxiliary workers. It was predicted that in the event of a full-scale war, civilians as well as soldiers might serve on the battle front; thus, nursing service would be as essential for civilians as for the armed forces. For this reason it was important to maintain a reasonable distribution of nurses throughout the country for both civilian and defense requirements.

The six national nursing organizations represented on the Joint Committee on Nursing in National Security recommended:

That all possible means be developed for recruiting more students for schools of nursing.

That a program be instituted immediately for encouraging inactive nurses to return to practice.

That as many practical nurses be trained and employed to help professional nurses as hospitals and other community agencies could utilize to good advantage.

That nurses be withdrawn systematically from the civilian services for military duty according to a plan that ensured their employment at the highest level of skill for which they were prepared.

That state and local advisory boards of nurses be organized and be given the authority by the government to review assignment of nurses to the armed forces and to civilian agencies.

That, if there was total mobilization, nurses be redistributed within the fields of nursing and within community agencies so that the most essential civilian needs would be taken care of first.

That major effort be directed to improving sound basic nursing education and to increase enrollment in schools of nursing that offered effective programs.

That selected nurses be encouraged to prepare for responsibilities as teachers, supervisors, and administrators, as well as for the special fields, in order to safeguard essential nursing service.

That administration of nursing services be improved so that nursing skills would be used to the best advantage and their full value would reach more people.

That nursing service be stabilized as much as possible and turnover of staff held to a minimum through the adoption and application of sound personnel policies for nurses and allied workers [7].

Despite these fears of an acute nursing shortage, military nursing services experienced only a limited build-up during the Korean War. During the three years of fighting, 2000 nurses volunteered or were recalled for service with the

Army Nurse Corps, which reached a peak strength of 5500. Only 10 percent, or about 500 members, however, received assignments in Korea.

Similarly, in June, 1950, there were 1950 regular and reserve Navy Nurse Corps officers on active duty assigned to 26 naval hospitals and dispensaries in and outside the continental United States—three hospital corps schools, two hospital ships, and eight Military Sea Transport Service ships. The Navy Nurse Corps attained its peak strength during the Korean War on June 30, 1951, when 3238 Nurse Corps officers were on active duty. Three hospital ships, *Consolation, Repose,* and *Haven,* rotated as station hospitals in Korean waters during the hostilities.

Before the war, on July 1, 1949, a total of 1199 Army nurses had been transferred from the Department of the Army to the new Department of the Air Force. As the Air Force Nurse Corps prepared to celebrate its first anniversary in July, 1950, it faced the grim but essential task of supplying, within a period of 48 hours, a large number of nurses to assist in the air evacuation of battle casualties from the Korean area. By mid-July, 1950, 200 Air Force nurses were actively engaged in the air-evacuation of patients.

Nursing in the Mobile Army Surgical Hospitals

There were periods in the Korean campaign when battle casualties ran exceedingly high. The difficulties in rescue and treatment of the wounded and injured were heightened by the extremes of weather and the mountainous terrain, but the fatality rates among these patients were surprisingly low. The major reasons for the decrease in fatalities were the availability of prompt and effective first aid treatment, rapid evacuation, and surgical treatment near the scene of action. A steady supply of whole blood and antibiotics also played a vital role. The use of Air Force and Marine Corps helicopters represented a significant advance in the evacuation procedure.

World War II had demonstrated to the military the need for a new type of hospital, as an adjunct to the existing methods for treating casualties in the field. Thus the Mobile Army Surgical Hospital (MASH) was organized and integrated into the line of evacuation of battle casualties. Designed to be highly mobile, this hospital provided expert care by physicians and nurses. It was to be located as close to the front line as was safely practicable—approximately eight to 20 miles.

Korea provided the first test for these mobile units, half a dozen of which supported front-line divisions throughout the Korean campaign. A typical Mobile Army Surgical Hospital was set up in tents; buildings were utilized, however, when available. Patients were first admitted to the receiving ward, where the medical officer and nurses surveyed the extent of the wounds and determined the presence or absence of shock. Immediately afterward they began resuscitative measures, ordered x-rays, and decided upon the course of therapy. In most cases this therapy included the administration of blood or

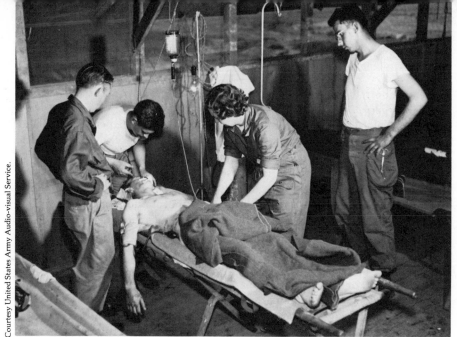

Nurse administering blood plasma to a wounded soldier in the 8063rd Mobile Army Surgical Hospital, July 21, 1952.

Captain Stella Basara, ANC, administers an anesthetic to a patient at the 44th Mobile Army Surgical Hospital in Korea.

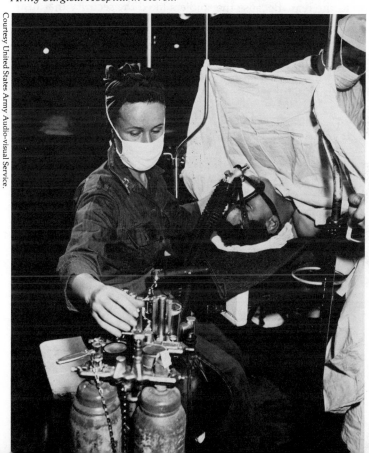

oxygen, or both, and general supportive measures designed to prepare the patient for surgery.

The typical MASH unit comprised approximately 156 personnel. There were about 15 medical officers, specializing in general surgery, thoracic surgery, orthopedic surgery, internal medicine, and anesthesiology. The nursing staff consisted of approximately 16: five nurses each for the preoperative and postoperative wards, four for the operating room, and two nurse-anesthetists. The remaining hospital complement consisted of about four administrative officers and 120 enlisted personnel who performed the various tasks necessary for the hospital to function smoothly.

Attached to each MASH unit was an Army helicopter detachment whose mission was to provide immediate means of evacuation for critically injured battle casualties or seriously ill medical patients. Rapid helicopter evacuation of the wounded contributed greatly to the marked decrease in mortality from wounds. When conditions were not suitable for air evacuation, patients were brought to the hospital from the battalion aid stations by ambulances, which were attached to all combat units. Evacuation from this hospital, in turn, might again be by helicopter or ambulance, depending upon the condition of the patient.

The MASH unit was the first hospital to which the wounded man was sent upon evacuation to the rear. Because the soldiers liked the security that near-

*A Korean setting provided the background for M*A*S*H, the popular film and subsequent television series, 20 years later. (Copyright © 1970 Aspen Productions, Inc. and Twentieth Century-Fox Film Corporation. All rights reserved.)*

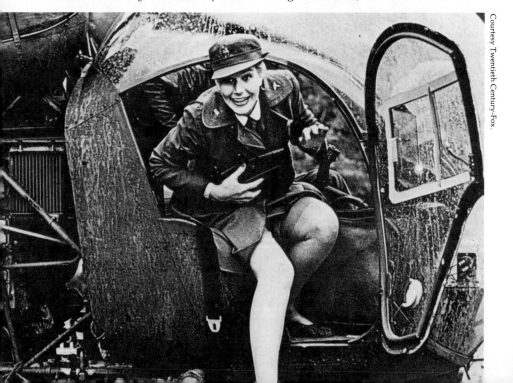

ness could provide, MASH units were a great factor in maintaining morale. The proximity of the unit to the front, its trained personnel, its adequate supply of whole blood, and its rapid helicopter and ambulance evacuation services all contributed greatly to the reduction of mortality rates in Korea as compared with those during World War II: the mortality rate among wounded soldiers who reached hospitals in Korea was half the corresponding rate during World War II.

Flight Nursing Matures

Along with advances in antibiotics and medical techniques, one of the major factors in reducing fatalities was the quick air delivery of patients to hospitals. Air evacuation of the wounded from the battlefields of Korea to military medical centers in Japan was the responsibility of the Military Air Transport Service and a unified Air Force-Navy complement of medical technicians and flight nurses. One flight nurse was assigned to each plane carrying ambulatory and litter patients. Flight nurses and medics worked around the clock, sometimes as long as 72 hours without a break, getting their only rest while en route back to Korea with a load of cargo. Nurses saved many lives during the summer of 1950 by supplying prompt medical attention and by advising pilots of the cruising altitudes suited to the individual requirements of seriously ill patients. Sometimes speed of delivery was vital; at other times a smooth flight was more important.

Wounded soldiers, direct from combat, dirty and disheveled, were happy to talk to American women again and proud of the bravery of the nurses who flew repeatedly into dangerous areas. One flight nurse and a medic were killed when a C-54 took off from Kimpo, near Seoul, crashlanding at night on the Sea of Japan not far from the Japanese coast. Another flight nurse was later awarded the Distinguished Flying Cross for helping other passengers on the plane to escape, even though she was severely injured herself.

Airlifting the wounded became an international venture as Australian, British, Turkish, and Filipino soldiers joined the fighting in Korea. Nurses learned an informal and international sign language of sorts that enabled them to help patients whose languages they could not understand. There were usually people on board who could help interpret a little. When the Chinese crossed the Yalu River and struck hard at American troops, air evacuation of the wounded stepped up considerably, reaching a high point in early December, when C-47s air-evacuated 4700 wounded and frostbitten Marines in four days. On December 5, 1950, flight nurses air-evacuated a record high of 3925 patients in a single day. At that time it looked as though the Chinese might overrun all of Korea, and Eighth Army medical officers decided to empty all Korean hospitals for safety's sake.

Sometimes the medical flight personnel included wounded Korean physicians and nurses who, disregarding their own disabilities, helped out with the patients. On the hurried and hazardous flights out of Wonju, flight nurses had little or no time to examine patients or give them serious medical attention.

Since the enemy was generally lurking nearby, it seemed more important to rush the loading and get the patients out fast. The C-47s were often incredibly crowded, with patients sitting or lying in the aisle.

Flight nurses assumed all the risks of the aircrews, taking their chances with the rugged terrain and weather, inadequate landing strips, possible enemy air attacks, frequent ground fire, and possible sabotage by patients. Nurses checking wounded prisoners on board one plane found that a North Korean had a live hand grenade stowed away in his clothes; they took away the grenade and let the POW fly with the other patients.

Gradually a systematic air evacuation pattern evolved. Wounded men whose total hospitalization was likely to require 30 days or less, with subsequent return to duty, were air-evacuated to southern Korea. Patients expected to be hospitalized for six months or less were moved by C-54s to Japan and returned to Korea to finish their tour of duty upon recovery. Patients whose probable recovery would take more than six months were airlifted back to the United States by the Military Air Transport Service in order to clear the hospitals in Japan for other patients. The general policy was to move the wounded as quickly as possible from the front lines to a rear-area hospital. Many of those airlifted to Korean bases were later evacuated to Japan and perhaps moved once more for eventual airlift home.

One result of air evacuation in the Korean War was the virtual elimination of the hospital ship as a means of transporting the wounded. During the early days of the war, Army medical officers were inclined to regard the hospital ship as the safest way to move large numbers of wounded. Gradually they came to agree with the Air Force that air evacuation of the wounded was the cheapest, most efficient, and most sensible method of transportation. Navy hospital ships off the Korean coast were used mainly as floating hospitals and were assigned to transport patients only when en route to Japan for overhaul or refitting.

A Day in the Life of a Flight Nurse

A typical trip into and out of Korea on a flight leaving from Japan was vividly described by Captain Janice Albert of the Air Force Nurse Corps:

Your alarm goes off at 0100. You are to be picked up at 0130 for a 0300 take-off. You're wide awake because you have a lot to do before your transportation arrives. You go about getting ready quietly while your roommate sleeps (she didn't get back from her flight until late that evening and is not scheduled to take off until much later). Before you went to bed, you checked and rechecked your medical supplies—ready for any emergency, since you do not know what type of wounded you'll be caring for until you load your patients aboard. You've slept in your "longjohns," so all you do is put on your flight suit and make-up, pick up your jacket and pocket-book, and you are on your way. Transportation arrives with your aeromedical technician. Together, you recheck your supplies—oxygen, medical kit, extra dressing, blankets, straps—they are all there and you proceed to the airplane that will take you to Korea. The plane is loaded with cargo. This time it is mail, but it could have been anything from blood plasma,

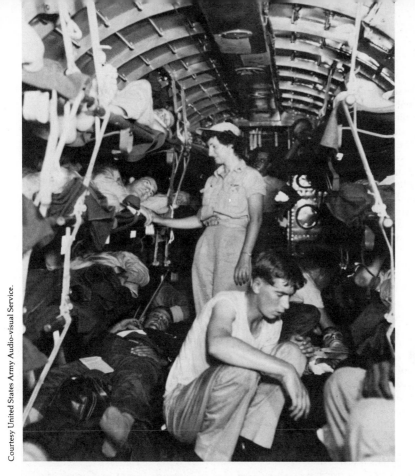

Flight nurse First Lieutenant Audrey H. Schoen of Long Island, New York, secures patients to litters in a C-47 cargo plane before an evacuation flight to rear areas from the 629th Medical Clearing Company, at an airstrip in Korea, on August 12, 1952.

whole blood, or medical supplies to ammunition, gasoline, airplane parts, jeeps, rifles—tools for waging war or preserving life—perishable foods, propaganda leaflets, or personnel returning or reporting to the fighting zone" [8].

Upon arrival and unloading in Korea, the aircraft was swept out, litter straps were unrolled, and the cargo plane became a hospital ward. Patients began to arrive from the Mobile Army Surgical Hospitals and the nurse made out her report of patients to be evacuated. The loading ramp—a converted jeep—pulled up to the plane and one by one the wounded were gently carried aboard on litters and secured to their proper spot. Miss Albert continued her story:

You and your aeromedical technician scarcely realize that you are 7000 feet above the ground as you go about your job. And though there is a language barrier, compassion serves as a universal tongue to bring understanding between you and your patients. You reassure a frightened private, redress the colostomy, give oxygen to the Turk with the penetrating chest wound, administer a narcotic to the boy who is still not fully aware of the absence of his left leg—a smile here, a gentle hand there, and soon the tension of the cabin is lessened, at least for the moment. The Frenchman shows you pictures of his wife and baby, and soon the rest want you to look at their pictures too. You light a cigarette for the Greek whose right arm is in a cast, you pass sandwiches, tuck in a blanket here, readjust the position of the man with a fractured leg, and check on the drainage bottle of the patient with a gunshot wound in his back.

Time passes rapidly and so far the trip has gone off smoothly. Suddenly, you become anxious about the Turk with the penetrating chest wound. After stepping up the oxygen, you consult with the pilot as to the position of the aircraft and find you are still an hour from your destination. You decide that the patient may not be able to stand that long a flight, so you ask the pilot to call the nearest airfield to have a doctor meet the plane. At your request he makes an emergency landing. The injured man is off-loaded and the plane continues its scheduled trip.

About an hour later, the plane has landed. Ambulances were waiting and the remaining patients were off-loaded. Nurse Albert further related:

Though your nose is shiny and you need lipstick, to these patients you look beautiful— you are the girl they left home, the one they expect to see soon.

Your trip is ended! You gather your medical supplies and head towards quarters. You have been on duty almost 16 hours. Tired? Yes, but a hot shower, a few hours sleep, and you are ready to do it again tomorrow if necessary. (Many times it is.)

As you reach the nurses' quarters, you feel a warm sense of spiritual satisfaction. You have once again contributed your small share toward easing and erasing the pains and anxieties of war's combat casualties [9].

The End of the War

In April and May of 1951 American and United Nations forces in Korea repelled two Chinese offensives, during which the attackers suffered staggering losses estimated in excess of one million casualties. On June 23, 1951, the head of the Russian delegation at the United Nations indicated that the war could be ended if both sides began discussions that would lead to "a cease-fire and an armistice providing for a mutual withdrawal of forces from the thirty-eighth parallel" [10]. Two years of negotiations, during which the fighting continued, took place before an armistice agreement was accepted. All fighting stopped on July 27, 1953. When the final casualty report for the 37 months of war was prepared, American losses totaled 142,091, of whom 33,629 were killed, 103,284 were wounded, and 5178 were missing or captured. The bulk of these casualties occurred during the first year of fighting. The war had witnessed great advances in medical care delivery to the wounded and nurses had made a tremendous contribution to this effort.

Accreditation Advances

Meanwhile the National League for Nursing's accreditation program was beginning to have a noticeable effect on nursing educational standards. Helen Nahm described the "poorer" school of 1952 as those having some or all of these characteristics [11]:

Very few full-time faculty members.

Unstable faculty.

High workload for faculty and students.

Much evening and night duty for students.

Little or no planned clinical or ward instruction.

Low service hours carried by graduate staff nurse or nonprofessional workers or both.

High withdrawal rates.

Low daily average patient census in one or more clinical areas.

Low score on state board examinations.

The temporary accreditation program in effect from 1952 to 1957 was geared toward helping the inferior schools find ways of improving themselves. Under this program, many special meetings were held, self-evaluation guides prepared, and consultations arranged. The purposes of these conferences were:

To learn more about the needs and problems of nursing schools throughout the country so that the professional nursing organizations could take steps to provide assistance in improving education programs.

The temporary accreditation program helped many schools improve their educational standards.

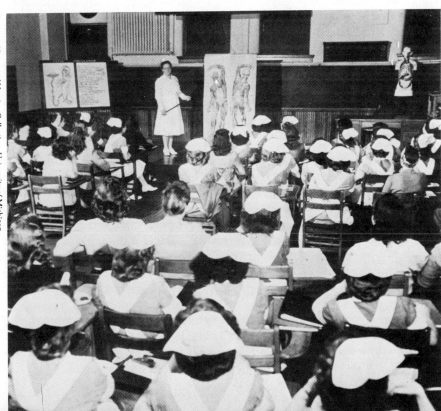

To assist nursing schools in interpreting information presented on the school profiles as well as other information sent to them following the meetings of the boards of review.

To discuss the criteria which were used by the boards of review in evaluating programs for temporary accreditation.

To discuss other criteria which probably should be used in evaluating nursing school programs.

To discuss steps which individual schools could take to improve their own programs.

To discuss measures which could be taken to help schools offering programs not approved for temporary accreditation.

To discuss whether a consultant service should be set up by the National League for Nursing through which schools of nursing could obtain individual assistance [12].

When this program terminated in 1957, the number of fully accredited schools had increased by 72.4 percent. In the meantime the total number of schools of nursing dropped from 1139 to 1115, but schools offering degree programs increased by 37 between 1952 and 1957, and 18 associate degree programs, representing an entirely new development, were established. In the same five-year period, the total number of diploma-granting schools was reduced to 936, or 79 fewer than in 1952.

Evidence of the positive effect of the temporary accreditation program was contained in the NLN publication *Report on Hospital Schools of Nursing, 1957*. Based on data collected in the last year of the temporary accreditation program, the report revealed the progress made by hospital schools and identified areas still presenting problems:

The hospital school of nursing of 1957 in most instances has come a long way toward achieving the characteristics of a truly educational institution. Although its students are to some extent still used for staffing the nursing services, its major concern is the development of its student. Preparation for nursing practice is . . . its primary aim . . . but its offerings extend beyond those required for technical or vocational training into those which provide the type of broad educational background that makes for personal as well as professional development [13].

There was concrete evidence of improvement in many areas. There were more full-time faculty members per school who were also better qualified than in 1949. The four-week annual vacation had become universal. Three-fourths of the schools reported students on a 40-hour week, and there was better planning of evening and night assignments. On the other hand, the report particularly emphasized the need for redefinition of clinical learning experiences, the area last influenced by school improvement. Finance was another area in which relatively little progress was noted: "In most schools of nursing . . . the curriculum is developed as an income-producing as well as a 'learning producing' operation . . . ." [14].

As professional nursing celebrated its seventy-eighth birthday and moved into the 1950s, prevailing feminine values strongly affected nurse career patterns. The high turnover among registered nurses helped to perpetuate a nurse shortage which was aggravated by the demands of the Korean War and the greater involvement of nurses in the psychiatric nursing field. Minimal qualifications demanded of nurses were significantly increased by the development and implementation of a common state board test pool throughout the United States. Educational standards were further upgraded by the launching of an aggressive school accreditation program.

Summary

An acute shortage of nurses throughout the nation characterized the midcentury years. Faced with rising life expectancy and expansion of the population, the growth of hospitalization and health insurance, and expanded opportunities for nurses, the nursing profession could not find solutions to the shortage.

Following World War II, marriage and childrearing enjoyed such a high priority that many young women withdrew from the nursing profession soon after graduation. Furthermore, because of the problems of living in the hospital and maintaining their own homes, married women were generally not accepted as nursing students.

A movement of the 1940s that did much to improve standards in nursing education was the development of the State Board Test Pool. From 1944 to 1950 the State Board Test Pool service expanded from the original six states that had employed it to all 48 states. Thus, nursing became the first profession for which a common licensing examination was used throughout the nation.

During the first half of the twentieth century the development of psychiatry had resulted in an increased recognition of the problem of mental illness in the United States. The number of patients in psychiatric hospitals had increased markedly over the past 50 years; yet the average mental institution only offered a minimal form of custodial care.

Although over 50 percent of all hospitalized patients were mentally ill, nurse preparation programs generally did not include psychiatric nursing content in their curricula.

The National Mental Health Act, which provided funds for research and training programs and assisted the states in establishing community mental health services, was passed in July, 1946. The Act enabled nurses to receive preparation in psychiatric nursing.

The Hospital Survey and Construction Act of 1946 and its amendments of 1949 laid the foundation for the development of an integrated and balanced system of hospitals throughout the country. Yet the new hospital movement was slow in reaching rural areas, and in 1947 an estimated 20 million people living in rural areas still did not have access to adequate hospital care.

The Social Security Act of 1935 and its amendments of 1950 led to the closing of public homes for the aged and the tremendous growth in the number of proprietary nursing homes.

At the 1950 ANA convention a restructuring of the nursing organizations was approved by the delegates whereby the NACGN would merge with the American Nurses' Association; and the NLNE, NOPHN, and the ACSN would join together as the National League for Nursing.

On June 25, 1950, the Korean War broke out. While the Army and Navy nursing services experienced only a limited build-up, the new Air Force Nurse Corps helped establish a new standard in mass air-evacuation of battle casualties.

The Mobile Army Surgical Hospital (MASH) received its first practical test in Korea. Located close to the front line, these MASH units offered expert care by nurses and physicians and resulted in a low fatality rate among wounded soldiers in Korea.

Flight nurses played a unique role in the evacuation of the wounded from Korea. Their work was both dangerous and demanding. The success of air evacuation virtually eliminated the hospital ship as a means of transporting the wounded.

The temporary accreditation program for nursing schools lasted from 1952 to 1957, during which time many special meetings were held, self-evaluation guides prepared, and consultations arranged. When the program was terminated in 1957, the number of fully accredited schools had increased by 72.4 percent.

References

1. Florida State Board of Nursing, *Registered Nurse Examination for 1939*. Jackson Memorial Hospital School of Nursing Archives, Miami, Florida.
2. "The State Board Test Pool Examination," *American Journal of Nursing*, vol. 52 (May, 1952): 613–615.
3. Karl Menninger, "The Future of Psychiatric Care in Hospitals," *Modern Hospital*, vol. 64 (May, 1945): 43–45.
4. M. O. Weiss, "The Skills of Psychiatric Nursing," *American Journal of Nursing*, vol. 47 (March, 1947): 174–176.
5. V. A. Turner, "American Nurses' Association Settles Important Issues," *Trained Nurse and Hospital Review*, vol. 124 (June, 1950): 260.
6. Alice Clarke, "Draft Nurses . . . A New War and Old Theme," *R.N.*, vol. 14 (March, 1951): 24–25.
7. Joint Committee on Nursing in National Security, "Mobilization of Nurses for National Security," *American Journal of Nursing*, vol. 51 (February, 1951): 78–79.
8. Janice Albert, "Air Evacuation from Korea—A Typical Flight," *Military Surgeon*, vol. 112 (April, 1953): 256–258.
9. *Ibid.*, pp. 257–258.
10. *New York Times*, June 24, 1951.
11. Helen Nahm, "Temporary Accreditation," *American Journal of Nursing*, vol. 52 (August, 1952): 997–1001.

12. National League for Nursing, Division of Nursing Education, *Report on the Program of Temporary Accreditation of the National Nursing Accrediting Service: Part I, Study of Basic Programs Offered by Schools of Nursing, 1952* (mimeographed).
13. National League for Nursing, *Report on Hospital Schools of Nursing, 1957* (New York: National League for Nursing, 1959), p. 5.
14. National League for Nursing, *op. cit*, p. 30.

17
Minorities in Nursing Strive for Recognition

In 1953, when births in the United States reached four million for the first time and filled hospital nurseries to the overflow level, business periodicals happily predicted that prosperity was ahead. Americans were growing older, with the over-65 bracket increasing more rapidly than any other age group, largely because the death rate had been cut in half since 1900. Life expectancy, which had been 63 years in 1940, had jumped to 67 in 1950, although it remained at 60 for nonwhites. For the first time a magazine was published exclusively for those preparing to retire. At the other end of the age scale, school enrollment boomed to an all-time high of 30 million and continued to climb.

But quite another story was buried under these cheering national averages. Nearly 3 percent of Americans over 14 years of age were illiterate, and among nonwhites the figure was four times higher. Despite wartime prosperity, black Americans were much worse off than whites with respect to level of education, life expectancy, housing, percentage of children who survived birth, and, most visibly, average annual income—$2000 for black workers in general and $815 for black women, as compared to $3500 for whites.

Outlawing Racial Segregation

One of the most important and difficult domestic issues in America during the mid-1950s arose out of the Supreme Court ruling in *Brown* v. *the Board of Education of Topeka* on May 17, 1954, which outlawed racial segregation in public schools. Despite improvements in the political, economic, and, to a lesser degree, social conditions among Northern blacks, no comparable progress had taken place for those living in the South, where rigid social barriers limited their opportunities and denied them the equality to which they were entitled under the Constitution and federal law. Nowhere was this more apparent than in the public school system, which adhered to the "separate but equal" doctrine set down by the Supreme Court in *Plessy* v. *Ferguson* in 1896.

In *Brown* v. *the Board of Education,* by unanimous decision, the Court overturned its old "separate but equal" doctrine by asserting that "separate educational facilities are inherently unequal," that "segregation in public education" denied the black students "equal protection of the law," and that separating black children "from others of similar age and qualifications solely because of their race generates a feeling of inferiority as to their status in the community that may affect their hearts and minds in a way unlikely ever to be undone" [1].

The editor of the *Nursing Outlook* noted this momentous court case in a vigorous editorial:

We rejoice with others when the Supreme Court of the United States handed down its decision on May 17. We were glad that the National League for Nursing had been a bit ahead of the times in its decision, reaffirmed by the Board of Directors in January, 1953, "that all activities [of the National League for Nursing] shall include all groups regardless of race, color, religion, sex . . ."

But the satisfaction we feel in the "rightness" of this step is only a beginning. We know that Negro nurses are employed by many hospitals and health agencies. We know that Negro nurses hold commissions in the armed services, that they receive all the benefits and carry all the responsibilities which go with those commissions. We know that 710 of our 1148 accredited schools of nursing accept qualified Negro students. We know, too, that some, although not many, Negro nurses hold administrative positions in hospitals and health agencies.

No, this is not enough. Is participation on the boards, on committees, and on staffs of all service groups extended on an equitable basis? Are all nurses free to take part in our organizations' programs, policy decisions, and conferences? There is much yet to be done. And we shall do it—slowly and quietly. What is most important just now is to look to the future and determine what this ruling will mean in the next few decades [2].

Slow Development of Black Nursing

In 1950 about 6 percent of all graduate and student nurses in the United States were black. It will be recalled that exactly 71 years earlier, in 1879, the first black trained nurse, Mary E. P. Mahoney, had received a diploma in nursing from the School of Nursing of the New England Hospital for Women and Children in Boston. The first school for black nurses, at the Provident Hospital, Chicago, had been organized in 1891. Advancement for the black nurse came slowly, because she was caught between two evolving processes in the social order. Racially, she was a member of an emerging group that had not been fully recognized on a merit basis by other groups; professionally, she was part of an emerging group whose worth to society had not been fully recognized by other groups.

Until after World War II black nurses could secure membership in the American Nurses' Association only through membership in the state nurses' associations in those states where black nurses were eligible for membership. Obviously, in certain southern states where black nurses were barred from admission to the state nurses' association, they were unable to belong to the American Nurses' Association, although they qualified for membership in every other respect. Partly as a result of this discrimination, the National Association of Colored Graduate Nurses was organized in 1908. At the first annual convention of the Association held in Boston in 1910, there were 26 charter members present

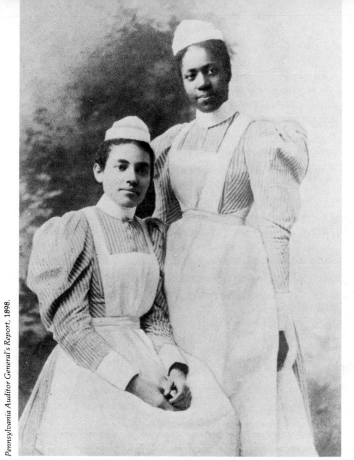

Two student nurses at the Frederick K. Douglass Memorial Hospital Training School for Nurses, Philadelphia, about 1896.

Second graduating class of the Colored Home and Hospital, New York City, 1902.

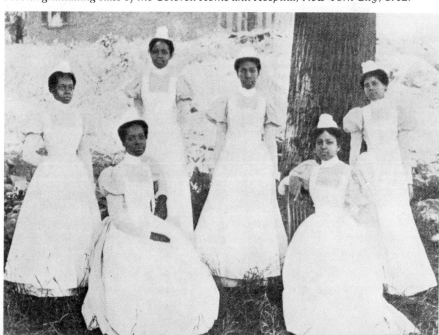

representing 10 states. From this nucleus the Association grew to a membership of over 1200 nurses by 1940, drawn from practically every state in the Union.

According to information in a report published in 1924 by the Hospital and Service Bureau of the American Conference on Hospital Service, only 58 state-accredited schools of nursing admitted black students, and most of these schools were located in black hospitals or in departments for the care of black patients in municipal hospitals. Twenty-eight states were found to offer no opportunity for education in nursing to the black woman. Of the 58 accredited schools, 39 —or 77 percent—were located in the South. This distribution closely followed the distribution of the black population of that time, 80 percent of which was in the South.

Black Nursing in the South

In a report entitled "Observations on Negro Nursing in the South" made by Nina D. Gage, Executive Secretary of the NLNE, and Alma Haupt, Associate Director of the NOPHN, in 1932, the following comments were made about some of these schools:

In the six states visited (Alabama, Georgia, Louisiana, Mississippi, Tennessee, and Texas) there are 23 Negro schools of nursing which are accredited by their respective

Students and faculty of the L. Richardson Memorial Hospital, Greensboro, North Carolina, 1932—one of the outstanding schools of nursing for blacks in the South during the 1930s.

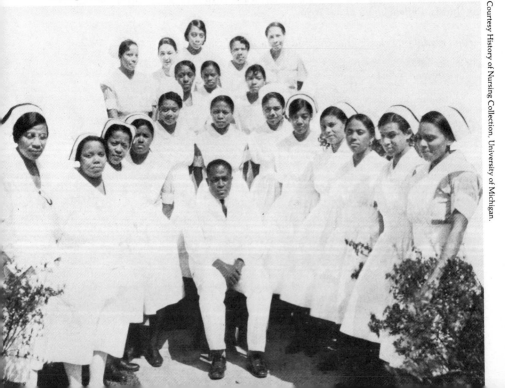

Boards of Nurse Examiners . . . . The schools of nursing themselves are of many varieties—some so poor as to make one question how they can possibly meet the standards
of a State Board of Medical Examiners. Others are pioneering in the field of education
with great success. [In one poor school] two shabby houses were used as a hospital of 35
beds and a nurses' home for 12 students. A colored nurse is superintendent of nurses
and the sole member of the faculty. A three-year course is given, every subject being
taught by the one nurse. With a wide range of subjects now necessary for the preparation of the nurse to meet the demands of the field, it is manifestly impossible, both physically and mentally, for one person to carry the entire teaching program of a school.
Without some specialization of the faculty the student cannot get the variety and different points of view needed to prepare her adequately for her future work. No public
health subjects are included in the curriculum of this school, but the students are frequently sent out to homes as private duty nurses, and the wages thus earned help to run
the hospital [3].

The critical lack of opportunities for preliminary education among black
youth in the South was highlighted in 1931, in *Brown America*, by Edwin R.
Embree:

The inadequacy of the schools and the low level of literacy and activity in the South are
such that not only Negroes but the whole population is retarded. . . . To the visitor,
colored schools seem not a system, but a series of incidents: bizarre, heroic, pathetic,
romantic . . . many of the schools run for only three or four months, with teachers paid
but $25 to $30 a month for these short terms. Studies of eight Southern states show an
average expenditure of $44.31 per capita for whites and only $12.50 for Negroes. In certain states with huge black populations, the discrepancies are even greater. Georgia
spends on the average $35.42 per white child and $6.38 per colored child. The figures of
Mississippi are $45.34 against $5.45. The inadequacy of these provisions for either race
is seen when one compared them with the average expenditure throughout the United
States as a whole, which is $87.22 per child [4].

Black women from better homes were not readily attracted to nursing. They
seemed to be more interested in teaching and music, as these careers offered
more immediate social prestige than did nursing. Although black schools of
nursing located in the South were in desperate need of qualified instructors,
the black nurse could not take graduate work in nursing in any university or
college in the South. This pointed very definitely to the need for the establishment of a graduate department in nursing education in one of the universities
that would admit blacks. Such lack of opportunity was especially unfortunate,
as there were, in the South, approximately 23,000 black midwives, wholly
unprepared by training for the work they were doing. If the midwife could be
replaced by the well-educated nurse who would combine midwifery with public
health nursing, one of the outstanding health needs of Southern blacks could
be met.

The United States census for 1930 listed 5728 graduate, registered black
nurses in a total black population of 11,891,143. Prior to World War II the
principal places of employment for black nurses had been black hospitals and
institutions, large public hospitals in the North, and local official and voluntary
public health agencies serving large numbers of black patients. Sixty-three per-

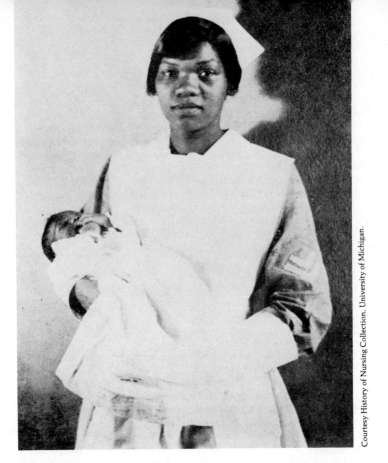

Black student nurse, about 1930.

Courtesy History of Nursing Collection, University of Michigan.

cent of active black nurses in 1941 were in hospital and institutional work, and 28 percent were in public health, as compared with 47 percent and 10 percent, respectively, of all active nurses. Private practice and industrial work offered little opportunity, if one were to judge by the fact that only 6 percent of black nurses were in private duty and 1 percent were in industrial nursing, as compared with the ratios of 27 percent and 3 percent, respectively, for all nurses. There were many opportunities in teaching and supervisory work, but such positions required graduate training—all but unavailable to black nurses.

Health Among Black Americans

Although authorities pointed to a remarkable decline in mortality among blacks, the black morbidity rate in 1930 was 18 per 1000 of the population while that of whites was 9.9. The urban black death rate was 95 percent higher than that of the urban white population. This fact assumed increasing importance as blacks migrated to cities. As a result of tuberculosis, heart disease, pneumonia, syphilis, and other preventable diseases, the death rates of blacks ranged from 1½ to eight times that of whites. Unhealthy living and working conditions, perpetuated by racial discrimination, fewer hospitals, clinics, physicians, and nurses, a relatively inadequate number of beds for black tuberculosis patients, inadequacy of public health nursing, and low economic status all combined to increase health hazards for blacks.

Health facilities for blacks lagged far behind demonstrated needs, which were rapidly increasing. Julius Rosenwald Fund administrators pointed out that while the black death rate had receded from an estimated 32 deaths per 1000 in 1890 to about 15 in 1940, the rate still exceeded the national average of 11.2. The inadequacy of hospital services for blacks in most states and the nonexistence of such services in some Southern rural areas accounted for much of this problem. The Fund reported that in some predominantly black rural areas, as few as 75 hospital beds were set aside for the use of one million blacks. In many cities, black patients were treated only through clinics. Even those able to pay for adequate hospital care encountered difficulty in obtaining it and were seldom permitted free choice of physicians. Restrictive hospital policies limited the number of black physicians and nurses and excluded them from important postgraduate experience.

The 110 black hospitals in the United States in 1940 had a total of only about 10,000 beds; and more than 70 percent of these hospitals were privately owned and dependent for support upon patients' ability to pay. Only 22 black hospitals were fully approved by the American College of Surgeons, with five others provisionally approved. There were only 20 black schools of nursing, and few others, governmental or voluntary, admitted black students. Even in northern cities, hospital accommodations were limited because of the restrictive policies of private institutions and segregationist practices in many public hospitals.

An American Dilemma

In 1937 the Carnegie Corporation of New York decided to sponsor "a comprehensive study of the Negro in the United States, to be undertaken in a wholly objective and dispassionate way as a social phenomenon" [5]. For nearly a century the whole question had been so charged with emotion that it appeared wise to seek as the responsible head of the undertaking someone who could approach the task as freshly as possible, uninfluenced by traditional attitudes or by earlier conclusions. For this reason Gunnar Myrdal, a distinguished Swedish scholar, was chosen to direct the study. Myrdal had already achieved an international reputation as a social economist and had served as a university professor, an economic adviser to the Swedish government, and a member of the Swedish Senate.

The "dilemma" analyzed and described by Myrdal was the failure of the American credo as it applied to the black. In the early 1940s Myrdal had suggested that numerous solidly entrenched beliefs about the black that were demonstrably false and loaded with emotion were used to excuse the white mistreatment of the black. As summarized by Myrdal, a caste system had been rationalized and defended by whites on the grounds that black people belonged to a separate race of mankind and were inferior in all important respects [6].

Myrdal conceded that there were inherent differences between the races, but he attributed these to environmental conditions. "When we approach these problems on the hypothesis that differences in behavior are to be explained largely in terms of social and cultural factors, we are on scientifically safe ground. If we should, however, approach them on the hypothesis that they are to be explained primarily in terms of heredity, we do not have any scientific basis for our assumption" [7].

Since first brought to this country as slaves, the black population had been heavily concentrated in the South. It was a curious phenomenon that, since the Revolution, each of the major wars had resulted in large black migrations. The movement did not reach a flood tide, however, until World War I. "The Great Migration," as Myrdal called it, starting in 1915 and, continuing in waves since then, had brought about dramatic changes in the distribution of blacks in the United States. World War II, in progress when Myrdal was writing, vastly accelerated the steady draft toward the North and the West. The black problem was no longer wholly Southern but had become national in scope. Furthermore, the shift from a rural to an urban environment had added to black unrest. In any case, Myrdal believed that "migration to the North and West is a tremendous force in the general amelioration of the Negro's position," but, at the same time, he stressed that a "solution" to the black problem was much too complicated to be effected by migration"[8].

Federal Efforts Aid Black Nurses

Blacks attained an impressive advance on June 25, 1941, when President Roosevelt issued Executive Order 8802, which declared:

The policy of the United States is to encourage full participation in the national defense program by all citizens of the United States, regardless of race, creed, color or national origin, in the firm belief that the democratic way of life within the Nation can be defended successfully only with the help and support of all groups within its borders [9].

While verbal affirmations of this principle had been made before, Roosevelt went much further and appointed the Fair Employment Practices Committee (FEPC) to investigate complaints and to take steps to redress grievances. The FEPC conducted public hearings and focused adverse publicity on discriminatory employers and unions. The effort to open up new areas of employment for blacks was well timed, since war production provided an almost unlimited demand for labor of all kinds. Between 1940 and 1944 the number of blacks employed in manufacturing and processing grew from 500,000 to around 1.2 million, and the number of blacks in government service increased from 60,000 to 200,000.

During the war a special staff member, Estelle Massey Riddle, supported by a grant from the General Education Board of the Rockefeller Foundation, was added to the National Nursing Council for War Service and was authorized to hold institutes and to visit schools of nursing and colleges to improve the preparation and utilization of black nurses in the war effort. The objective of this unit was to help integrate school of nursing enrollments as well as the military nursing services. Before this time, the program had been carried on largely by the National Association of Colored Graduate Nurses, under the leadership of Mabel Staupers, but its staff and budget had been greatly burdened by the steadily increasing load.

The subsidized program of the Cadet Nurse Corps proved a boon to black students, and by September, 1944, there were some 2000 black nursing cadets representing all but 500 to 600 of the total number of black students enrolled in all nursing schools. Of the nursing schools accepting black students, 20 were all-black schools enrolling 1600 of the 2000 students, while the remaining 400 black students were distributed among 22 integrated schools.

A larger number of black nursing schools participated in the United States Cadet Nurse Corps than had qualified for the use of federal funds before the Corps had been established. Under the 1941–1942 federal program only 12 black schools had been eligible to participate, while under the Bolton Act more than 20 schools for blacks were involved in the Cadet Nurse Corps.

Opportunities for black women to obtain a nursing education increased greatly during the war, first through scholarships made available through Public Health Service funds and later through the Cadet Nurse Corps. National Nursing Council consultants continually hammered away to break educational barriers for black women who wanted to become nurses. A list of schools admitting black nurses was prepared for use in the Council's Clearing Bureau, which answered letters from persons wanting to become nurses. It contained the names of 32 black and 14 mixed schools.

In 1943 the 32 black schools approved by the National League of Nursing Education admitted 1918 black students, but the bed capacity, patient census, and clinical facilities available in those 32 black hospitals with nursing schools presented a bleak picture. Obviously, there were not enough schools to educate black nurses, and those in existence were characterized by insufficient clinical facilities, lack of prepared instructors, and poor housing.

Seventeen of the schools for black nurses listed by the League were situated in the South. Many of the black applicants were graduates of nonaccredited high schools or poor accredited schools. Consultants reported that black educators and vocational counselors in high schools and colleges generally did not see nursing as a profession worthy of attracting their better students. It was believed that this attitude resulted chiefly from these educators' experience with poor nursing schools. A most helpful move was to include black colleges in the college field-program set up jointly by the National Nursing Council for War Service and the Division of Nurse Education of the United States Public Health Service. Orieanne Collins and Pauline Butler visited 82 campuses and talked with thousands of black women students about the leadership positions awaiting the college prepared nurse and about the free education offered through membership in the Cadet Nurse Corps.

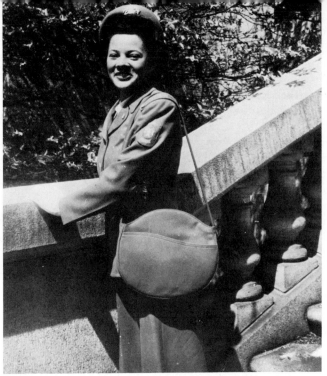

Cadet Nurse Natalie West of Freedmen's Hospital, Washington, D.C.

Cadet Nurses relax after a day on the wards at Freedmen's Hospital.

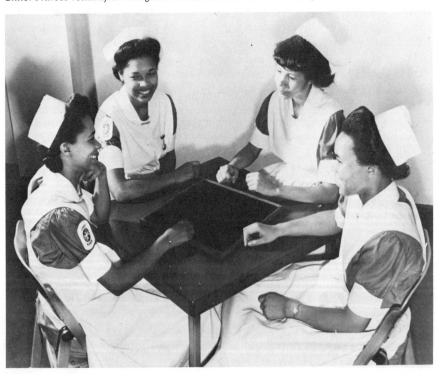

Racial and Ethnic Prejudice

In November, 1942, high school students representing a national cross-section were asked to respond to a survey of prevailing racial opinion among American teenagers. The results highlighted the special problems of blacks [10]:

Results of a 1942 Poll Identifying Racial and Ethnic Prejudice Among Teenagers

Ethnic group	Last choice roommate	Would not work with	Would not marry
Swedes	5	–	9
Protestants	4	–	9
Negroes	78	21	92
Catholics	9	1	16
Jews	45	7	51
Irish	3	–	5
Chinese	38	5	73
Makes no difference	5	69	1
Don't know	3	3	2
Total	190*	106*	258*

*Since the respondents were asked to name more than one group if they wished, the percentages add up to more than 100.

In May, 1944, and again in May, 1946, a cross-section of Americans were asked: "If you were sick in a hospital, would it be all right with you if you had a Negro nurse, or wouldn't you like it?" The results were as follows [11]:

Year	All right	Wouldn't like it	Don't know	Qualified answers
1944	53%	42%	1%	4%
1946	52%	47%	1%	–

1946 Results by Race

White	47%	51%	2%	–
Negro	97%	3%	–	–

Efforts to Promote Integration

In 1944, fighting such discrimination, 49 schools of nursing with black and mixed enrollments had admitted black students, as compared with 29 in 1941. Among those with mixed student bodies were some known to offer a variety of experience, such as the Philadelphia General Hospital and the Bellevue Hospital in New York. Gradually the list of mixed schools increased. By 1945 about 2600 black students were enrolled in schools of nursing, a 135-percent increase over that of 1939.

Enrollment in the all-black school of nursing of Freedmen's Hospital, Washington, D.C., showed a dramatic increase as it soared from 77 nursing students in 1939 to 166 students in 1944. This rapid expansion of the student body was repeated in other black nursing schools throughout the country. Only the wartime difficulties of securing adequately prepared instructors and supervisors as well as housing and clinical facilities prevented black enrollment from climbing still higher.

Executives of state boards of nurse examiners were slowly becoming aware that lower standards in nursing schools for blacks were neither desirable nor profitable in terms of health service. Standards set by black educators discouraged acceptance of lower standards for black educational institutions. Although there were signs of improvement, there was still a pronounced tendency to approve schools connected with hospitals that lacked the essential ingredients for a sound program. In a national survey of black nursing schools and black nurses conducted for the Public Health Service in 1944, Estelle Massey Riddle reported:

In talking with several executives, it was obvious that political pressure, real or imagined, has deterred positive action. For instance, in one school the State Board of Nurse Examiners had made some very important recommendations repeatedly about conditions which affected the welfare and education of the students, none of which have been

Students enrolling in the Cadet Nurse Corps at Freedmen's Hospital, 1944.

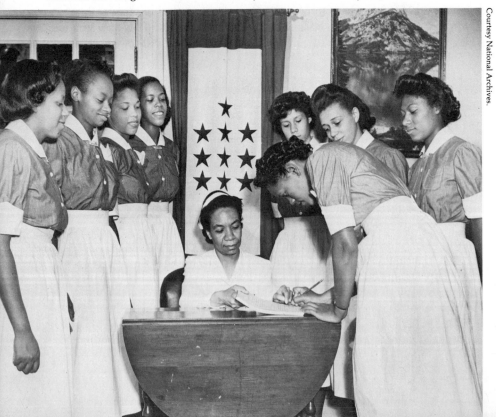

Courtesy National Archives.

complied with to date. The officials of the school have effective connections with the state politicians and seem to have no fear of disregarding the recommendations made by the State Board of Nurse Examiners.

In another instance, a state board executive asked for a recommendation from the National Nursing Council that a certain school for Negro nurses be closed. This was complied with. Within six weeks after the letter was sent, another visit was made to the school. The consultant was shocked at being told by the administrator that the state nursing executive had visited the school during the interim, at which time she expressed her displeasure at the "audacity" of the consultant for making a recommendation for closing the school. The school was moved from the tentatively approved to the fully approved list before any of the improvements had been made [12].

On the list of nursing schools distributed by the National Nursing Council for War Service, 12 of the 26 academic directors were white. Mrs. Riddle also observed that white directors of black nursing schools, with few exceptions, seemed indifferent or even hostile to their students. These attitudes were reflected in the nursing programs and in community reaction to the students. According to Mrs. Riddle, there was evidence of both subtle and overt diversion of black nurses with leadership abilities from the teaching and administrative fields. In the North, prejudice took the more subtle form of advancing the nurses who were least aggressive. In the South, the overt lack of respect for the personalities of the students and graduate nurses brought forth such expressions as "That's my school, but I would do anything before I would go back there to work," or "The instructor punished us for addressing our own Negro patients as Mr., Mrs., or Miss, even though some of these people are most highly re-

On the children's ward at Freedmen's Hospital.

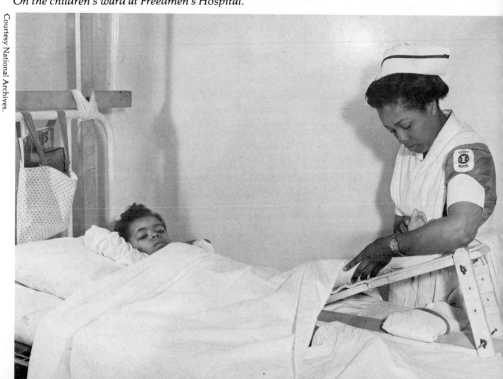

spected citizens of our community." As a consultant on official visits, Mrs. Riddle reported that she encountered the same lack of respect [13].

The Armed Forces Balk

By 1944 the number of black graduate nurses was estimated at 8000. The greatest gains for blacks in civilian service were reported to have been made in the hospitals of New York City, where in 1942 more than 1250 black nurses were serving under the Department of Hospitals. On the whole, nursing staffs in black hospitals were scarcely affected by the withdrawal of a few nurses who had been accepted into the Army Nurse Corps, even though the Procurement and Assignment Service had rated these hospitals as being overstaffed by hundreds of graduate nurses, according to established wartime standards.

The National Nursing Council for War Service urged that physically and professionally qualified graduate registered nurses, regardless of race, be appointed to military vacancies. Thus, as additional black cadets graduated, they were not only willing but encouraged to apply for commissions. Hundreds of Cadets and other black nurses received the following form letter from the Army [14]:

Dear Miss_____:

I am directed by the Surgeon General . . . to inform you that your application for enrollment in the Army Nurse Corps cannot be given favorable consideration because the quota of colored nurses required by the Corps has been filled.

The policy regarding the assignment for colored nurses is outlined by the War Department Planning Board and colored nurses are authorized for assignment only to those stations where colored troops predominate.

Your offered service is appreciated. . .will be given consideration at such time as vacancies occur.

Very truly yours

Before Pearl Harbor, Surgeon General James C. Magee of the United States Army Medical Corps stated that black nurses would not be used in the Army Nurse Corps. The American Red Cross and other leading nursing organizations, however, joined the National Association of Colored Graduate Nurses in protesting this situation. Partly as a result of this effort, a small number of black nurses were assigned to duty at Fort Huachuca, Arizona, Fort Bragg, North Carolina, Camp Livingston, Louisiana, and Maxwell Field, Tuskegee, Alabama. Although the Army Nurse Corps gradually increased the number of black nurses to 217, they were all confined, with one exception, to segregated areas in the South.

National nursing groups and friends of the National Association of Colored Graduate Nurses made repeated efforts to force a change regarding the restrictions pertaining to black nurses. Although Surgeon General Magee was adamantly opposed to appeals for increased use of black nurses, Surgeon General Norman T. Kirk, named to succeed Magee in June, 1943, was thought to be more flexible. On June 14, 1943, he received a strong protest from the National Nursing Council for War Service, to which he replied on June 28, stating that military policies were not unlike those used in civilian hospitals. As a result, the Council sent a carefully worded questionnaire to hospitals employing both black and white nurses in order to produce convincing evidence for the new Surgeon General. This effort resulted in the compilation of data covering 17 situations where black and white nurses worked together. The survey showed that working relations were harmonious even where integrated living and eating accommodations were provided.

Despite the persuasive information on civilian use of integrated personnel provided for the Surgeon General in the early summer of 1943, no immediate revision of Medical Department policy was made. Although the results of the survey were sent to Army and Navy officials concerned with nursing personnel, neither the Army nor the Navy acknowledged receipt of this report. In response to a pointed communication from the Council, the Navy sent the following letter to Executive Secretary Elmira Wickenden [15]:

My Dear Mrs. Wickenden:
Your letter of 1 March 1944 is hereby acknowledged.
Up to the present time there are no established billets for the appointment of Negro nurses in the Navy Nurse Corps.

Sincerely yours,
Ross T. McIntire
Vice-Admiral, USN
Chief of Bureau

Meanwhile, Surgeon General Norman Kirk had told Eleanor Roosevelt that the Army Nurse Corps' personnel difficulties lay not in professional use of black nurses on the wards, but in the many social complications related to quartering them and providing their off-duty subsistence allowances. As standing policy, the War Department accepted approximately 10 percent of the total troop strength in blacks, but this quota was impractical as applied to physicians, dentists, and nurses, he continued. The black population could not provide that proportion of fully qualified professionals, nor could that number be removed from civilian services without jeopardizing black health. General Kirk explained that the Army had adopted the policy of assigning black physicians and nurses only to those stations having a large complement of black troops. He thought that this arrangement provided reasonable workloads and felt that it solved recreation and off-duty entertainment problems.

By January, 1945, there were only one-tenth as many black nurses in the Army Nurse Corps, in proportion to the total Corps, as there were blacks in the Army as a whole. In contrast, if as many black nurses, in proportion to their numbers, had been accepted by the Army and the Navy as were white nurses, there would have been 1520 in the Army and Navy instead of only 330 in the Army at that date.

At the beginning of 1945 acceptance of more black nurses by the Army and

Navy was urged as an immediate step toward meeting increased nurse short-ages. In a joint statement by the National Nursing Council for War Service and the National Association of Colored Graduate Nurses, Elmira Wickenden and Mabel Staupers, the executive secretaries of the two organizations, emphasized that the 330 nurses then in the Army Nurse Corps represented less than one-tenth of the proportion of black soldiers in the Army. Rejections, and the fear of rejection, had kept down the number, they stated, although it had been esti-mated that at least 2000 out of the total of 8000 or more black graduate nurses then active in nursing might have been eligible for the military.

Assignment of more black nurses to the Army and actual admission of black nurses into the Navy was urged on the following grounds, among others:

It would add materially to military nursing resources in the present emergency.

It would demonstrate that as American men, regardless of race, creed, or color, are fighting for democracy, American women are being given the opportunity, equally without discrimination, to care for them when ill or wounded.

It would, if administered without segregation, carry over into military life the policy of integrating professional services, regardless of color, now being increasingly practiced in civilian life.

It would demonstrate to young Negro women who are considering nursing as a career the fact that opportunities to serve will not be denied them, thus paving the way for a greater contribution by Negro nurses after the war to the health not only of Negroes but of the whole population [16].

Although the Navy Nurse Corps had never accepted black nurses, on the grounds that there were no "billets" provided for them, on January 31, 1945, the following statement was authorized by the Surgeon General of the Navy:

There is no policy in the Navy which discriminates against the utilization of Negro Nurses. Each and every application for appointment in the Navy Nurse Corps or the Navy Nurse Corps Reserve is given full consideration provided the applicant meets the physical and other requirements for appointment [17].

Shortly thereafter, the first black nurse was sworn into the Navy Nurse Corps.

A Nurse's Role Helps Attack Racial Prejudice

Four years later a nurse was portrayed as the focus of the film *Pinky*, which was the first attempt by a major studio (20th Century-Fox) to dramatize the increasingly recognized problem of racial prejudice. Registered nurse Patricia ("Pinky") Johnson (played by Jeanne Crain) returns from Boston to the Deep South to visit her Granny (Ethel Waters), a black washerwoman who lives in a poverty shack on the outskirts of a large plantation. Because she looks white and had passed for white during her schooling in the North, Pinky is unused to the regional racial attitudes that become increasingly clear when she suffers the humiliations of being embarrassingly brushed off at the general store, of

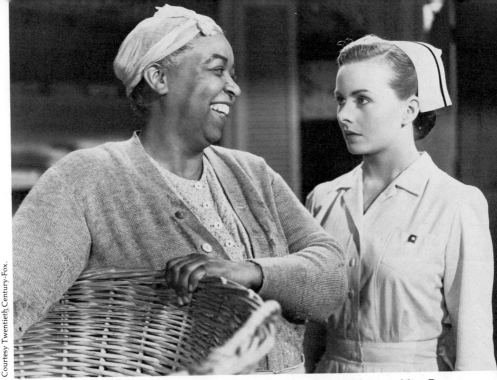

Granny (Ethel Waters) persuades Pinky (Jeanne Crain) to stay and nurse Miss Em.
(Copyright © 1949 Twentieth Century-Fox Film Corporation. All rights reserved.)

being falsely arrested by contemptuous white deputies, and being the victim of an attempted rape by two drunken townsmen.

Granny, who is fond of religious and folk aphorisms, argues, "Oh, Pinky child, when folks is real friends, there ain't no such thing as place." But the argument fails to convince her. Pinky is approached by a local black physician, Dr. Canady (Kenny Washington), who proposes that she stay in the area and help him set up a nursing school for blacks but Pinky dismisses the idea. She has packed to return North when Granny persuaded her to stay a bit longer as Miss Em (Ethel Barrymore), an aristocratic old spinster whom Granny has loved and served for years, is bedridden with a serious heart condition, and no nurse is available. Upon Granny's pleas, Pinky reluctantly dons her nursing uniform cap and begins free service at the plantation mansion, earning money during her off-hours by helping Granny wash clothes for white families.

Miss Em is a feisty, domineering matron, who never hesitates to order others about. Against the physician's orders, for instance, she demands coffee: "Make that coffee strong! I want the spoon to stand up in it!" She assigns Pinky menial chores such as housecleaning, washing dishes, and cooking. As Pinky begins to assert herself ("Nursing's my profession. In certain places, a nurse is treated with respect . . . . I'm a trained nurse, and I won't be spoken to like that!"), she seems to grow in Miss Em's estimation. Pinky becomes something of a confidante when Miss Em's vulturous cousin-in-law, Melba Wooley, comes calling ostensibly to inquire about Miss Em's health but actually to ask about her will.

Pinky's boyfriend, a young Northern physician, Thomas Adams, arrives on

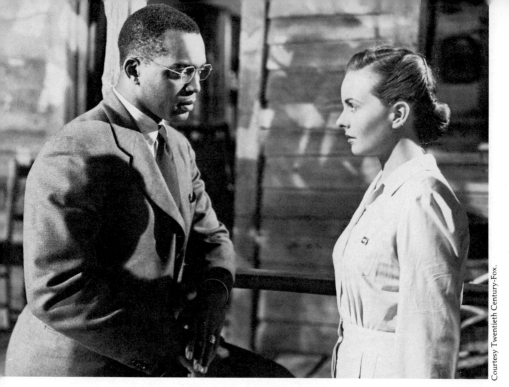

the scene and discovers her previously secret background. Stating that he does not believe in racial superiority ("What's rational about prejudice?" he asks), he proposes to Pinky, she accepts, and they make plans to settle in the North.

Miss Em dies and leaves the plantation and mansion to Pinky. In her will the matriarch maintains her full confidence in Pinky's judgment about how to use the inheritance. Cousin Melba files a legal suit contending that Pinky conspired to get Miss Em to leave her the property by drugging her so that she did not know what she was doing, and that the will should be declared void. Tom Adams suggests that Pinky avoid the unpleasant dealings she will predictably face in a Southern court, but Pinky insists that she has a certain moral obligation (from her slowly developing awareness of her racial identity) and an obligation to carry out Miss Em's wishes. Tom resigns himself to backing her throughout the trial.

The emotion of the townspeople rises to a fever pitch as the trial takes place in the sweltering heat of a small courtroom. At every turn in the case, Pinky seems to suffer prejudiced judicial setbacks, but the judge finally shocks the crowd of white spectators by ruling the will valid. Tom Adams then proposes that the couple sell Pinky's new property and start a new life together in Denver, where no one would know them. He argues that she could keep her racial background a secret and pass for his white wife. Pinky rejects the proposal and breaks off her engagement, maintaining that she must respect Miss Em's confidence in her management of the property. As a black, she notes to Tom, "You can't live without pride." With the help and encouragement of the black Dr. Canady and the elderly, white Dr. Joe, Pinky turns the plantation into a memorial: Miss Em's Clinic and Nursing School, a medical facility and nurse training school for blacks.

Pinky became one of the most publicized movies of the year. It garnered a cover story in *Life* (October 17, 1949) with nearly two pages of still photos. Popular mass-circulation weeklies were full of praise. *Time*, for instance, noted that "the story is told with considerable honesty and understated force . . . . it achieves a haunting character portrait." *Newsweek* called Ethel Barrymore's role "one of her finest screen characterizations" in "a cast of uniformly credible white and Negro players." Jeanne Crain was nominated for the Academy Award for best actress on the basis of her portrayal.

Gaining Acceptance for Black Students

In 1950 slightly over 200 schools of nursing had at least one black student enrolled. Within the group of schools having no black students were some that indicated a willingness to admit blacks, although they further stated that they had never had any black applicants or that black applicants did not meet entrance requirements. Also in this group were schools reporting that their policy prevented admission of blacks. Others stated that no policy existed. There had been a steady increase in the number of schools reporting that they would admit qualified blacks and a decrease in the number of schools reporting that their policy prevented such admissions or failing to make a definite response.

Schools that had changed admission policies between 1948 and 1952 included a number located in Kansas, Kentucky, Maryland, Oklahoma, and West Virginia. Of the few schools that reported that their policies prohibited black enrollment, the majority were located *outside* the Southern states. Some schools were forbidden by state law to admit blacks, and there were a few instances where city regulations made the admission of blacks impossible. Some schools, although willing to admit blacks, were located in areas not conducive to the welfare of the individual black student. In a locale where segregation was enforced, the black student could not be housed in the nurses' residence and could not use the cafeteria.

Other directors reported that acceptance of blacks had presented a difficulty only in scheduling social affairs for the students or in planning recreational activities. Schools in Wisconsin, Washington, Pennsylvania, Illinois, and Ohio found this to be true, as did schools in Kansas and Kentucky. In some areas if a mixed group entered a restaurant, no one was served. One school found it necessary to plan for a picnic at a private residence because the black students were not permitted in the public park where the activity was customarily scheduled.

Two schools reported difficulty in having black students accepted by agencies used for affiliation. A few schools found individual members of the medical staff reluctant to accept black students in the operating room or at their patients' bedsides. In one incident an RN refused to stay on duty with a black student. The director related that, "although we needed nurses, we let her [the RN] go rather than give in, and there has been no further difficulty." This attitude probably reflected the way many of the isolated incidents had been handled. There were also encouraging reports of black students being selected "campus queen," holding class offices, and being accepted into the nurses' homes with no difficulty. One director related that the parents of black students were given a somewhat indifferent reception at meetings of the parents' association of the school, but the attitude of the students themselves would probably help to break down prejudice in the parent group.

The comment was made repeatedly by school of nursing directors that success in the admission of blacks depended primarily on careful selection, a factor considered important in the admission of any student. A few schools had secured the support of their student bodies before accepting their first black students. Some had let it be known well in advance that blacks would be admitted. In contrast, other schools had made no effort to prepare any particular group for the first black student, in the belief that the more matter-of-fact the attitude of the faculty, the less difficulty would be encountered.

Unfortunately, not all integration efforts in nursing went smoothly among the student populations. In one border state, hospital service was carried on uninterruptedly although a group of graduate staff nurses walked out because the hospital refused to discharge three black nurses in the early 1950s. The number of nurses who had left their jobs was in dispute, according to newspaper reports. Representatives of the protesting nurses' group said that 23 of the hospital's 30 graduate nurses had withdrawn. The hospital, on the other hand, said that only 11 of the 23 "striking" nurses were employed at the hospital and that the others were in private practice, employed by industry, or retired. Following the walkout the hospital brought in graduate nurses from other communities to carry on patient services.

In January, 1951, the 42-year-old National Association of Colored Graduate Nurses was dissolved in order to merge with the American Nurses' Association. The dissolution, described as an "act of faith," created new responsibilities for the ANA, which it attempted to meet through its Intergroup Relations Program. One of the primary goals of this program was the removal of membership barriers in district and state associations.

Substantial progress was quickly made. Although before the war 15 state nursing associations had not admitted blacks, only the Georgia association retained race restrictions in 1954. Similarly, although in 1941 only 42 schools of nursing admitted blacks, by 1954 the number had risen to at least 710, including some of the nation's most outstanding hospital schools and collegiate programs.

The two decades following *Brown* v. *Board of Education of Topeka* saw black nurses fully integrated into virtually all health care settings in the United States. A much larger percentage of blacks entered nursing under the stimulus of federal programs to redress the underrepresentation of this group in the profession. The emergence of the black nurse into prominence might be exemplified

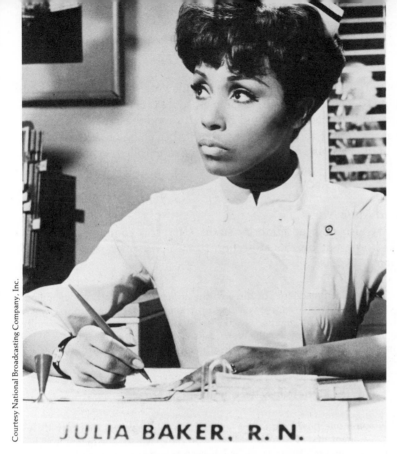

JULIA BAKER, R. N.

Diahann Carroll, star of the 1968–1971 television series Julia.

by the success from 1968 to 1971 of the television series, *Julia*, starring Diahann Carroll as a self-supporting registered nurse who attempts to readjust to life after the death of her husband and to raise her young son, Corey.

A School of Nursing for American Indians

The one school of nursing for American Indians during the 1940s and 1950s was located on a remote plateau in northeastern Arizona, at Ganado, 56 miles northwest of Gallup, New Mexico, in the heart of the Navajo Indian Reservation. Sage Memorial Hospital was the largest Indian hospital in the Southwest, with beds and ample clinical experience for the needs of the nursing school. The operating room, x-ray and clinical laboratories, and dietetic department were well equipped. Sage Memorial Hospital, built in 1929 by the Board of National Missions of the Presbyterian Church, was owned and operated by that organization primarily for the benefit of the Navajo Indians, although other tribes and white patients were cared for as well. This medium-sized hospital, although remotely located, was modern and had been approved by the American College of Surgeons.

The School of Nursing had been established in 1930, the first class graduating in 1933. The purpose of the school was to provide young Indian women with an opportunity to secure preparation as nurses, so that this profession could be open to them and so that they would be able to render a much-needed and intelligent nursing service to their people. From its beginning in 1930 the school had grown until, in 1945, 40 young women were enrolled, representing 25 tribes from 12 states.

The Harassed Male Nurse

The male nurse also suffered minority status. That this condition was long-standing was borne out by this quotation from a 1914 manual on hospital administration:

Those of us who practiced medicine, or directed the affairs of hospitals, under the old regime, when the trained woman nurse was unknown, and when the male nurse was a composite of drunkenness and genius, wonder whether the change that has wholly eliminated the trained male nurse is for the best. There is no doubt that there is something more virile, more substantial, and certainly less finicky in the male nurse than in the female.

On the other hand, the authors insisted that the male nurse:

. . . has usually some overpowering failing, some inherent weakness that forbids his success in any permanent line of human endeavor. In other words, the male nurse has been nearly always "a failure." Many times he has become a periodical drunkard. Sometimes he has been a bright young businessman or mechanic or clerk whose intemperate habits have brought him to the hospital, and, after repeated trials and repeated failures, he has found that his only safety lies in shutting himself out from the world, and subjecting himself to the discipline of the hospital or the eleemosynary institution. The most competent and reliable male nurse will oftentimes go along for weeks or months, attending conscientiously to his duties, taking most efficient care of patients, until in some unlucky moment he finds the whiskey bottle in the medicine cabinet and takes "just a drop to steady his nerves." The rest of the story is easily imagined. It has become a maxim that a trained nurse would not be a nurse if he were fit for any other occupation, and that is probably true [18].

Forgotten was that fully one-half the nursing of medieval times had been done by men and that the Knights Hospitalers, Teutonic Knights, Franciscans and many other male nursing orders had supplied excellent nursing care. It was Saint Vincent de Paul who had first conceived the idea of social service. Similarly, John Howard, Pastor Theodor Fliedner, Dr. Thomas Bond, Benjamin Franklin, and Henri Dunant had been oriented toward the value of men in nursing.

In World War I a large percentage of qualified men nurses had volunteered for military service. Many capable male nurses were absorbed into Army divisions where there was no opportunity for them to contribute effectively to the nursing needs of the service. For instance, some men nurses who were especially knowledgeable about psychiatric nursing had been utilized by National Guard

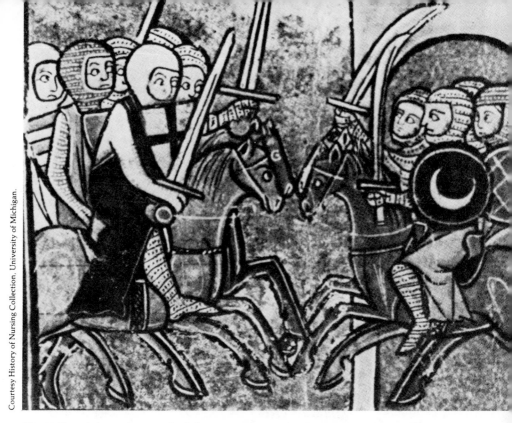

The image of the male nurse had deteriorated enormously since the thirteenth century when military-nursing orders such as the Knights Hospitalers had both battled for the Holy Land and supplied excellent nursing care.

units and assigned to a variety of menial tasks. They had not been made available to help in the tremendous task of caring for the thousands of psychiatric cases generated by the war.

During the 1930s Helen G. McClelland, Director of Nursing at the Pennsylvania Hospital, Philadelphia, commented on the effectiveness of male nurses:

> It was with definite misgivings on the part of the medical staff and a number of the nursing staff that the project of giving a year of training to the men studying nursing at the Department for Mental and Nervous Diseases was started in the General Hospital.
>
> However, it was only a short time before there was a realization on the part of all concerned that there was a decided improvement in the service given to the men patients when they were cared for by well-prepared men nurses.
>
> It was also found that the men seemed to have a better understanding of the psychology of men patients and, due to their previous psychiatric training, were better able to solve the problems of the patients during their period of adjustment to the various hospital routines. While this was true in all services to which they were assigned, the most marked improvements in nursing service to the men patients was noted in the genito-urinary wards [19].

According to the Department of Commerce, Bureau of the Census, in April, 1940, there were 7509 male nurses and students employed and 563 seeking employment. For the academic year 1939–1940 there were four accredited schools of nursing in the United States that admitted only men students. The total enrollment in these four schools was 212. At the same time there were 63 coeducational schools of nursing, with 710 men students and 3798 women students enrolled. The schools admitting men were geographically distributed approximately as follows: in the eastern states, 50 percent; in the southern states, 25 percent; in the midwestern states, 15 percent; in the western states, 10 percent.

The tentative Program for the new Men Nurses' Section of the ANA, as approved by the ANA Board of Directors in January, 1941, was as follows:

With few exceptions, men nurses have taken little part in nursing education, especially in the teaching of nursing arts and sciences and acting in the capacity of officers in the schools of nursing which do train men. Better candidates might be chosen if graduate men nurses had some part in selecting them. As a part of our program, we urge them to seek such positions when the opportunity arises.

If men nurses as students were encouraged to take part in all activities which might serve to stimulate the interest of the student in his profession, a continued or greater interest would be shown on graduation.

Men patients would receive much better care if attended by a graduate registered man nurse rather than by an orderly [20].

Male Nurses and Military Nursing

Since 1901 men nurses had been barred from the Army Nurse Corps because the law that had brought it into being designated it as the "Army Nurse Corps, Female." This fact was brought to the attention of the Board of Directors of the American Nurses' Association in January, 1941, by the Men Nurses' Section of the ANA, which sought repeal of this law and enactment of a law to give "men and women nurses equal opportunities in the military service." The Board of Directors voted that this request of the Men Nurses' Section of the American Nurses' Association be referred to the Surgeon General of the Army. On April 7, 1941, the following reply was received from Acting Surgeon General Albert G. Love of the Medical Department:

In the absence of General James C. Magee from the city, I am acknowledging the receipt of your letter of April 2, in which you refer to the desirability of legislation to place male nurses on the same military status as female nurses.

I regret that this office cannot concur in your opinion. It would be impracticable to employ male nurses in times of peace since such employment could complicate unnecessarily the administrative problems. We feel that we have provided a satisfactory and dignified position for such male nurses as may be employed during the military emergency. In addition, we feel sure that the Secretary of War would not approve the legislation suggested by you [21].

In early 1942 Edith Smith of the Federal Security Agency's Subcommittee on Nursing discussed the problem with Dr. James Crabtree of the Health and Medical Committee. Dr. Crabtree felt that unless the Army and Navy said that they would use these young men as nurses upon completion of their courses, there was no justification in requesting that they be granted student deferments. Miss Smith pointed out the need for these men in civilian life, but Dr. Crabtree said he felt that the need was so comparatively small and manpower requirements for the Armed Forces were so vast that, if it were necessary, schools of nursing for male nurses would have to be closed. He thought it a relatively minor problem and said that if draft boards were to exempt all the men who were taking any kind of training, the Army would be made up exclusively of boys under 17.

Miss Smith checked on the status of male nurses elsewhere around Washington. Pearl McIver said that she had recommended to the Venereal Disease Control Department of the United States Public Health Service that male nurses be employed in connection with government-sponsored venereal disease investigations. She persuaded that department to employ 10 men, but when three had been secured whose qualifications were satisfactory, the men were drafted. Miss McIver grew somewhat discouraged over the possibility of carrying out the plan, since the men were eligible for the draft.

A great need for male nurses had been reported at Saint Elizabeth's Hospital in Washington, D.C. This psychiatric hospital had employed 13 male nurses but had quickly lost seven to the military services. In June, 1942, the hospital had seven male nursing students but was not accepting any more, since it could not be certain that the men would not be drafted. The Veterans Administration thought that Saint Elizabeth's had about 10 men employed in the genito-urinary wards. However, those men were not very satisfactory. "They get drunk," said Superintendent of Nurses Mary Hickey, "and the doctors do not like them. They do not find them as good as female nurses in the psychiatric wards" [22].

Fighting such biases, at a meeting of the American Nurses' Association House of Delegates held in Chicago in May, 1942, the following resolution was adopted:

Whereas, the Army and Navy are in great need of the services of graduate, registered professional nurses; and whereas, the graduate, registered professional men nurses, members of the American Nurses' Association, are prepared to render this service; therefore, be it resolved: that the American Nurses' Association in convention assembled in Chicago, May 17–22, 1942, address a communication to the Surgeons General of the Army and of the Navy, respectfully requesting that graduate, registered professional men nurses, members of the American Nurses' Association, be given the opportunity to serve as nurses as soon as possible after induction or enlistment into the armed forces of the country [23].

Male Nurses Seek Recognition
Despite these appeals, arrangements continued to call for the induction of registered men nurses into the armed forces as privates in the Army or as pharmacist's mates third class in the Navy. The result was that men nurses who were employed in military service had no official status. They received no recognition as a professional group, no authority, and no distinctive marking to identify

them to the wounded or to other health workers. Reports from men nurses in the Army showed that their services as nurses were not utilized. Others revealed that while they were serving as nurses, they were doing it without nursing rank.

Several nursing groups appealed to the War Department to secure rank for men nurses, but such requests were consistently opposed by the Army Nurse Corps. One male nurse wrote in response to this attitude:

> Ever since Pearl Harbor, we men nurses have been striving for recognition as nurses in the armed forces. We are not seeking glory; rather, we wish to serve in a capacity in which we sincerely believe the greatest value would be gained from our highly specialized training and experience.
>
> We have intensified our efforts recently because of the critical shortage of nurses in the services. We want our fighting men to have the best care that medical science can give. We have received favorable replies from many Congressmen and other interested officials, yet the Army and Navy Medical Departments continue to offer the same objections to our recognition [24].

In an account of his personal experiences, Private Jacob Rose, R.N., asked that, if the Army needed nurses, what difference did it make if they were men or women as long as they were equally trained for a specific job? He recalled how the Army "cried for nurses, spent huge sums in advertising that urged nurses to volunteer, threatened a draft of all nurses, but a registered male nurse didn't merit recognition in the Medical Department. Instead, we continued to hear lectures from a non-medical officer on first aid, whose lectures made little sense." Rose related that during his basic training at Camp Barkley, Texas, there were five registered men nurses in two training companies alone, and four were Bellevue graduates. He did not know how many others whose nursing skill was going to utter waste were scattered throughout this tremendous training camp. However, they were together for almost five months, "marching, drilling, detesting the inevitable KP with its endless pots and pans—finally culminating in a 17-day bivouac" [25].

After almost 20 weeks of basic training these male nurses were separated and Rose went to the India-Burma theater. There he learned to drive a 12-ton bulldozer and leveled out a baseball field. He also filled in all the potholes in the road leading past the Twentieth General Hospital at Ledo. Such experiences were probably duplicated by hundreds of male nurses in the armed forces.

The effect of the war and of Selective Service was practically to wipe out the enrollment of men in schools of nursing. Men nurses believed that the prevailing policy was a serious error. It markedly affected the quality of nursing service, especially in psychiatric hospitals, and contributed to the later shortages of men nurses.

The Dilemma of Sex Stereotyping

After the war men nurses urgently recommended that the ANA Committee on Federal Legislation continue its efforts to obtain appropriate regulations under

Selective Service for the deferment of men nursing students. Men nurse veterans strongly urged that legislation be obtained to provide commissions for men nurses. They reiterated that their services had not been used effectively during the war. In 1946 Leroy N. Craig claimed that the ANA had been and remained in 100 percent support of military status for men nurses, but the proposed legislation was blocked because the Surgeons General of the Army and Navy believed that men nurses should not be allowed commissions in the Nurse Corps.

A 1946 survey showed that 27 states had a total of 68 schools that admitted men to the basic course but that 13 states had only one school each. New York topped the list with 22 schools. Eighteen of them were in state mental hospitals, which admitted men and women. From 1938 to 1946, 24 of the reporting schools admitted 853 men, of whom 633 went on to graduate. Lack of appropriate housing facilities was the primary obstacle to the admission of men to more schools. This was true also of affiliated institutions, and it tended to prevent men students from securing preparation in fields such as tuberculosis, communicable disease, and cancer nursing.

Existing barriers to the employment of men nurses appeared to be due more to sentiment and tradition than to any actual ineptitude based on sex. About

Male nurses have been engaged in a long fight for proper recognition and acceptance.

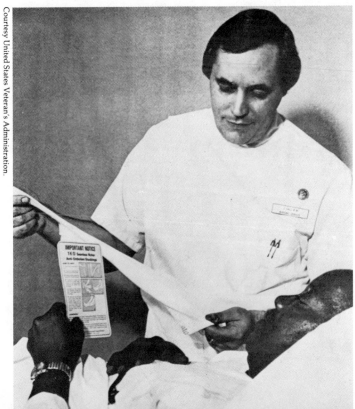

Courtesy United States Veteran's Administration.

Total Nursing Students, Males and Blacks Admitted and Graduated from 1945–1965 as a Percentage of all Admissions and Graduations.

	Admissions					Graduates				
Year	Male	%	Black	%	Total	Male	%	Black	%	Total
1945	42	.07	821	1.45	56,567	28	.09	520	1.64	31,721
1946	–	–	–	–	30,899	36	.10	540	1.49	36,195
1947	334	.87	1001	2.62	38,210	42	.10	592	1.45	40,744
1948	470	1.08	1262	2.91	43,373	28	.08	597	1.74	34,268
1949	398	.91	1383	3.17	43,612	136	.64	507	2.37	21,379
1950	508	1.15	1200	2.72	44,185	205	.79	583	2.26	25,790
1951	384	.92	1350	3.24	41,667	248	.86	782	2.72	28,794
1952	361	.85	1964*	4.61	42,562	271	.93	1035*	3.57	29,016
1953	332	.77	1928*	4.45	43,327	335	1.14	1045*	3.57	29,308
1954	400	.89	1843*	4.10	44,930	236	.83	1061*	3.72	28,539
1955	459	.99	2119*	4.56	46,493	230	.80	1151*	4.01	28,729
1956	484	1.07	1976*	4.37	45,255	224	.75	1151*	3.84	29,933
1959	690	1.40	1597	3.25	49,166	287	.95	1090	3.62	30,113
1962	856	1.73	1456	2.94	49,521	393	1.21	1081	3.34	32,398
1965	1076	1.77	1891	3.12	60,701	604	1.72	1050	2.99	35,125

*Includes all nonwhite students.

1950 Ruth Sleeper noted that at Massachusetts General Hospital there had been objection to male nurses from the medical staff, perhaps because physicians had found them a little more difficult to work with than women nurses. She also said that there had been some questions as to whether the relation of the male nurse to the patient had always been "right," and she had been requested in some instances not to employ a man as head nurse. On the other hand Katherine Densford related that she had employed male nurses in many capacities, including that of faculty member on her teaching staff, without any difficulty whatever. Two men nurses who had received their preparation for faculty positions in Minnesota had been able to use their education as a stepping stone to hospital administration. Miss Densford did not feel that the men's education was lost when applied later in hospital administration.

The male nurse would have a difficult road ahead in the coming decades, and the battle against feminine stereotyping of nurses would never really get off the ground until a massive effort could be launched at resocializing the general public. The strength of the link between women and nursing was perhaps one of the strongest in any occupation and consequently would only be overcome slowly as increasing numbers of men would undergo the unique interpersonal and social demands that all phases of nursing education and service would make upon their egos.

On the whole, the war had the effect of enhancing opportunities for black women in nursing while at the same time militating against male nurses. Perhaps this dichotomy is best explained in terms of professional and lay pressure. The cause of black women had adherents in the National Nursing Council for War Service and all the way to the White House and Eleanor Roosevelt. By contrast, the movement for fair treatment of men desiring a nursing education and male nurses entering the armed forces never really got started. Most nurses and the general public seemed to adhere to the view that the man's place in wartime was on the battlefield, and that at all times women alone should take care of the nursing. Consequently, men continued to constitute the smallest minority in nursing, amounting to only 1 percent of the 440,000 active nurses in 1960.

Summary

The 1954 Supreme Court ruling Brown v. *Board of Education of Topeka, which outlawed racial segregation in the public schools, was a long overdue step toward racial equality in America.*

Although the first black trained nurse, Mary E. P. Mahoney, had received a diploma from the School of Nursing of Boston's New England Hospital for Women and Children in 1879, progress for black nurses was slow. As late as 1954, for example, many black nurses were barred membership in the American Nurses' Association because their state associations would not admit them.

Prior to World War II, schools of nursing admitting large numbers of black students were generally located in southern black hospitals. Although some were considered first-rate schools, many were totally inadequate.

The average health status of blacks was markedly lower than whites, and available health care for blacks lagged far behind whites.

Certain World War II developments proved helpful to black nurses. The Rockefeller Foundation funded a project to help integrate school of nursing enrollments and the military nursing services. The subsidized United States Cadet Nurse Corps offered new opportunities for black women to become nurses.

Before Pearl Harbor the Surgeon General of the Army Medical Corps had stated that black nurses would not be used in the Army Nurse Corps. The American Red Cross and other leading nursing organizations joined the National Association of Colored Graduate Nurses in protesting this situation. Although the Army Nurse Corps soon accepted a limited number of black nurses, they were mostly confined to segregated military camps in the South.

A pioneering 1949 motion picture, Pinky, forcefully depicted racial prejudice through the experiences of a black nurse from the North who undergoes humiliation and degradation before successfully standing up to prejudice and founding a nursing school for blacks.

Many nursing schools claimed willingness to admit black students but pointed to state or municipal laws prohibiting integration or to the "problems" that integration of living quarters and school social activities would cause. Integration did not always go smoothly, but substantial progress was made during the 1950s, and virtually every school of nursing was integrated by the late 1960s.

In 1951 the 42-year-old National Association of Colored Graduate Nurses merged with the American Nurses' Association. The ANA took on new responsibilities through its Intergroups Relations Program which was aimed at removing the remaining membership barriers in certain district and state associations.

In 1930 Sage Memorial Hospital School of Nursing at Ganado, Arizona, was established to provide young Indian women with an opportunity to become nurses. By 1945, 40 women representing 25 tribes were enrolled in the school.

The status of male nurses had deteriorated markedly since the heroic exploits of the Knights Hospitalers in the Crusades. Both World War I and II saw qualified men nurses assigned to nonnursing duties with no opportunity to contribute to the nursing needs of the military.

During World War II appeals were made to the Army and Navy to afford male nurses their appropriate status, but they were still inducted as privates in the Army or as pharmacist's mates third class in the Navy. Men in nurse training *schools were not given student deferments and male enrollments dropped to almost nothing.*

During the 1950s little progress was made by male nurses who constituted only one percent of the active nurses in 1960.

References

1. *New York Times*, May 18, 1954.
2. "The Long View," *Nursing Outlook*, vol. 2 (August, 1954): 403.
3. Nina D. Gage and Alma C. Haupt, "Some Observations on Negro Nursing in the South," *Public Health Nursing*, vol. 24 (December, 1932): 674–680.
4. Edwin R. Embree, *Brown America: The Story of a New Race* (New York: Viking Press, Inc., 1931), pp. 88–104.
5. Gunnar Myrdal et al, *An American Dilemma: The Negro Problem and Modern Democracy* (New York: Harper and Brothers, 1944), p. ix.
6. *Ibid.*, pp. 137–153.
7. *Ibid.*, pp. 175–181.
8. *Ibid.*, pp. 191–201.
9. *New York Times*, June 26, 1941.
10. Hadley Cantril, *Public Opinion, 1935–1946* (Princeton: Princeton University Press, 1951), p. 477.
11. *Ibid.*
12. Estelle Massey Riddle, *National Report of Negro Nursing Schools and Nurses*, May, 1945. Unpublished manuscript, Federal Records Center, Cadet Nurse Corps Files, RG 90.
13. *Ibid.*
14. Ida W. Danielson to Negro Nurse Applicants to the Army Nurse Corps, undated. National Archives, War Manpower Commission, RG 211.
15. Ross T. McIntire to Elmira B. Wickenden, March 7, 1944 (copy). Densford Papers.
16. *Minutes*, Meeting of the National Nursing Council for War Service, February 21, 1945, New York City. Densford Papers.
17. *Ibid.*
18. J. A. Hornsby and R. E. Schmidt, *The Modern Hospital: Its Inspiration, Its Architecture, Its Equipment, Its Operation* (Philadelphia: W. B. Saunders Co., 1914), p. 335.
19. Leroy N. Craig, "Opportunities for Men Nurses," *American Journal of Nursing*, vol. 40 (June, 1940): 669.
20. *Report of Men Nurses' Section of the American Nurses' Association, May, 1942*. Unpublished manuscript, National Archives, RG 215.
21. Acting Surgeon General Albert G. Love to Leroy Craig, April 7, 1941. National Archives, RG 215.
22. Quoted in Memorandum from Edith Smith to Alma Haupt regarding drafting male nurses, July 10, 1942. National Archives, RG 215.
23. American Nurses' Association, Thirty-third Convention, Men Nurses' Section Reports, June 1, 1942, Chicago, Illinois. Unpublished manuscript, National Archives, RG 215.
24. Quoted in the *Congressional Record*, 1945, Appendix, p. 838.
25. Jacob Rose, "Men Nurses in Military Service," *American Journal of Nursing*, vol. 47 (March, 1947): 146.

18
Toward Professionalism

As America passed midcentury, fears of Communist infiltration, frustrations over the Korean conflict, and the conservative mood of voters provided the Republicans with a sweeping victory in the 1952 elections. Blessed with Republican control of both chambers of Congress, the new President, Dwight D. Eisenhower, recognized that much of the demand for change and reform that had created the social welfare programs and proposals of FDR's New Deal and Truman's Fair Deal had subsided. He did, however, establish the Department of Health, Education, and Welfare on April 11, 1953, an action that culminated more than 30 years' effort by citizens who believed that the federal government needed an agency of cabinet status to carry out effectively its constitutional responsibility for "promoting the general welfare." Only by such action could the health, education, and welfare interests of the American people receive their due consideration at the policymaking level.

Wonder Drugs

Before the 1940s few people had heard of antibiotics. In the 1950s, even with their short clinical history, these drugs had helped erase many infectious diseases from prominence. Mortality rates for tuberculosis, syphilis, whooping cough, and gastritis were at an all-time low, and the mortality rate for pneumonia was more than 40 percent below the average for the 1940s. Much of the credit for this belonged to antibiotics.

Although penicillin, in 1943, was the first to be given wide clinical use, antibiotics had been known long before then. Louis Pasteur, for example, had hinted that such substances might have medical value, and in 1928 English scientist Alexander Fleming discovered that a certain type of microorganism was somehow able to halt the growth of certain disease organisms. By 1939 hundreds of scientists, their scientific curiosity ignited by an apparent paradox, were concentrating on these drugs; they noted that, while disease organisms fell constantly upon the earth's soil, soil was often relatively free of disease bacteria.

The reason for this was found when researchers uncovered signs of a battle for survival being waged in the soil by millions of microorganisms, some of which employed a kind of chemical warfare, emitting a potent substance to kill or weaken neighboring organisms. Once these and other microscopic "battles" were understood, scientists turned their attention to the next logical question. Certain chemicals obviously destroyed certain microorganisms, including some that caused human disease. What would happen if one of these chemicals were given to a human being suffering from one of these diseases? Would the chemical still destroy, or help to destroy, the responsible agent? Would it also destroy the patient?

Answers to these questions were found in the amazing clinical record of antibiotics, or "wonder drugs," including penicillin, streptomycin, aureomycin, chloramphenicol, and terramycin, together with many others. Although no antibiotic proved entirely free of side effects or adverse reactions when given to people who were found to be abnormally sensitive to them, the relatively few patients so affected were outnumbered by countless millions of others whose health benefited or whose lives were saved. The use of antibiotics altered nursing-care requirements for some patients. Supportive nursing-care measures diminished in importance.

Antibiotics revolutionized the treatment of many diseases and saved millions of lives.

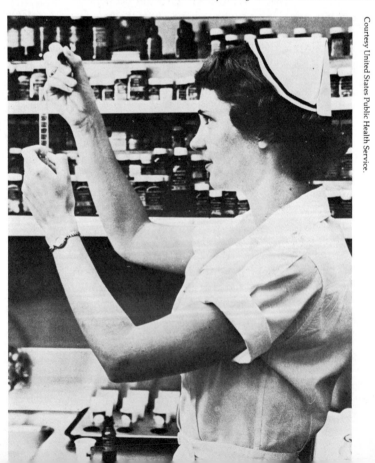

Hospitals in Transition

More than 6600 hospitals with over 1.5 million beds were listed in the census of the American Medical Association in 1952. In that year hospitals admitted nearly 19 million patients and cared for an average of 1.3 million inpatients each day. Approximately 1000 of these hospitals, with over half of all hospital beds and 60 percent of hospital patient-days, provided care exclusively for tuberculosis or psychiatric patients. Since the length of stay in mental and tuberculosis hospitals had to be measured in months or years, care in such institutions was beyond the financial resources of most people and had to be provided almost entirely through taxation. Ninety-six percent of the beds in these hospitals were supported by tax dollars.

Approximately 5600 hospitals provided general services or a special type of service usually associated with the general hospital. Although general hospitals and allied special hospitals contained fewer than half of all hospital beds and accounted for only 40 percent of patient-days, 98 percent of all hospital admissions were made by this group. In 1952, 55 percent of the general hospitals were owned and operated by churches, fraternal organizations, and other voluntary groups on a nonprofit basis, and 20 percent were proprietary hospitals operated by individuals or corporations on a profit basis. The remaining 25 percent were government hospitals: 16 percent municipal, 3 percent state, and 6 percent federal.

Typically, the patient entered the hospital confidently expecting that, during his stay, he would be cared for by professional nurses. Unless he was too sick to care, however, he was in for a shock: where was the familiar figure of the white uniform? He was bewildered by a succession of blue, gray, and striped uniforms. On any given day from 7:00 A.M. to 3:30 P.M. he would probably see a professional graduate nurse about six minutes. Moreover, he would see other professional personnel, including students, less than 15 minutes. During his entire stay he would average on the day shift 54 minutes of direct bedside care which would be divided as follows: six minutes from graduate nurses, 14 minutes from professional students, and 34 minutes from nonprofessional personnel.

In 1946 nursing students had made up 20.9 percent of the personnel in general hospitals; but by 1952 the percentage had dropped to about 12 percent nationwide. Relative to the number of patients served, the number of students of professional nursing had decreased markedly, from 40 per 100 patients per day in 1944 to 25 per 100 patients per day in 1952, a drop of nearly 38 percent. Although the total number of nursing students had increased slightly in the latter years of that period, it had not been able to match the increase in the number of patients. In addition, the amount of service provided by each student was decreasing. As a result of new standards in nursing education, nursing students were spending a higher proportion of their time in the classroom and laboratory and a lower proportion at the bedside. The growing emphasis on upgrading the educational experience was indicated by the fact that the number of full-time instructors had increased despite the decline in the number of students. In

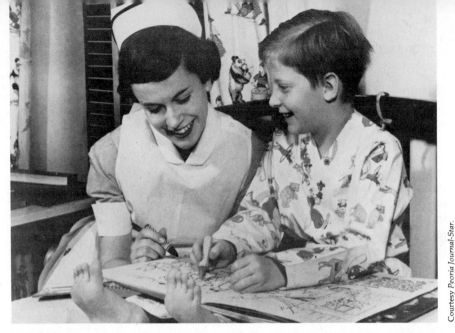

The presence of a student nurse at the bedside was no longer to be taken for granted.

1944 there were 37 students per instructor; in 1952 there were only 19.

Nearly 390,000 nurses were working in the United States in 1952. The number of hospital nurses, the largest single group, had increased by 15 percent in the previous four years to a total of 231,000. Private duty nurses, the next largest group, who were also at the bedside, numbered 74,000. Some 35,000 nurses working in physicians' offices, 25,300 public health nurses, 14,000 industrial nurses, and 8200 nurse educators in schools of nursing made up the remainder of the total, along with 1900 nurses in a variety of other fields.

The volume of nursing required for modern medical and health service and the expanding range of activities had introduced a large number of auxiliary workers who came to be classified as nursing personnel. In 1946 hospitals throughout the country employed 177,552 auxiliary workers, including maids. In early 1952 they employed 297,310. This, of course, had resulted in a changing pattern of nursing service. In New York hospitals, for example, registered nurses performed 75 percent of the nursing care in the early 1940s, but 10 years later they carried out 30 percent of the nursing care. The same thing was happening all over.

Hospital Staffing Patterns

An analysis of hospital staffing patterns indicated that in the typical 100-bed general hospital over half of all hospital personnel were in the nursing department. The dietary and housekeeping departments each accounted for slightly more than 10 percent of the personnel. Between 7 and 8 percent of the personnel were required for administration, business office, record-keeping, and related functions; 6 percent for laundry; 3 percent for plant operation and maintenance; 6 percent for the laboratory, x-ray, and other professional service departments.

From the point of view of maximal utilization, the personnel of the nursing department were considered by administration to be the most important, not only because they predominated numerically but because they served to coordinate the activities of personnel in other departments providing care directly to the patient. In many hospitals the nursing staff assumed responsibility for various activities customarily associated with the attending physicians, the "house" medical staff, housekeeping, dietary, laboratory, business office, and other departments. Increasingly, there was a tendency to shift responsibilities either to or from the nursing department, depending upon both the relative shortages of different types of personnel and the prevailing theories of organization of hospital service.

A 46 percent increase in the total number of paid nursing personnel per 100 patients per day among all nonfederal general hospitals from 1944 to 1952 was accompanied by significant shifts in the relative proportion of administrative and supervisory personnel, general duty nurses, and auxiliary nursing personnel—although each of these classifications had contributed to the increase. In 1944 there had been approximately one general duty nurse and three auxiliary nursing workers for each supervising nurse. By 1952 there were approximately two general duty nurses and four auxiliary workers for each supervisory nurse.

The average nurse spent more and more time managing personnel and administrative details. Some nurses and employers of nurses were convinced that the professional nurse of the future would have largely supervisory and managerial responsibilities and would direct patient care delegated to other, less extensively prepared members of the nursing team. This view was reflected in the task-oriented philosophies of some schools, while others sought to prepare the nurse for more patient-centered activity. Delegation was often praised as a management essential. The primary responsibility of the registered nurse had changed from direct nursing care and maintenance of the environment to administration of complex systems, supervision of workers with diversified skills, and provision of comprehensive nursing services.

Throughout the field of nursing the word "utilization" was being used more and more as hospitals conducted studies, aided by engineers in some cases, to find out how many functions of the nurse could be performed safely by others. The number was surprisingly large. In a Division of Nursing Resources, United States Public Health Service–assisted study at Harper Hospital in Detroit, for example, it was found that 42 percent of all treatments could be handled by practical nurses and 30 percent by nurses' aides. A New York State official estimated that from 30 to 50 percent of the nurse's time was spent in nonnursing functions. Hospitals everywhere, however, were reassigning nonnursing activities to nonnurses as a matter of necessity, not of theory.

A major effort was made to encourage more efficient use of professional nursing skills. The Division of Nursing Resources made hospital studies and

developed techniques to determine whether professional nurses were performing clerical, housekeeping, or other routine duties that could be assigned to
others. These findings were used as a basis for several handbooks to facilitate
written analyses of hospital nursing duties.

A manual, *How to Study Nursing Activities in a Patient Unit*, was developed
by the Division of Nursing Resources to help hospitals determine whether
nursing time was diverted from nursing care of patients to duties that other
employees could perform. The method, which adapted industrial work sampling techniques to the problems of utilization of hospital personnel, had been
tested in three hospitals. Results showed that staff nurses were actually spending about half of their time caring for patients, the remaining time being spent
on tasks that could be assigned to clerks, maids, and messengers.

Educational Deficiencies

According to 1954 estimates, about 20 percent of the positions held by registered
nurses entailed responsibilities that could be best fulfilled by persons who were
prepared in master's degree programs; for another 30 percent of these positions,

*The three leaders of nursing in the United States Public Health Service during the 1950s,
Pearl McIver, Lucile Petry, and Margaret Arnstein were recipients of the Lasker Award
in November, 1955.*

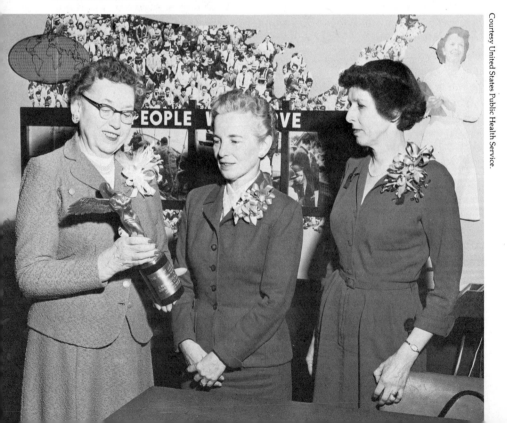

preparation at the baccalaureate level would be adequate. Against this estimate stood the actual situation, in which approximately 1 percent of all nurses held master's degrees and 7.2 percent held baccalaureate degrees—not all of which had been conferred in the field of nursing.

According to data on graduate nurse education in colleges and universities collected by the National League for Nursing, the enrollment in graduate nurse programs had remained about the same from 1947 to 1955. Although there was an increase in the number of students enrolled in advanced nursing programs between 1951 and 1953, there was a sharp decrease—from 1125 to 814—in the number who were graduated from baccalaureate programs preparing nurses for the specialty positions of administrator, supervisor, teacher, and consultant. At the same time, the number of nurses who had earned their master's degree in the specialty programs was no higher in 1953 than it had been in 1952. This meant that there were proportionately fewer nurses completing post-diploma training each year.

Private philanthropy answered this challenge first. Early in 1955 an NLN fellowship program for nurses working on master's and doctoral degrees was made possible through a grant from the Commonwealth Fund. The Fund supported this program in order to help overcome a critical shortage of nurses prepared for administration in nursing service and education, teaching, and nursing research. The grant provided opportunities for over 200 nurses to undertake master's or doctoral study during the years 1955–1963.

Federal support of psychiatric nursing education from 1947 to 1955 amounted to a total of about $5 million. During the fall of 1955, the 191 full-time students who held these scholarships accounted for the comparatively high ratio of full-time to part-time students enrolled in psychiatric nursing programs. From 1936 through 1955, 14,000 to 15,000 nurses received government assistance for academic study in public health nursing under provisions of the Social Security Act of 1935. Although these grants had diminished in number in recent years, this aid allowed nurses to complete programs leading to a baccalaureate degree; as a consequence, the percentage of public health nurses with baccalaureate or postbaccalaureate preparation was about three times greater than that of the general nursing population. In contrast was the small proportion of full-time students enrolled in programs in medical-surgical and maternal-child nursing. A larger program was desperately needed and only the federal government had the sizable resources required to implement it.

The Federal Nurse Traineeship Program

In 1956 the first appreciable step since World War II toward a major program of renewed federal aid to nurses was effected. The Health Amendments Act of 1956 was passed by Congress and signed by President Eisenhower on August 1, 1956. Title II authorized funds for financial aid to registered nurses for full-time study to prepare for administration, supervision, and teaching in all fields of nursing. The use of the funds was limited to tuition and fees, stipends, and allowances (including travel expenses for trainees). The law prohibited the federal government or any employee from exercising any direction, supervision, or control over the personnel or curriculum of the recipient training institutions. From 1957 to 1964 appropriations grew from $2 million to $7.3 million. A short-term program was initiated in 1960 whereby professional nurses, unable to study full-time but in need of additional skills to maintain their positions, could be financially supported in the necessary course work for periods of five days to one month.

During the first six months of the program, long-term traineeships were awarded to over 9000 nurses, and nearly half were 30 years of age or younger. Slightly more than 60 percent studied at the graduate level, some of these nurses earning a doctoral degree. Of the total, 55 percent were preparing for positions in teaching, 24 percent for supervision, and 21 percent for administration. Although data for earlier years are not available, of the 1447 graduate-level trainees in 1960–1961, 835 completed their programs of study during their traineeships.

Follow-up on the accomplishments of former trainees was conducted routinely through questionnaires sent six months after completion of the program. Replies from nurses who received traineeships during the period from 1957 through 1961 showed that 39 percent were teachers, 31 percent were in nursing service positions as head nurses or administrators, and 7 percent were continuing in school. In the 1960 and 1961 follow-ups, trainees were asked to provide additional information regarding any change in their level of responsibility following traineeship study. Fifty-six percent said that they were holding positions at a higher level. It was the general agreement of nursing leaders, however, that, even with this new influx of prepared nurses, the demand far exceeded the supply.

The short-term training provisions associated with the Title II program were begun in 1960 with $300,000, an amount that quickly tripled in the following two years. During the first three years of the short-term program, over 10,000 nurses had benefited from the courses, 500 of whom had had their training financed by sources other than the federal government. A total of 307 courses were supported through grants to 73 sponsoring agencies. Of these, 55 were colleges and universities, 10 were state leagues for nursing, four were hospitals, three were state departments of health, and one was a regional education commission. Since the number of approved applications for grants had exceeded available funds, it had been necessary to make awards on the basis of priority ratings set by a review committee. The large majority of short-term trainees had been supervisors and head nurses in hospitals. Data regarding the educational qualifications of the 10,184 federally aided trainees revealed that 65 percent had no degree, 26 percent had baccalaureate degrees, and 9 percent had master's degrees.

The program directors of short-term courses were required to submit an evaluation report at the close of each course. Some of the sponsoring agencies had studied the results of these courses as perceived by their students. There

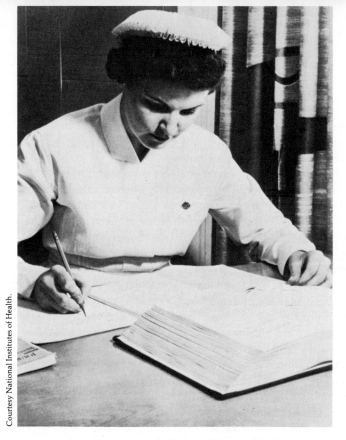

Short- and long-term United States Public Health Service traineeships supported additional study for thousands of nurses.

was evidence that the major value of the courses had been in the initiation of new ideas for the improvement of patient care, and subsequent employers reported that former trainees effected changes in work situations that resulted in improved nursing practice. Instances were also reported of nurses who, after having participated in a short-term course in a university setting, had gone on to enroll for full-time academic study. All but 12 states had at least one school offering traineeships under this program to registered nurses, and many schools had used training funds to support students on two or more academic levels.

Birth of Associate Degree Nursing

A project aimed at developing nursing education programs in junior and community colleges was announced in January, 1952, by Louise McManus, Director of the Division of Nursing Education at Teachers College, Columbia University. She explained that the purpose of the experiment was to determine if a two-year program, which would prepare bedside nurses for beginning, general duty positions, was feasible. Such an approach would help reduce the critical shortage of nurses throughout the nation by producing more nurses faster; it would also help move nursing education into the overall system of American higher education.

Commenting on the need for the project, Dr. McManus asserted that nursing education was largely outside the general system of education in the United States and, unlike education for other professions, had not had the benefit of research. She declared that the present system of nursing education had failed to produce the required number and types of nurses.

Ninety percent of the nation's nursing schools were owned and operated by hospitals, Dr. McManus pointed out. Their programs were mainly of the apprentice type, directed primarily at the immediate care of patients, without regard for the community and academic experiences the modern nurse should receive. She emphasized that the demands of the hospitals, as far as nurse education was concerned, required a three-year program which included repetitive practices believed to be considerably in excess of that needed for economical and effective learning. Mildred L. Montag, assistant professor of nursing education at Teachers College, was appointed project coordinator.

Seven community junior colleges were selected for inclusion in the five-year research project to develop and evaluate associate degree nursing education. The colleges represented different sections of the country, were of various sizes, had different sources of support, and different curriculum patterns. As these programs were established, general education accounted for one-third of the total curriculum while nursing courses accounted for about two-thirds. Of the nursing portion, 75 percent was clinical practice. Emphasis was placed on giving the student as much experience as possible through careful planning and instructional supervision yielding more effective use of time spent in the clinical area.

Students would qualify for the associate degree and would be eligible for the licensing exam of the state in which the college was located. Eight hundred and seven students were admitted to the programs. The dropout rate ran about 20 percent, with reasons resembling the pattern of college education rather than that of hospital schools.

In 1958 the results of the five-year study indicated that the two-year curriculum could prepare a registered nurse and that the program could become an integral part of a total college, financed as any other college program. One hundred and ninety-two associate degree graduates had taken state board licensing examinations by then, and 91.7 of these passed the examinations the first time. In nursing programs of all types, the figure was 90.5 percent. According to the study findings associate degree graduates were found by head nurses to be as good as or better than most of the graduates with whom they worked in 80 percent of the cases. The graduates themselves were satisfied with their preparation.

Diploma program advocates insisted that graduates of hospital schools of nursing were more competent in patient care than were those coming from collegiate schools. Hospital school diploma programs provided learning experiences that were more functionally and realistically related to the competencies, skills, and knowledge involved in patient care. Representatives of this group pointed out that the number of hospital schools had dropped from 1190 to 768 in the previous eight years. College and university graduates would not be sufficient to staff the hospitals of tomorrow. Some felt that the answer lay in setting up nurses' colleges, similar to teachers' colleges, built out of hospital schools of nursing. They would be licensed to grant the degree of bachelor of nursing. The entire curriculum would be tailored to the needs of the nurse as a bedside practitioner, with academic courses integrated into functional units of instruction related to the problems of patient care.

These hospital nurses' colleges would not offer graduate courses leading to master's or doctoral degrees. University schools of nursing would expand their graduate nursing education to provide programs for nursing instructors, researchers, public health workers, college professors, and organizational leaders. Such courses would be more meaningful if undertaken after the nurse had some experience and had shown interest and ability in a specialized area.

The diploma program in the hospital school of nursing had always been, and still was, the backbone of nursing education in the United States, but changes had to be made if this form of nursing education was to survive. Ruth Sleeper of Massachusetts General Hospital was convinced of the value of the diploma program but warned that those responsible for the three-year nursing schools must make many changes if the diploma programs were to hold respected places in the country's educational system. Unless changes were made, she said, "the hospital school will not continue to attract desirable candidates in sufficient numbers and a new system of preparing our nurses will be found."

Biomedical Research Booms

Public responsibility for biomedical research was assumed on a larger scale in the 1940s. It was now accepted public policy to use tax funds for supporting research in voluntary as well as public institutions, and many laws embodying these principles had been passed. General authority for research grants and fellowships in the entire health field had been given to the Public Health Service of the Federal Security Agency through the Public Health Service Act of 1944 and its amendments. Federal acts dealing with cancer (1937), mental diseases (1946), dental diseases (1948), heart diseases (1948), and hospital construction (1949) contained provisions for research.

In 1947 governmental agencies contributed about 28 percent of all funds expended on medical research, the federal government carrying by far the largest share; industrial companies were responsible for 45 percent, foundations for 13 percent, and other sources for the remainder. Leading among the civilian federal agencies was the Public Health Service, using the National Institutes of Health as its research arm, and administering research grants and fellowships to individuals affiliated with voluntary institutions.

The purpose of the Public Health Service Research Grants Program was to support research in medical and allied fields for which funds were inadequate or which could not otherwise be conducted in the grantee institution. The major objectives of the grants program were: (1) to expand research activities in universities and other institutions; (2) to stimulate the initiation of research in small colleges where previous research programs had been very limited or nonexistent; (3) to encourage investigators to undertake research in neglected areas; and (4) to provide training for scientific personnel. The vast volume of requests for research grants soon required the establishment of a priority system for determining funding awards. This priority system was established in order to permit all new applicants to compete for funds on an equal basis and to insure quicker response to an action on the applicant's request.

Medical research in the 1950s was necessarily concentrated more on man's bodily responses to his environment. To cope with the problems of chronic disease and other causes of death and disability, science needed to provide medicine and public health with innumerable facts about the growth, aging, and regeneration of living tissues. Research probed into such mysteries as the metabolism of cells and the molecular structure of body chemicals. The problems studied required scientists trained in many different fields, working in close association with scientists in other institutions, and utilizing a great variety of specialized equipment.

Nursing Research

Research into the practice of nursing was seen as more and more essential if the health needs of modern society were to be met. Increasingly, extension of health services and developments in medicine without adequate corresponding developments in nursing practice had resulted in a dilution in the quality of nursing. Opportunities for professional nurses to use their special knowledge and skill in generating new knowledge for the profession had not kept pace with the prevention of illness or with the health needs of society. Nursing research was concerned with the systematic study and assessment of nursing problems or phenomena and was aimed at finding ways of improving nursing practice and patient care through creative inquiry. It included studies of nursing practice, nursing services, nursing service administration, nursing education, the individual nurse, and involved every field of knowledge related to nursing.

In the early 1950s the scholarly journal *Nursing Research* had been launched, and the first issue went out to approximately 8500 subscribers all across the nation and in 22 other countries. This journal quickly emerged as the leading indicator of nursing's thrust into research and development and became essential reading for the expanding cadre of nurse-researchers.

A research program approved by the ANA House of Delegates in 1950 was designed to enable nurses, with the help of allied groups and social scientists, to study nursing functions in various settings and geographic locations and nurses' relationships with co-workers and associates. The American Nurses' Association depended entirely on membership dues for the financing of this series of studies. By 1954 grants for research had been made to institutions or organizations in 13 states, and nursing had been studied in more than 80 hospitals.

This scholarly look at the profession included surveys, interviews, attitude-role relationship studies, observation or "shadow" studies of nurses on the job, classification of activities, and time analyses revealing proportions of time spent by various personnel on different activities. In the first years of the ANA program most of the research was done by social scientists of various disciplines; later, many nurses had gained the qualifications to carry out studies as well. Under this program researchers learned that nurses performed over 400 functions. Other findings pointed out the extent to which functions carried out by the different categories of nursing personnel overlapped. Changes in the role of the professional nurse were confirmed by findings that indicated that many of the tasks once considered the sole province of the physician were now being assigned to nurses. The number of these tasks was found to vary from state to state, with some direction from the state laws governing the practice of nursing and medicine.

In 1955 the American Nurses' Association formed a membership corporation, the American Nurses' Foundation, organized exclusively for charitable, scientific, and educational purposes. The Foundation solicited tax-deductible grants and gifts from the general public and from other charitable organizations. The primary objectives of the Foundation were to increase public knowledge and understanding of professional nursing, practical nursing, and the arts and sciences upon which the health of the American people depended. The Foundation was to conduct studies, surveys, and research; provide research grants to graduate nurses; make grants to public and private nonprofit educational institutions; and publish scientific, educational, and literary work. The ANA board of directors donated $100,000 to the new corporation, to be disbursed during 1955 for studies of nursing functions.

The extramural grants program in nursing research of the United States Public Health Service Division of Nursing Resources originated in fiscal year 1956. In contrast to most of the extramural programs of the National Institutes of Health, which were focused on basic disease research, the Division of Nursing Resources program emphasized applied research. During the fiscal year ending June 30, 1956, the Public Health Service awarded nearly $500,000 to qualified researchers for projects in nursing. This was the first time that a specific grants program for nursing research had been made available from federal sources. Over the next two decades this program helped to nurture the embryonic growth of nursing research with support for individual research projects, faculty research development projects, and nine special national nursing research conferences held under the auspices of the ANA.

Federal support for research training for nurses was provided in two ways. In 1956 a program of special predoctoral fellowships was established by the Division of Nursing Resources. This program made individual awards to qualified nurses for training for individual research and collaborative interdisciplinary research and for the stimulation and guidance of research. In 1962 nurse-scientist graduate training grants were initiated to assist the institutions developing nursing research competence as well as to provide stipends for the graduate

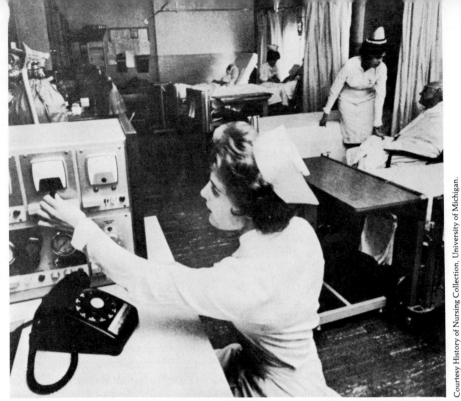

Although aided by electronic equipment, the heart of patient care was the quality of the nurse.

nursing students who were preparing for research. These grants were made to graduate schools of nursing and provided support for full-time students of nursing and anthropology, psychology, sociology, anatomy, physiology, and microbiology.

The first doctoral programs in nursing had originated within the schools of education at Teachers College, Columbia University, in the early 1920s and at New York University in 1934. The growth of the concept was extremely slow: it was 1954 before the University of Pittsburgh added a small maternal-child nursing Ph.D. program and 1960 before Boston University began a Doctor of Nursing Science (D.N.S.) program in psychiatric nursing. The first comprehensive doctoral-level movement came in 1964 at the University of California, San Francisco, with the establishment of D.N.S. degree in several nursing specialties.

Characteristics of the Health Services Industry in 1960

As a new decade got under way, the 1960 census provided data for an overall look at how nursing fit into the nation's health care picture. The United States Bureau of the Census divided the civilian labor force into 71 separate industries. Between the 1950 and 1960 censuses, the health services industry had gained almost one million workers, for a growth rate of 54 percent. Only seven of the

71 other industries had experienced a higher growth rate. The health services industry ranked third among these industries, employing over 2.5 million persons.

From 1927 to 1945, hospital costs per patient-day had increased 25 percent. The annual increase in patient-day costs over this period averaged 10 cents a day. By sharp comparison, from 1945 to 1960, hospital costs per patient-day had increased by more than 250 percent, and the annual increase in patient-day costs over this period averaged about $1.65 per day. Through health insurance and through greater use of local, state, and national tax funds, more and more hospital money was coming from healthy people. Healthy people did not pay for hospital care piecemeal as it was delivered to them; they paid for it, in whole or in part, through health insurance plans. By 1960 nongovernmental general hospitals received, on the average, nearly half their total income from insured patients. In many such hospitals, the proportion from insurance was two-thirds or more and growing fast.

Growth and diversification were the principal characteristics of the health occupations. In 1940 hospitals had had approximately one professional nurse for every 15 beds and one practical nurse, aide, attendant, or auxiliary for every ten beds. By 1960 they required one professional nurse for every five beds and one auxiliary person for every three beds. In addition to nursing personnel, hospitals had been increasing the number of personnel in other health occupations categories, at a rate exceeding the numerical growth rates of hospital beds and total annual admissions to short-term general hospitals. The direction of people with new levels of skills and abilities called for strong leadership.

A study of some 325 hospitals in 1961 showed that about 20 percent of the positions for professional nurses were vacant, as were 18 percent of the positions for practical nurses. In New York City over half of the positions for professional nurses in the public hospitals were unfilled. In all hospitals in Los Angeles, private as well as public, 25 to 30 percent of the positions for professional staff nurses were reported as unfilled. In a survey of all general hospitals in the state of Massachusetts, it was found that 20 percent of the positions for professional staff nurses were not filled. Because the need for professional and practical nurses was increasing so much faster than the supply, hospitals had employed ever-larger numbers of nursing aides, many of whom were inadequately trained. This pragmatic solution to the problem of shortages had produced an alarming dilution in the quality of service. In some hospitals the use of auxiliary workers had reached such extreme proportions that nursing aides gave as much as 80 percent of the direct nursing care.

How was the United States to secure the needed nurse supply when wages were so inordinately low? In 1959, of all professional women who worked from 40 to 49 weeks during the year, nurses had the lowest median income. For secondary school teachers, the median was $5200; for elementary school teachers, it was $4900; for librarians, $4200; for social, welfare, and recreation workers, $3700; and for professional nurses, $3200.

A number of other factors also militated against the probability of a larger proportion of women and men choosing nursing as a career. Relative to most of the other predominantly women's professions, particularly teaching, the working conditions and hours in nursing were unfavorable. Teachers worked fewer weeks of the year and had more hours in which to fulfill home and family responsibilities. What is more, the proportion of female high school graduates who later completed a nursing education was generally declining. From 1957 to 1960, 4 percent of the female high school graduates from three years previous had completed a program in professional nursing. In 1963 this had dropped to 3.35 percent.

Even hospital administrators, nursing directors, and members of hospital boards of trustees who believed that graduate nurses should be more realistically remunerated for their services had problems in finding the money. The cost of nursing care was the hospital's largest single expense and an important factor in determining room and board rates. Medical care was expensive, and its cost was rising at a rate greater than that of the cost of living.

As operating cost increased, hospitals had to pass most of it to consumers in the form of higher daily service charges. The hospital daily service charge was the fee for routine nursing care, room and board, and minor medical and surgical supplies and usually excluded the costs of laboratory work, x-rays, operating rooms, and special nursing services, which were additional charges made on the hospital bill. From 1946 to 1961, hospital daily service charges had risen 228 percent, over four times as much as the Consumer Price Index for all items.

Despite acute shortages of nurses, hospitals did their best to provide quality care.

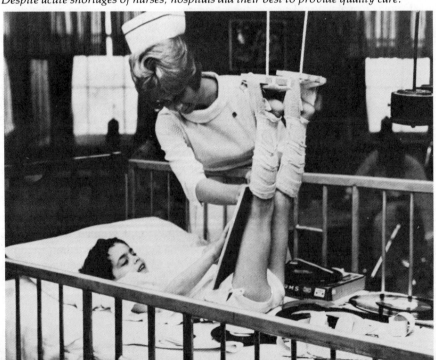

Several developments had contributed to the rapid rise in hospital costs. Improved medical technology, including new and expensive drugs and equipment, and new medical techniques such as open heart surgery, had caused the cost of hospital care to escalate. The most important factor, however, was the increased payroll expense, which accounted for 62 percent of the total expense of hospital operations in 1961. The payroll expense in short-term hospitals had increased by 521 percent between 1946 and 1961.

During 1961 an estimated 74,000 new students were admitted to schools of professional and practical nursing, compared to 71,297 in 1960. The 1126 professional nursing programs offered in hospitals, colleges, universities, and junior colleges admitted 49,487 new students in 1961, an increase of only 3000 since 1953. Among professional nursing schools, diploma programs in hospitals continued, as in the past, to enroll the largest number of new students, but their enrollment of 38,702, or about 78 percent of the total, marked the first time in history that diploma schools in the United States had admitted fewer than 80 percent of all professional nursing students. Both baccalaureate and associate degree programs showed a rise over previous years. Colleges and universities admitted 8700 nursing students (18 percent) to study for bachelor's degrees in nursing. Associate degree programs, usually in junior and community colleges, admitted the remaining 2085 new students (4 percent).

Financial Deficits of Diploma Schools

In the diploma schools the prevailing pattern of financing had changed very little over the previous half-century. There had been a few modifications here and there and moderately increased charges, but the pattern remained the same: apprentice-type financing, which hospitals had formerly exchanged for apprentice-type training. The real difficulty was that the cheap-labor component of the traditional hospital system had virtually disappeared. Higher standards had pushed almost all diploma programs far into the red. The outdated idea, still almost universally applied to fiscal practice, was that the student should pay for her education through service to patients. This conviction was strongly ingrained in the thinking patterns of most people and was not easily altered.

By 1960 few hospital administrators would deny that the operation of a modern school of nursing was an expensive proposition. Significantly, the official reports of some 30 hospitals operating schools of nursing in Ohio showed an average net cost per student of $963.21 in 1955. Another hospital had operated its school that same year at a net cost of $1517 per student. Yet another hospital school, with an excellent record of scholastic achievement and a high reputation among nurse educators, had 162 students enrolled and spent $304,000 more than it had received in tuition, fees, value of student service, and other credits.

Only highly reactionary policies by hospital administrators could halt such deficits. In 1960 Dr. Thomas Hales, administrator at Albany Hospital, Albany, New York, was able to boast that he still operated his school of nursing on the philosophy of a balanced budget. In order for hospitals to plan for this type of school operation, however, he insisted that it was necessary for the school and the hospital to agree to a list of basic principles:

Hospital and school must agree that their objective is to turn out a competent bedside nurse.

Hospital and school must believe in the "apprenticeship" philosophy of nurse education—that the student "learns by doing," and that she cannot learn nursing skills by spending most of her time in the classroom and laboratory.

They must agree that "repetitive practice" is valuable in the training of a student nurse, because every patient presents a different challenge.

They must be willing to cut to the minimum the assignment of students that take them away from the service areas where patient care is provided.

Vacation, holiday, and sick leave policies must be kept on a realistic basis. They cannot follow college campus patterns without bankrupting the school.

A work week of no less than 40 hours (preferably 44 hours) of combined classroom and ward experience is essential for the sound financial operation of the school.

A reasonable and fair evaluation of student services must be developed.

Strict accounting must be kept of the student's time on the wards when she is rendering the services to patients that justify the hospital in compensating for these services [1].

Hospital administrators were now anxious for federal dollars. One noted that federal subsidization was no longer as radical an idea as it had been in the United States over the past 200 years. Nursing was perhaps the only profession for which the government had not taken responsibility for education. There were state universities for the preparation of teachers, lawyers, veterinarians, engineers, pharmacists, physicians, and others, but only a few for the education of nurses. A program of federal grants to hospitals sponsoring diploma schools (with additional state matching funds) was proposed in Congress but met with little support.

Variables in Nursing Education

The improved quality of diploma programs at the end of the 1950s was well documented. The National League for Nursing's *Report on Hospital Schools of Nursing, 1957* was designed "to help hospital schools of nursing determine where they stood in relation to their goals and, on the basis of this stock-taking, to plan the emphasis and direction of their continuing efforts to improve their programs" [2]. Comparative data pointed out that about one-half of all hospital schools had, at the time of the study, demonstrated that they had met the NLN-accrediting criteria. A follow-up study, *Today's Diploma Schools of Nursing*, published in 1963, reported that "the majority of the diploma schools of nursing were full-fledged educational institutions, competent to identify their own problems and to determine for themselves the ways by which they

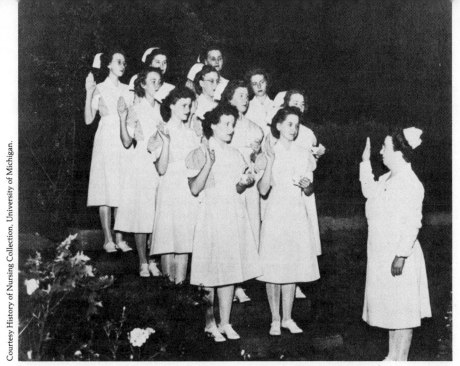

By the early 1960s operating a hospital school of nursing along highly authoritarian lines, such as those of 20 years earlier, was becoming increasingly difficult.

can best meet current criteria for educational excellence" [3].

One of the main obstacles to growth of baccalaureate nursing education during the 1950s could be attributed to the character of many of the so-called baccalaureate programs. In many instances these were really standard diploma programs that were offered in a collegiate setting, with a few science and general education courses added to the curriculum. The difference between baccalaureate preparation and diploma preparation was often too obscure to be recognized by the employers of the graduates, and the main difference noted by prospective students was probably financial. Thus, baccalaureate education for nursing was, in too many instances, of unknown quality.

Nurses for a Growing Nation, published by the National League for Nursing in 1957, projected nursing personnel and education needs to 1970 and pointed conclusively to the need for increasing the number of baccalaureate degree graduates and expanding facilities to meet this need. Viewing these programs as providing the foundational knowledge and skills for graduate study (and as the shortest and most economical preparation for teaching, administration, supervision, and clinical specialization), the report estimated that one-third of all nursing graduates should be from baccalaureate programs. Yet, in 1962, only 14 percent of nursing's basic students were being graduated from these programs.

During the six-year period 1956–1962 the number of baccalaureate nursing programs increased from 161 to 178, and the average enrollment in these programs increased from 116 to 132. On the surface this increase would appear to have been most encouraging, since it came at a time when more students, men and women, were entering college than ever before. Despite the increase in number and size of baccalaureate programs, however, there had not been a sufficient increase in the number of graduates from master's programs who were preparing for college teaching.

In the fall of 1962 enrollments in master's programs in nursing (of both full-time and part-time students) totaled 2472, while graduations from these programs totaled 1098 for the academic year 1961–1962. The dearth of candidates qualified for college teaching was reflected in statistics reported in 1962: only 4 percent of the nursing faculty members teaching in baccalaureate and higher degree programs held doctoral degrees, 76 percent held master's degrees, and 20 percent held baccalaureate degrees. Master's level preparation was acknowledged as the minimal base for quality instruction.

In addition to the 192 baccalaureate and higher degree programs seeking to attract master's graduates in 1962, there were 874 diploma and 84 associate degree programs that were also bidding for the potential candidates. In the same year the budgeted vacancies in these three types of programs totaled 1202. Added to the needs of the schools were the demands for administrative and supervisory personnel of some 6000 hospitals and 7800 health agencies and boards of education. It could readily be seen that the nursing administrator had to compete for a very scarce supply of well-qualified faculty.

Some of the responsibilities to be undertaken by any college or university that would offer a program in nursing education were identified by Margaret Bridgman in her study, *Collegiate Education for Nursing*:

Recognition of nursing as a subject comparable to others that are established as college majors and realization that it must be developed in the same way to justify a degree and give students the benefits they have a right to expect from college education for their chosen profession.

Recognition of the need to produce graduates really competent for the functions for which college-educated nurses are so urgently needed.

Establishment of an educational unit in nursing in the institution on a completely equal basis with other units of the institution, with a faculty adequate in number and well qualified in the various special types of nursing to teach all the courses in nursing, including faculty-guided clinical practice. A minimum number of faculty members is six, with specialists, respectively, in medical, surgical, obstetric, pediatric, psychiatric, and public health nursing.

Provision for the necessary facilities for education: classrooms, faculty offices, and library.

Provision of housing and all other student personnel services required for college students.

Provision of available and accessible hospital and other agency facilities for the practice of nursing, since it is here that faculty help students to develop professional skills and to use pertinent knowledge from all preceding academic and professional sources [4].

In other words, the university had to accept the same responsibility for this type of education as for any other in which it undertook to provide the kind, level, and quality of preparation that was characteristic of the institution and represented by its degree.

The Surgeon General's Consultant Group on Nursing

Assuming office in January, 1961, President John F. Kennedy declared in his televised inaugural that "the torch has been passed to a new generation of Americans—born in this century . . . and unwilling to witness or permit the slow undoing of those human rights to which this Nation has always been committed" [5]. Nurses, physicians, and hospital administrators waited, complacently, on the whole, to see how the new generation would handle federal aid to nursing.

Postwar federal legislation to assist basic nursing education had long been backed by many hospital, nursing, and public health officials. It was not until 1961, however, that the Surgeon General of the United States Public Health Service appointed the special Consultative Group on Nursing to advise him on nursing needs and to identify the appropriate role of the federal government in assuring adequate nursing services for the country [6]. Among the representatives were Lulu Wolf Hassenplug, dean of the UCLA School of Nursing; Marian Sheahan, NLN deputy director; Dr. James T. Howell, assistant director, Henry Ford Hospital, Detroit; William K. Turner, director, Newport Hospital, Newport, Rhode Island; Dr. William Willard, vice-president, University of Kentucky Medical Center; and Dr. Eleanor Lambertsen, director, Division of Nursing Education, Teachers College, Columbia University.

In his foreword to the group's report, *Toward Quality in Nursing*, chairman Alvin C. Eurich wrote: "In the opinion of the group, the nation faces a critical problem in ensuring adequate nursing services in the years ahead. The need for more nurses is urgent . . . . Lack of adequate financial resources is a basic problem . . . . In the judgment of the consultant group, if the nursing problem is to be solved, there is no alternative to federal aid."

The crux of the problem was contained in another paragraph of the foreword: "Today nursing education is at a crossroad. We need a careful examination of the existing types of nursing education programs, to determine how they can be merged into a pattern that will adequately prepare the nurse to render better patient care and allow her to advance professionally in an orderly manner." The passage went on to declare that "pending the outcomes of such an orderly study, we need immediate action to expand and improve nursing service within the evolving framework of education and patient care." Any timid, piecemeal approach to the nursing problem, warned Dr. Eurich, was "doomed to failure" [7].

As a basis for federal action, the major problems facing the nursing profession, according to the report, were identified as follows: (1) too few schools were providing adequate education for nursing; (2) not enough capable young people were being recruited to meet the demand; (3) too few college-bound young people were entering the nursing field; (4) more nursing schools were

Toward
Quality in Nursing
Needs and Goals

Report of the Surgeon Generals'
Consultant Group on Nursing

Public Health Service　　　　　　　　February 1963

U.S. DEPARTMENT OF HEALTH, EDUCATION, AND WELFARE

The Report of the Surgeon General's Consultant Group on Nursing established the framework for subsequent legislation.

needed within colleges and universities; (5) the continuing lag in the social and economic status of nurses discouraged people from entering the field and remaining active in it; (6) available nursing personnel were not being fully utilized for effective patient care, including supervision and teaching as well as clinical care; and (7) too little research was being conducted on the advancement of nursing practice.

The group reported that "the nursing education system faces a grave challenge" and that "the present educational structure for the training of nurses lacks system, order, and coherence." The group stated its conviction that the baccalaureate program should be but minimum preparation for nurses who were to carry out leadership responsibilities. "To create order out of the present confusion," the group advised, "a careful examination of the systems of nursing education [and a determination of] how these systems can be merged or related in a pattern that will adequately prepare the nurses of the nation to render better patient care" should be made [8].

As a goal for the decade ahead the consultants called for an estimated 680,000 professional nurses to be made available for practice by 1970—130,000 more than were then active. To reach the 1970 target, the consultants estimated that, by 1969, the basic professional nursing schools should graduate 53,000 nurses annually, a 75 percent increase over the number of 1961 graduates. The estimates of the increased number of graduates needed, by type of basic nursing school, were: basic baccalaureate degree programs, 8000 (4039 in 1961); diploma programs, 40,000 (25,311 in 1961); and associate degree programs, 5000 (917 in 1961).

Also needed, the consultants suggested, would be 3000 nurses with master's or higher degrees—a 194 percent increase over the comparable group in 1961—and 5000 post-RN baccalaureate graduates—an approximate 100 percent increase over comparable 1961 totals. The needs for LPNs were estimated at 350,000 by 1970, an increase of more than 50 percent over the current level. More than 6 percent of the nation's female high school graduates would have to be recruited into nursing, according to the consultant group, or an annual increase of at least 7000 over the existing recruitment rate.

To stimulate recruitment the consultant group recommended that the Public Health Service expand financial and other aid to state, regional, and national agencies concerned with nursing recruitment. It also suggested that low-cost loans and scholarships, supported by federal funds, be provided by both professional and practical nursing schools. To improve educational programs, the group recommended that federal funds be provided to construct additional nursing school facilities and to expand educational programs and services. It also suggested that the Public Health Service and the nursing profession develop prototypes of educational facilities most conducive to the effective teaching of nursing.

In addition, to assist professional nurses in obtaining advanced degrees, the group recommended that the federal program of Professional Nurse Traineeships be doubled within a five-year period. They thought that this program

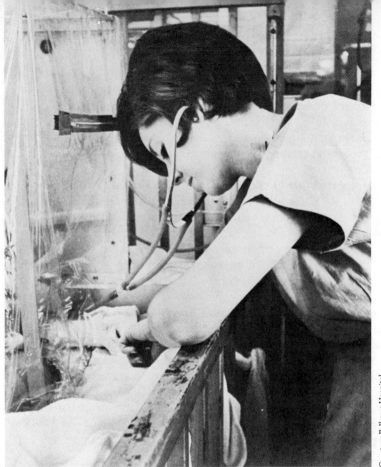

More and better-educated nurses were called for by the Surgeon General's Consultant Group on Nursing.

should be expanded to provide for the preparation of nursing specialists in clinical fields. Other aspects of training for which the group recommended provision of federal funds were short-term traineeships and baccalaureate study for diploma graduates.

To help hospitals improve utilization of nurses, the group suggested that federal funds be provided to conduct demonstrations, to experiment with new and improved methods, and to educate nurses in the use of these methods. Federal funds should be made available to expand consultative and other services designed to improve the quality and quantity of nursing care. Further, project grants should be made to nursing schools and other agencies to strengthen inservice education, on-the-job training, and continuing education of nurses. Finally, to increase support for nursing research, the consultant group recommended an immediate increase in funding for the Public Health Service nursing research fellowship program, in order to finance the establishment of 100 new full-time research fellowships. The group also favored action that would double the funds for the PHS's program of nursing research.

The Nurse Training Act of 1964

Based on these recommendations, a much-expanded program of federal aid for professional nursing education was proposed in a 1964 administration bill, H.R. 10042, the "Nurse Training Act of 1964." The bill, incorporating White House proposals for nursing school construction grants as well as for student loans and scholarships, was introduced in February by Congressman Oren Harris of Arkansas. Witnesses for the Department of Health, Education, and Welfare gave strong support to the bill. Boisfeuillent Jones, special assistant to the HEW Secretary, called H.R. 10042 "the logical next step in strengthening and coordinating existing programs aiding nurse education with a major new nationwide effort to alleviate critical shortages of nurses required for the health care of all citizens" [9].

Key supportive testimony at the House hearings came from the American Nurses' Association. The ANA emphasized aid for collegiate schools of nursing, including construction grants, on the basis that these schools educated teachers, who in turn would be needed in greater numbers if the shortage of practicing nurses was to be alleviated. Nurses testifying at the House hearings seemed content to support the administration bill as drafted. It authorized $346 million, over five years, for nursing school construction, special projects and planning grants, student loans and merit scholarships, and a continuation of the professional nurse traineeship program.

The House considered the professional nurse education bill on July 21, 1964. During the House floor debate, discussion centered on the proposed $41 million formula grants to diploma schools of nursing to help meet educational costs. Representative Kenneth A. Roberts of Alabama, a sponsor of the bill and its floor manager in the House debate, reported that the House Interstate and Foreign Commerce Committee had adopted this provision because "the committee was quite concerned by the trend that has been developing in recent years, under which the number of diploma schools of nursing has declined from 1134 in 1949 to only 875 today." Representative Roberts added that "a number of these 875 schools face the very real possibility of having to close their doors because they are unable to meet the additional costs to them for training nurses [and that] these schools run a continuing deficit, which, of course, is borne by increased costs to patients at hospitals" [10].

The House-passed version of the Nurse Training Act of 1964 was approved by the Senate on August 12, with a few technical amendments and one other that incorporated recommendations made by the American Hospital Association. The latter amendment added diploma schools of nursing to the five-year, $17 million program for special project grants to aid schools in meeting the cost of improved or expanded nursing education. The House-passed version of the bill had limited these grants to public and nonprofit private collegiate and associate degree nursing schools. This new assistance was made in addition to the House- and Senate-approved five-year program of formula grants, totaling $41 million, for training costs of public and nonprofit private diploma schools of nursing.

As finally approved for the President's signature, the five-year legislation authorized $283 million for five programs and an additional $4.6 million for administration of the programs. Ninety million dollars was authorized for construction of nursing facilities, including new, renovated, or replacement buildings. Of this total, $55 million was for diploma and junior college programs and $35 million was for collegiate programs. Another $17 million was authorized for "teaching improvement grants," or special projects, and would be available to all programs [11].

Also authorized was $50 million for the continuance of existing traineeship programs which had been instituted to increase the number of graduate nursing students with preparation for positions as administrators, supervisors, clinical specialists, and teachers in hospitals and related institutions, public health agencies, and schools of nursing" [12]. The bill provided $85 million for loans, not grants, to nursing students in order to help defray the cost of nursing education. For those graduates who worked for five years following graduation,

The Nurse Training Act of 1964 was aimed at rapidly expanding enrollments in schools of nursing.

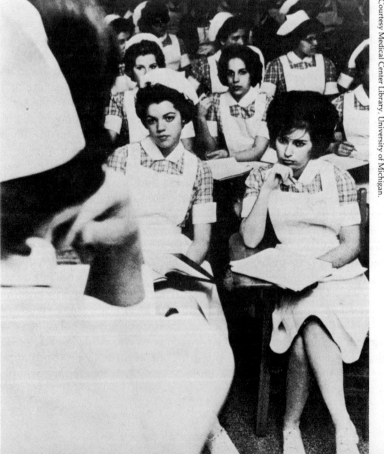

50 percent of the loan was to be deferred.

Significant to those concerned about the future of hard-pressed hospital nursing schools was the authorization, specifically for diploma programs, of $41 million "to improve the quality of instruction." The maximum payment to any one program would be based on a formula granting $100 per year per student enrolled. The legislation was to cover the five fiscal years 1965–1969 with the exception that construction grants were authorized to begin in fiscal year 1966. In the meantime, the Health Professions Educational Assistance Act of 1963 would continue to provide funds for the construction of collegiate facilities.

The loan program authorized by the Nurse Training Act of 1964 was designed to increase the number of nursing students by enabling the needy to finance their nursing education with long-term, low-interest loans. Approved diploma, associate degree, baccalaureate, and graduate schools of nursing were eligible for participation. Nursing schools utilizing loan funds requested and received allocation from the Public Health Service, determined the eligibility of student applicants for loans, decided the amount of the loans, administered the funds, and collected the repayments. The school was required to provide $1.00 for every $9.00 of federal contribution to the loan fund.

The dozen years from 1952 to 1964 were pivotal in the continued maturation of nursing. Fueled by biomedical advances such as the wonder drugs, the number of hospital admissions soared; Hill-Burton funds supported a concomitant increase in available hospital beds. The on-going shortage of nurses and the resultant wide-scale employment of auxiliaries took the nurse further away from direct patient care as she was required to assume managerial responsibilities. The student labor component of the total nurse staffing picture continued to diminish in importance. With the urging and assistance of the professional nursing associations, the federal government took important steps toward improving the quality of nursing education in America.

Summary
Advances in the use of antibiotics saved the lives of countless millions of persons, and the use of these "wonder drugs" altered the nursing care needs of many patients.

An influx of auxiliary hospital workers in the 1950s took the professional nurse further and further away from the bedside as she assumed management and coordinating responsibilities. As a result of new standards in nursing education, students spent a lower proportion of their time in direct care. These two forces drastically altered the pattern of nursing service.

In the early 1950s enrollment in master's degree nursing programs stagnated, while a sharp drop in nurses earning baccalaureate degrees was experienced. Private and federal funds to support nurses seeking advanced preparation were instrumental in reversing this trend.

In 1952 Teachers College, Columbia University, launched a project, directed by Mildred Montag, to determine the feasibility of a two-year nurse preparation program. Testing the idea in seven junior college sites throughout the country, the initial study results documented the success of the approach.

Federally supported biomedical research surged during the 1940s and 1950s. In 1956 a research grants program was launched by the Division of Nursing Resources of the Public Health Service which provided the major impetus for the development of nursing research in the United States over the next decades.

Throughout the 1950s and early 1960s, widespread shortages of nurses existed throughout the nation. Low pay and bad working conditions continued to divert young people from choosing nursing as a career.

As hospitals costs rose, the traditional method of financing hospital nursing education through the service provided by students clashed with the development of diploma schools of nursing into true educational institutions.

Baccalaureate prepared nurses were still a scarcity in the early 1960s. One obstacle to the growth of baccalaureate programs up to that time was that many of these programs were essentially standard diploma programs plus two years of general education, carried out in collegiate settings. The differences between generic baccalaureate and diploma graduates often were not valued by employers.

Following the election of President Kennedy in 1960, a new and favorable political climate promoted federal aid to the health professions.

In 1961 the Surgeon General appointed the special Consultant Group on Nursing to advise him on nursing needs and to identify the appropriate role of the federal government in assuring adequate nursing services for the country.

The Consultant Group developed a series of recommendations aimed at increasing both the quality and quantity of nursing practice, education, and research. Its report, Toward Quality in Nursing, won broad acceptance as a guiding document for planners in nursing for the following decade.

In 1964, based on the recommendations of the Consultant Group, a much-expanded program of aid for professional nursing education was proposed in an administration bill known as the "Nurse Training Act of 1964." As finally approved by the President, the legislation authorized the allocation of $283 million over a five-year period.

References

1. Thomas Hales and Elizabeth A. Bell, "How Schools of Nursing Can Break Even," *Modern Hospitals*, vol. 94 (April, 1960): 103–106.
2. National League for Nursing, Department of Diploma and Associate Degree Programs, *Report on Hospital Schools of Nursing, 1957* (New York: National League for Nursing, 1959), pp. 1–5.
3. National League for Nursing, Department of Diploma and Associate Degree Programs, *Today's Diploma Schools of Nursing: Report of the 1962 Survey of 728 Diploma Schools of Nursing* (New York: National League for Nursing, 1963), pp. 3–4.
4. Margaret Bridgman, *Collegiate Education for Nursing* (New York: Russell Sage Foundation, 1953), pp. 185–197.
5. *New York Times*, January 21, 1961.
6. U. S. Public Health Service, *Toward Quality in Nursing: Needs and Goals. Report of the Surgeon General's Consultant Group on Nursing* (Washington, D.C.: Government Printing Office, 1963), p. xiii.
7. *Ibid.*, p. xiv.
8. *Ibid.*, pp. 33–52.
9. U. S. Congress, House, Committee on Interstate and Foreign Commerce, Subcommittee on Public Health and Safety, Eighty-eighth Congress, Second Session. *Nurse Training Act of 1964.* Hearings before the Subcommittee. (Washington, D.C.: Government Printing Office, 1964), p. 27.
10. U. S. Congress, House, Committee on Interstate and Foreign Commerce, *Nurse Training Act of 1964.* Report to accompany H.R. 11241, Eighty-eighth Congress, Second Session. (Washington, D.C.: Government Printing Office, 1964), Report No. 1549, p. 3.
11. U. S. Congress, Senate, Committee on Labor and Public Welfare, *Nurse Training Act of 1964.* Report to accompany H.R. 11241, Eighty-eighth Congress, Second Session. (Washington, D.C.: Government Printing Office, 1964), Report No. 1378, pp. 1–24.
12. *Congressional Record*, August 12, 1964.

19
Politics, Health, and Nurses: The End of Innocence

By the mid-1960s health care had evolved into a complex, rapidly changing technological industry. Nursing practice had assumed progressively greater degrees of complexity and diversity as specialized roles, such as intensive and coronary care nursing, emerged and as the maturation of nursing as a scientific discipline affected both new and traditional dimensions of patient care. The emergence of numerous diagnostic and therapeutic technologic medical advances—radioactive isotopes, ultrasound and infrared machines, for example—also altered nursing practice and commanded the development of new modes of nursing practice.

The Balance Sheet in Attacking Causes of Death

It will be recalled that at the turn of the century the leading cause of death in the United States had been diseases that were essentially acute and communicable: the influenzas, tuberculosis, and gastritis. In 1900 these three diseases had a combined death rate of 540 per 100,000 and accounted for nearly one-third of all deaths. In 1960, however, the top three killers were diseases of the heart, malignant neoplasms, and vascular lesions—such as strokes—affecting the central nervous system. Accidents followed closely in fourth place. The first three killers accounted for 693 deaths per 100,000 persons and 70 percent of all deaths in 1963.

The American system of health care in 1965 was essentially a mosaic of public and private health programs that had grown, piece by piece, to meet national needs as they arose. For 200 million people there were 300,000 physicians in a variety of practices, 700,000 registered nurses, over three million other health workers, 7000 hospitals, 20,000 long-term health facilities, and many other private and public institutions. Between 1956 and 1965, admissions to short-term, nonfederal hospitals rose from 120 per 1000 population to 138. Factors that had increased the demand for all forms of medical care included demographic changes, rising incomes, greater expectations from the health industry, and wider insurance coverage.

Most experts agreed that several factors operated to increase the usage of hospitals rather than relying upon less expensive but perhaps equally effective

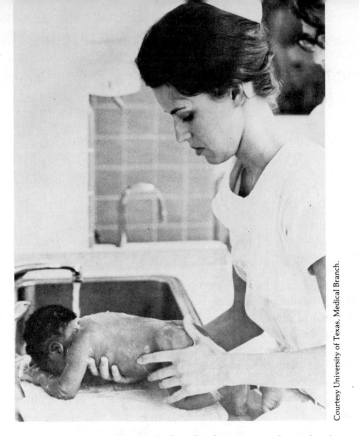

By the mid-1960s health care had evolved into a complex technological industry.

forms of medical care. More people carried hospitalization insurance than coverage for other forms of care. A physician might choose to place his patient in the hospital rather than to treat him at his home or at the office, since hospitalization was covered by the patient's insurance and house and office calls were not. In many cases, hospitals were overutilized to suit the physicians who found it convenient to have their patients available in one place. The relationship between physician and hospital was at the heart of the problem. Through real competence, seniority, or politics—usually a combination of all three—a physician became a member of a hospital staff, after which point, with almost no outside control, he could affect the largest component of hospital costs—labor—and seriously influence most other cost areas.

It was speculated that increased hospital utilization might be the result of increases in the number of hospital beds. Studies showed that physicians tended to keep patients in the hospital longer if beds were available and that the principal determinant of the level of hospital use was the availability of beds, not the price of the care or the characteristics of the patient population. Also, demand for hospital beds varied with the seasons and the day of the week.

From 1946 to 1966 the average length of hospital stay decreased from 9.1 to 7.9 days. Most of that decrease had occurred by 1950, however. While from

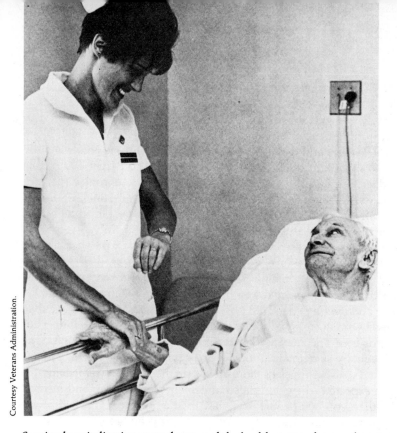

Soaring hospitalization costs threatened the health status of many Americans.

1950 to 1966 daily costs had gone up and the length of stay had not changed appreciably, the number of bed-days per 1000 population had increased. In 1950 the average daily hospital census was 2.4 inpatients per 1000 population. By 1965 this figure had risen to 2.9, an increase of about 12 percent. A more common measure of hospital utilization was admissions per 100,000. On this scale, the proportion had risen from 11,114 in 1947 to 13,885 in 1966, an increase of 25 percent. While hospital utilization and daily costs were rising, lengths of stay and occupancy rates in general community hospitals had remained about the same. From 1946 the occupancy rate of 72.1 percent had declined to a low of 70.9 in 1954, climbing again to 76.5 percent in 1966.

For low-income families, fee-for-service financing and the high cost of medical care acted as a deterrent to the early initiation of medical care. The tendency in many cases was to delay seeking care until the condition became intolerably serious; by the time care was sought, the benefits of early diagnosis and treatment had been lost. The disproportionate burden of the cost of health care for low-income people was demonstrated in a 1958 study of nationwide family health expenditures, which reported that the proportion of family income spent on health decreased steadily from 13 percent among families earning less than $2000 per annum to 4 percent among families earning $7500 or more.

Movement for National Health Insurance for the Elderly

The elderly were twice as likely to have had one or more chronic conditions as were those under 65. While some of these conditions such as sinusitis, hay fever, or bronchitis were relatively minor, many more were serious: high blood pressure, heart disease, and diabetes. The incidence of chronic conditions increased from 74 per 100 people in the age group 65–74 to 84 per 100 people aged 75 and over. Similarly, the extent of disability due to chronic illness increased with age. Well over half the aged with one or more chronic conditions had some limitation of activity, whereas, among younger people with chronic illness, only one of five had any limitations of activity.

The chief chronic illnesses of old age were arthritis, rheumatism, heart disease, and high blood pressure. Among the population aged 65 and over during the period July, 1957, to June, 1959, 149 per 1000 had heart conditions, 129 had high blood pressure, and 266 had arthritis or rheumatism. In 1959 people aged 65 and over averaged 6.8 physician visits per year, two more than those averaged by younger people. The rate of physician visits was higher for women than for men and increased with the size of family income. Among the aged with equally severe limitations of activity or chronic illness, persons with high incomes visited physicians more often than those with lower incomes.

As might be expected, the elderly also utilized health facilities and medical services more than younger people, and they used a greater volume of physicians' services and were admitted to hospitals more often and for longer periods. They were the primary users of nursing home and other long-term care facilities and received a greater amount of home care, part of which was provided by nurses. They needed and used more drugs.

Pressure for a national compulsory health care plan, mainly from Northern Democrats, labor, and liberal groups, had reached a high in 1949 and 1950. It will be recalled that hearings on the Wagner-Murray-Dingell bills, embodying the Truman proposals, had prompted criticism of the President and charges of socialism from the American Medical Association. In the end, the opponents of Truman's proposals won. Congress failed to act again in 1950, but did move to help states to provide medical care for welfare recipients under Old Age Assistance, Aid to Dependent Children, Aid to the Blind, and Aid to the Permanently and Totally Disabled. Although President Eisenhower had opposed compulsory health insurance during his 1952 campaign, in 1954, as President, he proposed that the federal government reinsure private insurance companies to protect them from losses on health insurance. The bill, supported by some insurance companies, was labeled inadequate by labor spokesmen, received criticism from the AMA, and underwent defeat that year.

Proponents of compulsory national health insurance had begun to suggest that an immediate step toward such an act would be payment, through Social Security Old Age Survivors Insurance, of hospitalization costs of people retired on OASI pensions. Such a bill was put forth in 1952 by Senator Murray, Representative John Dingell, and Representative Emanuel Cellar, but no action was taken on it or similar bills during the next several years. In the late 1950s,

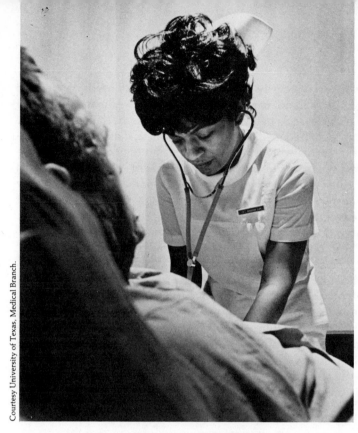

Older people were much more likely to have chronic conditions requiring nursing care.

in Congress, the OASI approach to health care for the elderly was sponsored by Representative Aimé J. Forand of Rhode Island. After a brief discussion, no action was taken on the 1957 Forand bill, but it was introduced again in 1959.

At that time the American Nurses' Association came out in favor of extension of social security to provide health insurance coverage for the aged, along with inclusion of payments for private duty and public health nursing care. The ANA also urged that careful attention be paid to the type of nursing home care covered in order to prevent the financing of substandard institutions. The ANA's position held that health insurance, especially for the aged, should cover more than the cost of hospital, nursing home, and surgical services as provided for in the Forand bill. Nursing was an essential component of modern medical care and should be made available if the benefits of science were to be provided for the aged and disabled. Beneficiaries of any health insurance should be insured for needed private duty nursing services no less than they were insured against surgical costs. Coverage should also include public health nursing care in the home as well as regular nursing home costs. This position had been established by the ANA House of Delegates at the 1958 convention when the organization had moved from the neutral position on the broader question of compulsory health insurance adopted in 1952.

The American Medical Association had gone on record, in 1957, in absolute opposition to use of social security for financing the health needs of the aged and had spared no words in doing so. President David B. Allman, addressing the AMA House of Delegates, had directed the opening barrage against the Forand bill. "This is socialized medicine," he said, adding that it was the beginning of the end of the private practice of medicine and the death knell for the young and growing voluntary health insurance industry. He further warned that the bill constituted a serious threat to the well-being and local autonomy of the voluntary hospital at the community level and heralded the advent of federally sponsored socialism.

Dr. Allman charged that the Forand bill prescribed a course of treatment before there had been diagnoses of "(1) the economic resources of our older population; (2) the present and planned programs of voluntary insurance; (3) indigent care at the state level; (4) the incidence of hospitalization and illness by age groups and other complex research questions which they did not even try to find the answers to." Dr. Allman insisted that in the field of old-age coverage the health insurance industry was beginning to make rapid and far-reaching strides and added that his own conviction was that "we are on the verge of giant achievements in furthering the well-being of our older population" [1].

The American Nurses' Association backed a health insurance program for the aged that would cover nursing services in the home.

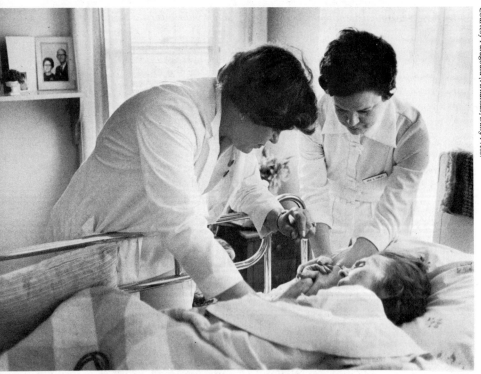

Courtesy Paragould [Arkansas] Daily Press.

An editorial in *The American Journal of Nursing* speculated on why nurses and physicians took opposite sides in this controversy:

Day after day nurses watch the numbers of the chronically ill increase. Necessarily sensitive to their patients' needs, they are acutely aware of the fright of many patients—and their families—who cannot foresee how they can continue to pay for decent medical care for an uncertain future. They know many of these patients cannot begin to pay for medical expenses with the income limits placed on them when they are drawing social security . . . .

Of less importance to them as nurses, but of equal importance as citizens, is the realization that they or members of their family might be facing the same situation.

The vast majority of nurses are in the income bracket where high medical expenses can toss them into serious debt; and voluntary medical insurance—especially beyond the work years—is relatively costly, or impossible to buy. Though increased salaries might relieve this, [the nurses'] efforts at acquiring them are blocked by the shaky economy of those same voluntary hospitals and public health agencies who are now subsidizing a large part of the cost of the care of the aging and chronically ill. And they are quite aware of the fact that the government is already in the health picture, for [it is] too often the inadequate reimbursement from local and state governments—not to mention Blue Cross—which is the usual reason for denying their requests for salary increases. They know that all of this cannot help but affect the nursing care of the people [2].

Although the 1959 version was defeated, the Forand bill had become a political issue. After much debate, in 1960, the House Ways and Means Committee rejected both the Forand bill and an Eisenhower administration proposal calling for federal matching grants to the states to help the needy meet the costs of illness. Although similar legislation was turned back in both 1961 and 1962, the proponents kept fighting. During 1963 and 1964 over 100 bills calling for provision of medical care for those 65 or over were introduced. In 1964 such a bill was passed by the Senate, representing for the first time passage of a health-care-for-the-aged bill by either house. The bill then went to conference committee, where a deadlock over its provisions lasted until Congress adjourned. Medicare, as it had come to be called, had once again failed to gain congressional approval.

When Lyndon B. Johnson was elected President in 1964, Medicare was high on his administration's priority list. Almost immediately after the Eighty-ninth Congress had convened, the new Medicare proposals (H.R. 1 and S.1) were introduced. On March 29, 1965, the Ways and Means Committee reported its recommendations in the form of a new bill, H.R. 6675, which established two coordinated health insurance programs under the Social Security Act for people aged 65 and over: (1) a basic plan of hospital insurance and related care under the social security program, with financing through a separate payroll tax and trust fund; and (2) a voluntary supplementary plan providing for physicians' fees and other medical and health services, financed by premium payments of $3 per month by each participant, matched from federal general revenues. Undergirding the two new insurance programs would be a greatly expanded medical care program, called Medicaid, for the financially and medically

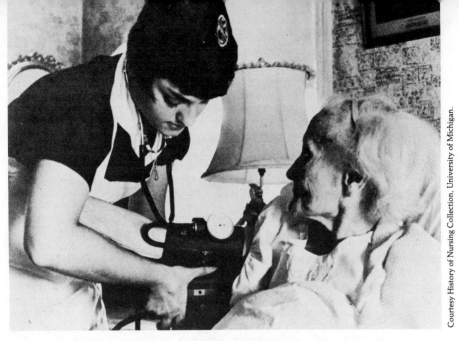

Medicare provided a comprehensive health program for the elderly.

needy. The bill also provided for an across-the-board 7-percent increase in social security benefits, for an increase in the taxable wage base from $4800 to $6600, and for a five-year program of "special project grants" to provide comprehensive health care and services for needy children.

The Congress was not unaware of the importance of this bill. Senator Russell B. Long, floor leader, opened debate on the measure:

Mr. President, the pending bill will be the largest and most significant piece of social legislation ever to pass the Congress in the history of our country. It will do more immediate good for more people who need the attention of their government than any bill that the Congress has ever enacted. We measure our accomplishments here by our association with those few pieces of legislation which clearly move the American people toward a better life . . . .

This Medicare program not only means dignity to the individual, but serves our country as an economic stabilizer while at the same time it provides for the whole of the free world a beacon reflecting the democratic way of achieving social progress. We are considering a bill which represents concern, consideration, and compromise in the best American tradition, and reflects the ideas of many men sitting here today [3].

After a 10-hour session and action upon numerous proposed amendments, the Senate, at 8:00 P.M. July 9, 1965, passed the bill by a vote of 68 to 21. The bill contained 513 changes from the version approved by the House. Most of them, however, were not substantial, and the major features of the two versions were the same.

The bill was sent to a conference committee for reconciliation of differences between the two versions. The conference committee convened for its first negotiating session on July 14 and promptly settled a major point of disagreement: 60 days of hospitalization would be provided, with the patient to pay a deductible of $40, and an additional 30 days would be added, with the patient to pay $10 a day. Agreement was also reached on the limits for nursing home or extended-care services and for home visits by nurses. The compromise bill, as signed by President Johnson, conformed in all basic respects to the Administration's specifications for a comprehensive medical care program.

The ANA Position Paper on Education for Nursing

During December, 1965, a conflict over the future role of diploma schools abruptly intensified. "Education for those who work in nursing should take place in institutions of learning within the general system of education," stated the ANA's first Position Paper on Education for Nursing. Prepared by the ANA Committee on Education and adopted by the ANA Board of Directors in September, 1965, the publication marked the beginning of what would become an ever-widening schism in nursing education. The statement pointed out that recognition of the need for improved nursing practice had led the Association to conclude that:

The education for all of those who are licensed to practice nursing should take place in institutions of higher education; minimum preparation for beginning professional nursing practice should be a baccalaureate degree; minimum preparation for beginning technical nursing practice should be an associate degree in nursing; education for assistants in the health service occupations should be short, intensive preservice programs in vocational education rather than on-the-job training [4].

In discussing the implications of the ANA position, the statement maintained that "responsibility for the education of nurses historically has been carried out by hospitals, and the graduates of hospital-based diploma programs comprise approximately 78 percent of nurses now in practice. However, economic pressures on the hospital, and other developments in society, are increasing the movement of nursing education programs into the colleges and universities . . . . It is reasonable to expect," the statement continued, "that many diploma schools of nursing will participate with colleges and universities in planning for the development of baccalaureate programs; others will participate with junior colleges in planning for the development of associate degree programs." Of course, both senior and junior college programs would need hospitals and other community resources for use as laboratories. The statement also noted that colleges and universities needed to provide improved education for nurses by offering new programs, by expanding existing programs, by determining the distinctions between programs of education that prepared either "technical" or "professional" nurses, and by carrying on programs for continuing education, advanced study, and research [5].

In line with the principle that all nursing education should take place in educational institutions, the ANA statement proposed that the nursing profession replace outside programs for practical nursing with junior college and community college programs in beginning-level technical nursing practice. The reasons given for this proposal were the major changes that had occurred in the nursing profession in the past few years: increasingly complex activities were being delegated to practical nurses, many of whom were now expected to carry job responsibilities beyond those for which they had been educated.

Changes in the Educational Plant

It will be recalled that the associate degree nursing program was a relatively new development, and only in the early 1960s did its impact begin to be felt. In 1955 there had been only 16 schools with such programs; by 1964 the number had risen to 130. As this potential giant began to develop, the quality of some programs became suspect to some nurses because of what was perceived to be a drastic shortage of clinical experience in the curricula.

The trend in nursing education away from diploma schools and toward colleges or universities became even more pronounced during 1966. Statistics gathered by the NLN indicated that the number of diploma programs had fallen from 821 in 1965 to 797 in 1966. At the same time, associate degree and baccalaureate programs had increased, respectively, from 174 to 218 and from 198 to 210. The decline in diploma programs was more than made up for by the increase in collegiate programs, with the total number of the latter increasing, in 1966, from 1193 to 1225. Of these programs, almost 61 percent were accredited by the National League for Nursing, including 72.4 percent of the diploma programs, 8.7 percent of the associate degree programs, and 70 percent of the baccalaureate programs. Three-fourths of all nursing students were enrolled in NLN-accredited programs.

The changing pattern in nurse education was reflected in student admission data. In 1966 diploma programs admitted 64.1 percent of the total 60,701 students newly enrolled in nursing programs, a decrease of 4.7 percent from the year before. Associate degree programs showed a marked increase in students, admitting 14.2 percent of all students, compared with 10.7 percent in 1965. Total admissions to baccalaureate programs increased from 20.5 percent to 21.7 percent.

The trend away from diploma schools was even more marked when traced over the 10-year period beginning in 1956, when 82.8 percent of all nursing students had been receiving their education in hospital schools (94,920 diploma students out of a total of 114,570). By 1966 the total number of students in diploma programs had decreased slightly to 90,651. In 1956 associate degree programs had enrolled 1 percent of all nursing students—a total of 1132—as compared with the 15,338 associate degree students of 1966. Baccalaureate program enrollment also increased, although not as dramatically, growing from a total enrollment of 18,518 in 1956 to 33,081 in 1966.

According to a study published by the National League for Nursing in 1964, the operation of schools of nursing cost hospitals in the United States an estimated $250 million a year. In a six-year study on costs in nursing education

Basic School of Nursing Programs, 1953–1976, and Percentage Change from Preceding Year.

Year	Diploma	%	AD	%	BS	%	Total	%
1953	1017		21		198		1236	
1954	992	−2.5	30	+42.9	214	+ 8.1	1236	0
1955	981	−1.1	34	+13.3	146	−31.8	1161	−6.1
1956	956	−2.5	20	−41.2	161	+10.3	1137	−2.5
1957	943	−1.4	28	+40.0	166	+ 3.1	1137	0
1958	935	−0.8	38	+35.7	172	+ 3.6	1145	+0.7
1959	918	−1.8	48	+26.3	171	− 0.6	1137	−0.7
1960	908	−1.1	57	+18.8	172	+ 0.6	1137	0
1961	883	−2.8	69	+21.1	174	+ 1.2	1126	−1.0
1962	874	−1.0	84	+21.7	178	+ 2.3	1136	+0.9
1963	860	−1.6	105	+25.0	183	+ 2.8	1148	+1.0
1964	840	−2.3	130	+23.8	188	+ 2.7	1158	+0.9
1965	821	−2.3	174	+33.8	198	+ 5.3	1193	+3.0
1966	797	−2.9	218	+25.3	210	+ 6.1	1225	+2.7
1967	767	−3.8	281	+28.9	221	+ 5.2	1269	+3.6
1968	728	−5.1	330	+17.4	235	+ 6.3	1293	+1.9
1969	695	−4.5	390	+18.2	254	+ 8.1	1339	+3.6
1970	641	−7.8	444	+13.8	270	+ 6.3	1355	+1.2
1971	587	−8.4	491	+10.6	285	+ 5.6	1363	+0.6
1972	543	−7.5	541	+10.2	293	+ 2.8	1377	+1.0
1973	494	−9.0	574	+ 6.1	305	+ 4.1	1373	−0.3
1974	461	−6.7	598	+ 4.2	313	+ 2.6	1372	−0.1
1975	428	−7.2	618	+ 3.3	329	+ 5.1	1375	+0.2
1976	390	−8.9	642	+ 3.9	341	+ 3.6	1373	−0.1

made under a grant from the Division of Nursing of the United States Public Health Service, the League had found that hospitals under public control spent more money to educate nursing students than did hospitals under private control, and that both types of schools spent more on noneducational functions, such as student maintenance, than they did on educational functions. By applying a uniform system of cost analysis to a representative sampling of the diploma program population, NLN researchers found that:

The median gross cost of educating one student for one year in a diploma nursing program was $2600; the median net cost was $2300.

The median yearly income to the hospital per student to defray the cost of the program was $250. This included tuition, fees for room and board, health services and student insurance, and income from contributions and gifts. The estimated value of the student's clinical experience to the hospital and other institutions in which she serves while learning was only $750 [6].

Of the $2600 gross cost of nursing education, $1500 went for noneducational functions of the school (including housing, meals, laundry, recreation, and

Admissions to Schools of Nursing, 1953–1976, and Percentage Change from Preceding Year.

Year	Diploma	%	AD	%	BS	%	Total	%
1953	36,947		609		5707		43,263	
1954	38,106	+ 3.1	741	+21.7	6017	+ 5.4	44,864	+ 3.7
1955	38,884	+ 2.0	629	−15.1	6931	+15.2	46,444	+ 3.5
1956	37,763	− 2.9	559	−11.1	6833	− 1.4	45,155	− 2.8
1957	37,571	− 0.5	578	+ 3.4	7094	+ 3.8	45,243	+ 0.2
1958	36,402	− 3.1	953	+64.9	6866	− 3.2	44,221	− 2.3
1959	37,722	+ 3.6	1266	+32.8	7275	+ 6.0	46,263	+ 4.6
1960	40,013	+ 6.1	1598	+26.2	7555	+ 3.8	49,166	+ 6.3
1961	38,702	− 3.3	2085	+30.5	8700	+15.2	49,487	+ 0.7
1962	38,257	− 1.2	2504	+20.1	9400	+ 8.0	50,161	+ 1.4
1963	36,434	− 4.8	3490	+39.4	9597	+ 2.1	49,521	− 1.3
1964	37,936	+ 4.1	4461	+27.8	10,270	+ 7.0	52,667	+ 6.4
1965	39,609	+ 4.4	6160	+38.1	11,835	+15.2	57,604	+ 9.4
1966	38,904	− 1.8	8638	+40.2	13,159	+11.2	60,701	+ 5.4
1967	33,283	−14.4	11,237	+30.1	14,070	+ 6.9	58,590	− 3.5
1968	31,628	− 5.0	14,870	+32.3	14,891	+ 5.8	61,389	+ 4.8
1969	29,267	− 7.5	18,907	+27.1	15,983	+ 7.3	64,157	+ 4.5
1970	28,996	− 0.9	23,797	+25.9	17,635	+10.3	70,428	+ 9.8
1971	28,980	− 0.1	29,889	+25.6	20,413	+15.8	79,282	+12.6
1972	29,801	+ 2.8	36,996	+20.0	27,357	+34.0	94,154	+18.8
1973	29,848	+ 0.2	44,387	+16.7	30,478	+11.4	104,713	+11.2
1974	26,943	− 9.7	48,596	+ 9.5	32,672	+ 7.2	108,211	+ 3.3
1975	24,696	− 8.3	50,180	+ 3.3	35,192	+ 7.7	110,068	+ 1.7
1976	23,622	− 4.3	53,033	+ 5.7	36,656	+ 4.2	113,311	+ 2.9

separate health services) and $1100 went for educational functions (including the instructional program, counseling, libraries, and educational records). The investigators found that the cost of nursing education per student was highest in programs with fewer than 70 students enrolled and was lowest in programs with more than 120 students enrolled. The cost of instruction per student was higher in the Northeast than in any other region of the country, was greatest in tax-supported programs of municipal governments, and was least in programs under the control of religious institutions.

More Help from the Federal Government

As the Nurse Training Act of 1964 would expire in 1969, Congressional hearings were held regarding bills to extend the grant program during the spring of 1968. The Senate Labor and Public Welfare Committee cut the Johnson administration's requested five-year authorization to three years, and the revised bill passed the Senate without debate on June 24, 1968. The House then further reduced the bill's authorization to two years, altered the authorizations slightly,

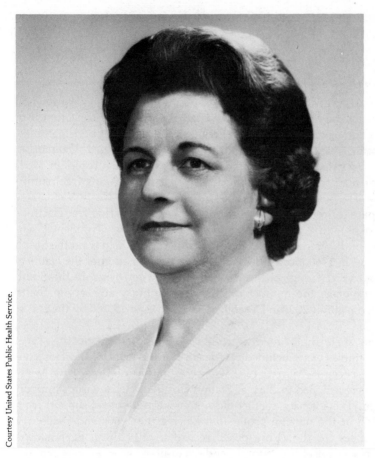

Jessie M. Scott, Director, Division of Nursing, and Assistant Surgeon General, United States Public Health Service.

and passed it unanimously on August 1, 1968. Thus, the Nurse Training Act of 1964 was extended through fiscal years 1970 and 1971, with authorized appropriations totaling $260 million. The Act extended the program of federal aid for school of nursing construction grants, special project grants, as well as the student assistance programs of loans, scholarships, and traineeships. The Act continued to be administered by the Division of Nursing of the United States Public Health Service under the direction of Jessie M. Scott, Assistant Surgeon General [7].

As Lyndon B. Johnson prepared to lay aside the responsibilities of the nation's highest office in January, 1969, he could view a national health care system that differed markedly in some respects from the system of only five years before. During this period broad changes had been made in financing health care for the aged and the poor, in educating health personnel, and in health research; the first steps had been taken in changing the methods of health care delivery;

and annual federal spending for health had tripled from $4.1 billion in 1963 to $13.9 billion in 1968.

Nursing in the Vietnam Era

Meanwhile the 12-year-long American troop commitment to Vietnam had made that conflict the longest in United States history. American interest in Southeast Asia had begun in 1950 when President Truman sent a 35-man military advisory team to aid the French in their fight against the North Vietnamese. After the French garrison at Dien Bien Phu fell to communist forces in 1954, France and North Vietnam agreed to partition Vietnam, pending free reunification elections. The South Vietnamese government refused a North Vietnamese request to prepare for reunification elections on the grounds that free elections would be impossible in North Vietnam. The following year President Eisenhower offered South Vietnam economic aid and agreed to help train the South Vietnamese army. In 1960 North Vietnam announced formation of the National Liberation Front (Viet Cong) of South Vietnam, and terrorism in the South increased. In response, the number of American military advisers in South Vietnam rose from about 2000 in December, 1961, to over 15,000 by the end of 1963.

It was at this stage that American military nurses arrived on the scene. Thirteen Army nurses were included on the staff of the Eighth Field Hospital, arriving at Nha Trang in March, 1962. Concomitantly, the first Navy Nurse Corps officers were assigned to duty at Station Hospital, Headquarters Support Activity, Saigon. The Vietnam conflict did not evoke widespread support from either the nation or the nursing profession. During the 1950s and 1960s, recruitment of nurses for the Army posed recurrent difficulties. Professional nurses were in chronically short supply, and the military services were obliged to recruit in direct competition with civilian nurse employers.

Extraordinary incentives were offered. In 1956 the Army established the Army Student Nurse Program. Student nurses received financial aid and in return served in the Army for a minimum of two years for a diploma in nursing or for three years for a degree. Students remained at their own nursing schools until they had completed the prescribed course and qualified for state licensure. Four months before completion of their nursing courses, the participants applied for commissions in the Army Nurse Corps Reserve. Upon receipt of notification of state licensure, they were commissioned and ordered to active duty.

Despite these incentives, the strength of the Army Nurse Corps dwindled, creating a gap between capability and mission. During the early days of the Vietnam conflict, the Army Student Nurse Program continued to be the major source for junior officers. Army Student Nurse Program participants represented 52 percent of the total Nurse Corps' growth in fiscal year 1962. Despite personnel policies disapproving resignations and voluntary requests for relief from active duty, the losses in the Corps exceeded the gains for that year, and the downward trend continued.

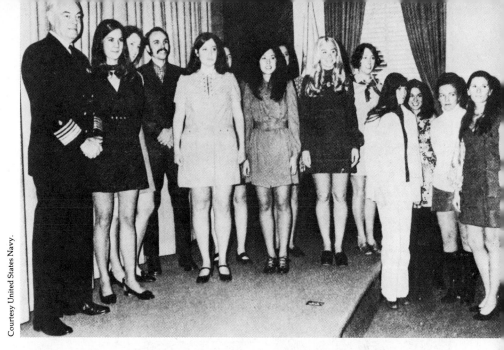

The Surgeon General of the Navy administers the oath of office to 13 student nurses on December 2, 1971.

It was thought that the difficulty encountered in recruiting Army nurses reflected the general shortage of professional nurses in civilian life, but specialization, increased demands for health services, and the development of new fields of practice also contributed to the problem. Recruitment of military nurses had become increasingly competitive: civilian hospitals were paying higher salaries, had improved working conditions and housing, and were offering other attractive inducements. The Army Medical Service had to employ hundreds of civilian nurses to fill military nursing requirements.

Within the context of a general military build-up, the Department of Defense, with Congressional support, approved the establishment of the Walter Reed Army Institute of Nursing. It was stated that the Army, by opening its vast resources to prepare qualified nurses, would make an important contribution to the fulfillment of military and civilian nursing needs. The goals of the new school of nursing were to increase the Army's number of degree-holding nurses and to increase the reenlistment rate of Army nurses.

The first large contingent of Air Force nurses for Vietnam reported in February, 1966, and were assigned to the Twelfth Air Force Hospital, Cam Ranh Bay. Soon after followed a rapid increase in the number of Army nurses serving in Vietnam, from slightly more than 200 in June, 1966, to more than 600 in June, 1967, to a peak of 900 in January, 1969. The military situation was discouraging, and by April, 1966, more Americans than South Vietnamese were being killed in action: in July the number of American dead reached 4440—more than the number of Americans killed in the Revolution, 10 times more than in the Spanish-American War. Four Navy nurses were wounded during a Viet Cong attack on the Brink Bachelor Officers' Quarters and became the

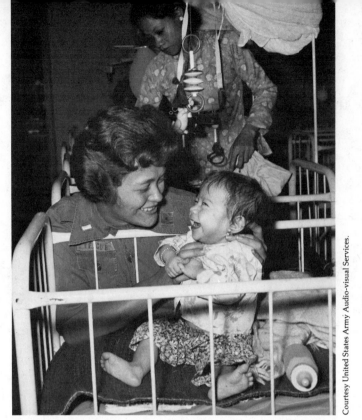

Courtesy United States Army Audio-visual Services.

Army nurse Shirley Teague of Houston, Texas, with a Vietnamese baby at the Sien Hoa Orphanage.

A new development in military nursing: Lieutenant Jeffrey C. Miller and his wife Joan both became members of the Navy Nurse Corps.

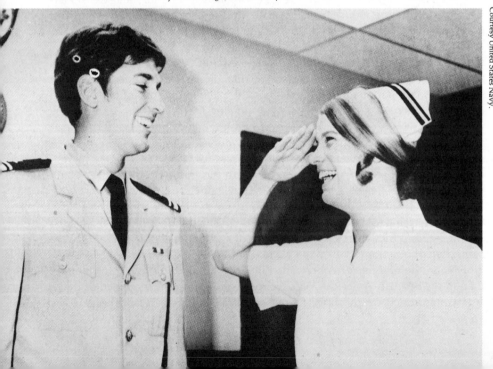

Courtesy United States Navy.

first women members of the armed forces to receive the Purple Heart for injuries sustained in Vietnam. In September, 1966, Navy Nurse Corps officers were assigned to Danang. The Navy hospital at Danang had become the largest combat-casualty treatment facility in the world. Designed originally as a 60-bed facility, it soon expanded to comprise 600 beds and eventually admitted more than 70,000 patients.

Two veteran hospital ships, U.S.S. *Repose* and *Sanctuary*, provided direct medical support, particularly to those units engaged in amphibious operations. *Repose* arrived at its assigned station in Vietnam in February, 1966, and was joined by *Sanctuary* on April 12, 1967. Both ships were staffed with highly specialized personnel (including 30 nurses aboard each), were equipped with the most modern medical equipment, and had the capability to provide optimal medical care to the wounded. The hospital ships offered many advantages over fixed medical facilities, including versatility, mobility, a better environment, more efficient use of medical personnel, and greater support in amphibious operations. Although responsible mainly for providing medical service support to Navy and Marine Corps personnel, the ships dispensed aid to all combat arms, and 28 percent of the workload involved patients other than members of the naval service.

A Congressional bill authorizing appointment of male nurses to the regular forces of the Air Force, Army, and Navy Nurse Corps was signed by the President on September 20, 1966, and the roster of male nurses in all the services soon multiplied. By the close of the 1967 fiscal year, 1032 male Army Nurse Corps officers made up 22 percent of the Army's nursing total. About half were in the clinical nursing specialties of anesthesia, operating room, and neuropsychiatry.

Meanwhile, the build-up of American forces in South Vietnam continued: by May, 1965, troop strength had increased to 35,000; by January, 1966, to more than 180,000; by December, to 380,000; and by the end of 1967, to nearly 500,000. As the fighting and the number of American casualties escalated, large-scale protests against the war erupted at home. Thousands of protesters marched in Washington in October, 1967, and hundreds were arrested trying to storm the Pentagon. Although student unrest erupted into violence on campuses all across the country, nursing students in general did not become involved. Despite mass protests at home, American troop commitment in Vietnam soon came to surpass the peak reached in Korea 25 years earlier.

The peculiar nature of counterinsurgency operations in Vietnam required modification of the usual concepts of hospital usage in a combat area. Because the Viet Cong, employing classic guerrilla strategy, declined to engage in set-piece battles against large enemy units, there was no "front" in the traditional sense. In reaction, American strategy dictated partitioning of the country into separate field zones, each patrolled from a central camp (fire base). Isolated, dependent upon helicopter supply, the base camps, normally tranquil, were prey to night attack and envelopment by light infantry. Thus, with few exceptions, no large, dramatic battles took place during the Vietnam war.

Semipermanent, air-conditioned, fully equipped hospitals were constructed in Vietnam. In contrast to World War II and Korea, when overrun territory could be occupied and held, the Vietnam-era hospital could not follow in direct support of tactical operations. Operating on much the same principles as the fire base, all the Army hospitals in Vietnam, including MUST (Medical Unit, Self-contained, Transportable) units, were fixed installations assigned to area-support missions. Since there was no secure road network in the combat areas of Vietnam, ground evacuation of the wounded was almost impossible.

Despite the obstacles, never before in the history of warfare had wounded received such complete, rapid health care. Even with the multitude of problems involved, including those of terrain and climate, almost 99 percent of the soldiers hospitalized for wounds, diseases, and injuries recovered, and about 90 percent returned to duty. Because of the courage and skill of nurses, physicians, medics, helicopter and ambulance personnel, a soldier wounded in the jungles or rice paddies of Vietnam stood a much better chance of surviving, with the possibility of complete recovery, than the soldier in Korea or in any earlier war.

The ability of medical personnel to adapt recent medical advances to the situation in Vietnam showed clearly in statistics. For example, of all those Americans wounded and hospitalized in World War II, 4.5 percent died. The percentage had been reduced to 2.5 during the Korean conflict. In Vietnam, this was down to about 1.5 percent, marking a significant increase in the number of lives spared.

Between January, 1965, and December, 1970, 133,447 wounded were admitted to Army medical treatment facilities in Vietnam; 97,659 of these were admitted to hospitals. The hospital mortality rate for this period was 2.6 percent. The very slight increase in hospital mortality in Vietnam over that in Korea (2.5 percent) was identified as the result of rapid helicopter evacuation, which brought into the hospital mortally wounded patients who by earlier, slower means of evacuation would have died en route. If one assumes that most of the hospitalized patients who died within the first 24 hours belonged to this class, the true rate would perhaps be much closer to 1 percent. The average length of stay per case for patients in Vietnam was considerably less than in earlier conflicts, amounting to 63 days, compared to 75 days for those in World War II.

Despite the constant threat of enemy attack, the highest quality of nursing care was given. All the hospitals, from the northern highlands at Pleiku to the delta town of Vung Tau, were vulnerable to mortar, rocket, and small arms fire. Several, such as the Forty-fifth Surgical Hospital at Tay Ninh, the Third Field Hospital in Saigon, and the Twelfth Evacuation Hospital at Chu Chi, were hit one or more times. First Lieutenant Sharon Anne Lane was killed by hostile fire on June 8, 1969, while on duty at the 312th Evacuation Hospital at Chu Lai.

The degree of sophistication of medical equipment and facilities everywhere in Vietnam permitted Army nurses and physicians to make full use of their

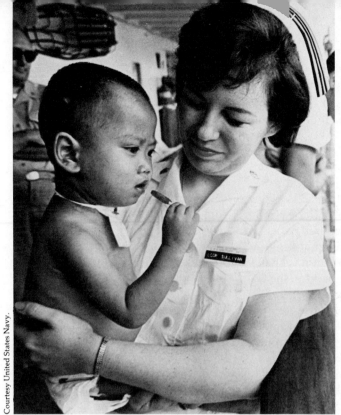

Navy nurse with a hospitalized Vietnamese baby.

First Lieutenant Kathie M. Weber administers intravenous fluid to Private Robert J. Vanaman, Company D, First Battalion, Seventh Cavalry Regiment, at the Twenty-fourth Evacuation Hospital at Long Binh, South Vietnam.

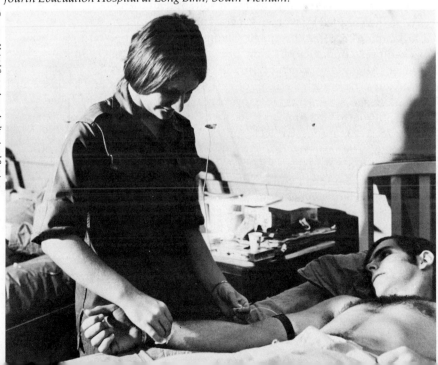

training and capability. As a result, the care that was available in Army hospitals in Vietnam was far better than any that had ever been generally available for combat support. It was now possible to take a wounded man from the field to a hospital facility, perform surgery, close his wounds, and transport him to a hospital in the continental United States within the same time it had taken to move a patient from France to a British hospital during World War I.

It became routine to travel from Clark Air Force Base in the Philippines to Andrews Air Force Base in Washington, D.C., in the same time it had taken a World War II casualty to be removed from the field to an aid station. It was possible to have an injured patient in a well-equipped operating room with up-to-date resuscitation equipment within 20 minutes from the time of injury. It was also possible to remove a patient 8000 miles from his point of injury to a definitive-treatment point in the United States within 72 hours, having paused along the way for major surgery.

As the war became more unpopular at home, peace talks opened in Paris on January 18, 1969. American forces in South Vietnam had reached a peak of 543,400 in April. By April 3, American battle deaths totaled 33,641, surpassing by 12 the number killed in Korea. Withdrawal of American troops began in July, and soon thereafter President Nixon announced a Vietnamization policy that would transfer the burden of fighting to South Vietnamese (ARVN) forces.

As the 1970s began, the federal government began to encourage women to play fuller roles in American society and to become more important in the extension of national policy. In June, 1970, Anna Mae Hays, Chief of the Army Nurse Corps, was promoted to the rank of brigadier general. Nurses were indeed proud to welcome General Hayes as the Corps' first general officer and as one of the first two women in American history to have attained that rank. The Navy and Air Force soon followed suit, and all the military nursing services were then headed by women generals or an admiral.

On January 25, 1972, President Nixon disclosed that secret peace negotiations had been conducted since the previous June by Secretary of State Henry Kissinger. After many interruptions, talks resumed January 8, 1973, and President Nixon ordered a halt to all offensive military operations against North Vietnam. Peace agreements were formally signed in Paris by the United States, North and South Vietnam, and the Viet Cong. A cease-fire was effected on January 28, 1973, and nearly 1600 American POWs were released by the North Vietnamese. The last American troops left Vietnam on March 29, officially ending any direct American military role. There had been 46,079 American combat deaths, and the number of wounded totaled 304,000, the latter figure exceeded only during World War II.

Nurses in Veterans Administration Hospitals noted that the uniqueness of the Vietnam War produced feelings in its veterans not experienced by veterans of other wars. No sooner had young recruits arrived in Vietnam than they became aware of the futility of American intervention. There was widespread resistance to fighting, extensive drug usage, and racial conflict among American troops. Profound guilt, feelings of stasis, impotence, psychic numbness, and a deeply embedded antiestablishment anger were common.

Coronary Care Nursing

Meanwhile, a new role for the nurse in attacking heart disease, one of the nation's leading causes of death, had been developed under a Division of Nursing research grant during the mid-1960s. Remarkable success was achieved in an experimental coronary unit set up at Presbyterian Hospital in Philadelphia. The essence of the project was to put myocardial infarction patients under continuous monitoring by electrocardiographs, with specially prepared nurses providing needed intervention, without delay, until a physician could be summoned. Co-principal investigators for the project, Rose Pinneo, R.N., and Lawrence E. Meltzer, M.D., reported that "the nurse is the most important factor in the coronary care unit—even more important than the doctor or electronic equipment." They pointed out that nearly one-third of all patients who were admitted to hospitals following an acute heart attack died during the period of hospitalization. They reported:

The system of intensive coronary care was conceived with the knowledge that as many as 40 percent of these deaths could be prevented if the potentially fatal attacks were detected instantly (by means of cardiac monitors) and treatment begun within a minute or two of their onset . . . . It is essential, therefore, that trained personnel be present

Nurses giving care in the Intensive Care/Coronary Care Pavilion at the Norwalk Hospital, Connecticut.

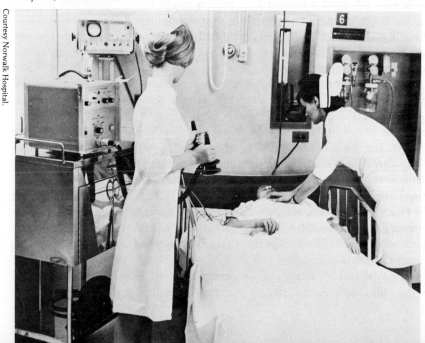

constantly so that life-threatening problems can be recognized and terminated before they are fatal . . . . We are convinced that nurses must assume this role. Our research unit was set up with the understanding that nurses would be taught not only to identify various derangements in heart rhythms from an electrocardiogram, but also to understand the treatment for each disorder. With such knowledge, in emergency situations she [the nurse] could be expected to initiate treatment, and if necessary, perform life-saving techniques—such as electric countershock—by herself. Unless the nurse is capable of undertaking these extraordinary duties and responsibilities, intensive coronary care has limited value [8].

The success of this experiment was underlined by the widespread acceptance of coronary care units by hospitals all across the nation.

Changes in Hospital Construction

During this time, hospital construction was undergoing marked changes. Most earlier hospital buildings had been built in urban centers. Postwar attention and federal assistance had been focused on rural shortages, leaving urban projects with low priorities. Physical deterioration and functional obsolescence had moved slowly but inevitably upon the older city hospitals. In many urban situations the problem had been intensified by population movement from the urban center to the suburbs, by industrial, commercial, and transportation changes, and by urban redevelopment. In 1960 a Public Health Service survey estimated the cost of modernizing or replacing obsolete general and mental facilities, *without* the addition of more beds, at $3.6 billion. This estimate was nearly four times the actual cost level of annual construction and modernization. The problem was particularly grave in the many metropolitan areas where hospitals had been unable to replace worn-out buildings and equipment. The 1960 survey indicated a cost of $2.2 billion solely for the modernization or replacement of general hospital facilities in metropolitan communities.

The Hill-Burton Act of 1946 had originally authorized state grants for surveying the needs and plans for construction of medical facilities, with authorized matching grants ranging from one-third to two-thirds of the construction and equipment costs. Since then, the Act has been amended four times to meet the changing needs of the nation's hospital system. In 1949 authorization was given for research, grants, experiments, and demonstrations relating to the effective use of hospital services, facilities, and resources. Specific authority to give grants for the construction of public and nonprofit nursing homes, diagnostic and treatment centers, rehabilitation centers, and chronic disease hospitals followed in 1954, and in 1958 authority was extended to permit eligible sponsors of projects to receive loans rather than grants. In October, 1961, the Public Health Service was authorized to increase appropriations for construction of nursing homes from $10 million to $20 million annually and to broaden the research program to include experimental and demonstration construction and equipment projects.

The Hospital and Medical Facilities Amendments of 1964, frequently referred to as the Hill-Harris Amendments, changed the Act in order to follow more

closely the changing concepts of hospital planning, construction, and operation. In addition to extending the program for five years, or up until fiscal
year 1970, the amendments established grants for the modernization and
replacement of health facilities, giving special consideration to hospitals situated
in urban areas. In the first fiscal year the grants totaled $20 million, with $35
million authorized for projects during the second year. This recognition of the
need to modernize and replace health facilities marked a shift in emphasis for
the Hill-Burton program, which, from its inception, had put priority on the
construction of facilities in rural areas where, in many instances, none had
existed previously.

To a degree not often true of federal health programs, the Hill-Burton program
came close to fulfilling its originally stated objectives. In the years between
1946 and 1970, it became increasingly apparent that those original objectives no
longer represented the real needs. A series of problems with the Hill-Burton
program could be recognized, some the result of particular Hill-Burton provisions and others the result of changes in society or in the organization and
financing of health services. A few of the more specific problems were:

A lack of effective planning and regionalization permitted the construction of too many
hospital beds in some locations and the overelaboration of services provided by many
other facilities.

The matching requirements for grants often prevented the construction of hospitals
high on the state's priority list because of lack of matching funds in poorer communities.

Improvements in transportation and the out-migration of population from rural areas
made surplus many of the small rural hospitals constructed under the program's original
priorities.

The establishment of need based on bed population ratios for large population aggregates
failed to recognize the variations in utilization of facilities within a community or of
particular services within an institution.

The use of a formula for establishing need based in part on the counting of current patient-days ignored the mounting evidence of an excess of acute hospital beds in some
areas.

The spread of third-party payment coverage for hospital costs made it possible for most
institutions to go directly to the capital market for construction financing, thereby
obviating much of the impact of Hill-Burton state plans on the distribution of facilities.

The emphasis in current health policies on reducing unnecessary hospital utilization in
order to moderate the increase of health care costs led to proposals for rationing the
supply of hospital beds as a means of controlling utilization [9].

Dilemmas in Health Care

Annual national health expenditures in the late 1960s approached $50 billion,
a figure representing roughly 6 percent of the gross national product and, pro-
portionally, the largest national health expenditure in the world. No other
nation spent so high a proportion of its gross national product on health. In
Sweden and the United Kingdom, so-called welfare states, the proportion of

the GNP directed to health was only 4.5 percent and 3.5 percent, respectively. Notwithstanding the large outlay, the pattern of financing in the United States had been predominantly private. Since the 1930s, the share from public sources had remained fairly steady at about one-quarter of the total amount. This relationship was altered as a result of Medicare and Medicaid, which increased the government's contributions to total health outlays from 26 percent in 1966 to 34 percent in 1967.

Unnecessary duplication of hospital and medical facilities was evident. The director of New York's Montefiore Hospital stated that the City had twice as many centers for cardiac surgery as it needed, with results that were "astronomical" financially and "miserable" qualitatively. According to the President's Commission on Heart Disease, Cancer, and Strokes, 30 percent of the 777 hospitals equipped to do closed heart surgery had had no such cases during the year studied. Of the 548 that had cases, 87 percent had fewer than one operation a week and 41 percent had fewer than one a month. Little of the surgery was of an emergency nature, and the mortality rate was higher in the institutions that performed such surgery relatively rarely—leading some to speculate that the reason for this might be that some of the expensive specialized units were not

More sophisticated hospital facilities, such as intensive care units, were less available to people in rural America.

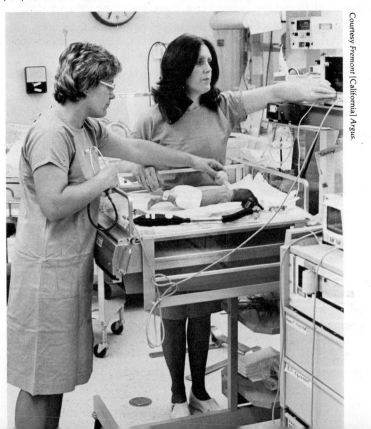

large enough or busy enough to give the staff practice in required techniques.

Over the years, most of the population of the United States had shifted to cities and towns. In 1910 about 65 percent of all Americans had lived in rural areas; by the 1960s, about 70 percent of all Americans lived in urban areas. Apart from congestion and pollution of the environment, perhaps the most serious problem associated with urbanization was that health services tended to be disproportionately concentrated and became less available to rural people. In the country, illness and disability had higher incidence rates, and, in terms of income, people living there could not afford the cost of health care. Because of the great middle-class exodus to the suburbs, many of the nation's cities had become ghettos for the poor, the aged, the uneducated, and other disadvantaged groups. Generally speaking, these groups could not afford to pay for health care and were frightened of, and discouraged from, seeking it.

The Passing of the Old Country Doctor

In earlier times, when most physicians were general practitioners and most graduate nurses served as private duty specialists; when physician and nurse had known firsthand each personal and family history, they had been able to function reasonably well by treating their patients symptomatically, by supporting morale, and by observing the injunction "First do no harm." There had been few barriers to access to the physician and the nurse who knew their patients and who were concerned with their needs and how they related to family and community. People did not expect miracles. They knew that tuberculosis and lobar pneumonia were dreadful diseases with high mortality rates; they knew that there was little that one could do about the childhood killers; and, in a prevailing spirit of fatalism toward those natural calamities, they accepted them, knowing that their physician and nurse were doing all that could be done.

The picture of the family doctor and the private duty nurse had become idealized during the early decades of the century. The image of this "golden age" persisted in a nostalgic wish to return to the era of the family doctor and the private duty nurse—good and all-knowing advisers embodied in countless novels, movies, and television shows.

The epitome of this image was forever implanted in the public conscience by the exploits of the radio and motion picture series, *Dr. Christian*, starring Jean Hersholt. The radio series which introduced Dr. Paul Christian to the public began on CBS network in the 1937 season, and the half-hour show was heard every Wednesday night at 10 P.M. for fifteen years. It was estimated that the show attracted a weekly listening audience of 20 million.

Like the radio series, the group of six black-and-white feature films centered around beloved Dr. Christian's practice in River's End, Minnesota, a storybook, small midwestern town filled with all the homey virtues and stereotypes of pre-World War II America. Devoted to humanitarian causes, the wise Dr. Christian was not only a superb country doctor (with almost miraculous medical and surgical prowess) but also an unflagging optimist as to the goodness of

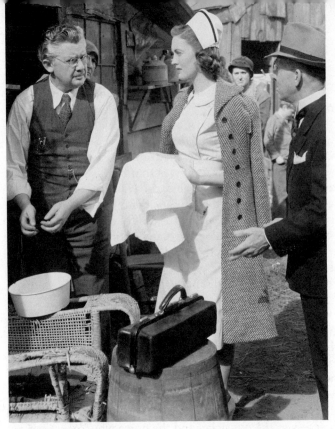

In The Courageous Dr. Christian, *the good doctor (Jean Hersholt) and his faithful nurse (Dorothy Lovett) effectively combat an epidemic of spinal meningitis among River's End squatters.*

mankind and the aspirations of his townfolk. Dr. Christian maintained a simple professional office at home, unhampered by neo-pharmaceutical equipment or smart medical terminology. Probably his most essential basic tool was the constantly stoked pipe which allowed him to puff and meditate on the ramifications of his patient's medical and emotional problems.

Medical practice in the United States had changed markedly since that time. The number of specialists had increased and the number of general practitioners had declined. Although, in 1934, 85 percent of all practicing physicians had been general practitioners, only 45 percent filled this role in 1960 and only 37 percent in 1965. By the late 1960s, society had numerous medical specialists such as internists, pediatricians, obstetricians, gynecologists, ophthalmologists, radiologists, pathologists, neurologists, and more in over 30 other specialties.

Although the trend toward specialization produced many benefits, a widely held opinion maintained that the loss of general practitioners had created problems in the delivery of health services. The concept of the family physician's office as the center for primary health care was no longer believed to be compatible with modern medicine. The physician of the 1960s felt that he needed ready, almost-immediate access to laboratory, radiologic, and other sophisticated facilities if he was to deliver high-quality medical care. Psychological needs of the patient, however, were not met as physicians concentrated their energies on biological aspects of diagnosis and treatment and referred the patient from one specialist to another, leaving little or no time to deal with patient problems in the psychosocial domain.

The nurse of the 1960s was imbued with the concept of comprehensive care of patients during her educational program but found upon graduation that time and system constraints made it difficult, if not impossible, for her to fully meet the psychosocial needs of her patients. Sometimes even physical needs had to be ignored because of limited staff. Following in the trend that had been existent since the early 1950s, the professional nurse's time was increasingly being consumed with administrative routine. Many of the nurse's traditional duties had been delegated to licensed practical nurses, to nurses' aides, and to a host of newly developed specialized health care workers such as respiratory therapists. Fragmented nursing and medical care prevailed and the patient suffered the consequences. Furthermore, as nurses began to be offered fewer opportunities for direct patient care and clinical decision-making, their personal satisfaction diminished. Many nurses felt a need to reclaim their professionalism in patient care and to reestablish the right and the opportunity to make, and act upon, clinical decisions.

Nurses needed to reclaim their professionalism in patient care.

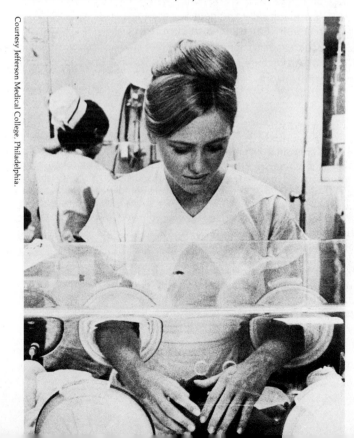

Need for Role Realignment

The gradual evolution of the nurse's role strained her traditional relationship with the physician. Many physicians seemed unaware of nursing's move toward professionalization; or if they were aware, they often ignored it in their working relationships with nurses. To fulfill the component of a profession, the professional person had to exercise independent judgment within his or her work; the function of professional education was to prepare the person to exercise such judgment. But many physicians still expected nurses to behave only as obedient extensions of their own professional judgment. The fiction seemed to be that the nurse was just the physician's helper.

So on the one hand, schools of nursing and professional nursing associations reinforced the nurses' self-image of an autonomous, professional person, sharing with substantial equality in appropriate judgments about health care. Yet, on the other hand, physicians, reinforced perhaps by neglect of the study of nursing, if not by contrary indoctrination within their professional education, ignored or controverted this image of the professional person and colleague that many nurses presented. The results were inner tension within nurses and resentment, if not open conflict. The physician generally had little interest in seeing the optimal utilization of the full potentialities and skills of the nurse. He wanted an assistant who would do what he told her to do. The physician wanted to make use of an extra pair of eyes and ears and hands, but he was not concerned with developing a pattern of work which would allow the maximum combined output of a nurse and himself to achieve better health care for patients.

There was general agreement that the health care delivery system must be massively reorganized to increase efficiency and control soaring costs. In 1967 the Report of the National Advisory Commission on Health Manpower summarized the case for reorganization:

Many of the serious problems discussed in this Report arise from the lack of an organizational framework for the multitude of disparate elements which provide medical care. Close cooperation and coordination among them is rare, and duplication of effort and actual conflict are all too common. Unfortunately, consumers of health care are unable to make the informed judgments required to assure an effectively operating market, and the sense of responsibility of most health professionals takes the form of concern for the individual patient rather than for society as a whole. As a result, there is limited effort to assure that resources are effectively coordinated and applied where they will be most useful.

In spite of the great complexity of modern medical care, independent practitioners and institutions continue to dominate the system. Individual practice has survived in medicine because it has features which are attractive both to the physician and to the public. We appreciate the advantages of independence but we are concerned about some of its associated disadvantages. Inadequate communication, coordination, and control links among practitioners and institutions contribute to gaps in quality and distribution, as well as to the inflation of medical costs [10].

Broadening the Talent Base

While there had been an impressive increase in the number of nurses with preparation for leadership during the 1960s, they were still in very short supply when considered in relation to the needs. These were the nurses responsible for teaching in all types of programs, for planning and directing the care given by all nursing personnel, for providing specialized care, and for the nursing research that would improve nursing practice and education. These were the nurses who would determine the quality of nursing care patients received. Only 111,000 of the 748,000 registered nurses in practice in 1972 had at least a bachelor's degree. Of this group, those prepared at the master's level or above were only 2.9 percent of the total employed registered nurses. Unlike that of other health professions, the cost of nursing education was not offset by one's eventual earning capacity. Since *federal* traineeships were awarded only for full-time academic study, nurses generally had to drop out of the work force to seek a master's degree. Virtually all had continuing financial obligations and many had responsibility for support of dependents.

A major thrust during the late 1960s and early 1970s was an attempt to broaden the base of potential nurses through recruitment efforts directed at minority groups, disadvantaged youth, men, and others who had not formerly considered nursing as a career. Education beyond high school was not a realistic goal for groups of people with low and moderate incomes. For these individuals, education was the way to enhance their self-image and raise their socioeconomic levels. To recruit successfully from this group, schools of nursing had to develop programs flexible enough to assist students who learned with difficulty

Federal scholarships and loans helped to broaden the base of recruits into nursing.

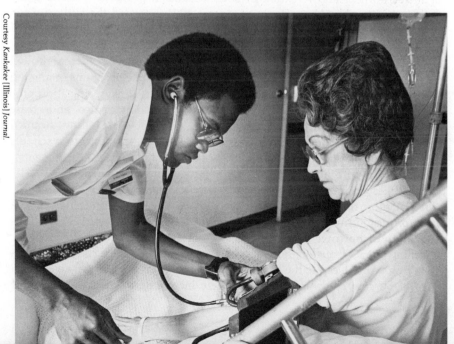

because of inadequate elementary and high school education. Imaginative ways to interest these young people in nursing, early counseling, remedial and tutorial work that began in high school and continued through the nursing curriculum—all helped to increase the number of practicing nurses.

The rising expense of education placed an increasing burden on the students and their families. Many highly motivated and well-qualified students were prohibited from pursuing a career in the health fields because of the expense involved. With the increasing need for nurses, it was unfortunate that any qualified student should be turned away for economic reasons.

The Nursing Educational Opportunities Grants (scholarships) had been authorized by amendment in 1966 and initiated in the summer of 1967. During the two years of the program, grants were awarded to an estimated 15,900 students who could not otherwise attend a school of nursing. The individual grants ranged from $200 to $800. The average grant was $530. The awards totaled $8.4 million.

The Health Manpower Act of 1968, Title II, had established a new program of scholarship grants to schools of nursing for full-time students of exceptional need. It provided greater support for the student than had the nursing educational opportunity grants and allowed the school greater flexibility in helping meet the student's need. The maximum annual amount of scholarship support a student could receive was $1500. No matching funds were required. The legislation provided no specific authorization of funds as the allocation formula was based on enrollment. In 1971, 64 percent of all programs awarded scholarships to 10 percent of all enrolled students. Eighty-six percent of the students who were awarded scholarships came from families whose gross annual income was less than $10,000. The availability of scholarships remained a critical factor in recruitment and retention of students and in programs providing for career mobility. The Nurse Training Act of 1971 extended the authority for scholarships and increased the maximum student scholarship per year to $2000 and revised the formula for scholarship grants to schools.

Meanwhile, the nursing student loan program had assisted students enrolled in diploma, associate degree, baccalaureate, and graduate programs of nursing education. The program had begun in 1965 with 426 nursing education programs participating. In 1971 an estimated 943 programs participated, an increase of 121 percent in six years. In the same period, the number of students awarded loans increased from 3645 in 1965 (3 percent of the total enrollments in schools of nursing) to an estimated 24,443 in 1971 (14 percent of the total enrollments). Seventy-seven percent of the students awarded nursing student loans came from families whose gross family income was less than $10,000.

In 1970 more than 5400 borrowers were taking advantage of the loan cancellation provision through full-time employment as registered nurses. With the graduation of borrowers from schools of nursing, the number of borrowers cancelling loans through employment had more than doubled each of the previous two years. Despite the benefits of this program, educational costs in all types of nursing education programs were increasing beyond the ability of students to meet them from their own or from their family's resources. The availability of this financial assistance was essential in making it possible for more individuals to enter and remain in schools of nursing.

The years from the mid-1960s to the early 1970s, dominated by the domestic and foreign conflicts brought about by the Vietnam War, were years of controversy for the nursing profession as well. The issue of medical care for the aged saw the ANA clash with the AMA, while the ANA position paper on education for nursing brought to a crisis the deep-seated dispute over the future role of traditional hospital diploma programs. Although Congress accelerated its efforts to increase the supply of nurses, shortages continued unabated as the enlarged arena of health care created thousands of new nursing jobs.

Summary

Hospitals of the mid-1960s had evolved into a complex technological industry. Major national health problems centered around chronic conditions such as heart disease and cancer, a major shift from the overriding concern over contagious disease at the beginning of the century.

The American health care system was distorted from its ideal configuration. Overuse of hospitals was due in part to the greater insurance coverage for hospital stays and to the convenience of a central location for the physician's work. Fee-for-service financing and high costs of medical care acted as obstacles to early initiation of health care, particularly among low-income families.

Congressional deliberations over various forms of national health insurance continued throughout the 1950s. The Forand bill proposed that Old Age Survivors Insurance be extended to cover the hospitalization costs of its recipients and was supported by the ANA. Although the bill was defeated, it opened the way for the eventual passage of Medicare and Medicaid in 1965.

The 1965 ANA position paper stated that nursing education programs should be situated in colleges or universities and intensified the controversy over the future of the hospital diploma program.

The number of diploma programs was falling rapidly while associate degree and baccalaureate programs were on the increase. American hospitals spent an estimated $250 million per year to operate diploma schools of nursing.

In 1968 the Nurse Training Act of 1964 was extended for two years (July, 1969–June, 1971), with authorized appropriations of $260 million for continued programs of loans and scholarships, construction, special projects and traineeships.

The Vietnam War was characterized by a shortage of nurses. The Army Student Nurse Program, initiated in 1956, formed the major source of new Army Nurse Corps officers during the early phases of the Vietnam conflict. In 1964 the establishment of the Walter Reed Army Institute of Nursing soon yielded an additional supply of baccalaureate-prepared nurses to meet military and civilian needs.

By the end of 1967, American troops in Vietnam had increased to almost 500,000. The peculiar nature of counterinsurgency warfare dictated modification of the military hospital from a mobile unit to a semipermanent structure. The Vietnam War-wounded received more effective nursing and medical care than in any previous war, as reflected in the all-time low mortality rates.

A research project supported by the Division of Nursing, United States Public Health Service, pioneered a new nursing role in coronary care. Coronary care units soon became an important service in most larger hospitals throughout the country.

Because postwar attention had been focused on rural hospital shortages, many urban hospitals underwent deterioration and gradual obsolence. The Hill-Burton Act of 1946 and its amendments authorized grants for hospital and nursing home construction. The Hill-Harris Amendments in 1964 gave special consideration to urban hospitals.

Annual health expenditures in the late 1960s soared to $50 billion, 6 percent of the Gross National Product. No other nation spent as high a proportion of its GNP on health yet many health needs of the American population were not being met, particularly those of inner city and rural dwellers.

Increases in medical specialization and decreases in the number of general practitioners created a dependence on larger, centralized facilities. Gone were the days of the reliable old country doctor and the ever-present private duty nurse.

Nurses became increasingly more involved in management activities and less involved in direct patient care. An opportunity for nurses to reclaim their former professionalism in patient care was beginning to emerge as part of the increasing recognition that massive reorganization would be necessary in the health care delivery system.

With federal assistance, a concerted effort was made to recruit more minority students into nursing. This program yielded a marked increase in minority representation and helped enhance the effectiveness of nursing education and practice.

References

1. American Medical Association, House of Delegates, *Proceedings of the 105th Annual Session of the House of Delegates, June, 1957* (Chicago: American Medical Association, 1957), pp. 15–24.
2. "Taking a Stand," *American Journal of Nursing*, vol. 59 (September, 1959): 1245.
3. *Congressional Record*, July 9, 1965.
4. "American Nurses' Association's First Position on Education for Nursing," *American Journal of Nursing*, vol. 66 (March, 1966): 515–517.
5. *Ibid.*, pp. 516–517.
6. National League for Nursing, *Study on Cost of Nursing Education. Part I. Cost of Basic Diploma Programs* (New York: The League, 1964), pp. 1–7.
7. U.S. Congress, House, Committee on Interstate and Foreign Commerce, Subcommittee on Public Health and Welfare, Ninetieth Congress, Second Session. *Health Manpower Act of 1968*. Hearings before the Subcommittee. (Washington, D.C.: Government Printing Office, 1968), pp. 41–43.
8. *Philadelphia Inquirer*, June 18, 1967.
9. U.S. Congress, Senate, *National Health Planning and Development and Health Facilities Assistance Act of 1974*. Report on S. 2994, November 12, 1974. (Washington, D.C.: Government Printing Office, 1974), pp. 19–25.
10. U.S. President, National Advisory Commission on Health Manpower, *Report of the National Advisory Commission on Health Manpower* (Washington, D.C.: Government Printing Office, 1967), Vol. 1, p. 72.

20
Toward a New Era in Nursing

As the 1970s dawned, health was still the third largest industry in the United States. In 1970 it occupied 5 percent of the nonmilitary labor force—4.5 million people—an 80 percent increase from 1960. The principal increase had been in the number of nurses and allied health professionals. This phenomenal growth had occurred largely in hospitals, which employed 60 percent of all health care workers. In 1910 each physician had been supported by two other health care workers. In 1970 each physician had 11. Hospitals had once managed with sometimes fewer than two employees per bed; in 1970 in many of the medical centers there were four, five, or even more.

Nurses in the 1970s
In 1972 the number of practicing registered nurses had reached 778,000—228,000 more than the number in practice before passage of the Nurse Training Act in 1964. Since publication in 1963 of the report *Toward Quality in Nursing*, the number of registered nurses with bachelor's degrees had increased by 90 percent and those with master's degrees by 70 percent. Those with doctorates had doubled to a total of more than 700. More than 500,000 nurses were working in hospitals, about 54,000 were employed in nursing homes and related institutions. Approximately 39,000 were private duty nurses caring for patients in hospitals and private homes, and about 52,000 were office nurses. Public health nurses in government agencies, schools, visiting nurse associations, and clinics numbered more than 69,000; nurse educators in nursing schools, about 29,000; and occupational health nurses in industry, approximately 19,000. Most of the others were on the staffs of state boards or other professional nurse associations or were employed by research organizations. More than one-fourth of all nurses employed worked part-time.

In the late 1940s and early 1950s women were interested primarily in the home, husband, and children, and only secondarily in careers. Under these circumstances professional ambition was scarcely evident in the nurse. The "feminine mystique" which pressured nurses to remain at home, produced a sense of guilt in those who were gainfully employed, especially if they enjoyed working. Popular women's magazines contributed greatly to this feminine

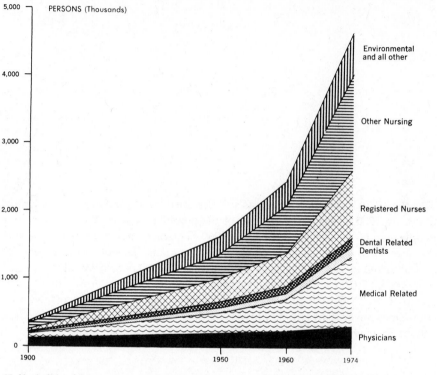

PERSONS (Thousands)

5,000

4,000

Environmental
and all other

3,000

Other Nursing

2,000

Registered Nurses

Dental Related
Dentists

1,000

Medical Related

Physicians

0

1900   1950   1960   1974

Half of all health care personnel provided nursing related services in the early 1970s.

image by limiting the subject matter of articles to home and family and by refusing to admit that women had any interest in outside affairs. Adolescent
daughters who were also exposed to the views put forth in these magazines
generally accepted the feminine role as centered entirely around husband and
children, with no place left for a career.

Yet between 1947 and 1972 the female labor force almost doubled, increasing
from 16.7 million to over 32 million. During the same period the adult female
noninstitutional population increased by only about 40 percent, from 52 million
to 74 million, a statistic which indicated that the numbers of women with gainful employment were increasing at a pace far exceeding the overall population
growth. Participation by women in the labor force followed an uneven pattern
during the postwar years. Between 1947 and 1960 the female labor force grew
by about 6.5 million. About two-thirds of this expansion reflected a greater
propensity for working among women between the ages of 35 and 64, with the
sharpest increase shown among women 45 to 54 years of age or among those
whose childbearing and childrearing tasks were finished. This growth of participation in the labor force by older women was also consistent with the rapidly
rising demand for workers in female-dominated occupations such as teaching,
clerical work, and nursing. Women in their middle years were the principal

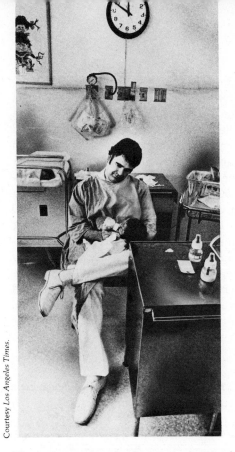

The nation was employing more nurses to look after patients than ever before. Nurse Tom Walsh feeding baby at County-USC Medical Center.

group responding to that demand.

Virtually all the increases in female employment between 1960 and 1971 were in either white collar or service sectors, continuing the patterns established between 1947 and 1960. The growth in the female labor force between 1960 and 1971 amounted to over nine million, fully one-third larger than the increase during the preceding 13 years. Significantly, women under 25 accounted for one-half of this increase, indicating that the postwar baby-boom generation had reached working age. These figures revealed that women were now much more interested in working and in avoiding interruptions in their careers.

The desire to be home with their children was a prime reason why many nurses were inactive, according to a research study supported by the United States Public Health Service, Division of Nursing. The results of a questionnaire answered by some 10,000 registered-but-inactive nurses in 12 states showed that most nurses believed that "a mother should be in the home while her children are young." The second most important reason for inactivity among nurses was the difficulty in making suitable arrangements for care of children. Other major reasons included low salaries and inability to arrange working hours compatible with domestic responsibilities. This study, conducted in cooperation with the state boards of nurse examiners, found that

4500 respondents expected to return to nursing, either full-time or part-time. The majority of those who intended to return within the next three years hoped to take refresher courses. The Division of Nursing suggested that working schedules be developed to allow for the part-time availability of nurses and that day-care centers be established for preschool and school-age children. In 1969 the Division of Nursing made available nearly $1.5 million for refresher training activities in order to increase the number of professional nurses returning annually to active practice from 20,000 to 30,000 by 1973.

Male nurses continued to represent a very small minority. Although in 1970 they constituted less than 2 percent of the nation's nursing force, increasing proportions of the students admitted to schools of nursing were male: 1.7 percent for the 1962–1963 academic year, 5.5 percent for 1971–1972. The majority of the males (2444) entered associate degree programs; 1340 enrolled in three-year diploma programs, and 1386 entered baccalaureate programs. The 1694 men of the 51,784 students who graduated in 1972 were four times the total number of males who had graduated in 1963.

Graduations from Programs of Nursing, 1953–1976, and Percentage Change from Preceding Year.

Year	Diploma	%	AD	%	BS	%	Total	%
1953	26,824		260		2171		29,255	
1954	25,797	− 3.8	344	+32.3	2352	+ 8.3	28,493	− 2.6
1955	25,826	+ 0.1	199	−42.2	2648	+12.6	28,673	+ 0.6
1956	26,828	+ 3.9	252	+26.6	3109	+17.4	30,189	+ 5.3
1957	26,141	− 2.6	276	+ 9.5	3478	+11.9	29,895	− 1.0
1958	26,314	+ 0.7	425	+54.0	3650	+ 4.9	30,389	+ 1.7
1959	25,907	− 1.5	462	+ 8.7	3943	+ 8.0	30,312	− 0.3
1960	25,188	− 2.8	789	+70.8	4136	+ 4.9	30,113	− 0.7
1961	25,311	+ 0.5	917	+16.2	4039	− 2.4	30,267	+ 0.5
1962	25,727	+ 1.6	1159	+26.4	4300	+ 6.5	31,186	+ 3.0
1963	26,438	+ 2.8	1479	+27.6	4481	+ 4.2	32,398	+ 3.9
1964	28,238	+ 6.8	1962	+32.6	5059	+12.9	35,259	+ 8.8
1965	26,795	− 5.1	2510	+27.9	5381	+ 6.4	34,686	− 1.6
1966	26,278	− 1.9	3349	+33.4	5498	+ 2.2	35,125	+ 1.3
1967	27,452	+ 4.5	4654	+39.0	6131	+11.5	38,237	+ 8.8
1968	28,197	+ 2.7	6213	+33.5	7145	+16.5	41,555	+ 8.7
1969	25,114	−10.9	8701	+40.0	8381	+17.3	42,196	+ 1.5
1970	22,285	−11.3	11,678	+34.2	9105	+ 8.6	43,068	+ 2.1
1971	22,334	+ 0.2	14,754	+26.3	9913	+ 8.9	47,001	+ 9.1
1972	21,592	− 3.3	19,165	+29.9	11,027	+11.2	51,784	+10.2
1973	21,445	− 0.7	24,850	+29.7	13,132	+19.2	59,427	+14.8
1974	21,280	− 0.8	29,299	+17.9	17,049	+29.8	67,628	+13.8
1975	21,673	+ 1.8	32,622	+11.3	20,241	+18.7	74,536	+10.2
1976	19,861	− 8.4	35,094	+ 7.6	22,678	+12.0	77,633	+ 4.2

Federal Dollars for Nursing

The federal government spent more than $380 million during the fiscal years 1965–1971 to promote the education of professional nurses. Students received about half of these funds, $123 million of which was allocated for loans and scholarships. About $68 million was awarded under the Professional Nurse Traineeship Program to 48,000 nurses to assist them in preparing for positions as teachers, supervisors, administrators, or clinical specialists. From 1965 to 1971 the annual number of nursing program graduates increased from 34,686 to 47,000. On January 1, 1972, there were about 748,000 nurses in practice, a ratio of 361 nurses to every 100,000 people.

Federal aid to schools of nursing also helped to increase the extent of professional nurse preparation and to improve its quality. The more than $97 million that was awarded during the fiscal years 1965–1971 to build, replace, modernize, expand, and equip educational facilities for nurses resulted in the addition of 6200 new first-year students and the maintenance of 20,000 others. Assisted by almost $34 million in federal funds during these years, nursing schools and

Federal assistance to schools of nursing and students increased both the quantity and quality of nurses. Associate degree nursing students at Palomar Community College, San Marcos, California, receive a course in Basic Principles of Aseptic Technique at Tri-City Hospital, Oceanside, California.

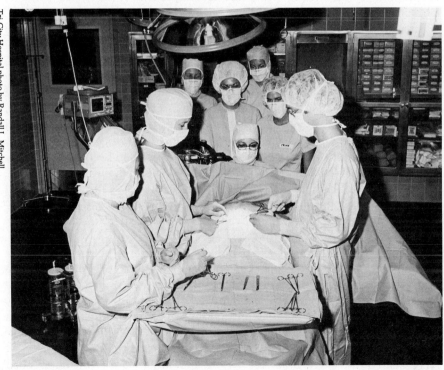

Tri-City Hospital photo by Randall L. Mitchell.

educational organizations undertook 343 special projects, among which were programs tailored to the needs of the disadvantaged and projects to recruit policemen and firefighters for nursing.

From the very beginning the Nixon administration displayed an unwillingness to take vigorous measures for extending the expensive federal nurse training program. Contrary to the President's policy decision to lump health manpower legislation into a single bill, the House Subcommittee on Public Health and Environment drafted two bills: the one pertaining only to nursing and the other to the remaining health professions. On July 12, 1971, the Senate Labor and Public Welfare Committee followed suit. Both bills subsequently passed the House and Senate by unanimous votes.

The three-year Nurse Training Act of 1971 authorized the following expenditures: $257 million for fiscal year 1972, $285 million for fiscal year 1973, and $313 million for fiscal year 1974, for a total of $855 million. By contrast, the combined seven-year authorizations under the Nurse Training Act of 1964 and the Health Manpower Act of 1968 had amounted to only $573 million. The new Act was designed to attack the nurse shortage. Especially welcome in the new program were capitation grants (based on an enrollment formula), which constituted the first large general support funds that most schools of nursing had obtained from the federal government. Although appropriations did not come close to matching the massive amounts authorized by the Act, they were at least maintained at a fairly respectable level, thanks to an aggressive ANA lobbying effort in Congress.

After the election of 1972, a landslide victory for President Nixon, the federal government began a concerted effort to downgrade and dismantle its educational programs for nursing. Under the direction of the new HEW Secretary, Caspar W. Weinberger, the Nixon administration adopted a reactionary policy toward nursing. Over $70 million of the 1973 nursing appropriation budget was illegally impounded by the President's Office of Management and Budget. This appropriation had been secured through the mechanism of Congressional continuing resolutions after President Nixon had twice vetoed the 1973 Labor-HEW appropriations bills. But even though the funds had been authorized by these continuing resolutions, the President refused to spend much of the money. Meanwhile, the President's 1974 budget declared that "categorical support for . . . nursing will be phased out. States and localities have the option to support these institutions with funds available through general revenue sharing" [1].

In short, federal support for nursing was scheduled to be cut from nearly $160 million in fiscal year 1973 to $52 million in fiscal year 1974 on its way to a nearly complete phase-out. Roused to action by the ANA, the NLN, and concerned nurses, Congress sufficiently offset the administration's reactionary policy toward nursing by voting appropriations for educational programs at the more realistic level of $146 million for fiscal year 1974, the last of the three authorized by the 1971 Training Act. Moreover, successful legal action by the NLN secured the release in January, 1974, of a large share of the impounded 1973 appropriations.

Nurse Staffing Patterns

There had been a tremendous growth in voluntary health insurance in the United States since World War II. Part of this growth was due to increasing pressure by labor groups for better fringe benefits and the general increase in funding of union-management health and welfare plans. By 1972 about 80 percent of the population had hospital or surgical health insurance or both. The percentage of people over age 65 who had private health insurance was substantially lower, however, since they were eligible for Medicare. Seventy-four Blue Cross plans covered about 74 million people for hospital care, and 70 Blue Shield plans insured about 67 million people for medical and surgical care. Some 1000 commercial insurance companies wrote group and individual policies covering 130 million people for hospital care. There were about 500 independent plans, which had 8,500,000 people enrolled.

Each year 34 million Americans were admitted to hospitals, and each person could expect to be hospitalized 11 times before he died. While the nation spent

Thirty-four million hospitalized Americans each year were entitled to a high level of nursing care.

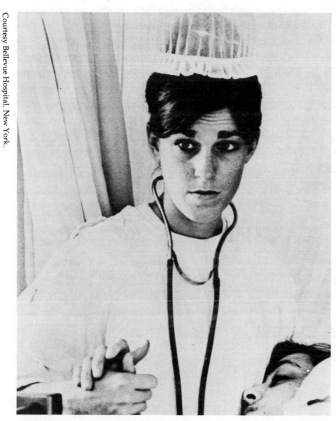

Courtesy Bellevue Hospital, New York.

almost $40 billion annually on hospital care, many patients were dissatisfied with the impersonal, condescending hospital treatment that they too-often received. Such behavior on the part of nurses, physicians, and other health care providers both undermined the human rights of patients and perpetuated consumer ignorance of medical treatment and health care.

Many hospitals could not function without licensed practical nurses and nurses' aides. As nursing positions remained unfilled, hospitals were hiring more and more aides and LPNs to fill the gap. Aides received on-the-job training, while practical nurses completed a one-year course and were then licensed by the state. As of January 1, 1973, employed licensed practical nurses numbered 459,000. The distribution of licensed practical nurses by field of nursing was as follows: 80 percent in hospitals, nursing homes, and other health care institutions; 19 percent in private duty, physicians' offices, and other fields; and 1 percent in community settings.

Compounding the problem for RNs was the inability of many patients to distinguish between RNs, LPNs, and aides. This difficulty was illustrated by patient responses in one study, which revealed that 58 percent could not differentiate between RNs and LPNs, although 70 percent could identify the aide. Whether ease in identifying the aide stemmed from her wearing a uniform other than white or from her frequent presence in the patient's room was unknown. While the patients indicated that nurses' aides were seen most frequently, they also seemed to realize who was more capable of providing high-quality care. Whereas the RNs were mentioned as having "more concern for the patient," the attitude of the aide was thought to be determined more by "concern for her

Skilled nursing practice began to receive renewed emphasis during the early 1970s.

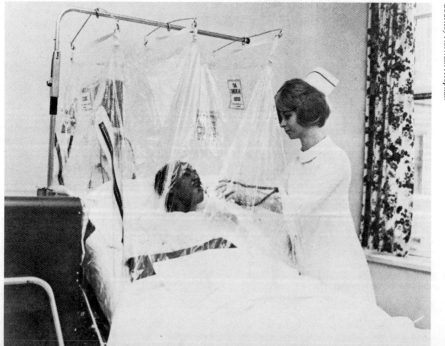

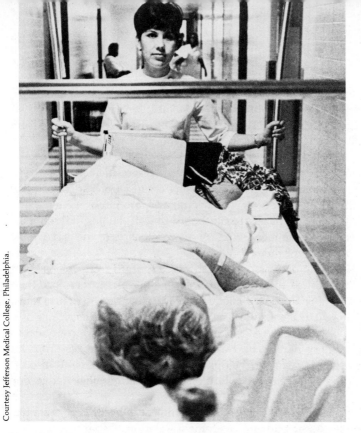

Forceful action was necessary to prevent a breakdown in the delivery of health care.

job." All patients participating in the study were asked, "What is your opinion about the number of nursing personnel staffing this floor?" Forty-three percent replied that more personnel were needed, 55 percent thought that the floors were adequately staffed, and 2 percent felt that fewer personnel were needed [2].

The federal government had become the focal point for action to correct abuses in the health care system, the state of which was the subject of a report by HEW Secretary Robert Finch on July 10, 1969:

This Nation is faced with a breakdown in the delivery of health care unless immediate concerted action is taken by Government and the private sector. Expansion of private and public financing for health services has created a demand for services far in excess of the capacity of our health system to respond. The result is a crippling inflation in medical costs causing vast increases in Government health expenditures for little return, raising private health insurance premiums, and reducing the purchasing power of the health dollar of our citizens [3].

An HEW white paper entitled *Towards a Comprehensive Health Policy for the 1970s* listed the main factors in the health care crisis as: (1) poor distribution of physicians, both in geographic location and in type of practice; (2) poor utilization of manpower resources; and (3) financial difficulties of health professional schools.

Developments in the Professional Associations

The American Hospital Association voted in August, 1967, to set up a special membership category for hospital schools of nursing. The proposal came from the more than 500 administrators and others who met in New York for the second AHA Conference of Hospital Administrators Conducting Hospital Schools of Nursing. Edwin L. Crosby, executive vice-president of the AHA, said that it was "obvious that the national nursing organizations are attempting to move all nursing education out of the hospital and into junior colleges, and universities . . . . It is now apparent to our board that, if the hospital school is to be strengthened and to be recognized by academic circles, the AHA must provide a strong program for them."

In October, 1969, a national association of nursing deans from colleges and universities was established to seek membership from among the more than 250 deans and directors of accredited baccalaureate nursing education programs. An initial meeting of 80 deans resulted in the formation of the American Association of Colleges of Nursing (AACN). The purpose of this new group was to provide administrators of nursing baccalaureate and graduate degree programs with a forum in which to review developments in the health fields. It also offered a means of designing concerted action on issues affecting higher education for nursing.

Perceiving the growing role of the federal government in health care planning, the American Nurses Association's Government Relations Department moved to Washington in January, 1971. The new department director, Constance Holleran, immediatey launched an aggressive campaign to represent the nursing profession more forcefully on Capitol Hill.

A year later, Nurses for Political Action was organized as a nonpartisan, nonprofit association with the avowed aim of attaining for nursing the support of legislators, government officials, and the general public. It was the first national organization of nurses to enter the political arena. In an official statement, the organizing group noted that although nurses, who now numbered nearly one million, were living at a time when a new national health care delivery system was being developed, their advice or opinion was rarely, if ever, sought.

The organization listed as its first priorities the achievement of substantive political influence on national policy relating to the delivery of health care, the inclusion of nurses in those groups responsible for the drafting of health care legislation, and recognition of their collaborative and independent functions as nurses in the total health system. This organization, which was soon affiliated with the ANA, subsequently changed its name to Nurses' Coalition for Action in Politics (N-CAP).

The Lysaught Report

The formation of the National Commission for the Study of Nursing Education in the United States had been announced jointly by the National League for

Nursing and the American Nurses' Association in 1967. Supported by $500,000 in foundation funds, this 15-member autonomous group was headed by W. Allen Wallis, president of the University of Rochester, and included leaders in nursing and other experts. A direct outgrowth of the report issued by the Surgeon General's Consultant Group on Nursing in 1963, it was charged with several basic tasks: to delineate reasonable community expectations for nursing care, to assess the resources required for effective and economical nursing and nurse education, and to recommend procedures for making quality nursing service more accessible.

The Commission's final report, *An Abstract for Action*, was published in 1970. Often called the "Lysaught Report on Nursing"—because the Commission's director was Dr. Jerome P. Lysaught of the University of Rochester—the publication offered four major recommendations, as follows:

Reestablish practice as the first and proper end of nursing as a profession.

Increase research efforts and funds for investigating the impact of clinical nursing practice on the quality, effectiveness, and economy of health care.

Encourage preparation of more nurses for expanded practice roles in the future by organizing state member planning committees to facilitate nursing education.

Establish a national Joint Practice Commission, with state counterpart committees to promote dialogue between medicine and nursing concerning congruent health care [4].

New Nursing Roles

One possibility of increasing the amount of health care available to the nation was to extend or expand the nurse's role. It was especially important to raise the level of responsibility of the registered nurse, since combining the selected areas of expertise of nurses and physicians in the delivery of primary health care would meet more of the health care needs of patients.

In the 1960s a number of research studies had explored the potential for expanding and extending the nurse's role. Dr. John Hathaway of Yale University, for example, conducted a study of "The Role of the Nurse in the Preventive Services of a Student Health Clinic," which showed that a nurse in the college health service could safely replace the physician in taking the medical history. Charles Lewin, Barbara Resnik, and Thelma Ingles carried out studies that lent additional credence to the view that traditional nursing roles could be expanded.

At the same time, the nursing profession, which was growing more concerned over the gaps in health care, began experimenting with the role of the clinical nurse specialist or nurse clinician. Emphasizing advanced nursing practice, knowledge in depth, and a recognition of the full spectrum of patient needs, this new concept offered the nurse the opportunity to fully utilize her expertise. Unfortunately the new role failed to achieve its objective of significantly upgrading the quality of patient care because hospital administrators and those who influenced them were frequently unwilling to pay for such services. Instead,

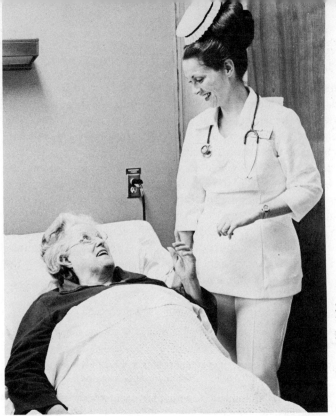

It takes more than medicine to cure a patient, says Linda Bryan, R.N., who talks with her patient, Dorothy Johnson, at Tarpon Springs General Hospital.

hospitals often assigned the clinical nurse specialist with staff or head nurse responsibilities, which prevented her from discharging her clinician's role.

Another evolving role was that of the "nurse practitioner." This title was first used in a special demonstration funded by the Commonwealth Foundation at the University of Colorado in 1965. This demonstration was designed to prepare professional nurses to give comprehensive well-child care in ambulatory settings and to serve as a research study for future changes in traditional collegiate nursing programs. Nurses were taught to make sophisticated clinical judgments on conditions of acutely ill or chronically ill children and to perform adequately as primary practitioners in childhood emergencies.

The nurses received instructional theory and clinical practice in the assessment of the physical and psychosocial development of children; in the management of common childhood problems; in counseling and teaching patients; in the performance of certain developmental, immunologic, and evaluative procedures; and in the utilization of appropriate community resources. Emphasis on family dynamics and community cultural values formed an integral part of the program.

A study to evaluate the program, undertaken by the Bureau of Sociological Research at the University of Colorado, confirmed the value of the new role. Pediatric nurse practitioners were found to be highly competent in assessing

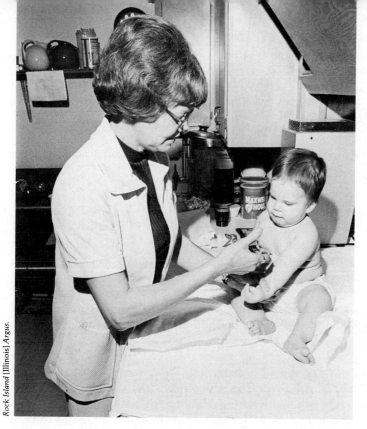

By the early 1970s the nurse practitioner had assumed national visibility to consumers.

normal and abnormal physical conditions in children and capable of caring for three-fourths of the well and ill children coming to community health stations. Pediatricians in private practice who utilized PNPs on their office staffs found that one-third more patients could be seen.

By the late 1960s and early 1970s, the nurse practitioner had assumed national visibility to consumers, other health professionals, and legislators. She differed from the traditional nursing model in the autonomy of her practice patterns, in her status in the delivery of health care, and in her relationship to patients, physicians, and health care agencies.

Actually, the concept of the expanded role for the nurse was not totally new. Some public health nurses had always engaged in many practices that belatedly came to be recognized as legitimate nursing functions. In many public health agencies, especially in rural areas, nurses had traditionally functioned in a relatively independent manner, in collaboration with physicians. For example, since 1926, nurses in the Frontier Nursing Service in Kentucky had performed many functions commonly considered as part of the physician's domain.

In a 1971 editorial, the editor of the *American Journal of Nursing* observed:

The kind of health care Lillian Wald began preaching and practicing in 1893 is the kind the people of this country are still crying for. She demonstrated, with no need to rest on formal research, that nursing could serve as the entry point—not only for health care, but for dealing with many other social ills, of which sickness is only a part. She felt that nurses should go *to* the sick, instead of expecting the sick to come to them (and waiting for physicians to refer them); that care of persons in the home, especially children, was far more effective and much less expensive, except perhaps for those needing, to use her own word, "intensive" care; that the nurse was also a teacher, who respected the capacity of the disadvantaged to learn, just as she always respected their right to human dignity. And, as for reaching the disadvantaged, Lillian Wald went to live among them a good half-century before the Peace Corps and Vista were conceived [5].

This movement to expand the traditional nursing role gained speedy momentum in the early 1970s after HEW Secretary Elliott Richardson requested a group of leaders in the field of health care to examine the possibilities of such an expansion. The resulting report, *Extending the Scope of Nursing Practice*, concluded that enlarging the nurse's role was absolutely essential for providing equal access to health services for all citizens. The committee warned, however, that "to attempt a definitive statement of the nature and scope of extended roles for nurses would go beyond the function of the committee and, moreover, may not even be possible."

Despite widespread agreement among various health professionals that the scope of nursing practice should be extended, there was no consensus about how this could best be achieved. The committee admitted that "it would be naive to gloss over the fact that working relationships between physicians and nurses are often less than ideal, with results that are disadvantageous to both professions but, more importantly, to their patients." Moreover, many nurses were unprepared or reluctant to assume extended roles in patient care, and physicians were rarely trained to work with nurses who were qualified to function in such roles. "We are convinced, however, that attitudinal barriers can be lowered, educational deficiencies corrected, real and imaginary legal restrictions of nursing practice can be dealt with, and other impediments to the extension of nursing can be overcome," the committee said, urging establishment of curricular innovations by health education centers and increased financial support for nursing education.

While acknowledging that the implementation of expanded roles for nurses would require careful legal evaluation, the report noted that state licensure laws affecting nursing would not present an obstacle: "An orderly transfer of responsibilities between medicine and nursing has proceeded over many years, and there is no reason to assume that questions of law might impede this process" [6].

"Increased attention should be paid to the commonality of nursing licensure and certification and to the development and acceptance of a model law of nursing practice suitable for national application throughout the states," the report noted. It also urged that the nursing profession undertake a study of recertification as a possible means of documenting new or changed skills among nurse practitioners and called for cost-benefit analyses and attitudinal surveys of providers and consumers to measure the impact of extended nurse practice on the health care delivery system.

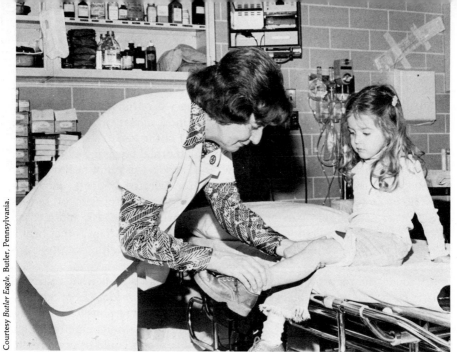

The Secretary's Committee to Study Extended Roles for Nurses recommended a major effort to expand the nurse's responsibility in identifying, assessing, and resolving health problems.

Nurse practitioners were performing many functions traditionally carried out by physicians.

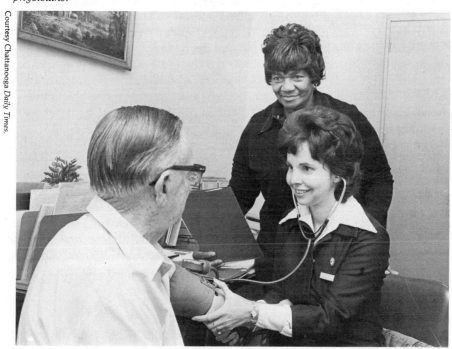

In specifying how the roles of nurses could be extended, the committee pointed out that there were a number of primary care functions which many nurses were already performing and for which more nurses could be prepared. Such functions included: (1) routine assessment of the health status of individuals and families; (2) provision of care during normal pregnancies and deliveries, provision of family planning services, and supervision of health care of normal children; (3) management of care for selected patients, including prescribing and providing care and making referrals as appropriate; (4) screening patients with problems requiring different medical diagnosis and medical therapy; and (5) consultation and collaboration with physicians, other health professionals, and the public in planning and instituting health care programs [7].

Although the report observed that nurses had had a somewhat restricted role in clinical settings, it predicted that their increasing freedom from administrative functions would enable them to assume greater responsibility for the clinical management and care of patients. In addition, the committee noted that many nurses were already prepared and that others could be prepared to perform such acute care functions as: (1) securing and recording a health and developmental history and making a critical evaluation of such records as an adjunct to planning and carrying out a health care regimen in collaboration with medical and other health professionals; (2) making prospective decisions about treatment in collaboration with physicians; and (3) initiating actions within a protocol developed by medical and nursing personnel, such as making adjustments in medication, ordering and interpreting certain laboratory tests, and prescribing certain rehabilitative and restorative measures [8].

The success of the initial programs and the financial support of federal and private funding agencies stimulated the development of training programs for the preparation of family nurse practitioners, school nurse practitioners, adult nurse practitioners, rural nurse practitioners, emergency nurse practitioners, geriatric nurse practitioners, OB/GYN nurse practitioners, and maternal nurse practitioners. Several federal agencies—Maternal and Child Health Service, Regional Medical Programs, and the Division of Nursing of the United States Public Health Service—supported these programs. The Nurse Training Act of 1971, which provided broadened authority for special project grants and contracts, specifically stated that funds could be used to "develop training programs for the training of pediatric nurse practitioners or other types of nurse practitioners." The National Center for Health Services Research and Development initiated programs in fiscal year 1972 to prepare family nurse practitioners under the general title of "Primex." By 1977 there were over 150 nurse practitioner programs in existence and some 7000 nurse practitioner graduates.

Nurse Midwives

Although nurse midwifery had been practiced on a limited basis in the United States for several decades, it was not until the 1970s that interest in this form of maternity care heightened. The role of the nurse midwife—management of prenatal care, labor and delivery, postpartum care and care of the normal newborn and family planning—was found to be both cost-effective and qualitatively effective. Nurse midwives of the 1970s generally delivered babies in hospitals with medical backup rather than in the homes of patients, although some hospitals had developed normal delivery areas adjacent to the high-risk units, which provided a home-like setting at a lower cost. Normal mothers needed neither the technology nor the awesome institutional environment found in acute health care settings. A 1976 New York City study showed that use of midwives reduced birth costs from $2000 to $899. Qualitatively, nurse midwives provided aspects of care that had been deemphasized by busy obstetricians such as empathic counseling about problems experienced during pregnancy and teaching the prospective mother about activities of daily living such as nutrition and exercise.

The American College of Nurse Midwives, the professional organization which certified nurse-midwives graduating from accredited programs, had 1300 members in 1977 and estimated an additional 500 uncertified nurse midwives in the country. One of the chief aims of the organization in the 1970s was to lobby for third party reimbursement for the services of the nurse midwife, an essential ingredient to fostering the development of this type of service to the American people.

Need for New Nurse Practice Acts

Unlike the medical licensure laws, which had originally been necessary to combat widespread quackery, state licensure statutes for nursing personnel were not enacted to correct abuses of independent, entrepreneurial practice. Instead, they usually provided "friendly" regulation. Enacted with the cooperation of the nursing profession itself, they were designed to protect both the regulated personnel and the public from unqualified, unethical practitioners. The forms of licensure, however, were generally similar to those for medical practice, except that, in some 20 states, licensure was permissive or optional rather than mandatory.

In 1970 every state licensed professional nurses. Whereas permissive licensure statutes merely prohibited unlicensed professional nurses from using the title "RN" or otherwise claiming to be licensed, mandatory licensure statutes established a precise definition of a licensed nurse and barred all unauthorized persons from nursing practice. By assuring minimum personnel qualifications, mandatory licensure had the obvious advantage of facilitating resolution of scope-of-practice and delegation problems. Objection to it came chiefly from nurse employers, who feared that the loss of practicing unlicensed nurses would cause serious personnel shortages.

Even in those states where licensure was mandatory, the nursing practice acts were filled with exemptions from licensure requirements. Throughout the 51 jurisdictions there were at least 13 different exemptions to the statutory definitions. Gratuitous nursing services were exempted from licensure in 46 jurisdictions; care provided by domestic servants was exempted in 23 states. Other exemptions included those for emergency care, federal employees, nursing students, recent graduates, nurses licensed in other states pending passage of the licensure examination, nurses licensed in neighboring states with overlapping practices, nursing in special facilities, services performed by auxiliary personnel, nursing under physicians' orders, and, in one state, nursing performed in a licensed facility.

In 1973 the efforts of the New York State Nurses' Association were instrumental in the passage of a revised nurse practice act that recognized nursing as an autonomous profession. This act distinguished between nursing practice and medical practice and described nurses' independent functions and defined nursing as "diagnosing and treating human responses to actual or potential health problems through such means as case finding, health teaching, and counseling." This definition was significant because it established, for the first time, a statutory authority for the practice of nursing.

Due to bitter opposition from both the state medical society and the state hospital association, the new practice act for New York State was passed only after a prolonged struggle. Although the hostility of the medical society had been expected, that of the hospital association came as something of a surprise. At one point it even issued a memorandum to state legislators charging that nurses were seeking unwarranted authority to practice medicine. Even though this memorandum temporarily killed the revised definition of nursing, the nurses persevered and finally obtained statutory independence for the nursing profession in New York State.

Revised nurse practice acts were necessary to allow new graduates to fulfill their potential in maximizing the delivery of quality nursing care.

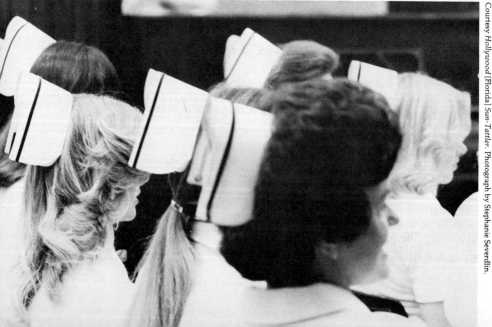

Courtesy *Hollywood [Florida] Sun-Tattler.* Photograph by Stephanie Severdlin.

Soaring Costs of Medicare and Medicaid

Through the federal-state Medicaid programs enacted in 1965, Congress had attempted to meet the health care needs of the poor, but it soon became clear that major reforms were needed. Benefits and eligibility varied widely from state to state, and the conflict of state and federal regulations resulted in waste and inefficiency. State budgets were increasingly unable to cope with rising patient costs. Medicaid was covering only half of all poor children nationwide, and in Southern states like Alabama, Mississippi, South Carolina, and Texas, no more than one poor child in 10 was receiving Medicaid services. Of the $11.3 billion in Medicaid payments made in 1974, over 40 percent went to California, New York, and Illinois, and an additional 30 percent went to eight other largely urban states.

Similarly, by 1970, Medicare was costing taxpayers $7 billion a year, twice as much as government planners had predicted. One reason for these unexpectedly high costs was the blatant opportunism exhibited by many physicians. According to a tabulation by the Senate Finance Committee, in 1968, 18 physicians each collected $150,000 or more from Medicare and more than 4000 collected $25,000 or more. There was clear evidence that these physicians were fattening their earnings by billing the government for unnecessary injections, blood tests, and x-rays. Some physicians had also developed the lucrative habit of making what the committee called "gang visits" to nursing homes, where they saw 40 or 50 patients in a single sweep and billed Medicare for their services at five to ten dollars per head. Relatively few physicians, of course, were cheating the government in such an outrageous fashion, but most did take advantage of the new funds pouring into the medical market and of the gratifying flexibility of Medicare's payment formula. In the four-year period after Medicare's enactment—a time when the general price index rose only moderately— the average family physician raised his fees by nearly one-third. Hospitals receiving Medicare money were required to have utilization review committees to prevent unnecessary use of hospital beds at government expense, but in 1970 a report by the Senate Finance Committee concluded that the work of these bodies was, by and large, "of a token nature" and "more form than substance".

In 1972 Congress enacted the most sweeping package of reforms in the Medicare and Medicaid programs since their inception in 1965. The final version of the Social Security Amendments of 1972, H.R. 1, was agreed upon by House and Senate conferees on the eve of Congressional adjournment and contained a total of 95 changes in the Medicare-Medicaid laws, including the controversial Bennett Amendment to establish Professional Standards Review Organizations (PSROs). Due in part to pressure from the Nixon administration and from American Medical Association lobbyists, the conferees agreed to limit the effect of the Bennett Amendment (originally to have regulated all Medicare and Medicaid service) to institutional review.

The PSRO provision of the new act (Section 249F) required that the HEW Secretary establish a nationwide network of voluntary, nonprofit groups of local physicians to regulate the quality and costs of health care services provided to recipients of Medicare, Medicaid, and Maternal and Child Health programs. The PSRO intended to achieve this objective by applying sophisticated concepts of peer review through a system of voluntary local organizations, state councils, and a national council, all regulated by the federal government.

By 1975 state Medicaid costs had risen to $4.5 billion, a startling 583-percent increase over 10 years. Federal expenditures for Medicare and Medicaid benefits had also skyrocketed. Their combined annual increase of about $5.2 billion in fiscal year 1977 exceeded the rest of the HEW health budget, including that of the National Institutes of Health. In many cases, primary care nurses could provide Medicare and Medicaid services much more cost-effectively and with much greater quality than could physicians. A strong move got underway to induce Congress to amend the Social Security Act to allow direct reimbursement to nurses providing Medicare and Medicaid services rather than in continuing to require the presence of a physician in order to qualify for such reimbursement.

Success came on December 13, 1977, when President Jimmy Carter signed the rural health clinic services bill (P.L. 95-210) which requires Medicare and Medicaid programs to reimburse clinics in health manpower shortage or underserved areas where primary care is delivered by nurse practitioners or physician assistants. When signing, Carter said, "At its best, the American health care system is unsurpassed, but its uneven distribution leaves millions of our people without access to adequate care. This problem affects urban and rural areas, but is widespread in the latter; two-thirds of the people in areas without adequate health care live in rural America." Private and public health insurance programs have failed to support nurse practitioners and the clinics that employ them, Carter said. The lack of insurance has been a major obstacle "to the

Nurses were highly cost effective in providing primary care.

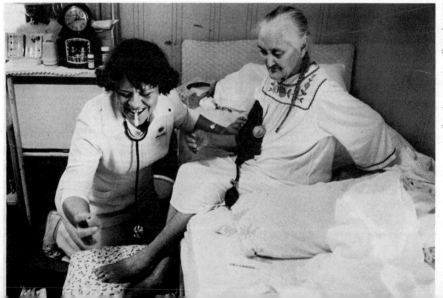

Courtesy *Paragould [Arkansas] Daily Press.*

healthy growth of these clinics." A vast field of opportunity for the establishment of nursing clinics was opened.

Nurses and Nursing Homes

The health care system had no ongoing mechanism for the systematic monitoring of patient outcome, nor was any provider accountable for patient health
beyond the success of the specific services rendered. The health care system
had little knowledge of or accountability for total health—ostensibly its final
aim and product. Each provider could choose, without accountability, the
type of services he would render. Moreover, once the provider had rendered a
series of services, he tended to lose track of the patient. There was no incentive
to insure that the patient had received from other providers all additional services necessary for an optimal state of health.

One study, for example, showed that it was three times more expensive to
care for a person in an institution than to provide the same medical care, social
services, rent, and food for the person at home. Since Medicaid did not pay for
at-home care, many elderly people who could remain at home were being
forced to live in institutions where the per-month cost in 1975 was about $800.
The elderly themselves maintained, in general, that institutional care should be
a last resort.

The origin of nursing homes in the United States can be traced to the Social
Security Act of 1935. Because of the tremendous public outcry against the public poorhouses of the Depression era, Congress stipulated that persons in public
institutions should not receive old-age assistance funds. Such funds were still
available, however, to the aged in private boarding homes. As a result there
ensued a sharp increase in the number of boarding homes throughout America.
After these homes began hiring nurses to care for the infirm aged, they were
more and more frequently referred to as "nursing homes." Because physicians
tended to overlook nursing home patients, many of whom had been transferred
as "chronic" cases from hospitals, they imposed a heavy burden on nurses
working in these homes.

The number of nursing home employees increased 405 percent from 1960 to
1970. In 1970, about 215,000 (43 percent) were aides and orderlies, 7 percent
were professional nurses, and 8 percent were licensed practical nurses. The
annual turnover for nursing home employees averaged 60 percent. In 1970
nursing homes employed a disproportionate number of aides (26 percent of the
830,000 national total), few LPNs (10 percent of the nation's 370,000), and a
minuscule number of the nation's RNs (.05 percent of 700,000). That same
year, registered nurses received an average wage of $3.75 per hour and had a
turnover of 71 percent.

There were many reasons for the limited number of professional nurses in
nursing homes. Federal regulations required the presence of registered nurses
in some 7300 skilled nursing facilities, and even then, with exceptions in rural
areas, only one RN was required to be on duty at all times. Significantly, about

90 percent of the nation's nursing homes were being operated as profit-making business ventures, in sharp contrast to the overwhelming nonprofit nature of short-term care facilities. Some nursing home operators, intent on reducing costs and increasing profits, refused to hire more than the minimum number of nurses required by law. Instead, they sought to "make do" with unlicensed aides and orderlies, whom they paid only the minimum wage. Other reasons for the comparative absence of nurses in nursing homes included the poor image of these homes, wretched working conditions, low job satisfaction, inadequate wages, and few fringe benefits. At the same time, schools of nursing and federal government programs had failed to stress geriatrics in nurse education.

Federal investigations disclosed that routine medical and nursing procedures, designed to insure the maintenance and well-being of the patient, were not being carried out. A 1971 study of 75 nursing homes conducted by the Department of Health, Education, and Welfare revealed that:

Thirty-seven percent of the patients taking cardiovascular drugs (digitalis or diuretics or both) had not had a blood pressure reading in over a year, and for 25 percent of these there were no diagnosis of heart disease on the chart.

Most of the patients reviewed were on one to four different drugs and many were taking from seven to 12 drugs; some were on both psychotropic "uppers" and "downers" at the same time.

Revised treatment of medication orders had been written for only 18 percent of the patients in the past 30 days, and 40 percent had not been seen by a physician for over three months.

Eight percent of the patients had decubitus ulcers, and 15 percent were visibly unclean.

Thirty-nine percent of the patients reviewed were inappropriately classified and placed.

No nursing care plans existed with respect to diets and fluids for 19 percent of the patients; personal care for 23 percent; activities for 14 percent; and individual treatment needs for 18 percent [9].

The National Health Service Corps

As the situation in nursing homes illustrated, medical facilities and services were often neither readily accessible nor evenly distributed. Whereas hospitals, clinics, and other medical care institutions and services were crowded into relatively tiny sectors in many urban areas, other large (particularly rural) regions had little or no access to physicians and other health care services.

After years of unsuccessful efforts to attract more doctors and nurses to rural America and despite millions of dollars spent on various federal and state programs, the health care shortage in small towns and rural areas appeared to be growing worse every year. In 1963, 98 counties in the United States had no doctors; in 1975 the number of such counties had risen to 135. Based on a 1975 goal of one physician for every 100 people, the shortage of physicians in rural areas was estimated at 20,000, a figure that was expected to reach 30,000 by

1985. The average age of practicing rural doctors was 54. The problem, as always, was that young doctors and nurses preferred to practice in comfortable metropolitan areas rather than in small towns where the work load was heavy, cultural and educational opportunities limited, and medical facilities often inadequate.

In an attempt to alleviate this critical health manpower shortage in medically disadvantaged communities, the National Health Service Corps had been established on December 31, 1970. The Corps hoped to recruit nurses with training or experience in the expanded role of nurse practitioner or those with strong public health backgrounds and experience in community development and program planning. By 1975 there were 405 Corps-appointed health care professionals (264 doctors, 71 dentists, 62 clinical nurses and nurse practitioners, and eight other allied health care personnel) assigned to 180 communities in 40 states. The purpose of these National Health Service Corps programs, which promoted improved systems of health care and developed professional and personal relationships, was to increase significantly the numbers of health care providers in medically underserved communities. In 1975 the Corps' retention rate was 26 percent, compared to 20 percent in 1974 and 3 percent in 1973.

Economic and General Welfare

In the period before the Depression, various employers had effectively used several antilabor instruments developed before World War I. They utilized discriminatory hiring and firing practices against employees who had joined organized unions. The "yellow-dog contract" (which forbade an employee from joining a union) was commonly used to prevent union membership and as a basis for civil suits against unions that persuaded employees to violate their contracts. The most useful of all weapons was the injunction, by which a court could forbid, at least temporarily, such practices as picketing, secondary boycotts, and the feeding of strikers by the union.

Section 7a of the National Industrial Recovery Act of 1933 contained the first positive assertion of the right of labor to bargain collectively but provided no means of enforcing this principle. Two years later, when the NIRA was declared unconstitutional for reasons that had nothing to do with the labor section, Congress replaced Section 7a with the much more elaborate National Labor Relations Act of 1935, usually referred to as the Wagner Act after its sponsor, Senator Robert F. Wagner of New York.

The Wagner Act proceeded from the premises that inequality of bargaining power between individual employees and large business units depressed "the purchasing power of wage earners in industry" and prevented "stabilization of competitive wage rates and working conditions" and that denial of the right to self-organization created industrial strife [10]. The Wagner Act established the principle of collective bargaining as the cornerstone of industrial relations in the United States and imposed upon management the obligation to recognize and deal with a legitimate labor organization in good faith. Furthermore, it guaranteed workers the right to form and join labor organizations, to engage in collective bargaining, to select their own representatives, and to engage in labor organization activities. The Wagner Act also outlawed a list of managerial practices that had had the effect of denying workers their rights. Henceforth, employers could not:

interfere with, restrain, or coerce employees in the exercise of their rights of self-organization and collective bargaining; dominate or interfere with the formation or administration of any labor organization or contribute financial or other support to it; encourage or discourage union membership by discrimination in regard to hiring or tenure of employment or condition of work, except such discrimination as might be involved in a closed-shop agreement with a bona fide union enjoying majority status; discharge or otherwise discriminate against an employee for filing charges or testifying under the act; refuse to bargain collectively [11].

The Wagner Act established the three-member National Labor Relations Board (NLRB) to enforce the above-mentioned clauses. After conducting hearings to determine the validity of union complaints, the Board could issue cease-and-desist orders to employers judged guilty of unfair labor practices. If employers did not comply with these orders, the NLRB could turn to a United States Circuit Court of Appeals for enforcement. The Board also had the power, on its own initiative or at the request of a union, to supervise a free, secret election among a company's employees to determine which union, if any, should represent the workers.

A decade later, in 1946, the American Nurses' Association took a step forward by adopting an economic security program, which endorsed state professional nurses' associations as exclusive spokesmen for their members in all matters affecting employment conditions and as their collective bargaining agents. According to the platform adopted at that time, the ANA was committed to obtaining wider acceptance of the 40-hour week with no decrease in salary, minimum salaries sufficient to attract and retain nurses of quality and to enable them to maintain standards of living comparable with those of other professions, and the expansion of nurses' professional associations as exclusive spokesmen for nurses in all questions affecting their employment and economic security. "Such a development," it was stated, "should be based on past successful experience of professional nurses' organizations in collective bargaining and negotiation" [12].

One of the main principles of this economic security program was its exclusive control by nurses. Nurses would represent themselves through state nurses' associations in collective bargaining with their employers. Immediately after acceptance of this principle, several state nurses' associations adopted programs and were fairly successful in representing their members in collective bargaining.

The most successful of these early efforts to obtain economic security occurred in California under the leadership of Shirley C. Titus, executive director of the California State Nurses' Association. A native of the state, Miss Titus was born in 1892 and spent her early years in San Francisco, where she received a diploma from St. Luke's Hospital School of Nursing in 1915. Immediately thereafter she assumed the position of Assistant Principal of her training school. Two years later she went to Washington, D.C. to work with Julia Lathrop as Assistant in the Prevention of Infant and Maternal Mortality in the United States Children's Bureau. After World War I she worked as Assistant Superintendent of Nurses at Barnes and St. Louis Children's Hospitals.

In 1924 Miss Titus entered Teachers College, Columbia University, where she earned a bachelors degree in nursing in 1925. Immediately thereafter she assumed the position of Director of the School of Nursing and Director of Nursing Services at the University of Michigan Hospital. Despite working long hours at this job, she still found time to pursue a masters degree in philosophy at Michigan, where she developed a deep sense of responsibility for the social and economic conditions of student and graduate nurses. This commitment inspired her to produce a flood of articles with such titles as "Is the Hospital Administrator Fulfilling His Responsibilities Toward His Nurses?", which ad-

Shirley C. Titus.

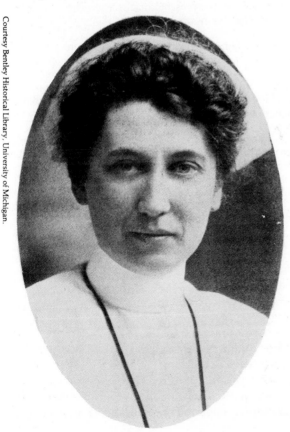

vocated using public taxes to support schools of nursing, and "The Pre-professional Education of the Nurse," which sought to explain why physicians objected to the establishment of minimum standards for school of nursing admissions.

During her tenure as Dean of the School of Nursing at Vanderbilt University from 1930 to 1939, Miss Titus embarked upon a campaign to realize some of her ideals. After becoming Executive Director of the California State Nurses' Association in 1940, she launched a vigorous campaign to improve the economic status of nurses. It was largely due to her efforts that the ANA economic security resolution won acceptance at the 1946 convention. Afterwards, she made the following comments about this new nurses' movement.

Although the workweek of all other workers has been markedly reduced during the past two or three decades, the professional nurse in many states today still works a 48-hour week or even longer. On the whole, because of long hours, the nurse's life is still pivoted on work, and this has tended to restrict her social horizon. Also, her low income has further restricted her social experience and her social outlook on life. Both organized medicine and the hospital have always sought to assume active and positive direction of nursing affairs in order that both nurses and nursing should function in a way that would best serve their special interests. These controls have prevented nurses from securing that background and experience which would have prepared them to live more fully and function more effectively in the present social scene. These controls have also seriously retarded and deflected the normal evolution of nursing from the status of a craft to that of a profession.

Because the nurse spends most of her waking hours in an environment which is dominated by hospital management and the doctors, she has remained far more docile, if not actually subservient, than perhaps any other American worker. Hospital management and organized medicine have not only shaped in part the world of nursing but they have also conditioned the thinking of nurses. And the nurse has accepted the thinking of these two groups—especially in regard to her status, her function, and her social and economic welfare—with amazingly little demur or question.

The result has been that during the last twenty-five or fifty years when other groups have been demanding their "place in the sun" and have been insistently and persistently striving to improve their economic world, nurses have continued to accept the status quo and to embrace the laissez-faire philosophy of life that rests on the principle that things as they are, however unsatisfactory and disagreeable they may be, must be accepted.

As I have given thought to the situation, it has seemed to me that the nurse within the four walls of her job—and her job has practically constituted her whole waking life—has been like a sleeper who has slept serenely on while a great battle—a battle for human freedom and the rights of the common man—was being waged. But eventually the sleeper awakens [13].

The Taft-Hartley Act

During the postwar era, however, the fortunes of labor took a turn for the worse, and the hospital lobby succeeded in blocking the nurses' drive to secure greater economic benefits. In 1947 Representative Fred Hartley introduced into the House a bill to exempt from the provisions of the 1935 Labor Relations Act "institutions that qualify as charities under our tax laws," such as churches, hospitals, schools, colleges, and societies for the care of the needy. The only opposition to this proposal came from Representative Arthur Klein of New York, who objected to excluding charitable and educational organizations from the ranks of "employers." Although the number of workers who would thus be deprived of Wagner Act protection was not large, Klein considered it ironic to exempt organizations devoted to social welfare from bargaining with their own, often-underpaid employees. Despite his opposition, however, the bill passed the House and went to the Senate, where there was no comparable committee report or proposal. Instead, Senator Joseph Tydings of Maryland simply offered a floor amendment to release nonprofit hospitals from the restrictions of the Wagner Act. During the scant debate that ensued, Senator Tydings justified his amendment as "designed merely to help a great number of hospitals which are having very difficult times. They are eleemosynary institutions, no profit is involved in their operations, and I understand from the Hospital Association that this amendment would be very helpful in their efforts to serve those who have not the means to pay for hospital service." Senator Robert Taft then explained that his Labor and Public Welfare Committee "considered this amendment, but did not act on it, because we felt it was unnecessary. The committee felt that hospitals were not engaged in interstate commerce and that their business should not be so construed. We felt it would open up the question of making further exemptions. That is why the committee did not act upon the amendment as it was proposed."

The remainder of the debate, between Senators Glenn Taylor of Idaho and Joseph Tydings, was very brief:

Mr. Taylor: What does the amendment do? Does it prevent hospitals' employees, particularly nurses, from organizing? Is that the sense of the amendment?
Mr. Tydings: It simply makes a hospital not an "employer" in the commercial sense of the term.
Mr. Taylor: Would nurses be prevented from organizing—they are poorly paid?
Mr. Tydings: I ,don't think so. They [the hospitals] should not have to come to the National Labor Relations Board . . . . A charitable institution is a way beyond the scope of labor management relations in which profit is involved.
Mr. Taylor: These may not be profit-making institutions, but even so I feel that simply because an institution, even one like the Red Cross, is kept up by popular subscription, the professional workers being employees of the Red Cross should be permitted a decent living and should not be hamstrung in their efforts to obtain it.
Mr. Tydings: I agree with the Senator [14].

The bill then passed the Senate. The conference committee accepted the Senate version, which became part of Section 2 of the National Labor Relations Act. Passage of the Taft-Hartley Act, with its provision exempting nonprofit hospitals from the obligation to bargain collectively, encouraged many employers to refuse to meet with their nurse employees to discuss working conditions or other matters affecting patient care. Some hospitals interpreted this exemption as a legal sanction for their *refusal* to engage in collective bargaining with nurses, a view which had been expressly denied on the floor of the Senate.

At other times, hospitals seemed to regard the exemption as the equivalent of an outright prohibition of collective bargaining.

The Fight for Collective Bargaining

As soon as this exemption became law the ANA began efforts to secure its repeal. In 1949 two bills relating to the Taft-Hartley Act were introduced in Congress. The ANA presented testimony before the Senate Committee on Labor and Public Welfare, and ANA representatives personally contacted many influential senators of both parties. Both bills, as well as a compromise proposal that finally passed the Senate, would have repealed the exemption of nonprofit hospitals and included them in the provisions of an amended National Labor Relations Act. Unfortunately, the House of Representatives killed this compromise bill by failing to act on it before the adjournment of the Eighty-first Congress.

Five years later improvement of working conditions through strengthened economic security programs and extension of the Federal Social Security Act shared the spotlight as key planks in an 18-point platform adopted by the American Nurses' Association at its 1954 convention in Chicago. More than 9400 registered graduate nurses and students witnessed the defeat of a motion that would have struck the phrases "collective bargaining" and "labor legisla-

Collective bargaining rights were likely to speed the process of change in the nurse's professional life.

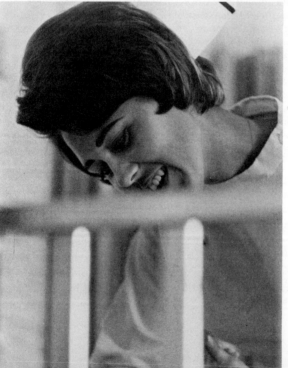

tion" from a platform supposedly endorsing a stronger economic security program. In voting against the motion the ANA's House of Delegates pointed out that the economic security program had too often been regarded as an emergency tool to be used only as requested by small groups of nurses in crisis situations. The House of Delegates appealed to the states nurses' associations to organize movements for the improvement of personnel conditions for nurses.

In the following year a study comparing the earnings and working conditions of nurses with those of other professional and nonprofessional groups amply demonstrated the inferior economic status of nurses. In 1955 the average gross monthly starting salary for a general duty nurse amounted to $253, which included the estimated cash value of any maintenance items provided by hospitals. Nurses' incomes fell below those of accountants, draftsmen, teachers, social welfare and recreation workers, and librarians. In some cases nurses' educational requirements and professional responsibilities exceeded those of higher-paid groups. Most startling was that the average factory worker earned about $70 more per month than the average nurse. Nursing also suffered in economic comparison with secretarial workers, who earned approximately $62 per month more than the average general duty nurse. Besides lower salaries, nurses received far fewer benefits than most other employees and often worked longer hours, which in many cases surpassed the then-standard 40-hour week.

Two years later resolutions urging the amendment of state and national labor laws were adopted in Chicago at the fortieth convention of the American Nurses' Association. The House of Delegates unanimously passed a resolution advocating amendment of the Taft-Hartley Act of 1947 "to remove the exemption granted to nonprofit hospitals in order that the protections and benefits of the act can be extended without discrimination to hospital employees." Nonprofit hospitals had "relied on the exemption to refuse to meet salary and other demands of nurses over the bargaining table," the resolution stated. An accompanying resolution urging state associations to take similar action regarding state labor laws also passed unanimously [15].

At that time, on the assumption that employers would deal with them fairly, the ANA publicly announced that nurses had voluntarily relinquished the right to strike. However, as Barbara Schutt, chairman of the Committee on Economic and General Welfare, pointed out to the delegates, many hospital administrators were refusing to discuss working conditions with nurses.

In 1959 the American Hospital Association House of Delegates approved a statement reaffirming the AHA position that voluntary nonprofit hospitals remain exempt from the provisions of the Taft-Hartley Act and from all laws requiring compulsory collective bargaining. This statement also reiterated the AHA position "upholding a strong and positive personnel policy in hospitals to provide for all hospital employees compensation, working conditions, and other personnel practices at least at levels prevailing for equivalent work in the community" [16]. This position had previously been expressed in the AHA *Statement on Hospital Management-Employee Relations* of 1956.

A hospital wage survey conducted by the Bureau of Labor Statistics revealed that salaries for general duty nurses in 1960 ranged from $65 per week in Atlanta to $89 per week in the Los Angeles area. The city average was $79.50 per week. Nurses earned $25 to $30 less per week than office, clerical, and maintenance crew employees in the 15 cities covered by the surveys. Accounting clerks and secretaries with skills usually acquired in high school or on the job averaged $4.00 to $8.00 per week more than the general duty nurse. Such hard economic facts provided little encouragement for prospective nurses.

The outlook was no more promising for the registered nurse who had obtained a baccalaureate degree. The highest salaries for women college graduates went to beginning chemists, mathematicians, and statisticians, who earned an average of $95 to $98 per week. Nurses with baccalaureate degrees commanded salaries identical to those for home economists, research workers, and therapists—approximately $78 per week. In contrast to those entering these other professions, however, the vast majority of college-educated nurses were by no means untried beginners. After acquiring their basic nursing education in dipploma schools, they usually completed a year or more of nursing practice before starting college programs leading to degrees.

Inadequate levels of compensation obviously discouraged the practicing nurse from acquiring further education. Although the growing complexity of the health care delivery system and the expansion of medical knowledge made additional academic training imperative, such advanced study was usually beyond a nurse's financial means. Moreover, the slight salary differential hardly made this financial investment worthwhile. Significantly, even a director of nursing with administrative responsibility for all nursing care in a hospital earned only from $118 to $158.50 per week in the cities surveyed by the Bureau of Labor Statistics—only $59 a week more than a general duty nurse.

Reinvigoration of Economic and General Welfare Programs

In 1960 the ANA continued to push its economic security program by approving a resolution introduced by the Michigan State Nurses' Association, the purpose of which was to initiate a strong public information campaign for the economic security program. In her call for action, Anne Zimmerman, chairman of the ANA Committee on Economic and General Welfare, urged the delegates to have "enough humility to acknowledge the economic poor health of the nursing profession and to continue to speak out courageously through our professional organizations to improve it." Supporting this position, Matilda Young, a member of Mrs. Zimmerman's committee, urged the House of Delegates to fight for the elimination of "legislative discrimination against nurses." It was shocking, she said, that 40 percent of nongovernmental hospitals in the United States were not covered by the Old Age Survivors Insurance System. Arguing for collective bargaining, Miss Young reminded the audience that the efforts of the ANA would be greatly facilitated "if each state nurses' association would make it clear to their congressmen that the exemption of nonprofit hospitals from the Taft-Hartley Act has created a most unfavorable climate" [17].

The proposed ANA platform for 1960–1962 was fortified by the retention of a plank committing the ANA "to assist nurses to improve their working conditions through strengthening economic security programs, using group techniques such as collective bargaining" [18]. All attempts to amend the plank from the floor, including a proposed deletion of the words "using group techniques such as collective bargaining," were defeated after a heated debate.

During the 1960s nurses' salary raises continued to lag behind general increases around the country. The Bureau of Labor Statistic's survey figures for 1963–1964 showed that teachers averaged $6325, secretaries, $5170, factory workers, $5075, and the general duty nurse in nonfederal city hospitals, $4500.

Nurses on Strike

In 1966 some 2000 dissatisfied nurses in 33 San Francisco Bay area hospitals resigned during a dispute over salary demands. This dispute was temporarily resolved when the hospitals and representatives of the California Nurses' Association agreed to submit the question of nurses' salaries to a fact-finding committee. This kind of militant action on the part of the nurses placed the California Nurses' Association in an untenable position. "If we put our foot down about the mass resignation technique, they would go ahead anyway," remarked an association executive. "We firmly believe that resignations on the part of nurses are a more serious step than strike," she added [19].

Soon afterward, the board of directors of the California Nurses' Association broke with tradition and with the policy of the national organization by en-

California nurses established the strike as a viable collective bargaining tool.

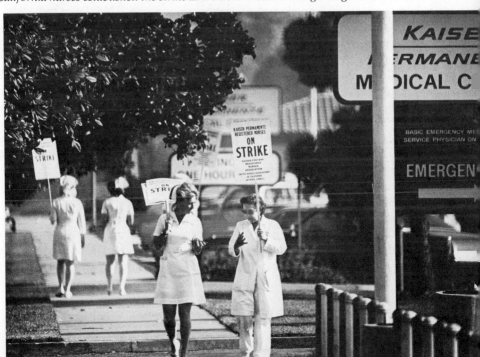

Courtesy Riverside [California] Press.

dorsing the strike as a weapon for attaining economic objectives. It was not an easy decision to make according to the associate executive director of the CNA, A. Lionne Conta, who observed that there had been a "total change in the attitude of the nurses" in recent months. Referring to "powerful and active" unions in California, she noted, "We felt that if we did not take action, they [the nurses] would turn to other organizations" [20].

Nursing incomes improved somewhat in the late 1960s. A survey made by the Bureau of Labor Statistics in March, 1969, reported an average hourly wage of $2.44 for nonsupervisory employees in nongovernmental hospitals, ranging from a high of $2.67 in the West to $2.13 in the South. National averages of earnings for a 40-hour week for selected occupations in non-federal city hospitals, on that date, were as follows [21]:

Full-time general duty nurses	$141.00
X-ray technicians	120.50
Switchboard operators-receptionists	78.00
LPNs	99.00
Nursing aides	76.00

These figures could be compared with the $129.51 weekly average of all American production workers in the same year, 1969. Nurses achieved additional gains in starting salaries during the early 1970s, although the increases were moderate compared to the successes of the nation's school teachers. Nurses could not expect any substantial salary increments for longevity of service, even in the best-paying hospitals.

Because of the belief that nurses should be represented by their professional association rather than by outside labor unions, the ANA launched in late 1973 an aggressive campaign to organize the nation's 800,000 registered nurses. Several months later, in June, 1974, two days before a record ANA conference crowd of more than 10,000 nurses gathered in San Francisco, 4400 members of the California Nurses' Association walked off their jobs at 43 Bay area hospitals and clinics when contract negotiations broke down between the CNA and Kaiser Foundation Hospitals, Affiliated Hospitals in San Francisco, and Associated Hospitals of San Francisco and the East Bay. Responding to the opportunity to dramatize the ANA's new cohesion and militancy, convention attenders manned picket lines and donned blue armbands in support of the striking nurses. "Take a striking nurse to lunch!" was the battle cry as convention goers lent moral and financial support to their picketing colleagues.

The San Francisco strike attracted national attention and focused interest on the issues involved in collective bargaining with health care agencies. The ANA's 980-member House of Delegates passed a resolution stating that "[the ANA] fully supports and encourages actions of the California Nurses' Association . . . in strike action," and that the walk-out did not endanger "the safety and well-being of hospital patients." A fund was created for voluntary strike support donations [22].

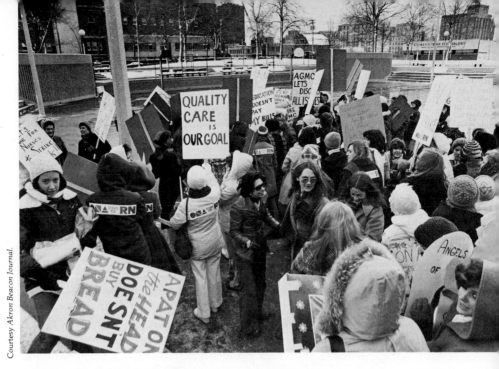

Courtesy Akron Beacon Journal.

Nurses are demanding a voice in promoting quality patient care.

Six weeks later, on July 26, 1974, President Nixon signed into law amendments to the Taft-Hartley Act that permitted nurses in 3500 nonprofit hospitals to engage in collective bargaining. They joined employees in profit-making hospitals and nursing homes, which had come under National Labor Relations Board jurisdiction in 1967, and those in nonprofit nursing homes, which had come under Board jurisdiction in 1970. Federal employees, including those in federal health care institutions, had enjoyed the right to bargain collectively since 1962, under provisions of an executive order signed by President Kennedy. Moreover, in 1967 the federal government had granted the American Nurses' Association and its constituent state associations the right to represent registered nurses in Veterans Administration hospitals during collective bargaining. In August that year the Iowa Nurses' Association had signed the first contract with the Veterans Administration in Des Moines.

As soon as Congress repealed the exemption of nonprofit hospitals from provisions of the National Labor Relations Act in 1974, the American Nurses' Association embarked upon an energetic campaign to organize the nurses in the nation's hospitals. By raising additional sums of money, increasing the number of field workers, enlarging staff at its Kansas City headquarters, and conducting a series of educational collective bargaining programs for its 53 constituent state and territorial nursing associations, the ANA succeeded in greatly revitalizing its economic and general welfare program. Under the banner of "collective professional action," the ANA began striving for recognition as a distinct professional group and as the primary advocate for the patient. One year later, in 1975, the ANA groups represented 200,000 of the 800,000 practicing RNs, including 70,000 RNs for whom state nursing associations had negotiated 515 bargaining contracts. Both the Taft-Hartley amendment and the women's liberation movement, which instilled in nurses a sense of worth as individuals and as professionals, promised to accelerate this process of change within the nursing profession.

The Nurse and the Modern Health Care Industry

As the nurse considered the economic aspects of the health care industry in the United States in the mid and late 1970s, two features stood out above all others— its vastness and its phenomenal rate of growth. This industry was clearly one of the largest in the country. In 1976, when the Consumer Price Index rose about 7 percent, health care costs increased at double that rate. In 1950 hospital care costs averaged $16 a day. By 1966 that figure had risen to $48. By 1976 costs were approaching $175 a day. Twelve cents of every dollar spent by the federal government in 1976 was allocated for health care. In the previous ten years total health expenditures for the nation had grown from $42 billion to $140 billion, or from 5.9 to 8.6 percent of the Gross National Product. At this rate, even if the government undertook no new programs, the amount would increase to $240 billion, or over 10 percent of the GNP by 1982. In 1977 the cost of health care was estimated to be $640 per person, or $2560 for a family of four. This figure represented 18 percent of the gross annual income for a family with the national median income of $13,700.

In 1960 the health care industry, employing 2.5 million persons, was the third largest in the United States. By 1977 the number employed in this field rose to an estimated 5.1 million persons or 5.2 percent of the nation's work force. By early 1978, there were more than one million active registered nurses, more than 500,000 active licensed practical nurses, and more than 375,000 practicing physicians in the United States.

For more than two decades hospital costs, which accounted for 40 cents of every 1977 dollar spent on health care, had been escalating far faster than the overall cost of living. From 1950 to 1977 the cost of one day's stay in a hospital increased more than 1000 percent compared with a 143 percent climb in the Consumer Price Index. The past decade had witnessed a particularly noticeable acceleration of this inflationary trend in hospital costs. For example, since 1965 the average cost of a day's hospitalization had increased more than 300 percent—from $41 to more than $167—while the cost of an average hospital stay climbed from less than $300 to more than $1300. The nation's total hospital bill jumped to $55.4 billion—an average of $254 per person and more than $1000 per family. An itemized breakdown of the 1977 average daily rate of $167 for hospitalization revealed the following costs:

Nursing care, $95.25 a day. This charge covered the services of professional and licensed practical nurses, technicians, aides, orderlies and students.

Meals, $19.82 a day. Three meals, brought to the room.

Cleaning, $8.06. Covered cleaning of rooms, corridors, elevators and lobby.

Fee to offset the operating loss of clinics and emergency rooms, $7.72.

Medical records, $6.55. Included transcription of doctor's notes and filing.

Interns and residents, $6.04. Physicians who are available around the clock.

Administration, $5.04. Included admission, handling of visitors, and processing of inquiries.

Building depreciation, $4.70.

Linen, $4.36. Included sheets, towels, hospital gowns.

Heat, power, and light, $3.52.

Repairs, $3.52.

Social services, $2.68. Counselors to help with problems related to illness.

The total amounted to $167.26.

The more than 7200 domestic hospitals constituted one of the nation's largest businesses. In 1977 they had a total capacity of 1.5 million beds and overall assets of more than $55 billion. As a rough measure of this industry's output, hospitals handled nearly 40 million admissions and more than 260 million outpatient visits at operating costs of more than $55.4 billion. Approximately 10.7 percent of the population was hospitalized at least once in 1977; this figure represented at least one hospital visit for 8.8 percent of the male population and 12.5 percent of the female population. While only 5.7 percent of the persons under 17 were hospitalized, 16.8 percent of the population 65 and over received such care.

In 1977 hospitals employed the equivalent of more than 3.3 million full-time employees with a total payroll of more than $29.6 billion. At the same time, the number of employees needed to care for the average patient increased significantly—from 1.8 in 1950 to 3.4 in 1977. Changes in treatment methods had tended to require additional equipment and skilled laborers to operate it—without eliminating the need for previous personnel.

This increased use of equipment reflected the many more laboratory services being performed. The number of laboratory tests for hospitalization increased by over 8 percent annually—from 2.9 billion tests in 1971 to more than 6 billion tests in 1977. The cost of these tests rose during this same period from $5.6 billion to more than $18 billion—a 10 percent annual growth. By 1977 laboratory services accounted for 11 percent of total health expenditures.

The usual economic relationship between supply and demand did not seem to prevail in the health care industry, where increases in the supply of hospital beds and number of physicians led to corresponding increases in the amount of health care sought. The reason for this phenomenon was not readily apparent. One explanation was that access to physicians was easier in areas where they were more concentrated. Another possible reason was the freedom of physicians to determine the scope and intensity of therapeutic procedures and health care services.

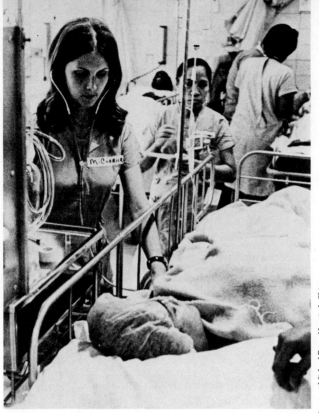

The number of hospital employees needed to care for the average patient increased from 1.8 in 1950 to 3.4 in 1977.

The well-informed consumer purchasing health care was the exception rather than the rule. As a result, physicians acted as suppliers who determined the demand for care. Because insurance coverage for hospital costs made health care seem free to many patients, the cost of services often received little consideration at the time of purchase. Physicians, therefore, had sidestepped the laws of supply and demand by doing little to restrict demand. Since most hospitals were reimbursed without question by insurance or other third-party payers for the full amount of their services, they had absolutely no incentive for lowering prices. Raising prices, on the other hand, usually resulted in a comparable increase in revenues. Due to this reversal of normal economic conditions, the usual market signals that accompanied excess supply—lower revenues and prices—failed to emerge.

The nation's third largest industry, health care continued among the least efficient. During 1976 America's health bill rose to $139.3 billion, a 14 percent increase over the $122.2 billion spent in 1975. These figures included personal health care, such as hospital care and physician services, as well as public health programs, biomedical research, and construction of new facilities. During 1974 and 1975, expenditures for health care climbed 31 percent, a far more rapid rate of increase than for the overall economy. As a result, health expenditures have assumed an increasingly larger proportion of the Gross National

Trends in National Health Expenditures for Selected Fiscal Years: In Billions of Dollars

Year	All Health Expenditures	Percent of GNP	Personal Health Care Expenditures			Federal Portion of Public	Medicare & Medicaid Portion of Federal
			Total	Private	Public		
1950	12.0	4.5	10.4	8.3	2.1	1.0	–
1960	25.9	5.2	22.7	17.8	4.9	2.1	–
1965	38.9	5.9	33.5	26.5	7.0	2.8	–
1970	69.2	7.2	60.1	39.6	20.5	13.4	9.4
1975	122.2	8.4	105.7	63.8	42.0	28.9	21.2
1976	139.3	8.6	120.4	72.0	48.4	33.7	25.2

Product: 4.5 percent in 1950, 7.8 percent in 1974, 8.4 percent in 1975, and 8.6 percent in 1976. Hospital charges increased 13.4 percent in 1976 alone and accounted for the most significant portion of this rise in the percentage of the GNP. In addition, physicians' fees, which hitherto had never registered a greater annual increase than 7.5 percent, leaped an unprecedented 12.8 percent in 1975 and 11.4 percent in 1976.

Because the nation's health care system had failed to meet the needs of the people despite these ever-rising costs, it was generally described as "the fastest growing failing business in the nation" and was coming under increased scrutiny. This failure to provide adequate health care was attributed to the need for a high concentration of health care personnel, the lack of incentives for im-

Clinical specialist in cancer nursing, Susan Herbst, shown with a 14-year-old patient, provides primary care to the chronically ill.

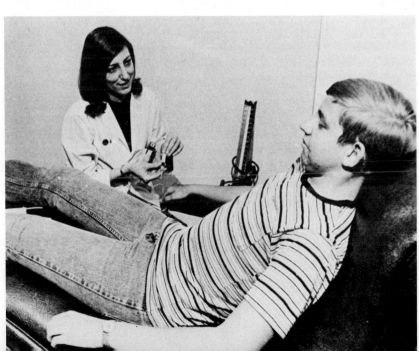

proved management of health care facilities, the use of expensive procedures and devices that supported vital functions but did not effect cures, the expensive health regulatory activities of the federal government, and the general inflationary trend in the nation's economy. To improve the health care delivery system it was necessary to bring these cost factors under control, to make health services more uniformly accessible, and to decrease the disparity between public expectations and the treatment offered by traditional medical science. Furthermore, the supportive services and preventive care, which were the strengths of the nursing profession, could no longer be overlooked.

Stimulated by the program of federal aid under the Nurse Training Act, the number of active registered nurses jumped 200 percent between 1950 and 1978. Projections made by the Bureau of Health Manpower, Health Resources Administration, United States Public Health Service, indicated that the supply of all types of health manpower would grow sharply over the next 15 years, both in absolute numbers and in relation to the population. The ratio of registered nurses to the population was expected to increase by about 46 percent and that of licensed practical nurses (LPNs) by about 29 percent. The ratio of physicians per 100,000 population was projected to rise from about 176 per 100,000 in 1975 to 241 per 100,000 in 1990, a 37 percent increase. The corresponding increase in the dentist-population ratio was estimated at 24 percent.

Supply of Selected Health Manpower per 100,000: Estimated 1970 and 1975, Projected 1980, 1985, 1990

Year	Physicians (M.D. & D.O.)	Per 100,000	Dentists	Per 100,000	Registered Nurses	Per 100,000
1970	323,200	157.6	102,200	49.8	722,000	356
1975	375,300	175.8	112,000	52.5	906,000	427
1980	446,100	200.2	127,000	57.0	1,166,000	523
1985	517,200	221.0	143,400	61.3	1,372,000	586
1990	589,700	240.6	159,000	64.9	1,532,000	625

During the late 1970s the major directions of the health care system in general and of the nursing programs in particular were subjected to a serious and thorough reevaluation. No aspect of the nursing profession escaped this review, which will undoubtedly increase in intensity in the future. The old questions were still valid: how many nurses does the nation need, and what sort of nurses should they be? How can the nation best utilize the services of the existing supply of nurses? To these questions new ones had to be added: to what extent can the traditional medical role be handled more qualitatively or more economically by a nurse?

The requirements of the modern health care system have significantly upgraded the quality of nursing education and practice. For example, according to Rachel Rotkovitch, Associate Administrator and Director of Nursing Services at Long Island Jewish-Hillside Medical Center, Hyde Park, New York, "for the last

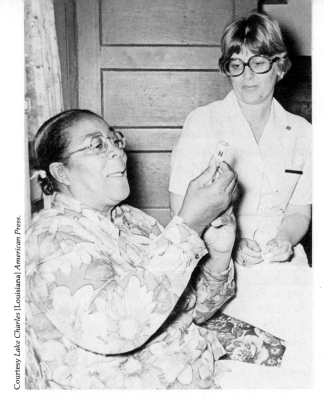

Treatment of chronic disease depends much more upon personal behavior and thus requires the participation of individuals.

The 20-year-old 1977 president of the National Student Nurses Association, Helen Archer, sees the registered nurse as an advocate for the patient.

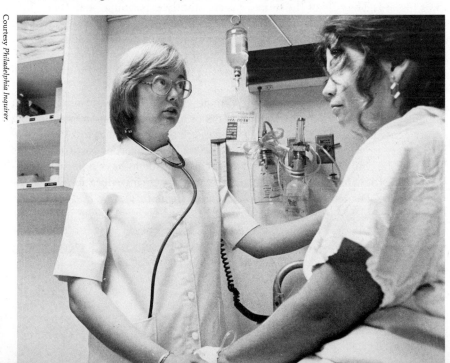

twenty years, nurses have been preparing themselves through additional education and better education for a primary role in dealing with patients." She further notes that "dedication and tender loving care have not disappeared from nursing, but now we have more in our armamentarium with which to fight the battle against illness." Moreover, nurses are eager "to put those weapons at the service of the public. The public is not aware of the potential for benefit we have for them."

To support her contention that "in many situations the nurse can serve as the primary provider in treating the patient," Mrs. Ratkovich had established a "my patient, my nurse" approach to patient care at the Long Island Jewish-Hillside Medical Center. This new nursing model represented a radical departure from the traditional, assembly line approach in which a nurse was either administering drugs or taking blood pressures, but not both, and never to a few patients, but to a whole ward. Primary nursing was based on the principle that the professional nurse must meet the patient, assess his needs, and deliver the necessary health care with her own two hands. The nurse would then know the patient as "my patient," for whom she would be "my nurse" [23].

This example typified the demand of nurses for a more direct role in patient care, a demand which resulted from a changed self-image. No longer content with their traditional subservient, dependent role, nurses now wanted to be considered as independent professionals and as full-fledged colleagues of the physician. Among the forces in society that helped to promote this change of attitude on the part of the nursing profession were the women's liberation movement, the soaring cost of health care, and consumer dissatisfaction with the health care.

In the late 1970s nursing was passing through one of the most exciting periods in its history. The role of the nurse was constantly expanding, and the quality of nurses, who were upgrading their knowledge and skills, stood at a new high. As history has shown, the advance of the nation's health care system depends to a large extent upon the number of qualified nurses providing the health service in question. In the final analysis, the state of health care in the United States has always been and will continue to be strongly influenced by nursing. Highly developed nursing talent will remain essential for performing civilian nursing service, satisfying the requirements of national defense, and educating future generations of nurses. Because nurses are the largest and most inclusive health care providers, the nation's decision-makers, in order to promote the health of the United States, have had and will continue to have a particular responsibility to maintain the stability and advance of nursing education, research, and practice. For its part, nursing must define its goals clearly and then must develop careful political strategies for pursuing these goals. The investment made today in nurses and nursing and in the development of the future nursing talent is an investment in tomorrow—an investment which will have a tremendous impact on the basic quality of the lives of all Americans.

Summary

By the beginning of the 1970s, the health industry was the third largest in the United States, and the number of professional nurses in practice had reached 722,000.

The federal government spent more than $380 million from fiscal year 1965 through fiscal year 1971 to advance the education of professional nurses, with about half that amount going for student aid and the remainder for school of nursing assistance.

The three-year Nurse Training Act of 1971 helped alleviate the nurse shortage by authorizing enlarged expenditures, despite resistance from the Nixon administration.

Appropriations under the new Act did not come close to matching the large authorizations approved, but they were maintained at a fairly respectable level, due partly to an aggressive ANA lobbying effort. Especially welcomed were the new capitation grants, the first flexible funds that most nursing schools had ever received.

There had been a tremendous growth in voluntary health insurance in the United States, and, by 1972, Blue Cross plans covered 74 million people for hospital care and 67 million for medical and surgical care.

Many hospitals were hiring large numbers of aides and LPNs to staff patient care units, but patients' inability to distinguish registered nurses from LPNs prevented consumer assessment of inadequate care that might result from overstaffing with nurses of insufficient preparation.

Developments among the professional nursing associations included the establishment of the American Association of Colleges of Nursing (AACN) and a special membership category for hospital schools of nursing in the American Hospital Association.

Greater political effort was initiated among nursing organizations. The ANA's Government Relations Department became more active in lobbying, and the Nurses Coalition for Action in Politics (N-CAP) was formed.

In 1970 the final report of the National Commission for the Study of Nursing in the United States (the Lysaught Report) recommended the reestablishment of practice as the primary focus of nursing, an increase in clinical nursing research, the establishment of state planning committees, and the formation of a commission to help articulate the roles of physicians and nurses.

Expansion of the nurse's traditional role was recommended by many authorities. Clinical nurse specialists were experimenting with new practice dimensions, but graduate education was considered necessary for this role and frequently resulted in alleged prohibitive costs to hospitals employing the nurse clinicians.

The new role of pediatric nurse practitioner emerged. PNPs were found to be highly competent in assessing the health status of children and managing minor problems. Their role represented a legitimization of some of the tasks nurses had traditionally performed independently, particularly in rural areas.

In the early 1970s HEW Secretary Elliott Richardson requested an investigation into the possible extension of nursing practice. The Secretary's committee found that nurses could perform primary care functions such as routine assessment of health status, care in normal pregnancies and deliveries, and prescription, provision of care, and referrals for selected patients. The committee also identified provision of family planning services and supervision of the health care of normal children as logical domains of the nurse.

In 1970 nurse licensure was optional rather than mandatory in about 20 states. Licensure statutes merely served, in these states, to protect the meaning of the RN's title. A strong push for mandatory licensure began in many of the states where it was still optional and substantial progress was achieved.

In New York State in 1973, nurses were ultimately successful in gaining passage of a revised nurse practice act that recognized nursing as an autonomous profession.

The Medicare and Medicaid programs instituted by the government in 1965 were fraught with problems. Medicaid benefits varied widely among states. In Southern states, coverage of poor children was minimal, and of the $11.3 billion in Medicaid expenditures in 1974, over 40 percent went to three urbanized states: California, New York, and Illinois.

By 1970 Medicare was costing twice as much as had been expected. This was due, in part, to some physicians' taking advantage of the flexible payment formula. Hospital review committees were not effective in controlling misuse of Medicare funds.

Even with reforms in Medicare, statistics indicated that the American health care system was failing to reach all segments of society equitably. Infant mortality and life expectancy rates compared unsatisfactorily with those of certain European countries, and dissatisfaction was exacerbated by the rising costs of health care. Health care providers were not accountable for the provision of health, but only for specific services.

Long-term care for the aged was becoming more and more prevalent. Nurses had heavy work burdens in nursing homes, where physicians tended to overlook patients and employee turnover was high. The number of professional nurses on nursing home staffs was minimal, partly because of general dissatisfaction with the nurse's role in the nursing home setting and partly for financial reasons. Geriatrics had not been stressed in nurse education, and studies indicated that nursing homes were lax in performing nursing and medical procedures.

To promote better distribution of health services to poorly served areas, the National Health Service Corps was formed in 1970. It attempted to recruit nurse practitioners and nurses with extensive public health experience.

In 1946 the ANA established its economic security program to encourage the development of state nursing associations to serve as exclusive representatives for their members and as their collective bargaining agents.

The Taft-Hartley Act of 1947 contained a provision exempting nonprofit hospitals from the obligation to bargain collectively with their employees. Many hospitals refused to meet with employees and encouraged other employers to refuse to meet with their nurses.

The San Francisco nurses' strike in 1974 focused national attention on the issues involved in collective bargaining in health care agencies. Several weeks later, President Nixon signed amendments to the Taft-Hartley Act that opened the way to collective bargaining for nurses in 3500 nonprofit hospitals.

Skyrocketing health care costs, especially for hospitalization, impelled a strong move to reorganize the health care industry. Although health care was absorbing an increasing percentage of the nation's gross national product, it was not yielding commensurate benefits to the public. An expanded supply of nurses, utilized in innovative roles, showed promise of higher quality care at a more cost effective rate.

References

1. Executive Office of the President, Office of Management and Budget, *The Budget of the United States Government, 1974* (Washington, D.C.: Government Printing Office, 1973), appendix.
2. Charles M. Ewell, "What Patients Really Think About Their Nursing Care," *Modern Hospital*, vol. 109 (December, 1967): 106–108.
3. *New York Times*, July 11, 1969.
4. National Commission for the Study of Nursing and Nursing Education, *An Abstract for Action* (New York: McGraw-Hill, Inc., 1970), pp. 86, 89, 92, and 107.
5. "A Prophet Honored," *American Journal of Nursing*, vol. 71 (January, 1971): 58.
6. U.S. Department of Health, Education, and Welfare, Secretary's Committee to Study Extended Roles for Nurses, *Extending the Scope of Nursing Practice: A Report of the Secretary's Committee* (Washington, D.C.: Government Printing Office, 1972), pp. 3–6.
7. *Ibid.*, pp. 7–9.
8. *Ibid.*, pp. 3–9.
9. U.S. Congress, Senate, Special Committee on Aging. Ninety-fourth Congress, First Session. *Nursing Home Care in the United States: Failure in Public Policy; Supporting Paper No. 4—Nurses in Nursing Homes: The Heavy Burden* (Washington, D.C.: Government Printing Office, 1975), p. 369.
10. U.S. Congress, House, Committee on Labor, *Labor Disputes Act, Hearings Held March 13–April 4, 1935* (Washington, D.C.: Government Printing Office, 1935), pp. 1–9.
11. *Ibid.*, pp. 5–12.
12. "The Biennial," *American Journal of Nursing*, vol. 46 (November, 1946): 729.

13. Shirley Titus, "Economic Facts of Life for Nurses," *American Journal of Nursing*, vol. 52 (September, 1952): 1109–1110.
14. *Congressional Record*, May 12, 1947.
15. "ANA Platform for 1956–1958," *American Journal of Nursing*, vol. 56 (July, 1956): 882.
16. "Statement of AHA Concerning Collective Bargaining in Hospitals," *Hospitals*, vol. 33 (September 16, 1959): 98.
17. "ANA Platform, 1960–1962," *American Journal of Nursing*, vol. 60 (August, 1960): 1100.
18. *Ibid.*
19. M. D. Kossoris, "San Francisco Bay Area 1966 Nurses's Negotiations," *Monthly Labor Review*, vol. 90 (June, 1967): 8–12.
20. "California Nurse Group Endorses Strike as Acceptable Bargaining Technique," *Hospitals*, vol. 40 (September 15, 1966): 201.
21. U.S. Department of Labor, Bureau of Labor Statistics, *Industry Wage Survey— Hospitals: March, 1969* (Washington, D.C.: Government Printing Office, 1971), pp. 1–11.
22. "American Nurses' Association Convention '74," *Nursing Outlook*, vol. 22 (August, 1974): 506–514.
23. Portland Oregon *Community Press*, April 27, 1977.

Bibliography

Adams, N., "Why Opinion Polls on Socialized Medicine Don't Agree." *Medical Economics* 24:72, 1947.

Adams, S. H., *The Great American Fraud*. Chicago: American Medical Association, 1907.

_____, "The Vanishing Country Doctor." *Ladies' Home Journal* 40:23, 1923.

Aikens, C. A., *Hospital Management*. Philadelphia: W. B. Saunders Co., 1911.

_____, *Hospital Training-School Methods and the Head Nurse*. Philadelphia: W. B. Saunders Co., 1907.

_____, *A Text-book for First Year Pupil Nurses, Containing Courses of Studies in Anatomy, Physiology, Hygiene, Bacteriology, Therapeutics and Invalid Cookery*. Philadelphia: W. B. Saunders Co., 1909.

_____, *Studies in Ethics for Nurses*. Philadelphia: W. B. Saunders Co., 1916.

Albert, J., "Air Evacuation from Korea—a Typical Flight." *Military Surgeon* 112:256, 1953.

Alcott, L. M., *Hospital Sketches*. Boston: Roberts Brothers, 1885.

_____, *Hospital Sketches, Camp and Fireside Stories*. Boston: Redpath, 1963.

Alford, R. R., *Health Care Politics: Ideological and Interest Group Barriers to Reform*. Chicago: The University of Chicago Press, 1975.

Alger, R. A., *The Spanish-American War*. New York: Harper and Brothers, 1901.

Allbutt, T. C., "Medicine in the Nineteenth Century." *Johns Hopkins Hospital Bulletin* 9:277, 1898.

Allen, W. H., *Civics and Health*. Boston: Ginn & Co., 1909.

Allenson, M., "My Impressions as a Post-Graduate." *American Journal of Nursing* 5:100, 1904.

Allison, G. E., "Some Experiences in Active Service; France." *American Journal of Nursing* 19:268, 1918–1919.

_____, "What the War Has Taught Us About Nursing Education." *American Journal of Nursing* 16:834, 1918–1919.

Almy, L. B., "The Nineteenth Century in Medicine, with a Glance into the Twentieth." *Yale Medical Journal* 8:31, 1901–1902.

Amadeo, M., "Achievements of Sisterhoods in Nursing-Case Activities." *Hospital Progress* 2:188, 1941.

American College of Surgeons, *Manual of Hospital Standardization: History, Development and Progress of Hospital Standardization; Detailed Explanation of the Minimum Requirements*. Chicago: The College, 1938.

American Foundation for Mental Hygiene, *The Mental Hygiene Movement; Origin, Objects and Work of the National Committee and of the American Foundation for Mental Hygiene*. New York: The Foundation, 1938.

American Hospital Association, "Constitution and By-Laws." *Transactions of the American Hospital Association* 25:605, 1923.

American Hospital Conference, *Conference on Hospital Standardization*. Chicago: American Hospital Association, 1919.

American Medical Association, Council on Medical Education and Hospitals. *Growth and Distribution of Hospital Facilities in the United States*. Chicago: The Association, 1938.

_____, *Hospitals, Sanatoriums, State and Charitable Institutions of the United States and Canada*. Chicago: The Association, 1922.

_____, House of Delegates, *Proceedings of the 105th Annual Session of the House of Delegates,*

June, 1957. Chicago: The Association, 1957.

———, *Proceedings of the 81st Annual Session of the House of Delegates, June, 1930*. Chicago: The Association, 1930.

American Nurses' Association, Commission on Nursing Research, *Priorities for Research in Nursing*. Kansas City: The Association, 1976.

———, *Inventory of Professional Registered Nurses, 1949 Edition*. New York: The Association, 1949.

———, *Inventory of Professional Registered Nurses, 1951 Edition*. New York: The Association, 1951.

———, *List of Schools of Nursing Accredited by the State Boards of Nurse Examiners*. New York: The Association, 1926.

———, Nursing Information Bureau, *Some Facts About Nursing: A Handbook for Speakers and Others*. New York: The Bureau, 1935.

———, *Report of 1956–58 Inventory of Professional Registered Nurses*. New York: The Association, 1963.

———, *Schools of Nursing Accredited by the State Boards of Nurse Examiners*. New York: The Association, 1918–1928.

American Nurses' Association and National League of Nursing Education, *Nurse Practice Acts and Board Rules: A Digest*. New York: The Association and the League, 1940.

"American Nurses' Association Assigns 'Top Priority' to Economic Security." *Modern Hospital* 48:71, 1962.

"American Nurses' Association Convention '74." *Nursing Outlook* 22:506, 1974.

"American Nurses' Association's First Position on Education for Nursing." *American Journal of Nursing* 66:515, 1966.

"ANA Platform for 1956–1958." *American Journal of Nursing* 56:882, 1956.

"ANA Platform, 1960–1962." *American Journal of Nursing* 60:1100, 1960.

American Public Health Association, *Report of the Committee on Municipal Health Department Practices*. Washington, D.C.: Government Printing Office, 1923.

"American Women and Our Wounded Men." *Washington Post*, 1944.

Amerman, B. E., "Public Health Nursing: A Profession." *Public Health Nurse* 6:22, 1914.

"An All-Out Effort to Recruit 48,000 Student Nurses." *Hospitals* 21:36, 1947.

Anderson, J. S., *Medical Nursing*. New York: Macmillan Co., 1888.

Andrus, L. H., and Fenley, M. D., "Evolution of a Family Nurse Practitioner Program to Improve Primary Care Distribution." *Journal of Medical Education* 51:317, 1976.

"Angel in War: Miss Nightingale and Her Nurses." *Contemporary Review* 106:420, 1914.

Angell, E. B., The Modern Hospital: Its Value to the Patient and to the Physician." *American Journal of Nursing* 1:703, 1900–1901.

"Angry Women in White." *Newsweek* 29:62, 1947.

Anscombe, E. M., "Methods of Ascertaining the Value of Student Services." *Transactions of the American Hospital Association* 39:631, 1937.

"Answering Dr. Catlin." *Trained Nurse* 16:121, 1896.

Arber, E., ed., *Thomas Watson Poems*. Westminster: A. Constable & Co., 1895.

"Are Nurses Hard to Find?" *Modern Hospital* 55:75, 1940.

"Are Nurses in Hospitals Underfed?" *Trained Nurse and Hospital Review* 51:364, 1913.

Ashley, J. A., *Hospitals, Paternalism, and the Role of the Nurse*. New York: Teachers College Press, 1976.

Atherton, A. B., "The Progress of Medicine and Surgery During the Last Third of the Nineteenth Century." *Maritime Medical News* 11:253, 1899.

Austin, A. L., *The Woolsey Sisters of New York: A Family's Involvement in the Civil War and a New Profession (1860–1900)*. Philadelphia: American Philosophical Society, 1971.

Aydelotte, M. K., and Hudson, W. R., "A Socio-engineering Problem—the Nursing Profession." *Nursing Outlook* 10:20, 1962.

Aynes, E., *From Nightingale to Eagle: An Army Nurse's History*. Englewood Cliffs: Prentice-Hall, 1973.

Bache, D., "The Place of the Female Nurse in the Army." *Journal of the Military Service Institution* 25:307, 1899.

Bachman, G. W., et al., *Health Resources in the United States: Personnel, Facilities, and Services*. Washington, D.C.: The Brookings Institution, 1952.

Bachman, G. W., and Meriam, L., *The Issue of Compulsory Health Insurance*. Washington, D.C.: The Brookings Institution, 1948.

Bachmeyer, A. C., "Systems of Accreditment for Schools of Nursing." *American Journal of Nursing* 36:375, 1936.

Bachmeyer, A. G., and Hartman, G., *Hospitals in Modern Society.* New York: The Commonwealth Fund, 1943.

_____, *Hospital Trends and Developments 1940-1946.* New York: The Commonwealth Fund, 1948.

Bacon, C. S., *Obstetrical Nursing: A Manual for Nurses and Students and Practitioners of Medicine.* Philadelphia: Lea, 1915.

Bacon, F., "Founding of the Connecticut Training School for Nurses." *Trained Nurse* 15:187, 1895.

Baker, N. B., *Cyclone in Calico: The Story of Mary Ann Bickerdyke.* Boston: Little, Brown and Company, 1952.

Baker, R., *America's First Trained Nurse, Linda Richards.* New York: Julian Messner, Inc., 1959.

_____, *The First Woman Doctor: The Story of Elizabeth Blackwell, M.D.* New York: Julian Messner, Inc., 1944.

Baker, T. H., "Yellowjack: The Yellow Fever Epidemic of 1878 in Memphis, Tennessee." *Bulletin of the History of Medicine* 42:241, 1968.

Bankoff, G. A., *Conquest of Pain: The Story of Anesthesia.* London: MacDonald & Co., 1946.

Bards, R. O., "The Education of the Nurse in America." *Transactions of the American Hospital Association* 12:345, 1910.

_____, "The Social, Economic, and Educational Status of the Nurse." *American Journal of Nursing* 20:955, 1919-1920.

Barrus, C., *Nursing the Insane.* New York: Macmillan Co., 1908.

Barton, G., *Angels of the Battlefield: An History of the Labors of the Catholic Sisterhoods in the Late Civil War.* Philadelphia: Catholic Publishing Co., 1897.

Bauer, W. W., "The Nurse in Industry." *American Journal of Public Health* 22:875, 1932.

Beard, M., "Nurse Emma: A Day with a Rural Nurse." *Survey* 62:113, 1920.

Beck, H. G., "The Evolution of Nursing." *Maryland Medical Journal* 59:157, 1916.

Beecroft, E. G., "The Eight-hour Day for Nurses." *Trained Nurse and Hospital Review* 62:277, 1919.

Bellevue Training School for Nurses, *Bellevue School of Nursing Procedures.* New York: Macmillan Co., 1923.

Berg, R. H., "Where Did All the Nurses Go?" *Look* 32:26, 1968.

Bernheim, B. M., "Hospital Beds: Sociological Problem." *American Scholar* 10:145, 1941.

Berry, J. M., "The New X-ray Laboratory at the Albany Hospital." *Modern Hospital* 15:264, 1920.

"The Biennial." *American Journal of Nursing* 46:728, 1946.

Billings, J. S., "A Century of American Medicine, 1776-1876." *American Journal of Medical Science* 72:439, 1876.

_____, "Medicine in the United States and Its Relations to Cooperative Investigation." *New York Medical Journal* 44:169, 1886.

_____, "The Plans and Purposes of the Johns Hopkins Hospital." *Medical News* 54:505, 1889.

_____, "The Relations of Hospitals to Public Health." *Lend a Hand* 11:168, 1893.

Billings, J. S., and Hurd, H. M., eds., "Hospitals, Dispensaries, and Nursing." *International Congress of Charities, Correction, and Philanthropy, Sec. III.* Baltimore: Johns Hopkins Press, 1894.

Billroth, T., *Care of the Sick at Home and in the Hospital.* New York: Scribner, 1898.

"Binghampton Is Over-Crowded, So Is Birmingham, So Is Colorado Springs." *American Journal of Nursing* 30:97, 1930.

Binhammer, H. M., Loveland, D. K., and Ellis, R., "Our Patients Require More Care." *American Journal of Nursing* 48:366, 1948.

Blackham, G. E., "The Place and Work of the Smaller Hospitals and Training Schools." *National Hospital Record* 9:52, 1906.

Blackwell, Elizabeth, *Pioneer Work in Opening the Medical Profession to Women: Autobiographical Sketches.* New York: Longmans, Green & Co., 1895.

Blake, E., "Graduate Nursing in the Modern Hospital." *Hospitals* 10:65, 1936.

Bliss, A. R., and Olive, A. H., *A Textbook of Physics and Chemistry for Nurses.* Philadelphia: J. B. Lippincott Co., 1918.

Block, L., "Analyze Costs Before Investing More in Nursing Education." *Hospitals* 20:70, 1946.

Blumgarten, A. S., *Materia Medica for Nurses.* New York: Macmillan Co., 1916.

Blythe, L., *38th Evac: The Story of the Men and Women Who Served with the 38th Evacuation Hospital in North Africa and Italy.* Charlotte, North Carolina: Heritage Printers, Inc., 1966.

Boardman, M. T., "Rural Nursing Service of the Red Cross." *American Journal of Nursing* 13:937, 1913.

_____, *Under the Red Cross Flag at Home and Abroad*, 2nd ed. Philadelphia: J. B. Lippincott Co., 1917.

Boas, E. P., *Unseen Plague: Chronic Disease*. London: Augustin, 1940.

Bohman, W. O., "Augmenting the Supply of Nurses." *Southern Hospitals* 18:36, 1950.

Bolton, F. P., "Report to Congress on the Nursing Shortage: Crisis in Health Care." *Hospitals* 28:83, 1954.

_____, "Why We Need a National Commission on Nursing Service." *Hospital Management* 81:76, 1956.

Bond, L. A., "Student Nurses Earn Their Keep and the Salaries They Don't Get." *Modern Hospital* 68:59, 1947.

Bonner, H. R., "Statistics of Nursing Training Schools, 1919–1920." *U.S. Bureau of Education Bulletin* 51:1, 1921.

Bonnet, P. D., "Why Not Start Over on Nurse Education?" *Hospitals* 21:25, 1947.

Boston City Hospital Training School for Nurses, *Circular of Information for Candidates and Probationers on the Necessary Outfit on Entering Service, Course of Training with a List of Questions to Be Answered by the Candidate, and a Form of Agreement to Remain Two Years as a Pupil of the School*. Boston: City Hospital, 1889.

Bowditch, N. I., *A History of the Massachusetts General Hospital, 1810–1851; with a Continuation, 1851–1872, by George E. Ellis*. Boston: Bowditch Fund, 1872.

Boyd, L. C., "Colorado School for Nurses 1887–1924: A Bit of Western Nursing History." *Trained Nurse and Hospital Review* 72:433, 1924.

Brainard, A. M., *The Evolution of Public Health Nursing*. Philadelphia: W. B. Saunders Co., 1922.

Brent, K. A., "Are Nurses Getting Too Much Education?" *Hospital Management* 67:68, 1949.

Brewster, F. S., and Smith, M. J., "An Experiment in Community Nursing." *Public Health Nurse* 10:176, 1918.

Briddon, C. K., "Reminiscences of Nearly Half a Century in Medicine and Surgery." *Medical News* 81:1010, 1902.

Bridge, H. L., *Manual of Practical Nursing*. St. Louis: C. V. Mosby Co., 1917.

Bridgman, M., *Collegiate Education for Nursing*. New York: Russell Sage Foundation, 1953.

Brines, W. S., "What Lights the Lamp—an Administrator Thinks the Emphasis in Nursing Education Belongs on Sympathy Rather Than on Science." *Modern Hospital* 79:83, 1952.

Bristow, A. T., "Is the Present System of Training Fair to the Pupil Nurse?" *American Journal of Nursing* 7:447, 1907.

Brittain, V., *Testament of Youth: An Autobiographical Study of the Years, 1900–1925*. New York: Macmillan Co., 1933.

Brockett, L. P., and Vaughan, M. C., *Woman's Work in the Civil War: A Record of Heroism, Patriotism, and Patience*. Philadelphia: Seigler, McCurdy, 1867.

Bromley, D. D., "The Crisis in Nursing." *Harper's Magazine* 161:159, 1930.

Brown, C. A., *Junior Nurse*. Philadelphia: Lea, 1914.

Brown, E. L., *Nursing as a Profession*. New York: Russell Sage Foundation, 1936.

_____, *Nursing for the Future*. New York: Russell Sage Foundation, 1948.

Bullock, R. P., *What Do Nurses Think of Their Profession?* Columbus: The Ohio State Research Foundation, 1954.

Bullough, B., "The Law and the Expanding Nursing Role." *American Journal of Public Health* 66:249, 1976.

Bundy, E. R., *Textbook of Anatomy for Nurses*. Philadelphia: P. Blakiston's Son & Co., 1906.

Burdett, H. C., *Hospitals and Asylums of the World*. London: J. & A. Churchill, 1891.

_____, *Hospitals and the State, with an Account of the Nursing at London Hospitals, and Statistical Tables Showing the Actual and Comparative Cost of Management and Maintenance, and of Work Done by the Principal Hospitals, Convalescent Institutions and Dispensaries Throughout Great Britain and Ireland*. London: J. & A. Churchill, 1881.

Burdick, A. S., "Perspectives of Medical Men and Medical Progress During the Nineteenth Century." *Medical Standard* 23:452, 1900.

Burgess, M. A., *Five-year Program for the Committee on the Grading of Nursing Schools*. New York: The Committee, 1926.

_____, "The Hospital and the Nursing Supply." *Transactions of the American Hospital Association* 29:400, 1927.

_____, *Nurses, Patients, and Pocketbooks.* New York: Committee on the Grading of Nursing Schools, 1928.

_____, "Nurses, Patients, and Pocketbooks," *Proceedings of the 34th Annual Convention of the National League of Nursing Education* 34:237, 1928.

_____, "What the Cost Study Showed." *American Journal of Nursing* 32:427, 1932.

_____, "Where Does Nursing Want to Go?" *American Journal of Nursing* 28:481, 1928.

Burks, C. R., "Changes in Diseases and Their Treatment in the Last Forty Years." *Transactions of the Medical Society of Virginia* 27:189, 1896.

Burrow, J. G., *AMA: Voice of American Medicine.* Baltimore: Johns Hopkins Press, 1963.

Bush, L. P., "Reminiscences of the Philadelphia Hospital and Remarks on Old-Time Doctors and Medicine." *Philadelphia General Hospital Reports* 1:68, 1890.

Butler, I. F., "How to Nurse the Nursing Profession." *Ladies' Home Journal* 38:12, 1921.

Cabot, R. C., "The Motive of Nursing." *Boston Medical and Surgical Journal* 182:355, 1924.

Cades, H. R., "Are There Too Many Nurses? Twelve to Twenty Talk on Jobs." *Woman's Home Companion* 57:39, 1930.

"California Nurse Group Endorses Strike as Acceptable Bargaining Technique." *Hospitals* 40:201, 1966.

Campbell, A. F., "Two Chicago Hospitals and Training Schools." *Trained Nurse and Hospital Review* 23:130, 1899.

Cantril, H., *Public Opinion, 1935–1946.* Princeton: Princeton University Press, 1951.

Carey, H. W., *A Textbook for Nurses in Bacteriology.* Philadelphia: F. A. Davis Co., 1915.

Carlisle, R., *Account of Bellevue Hospital.* New York: The Hospital, 1893.

Carter, F. G., "Hospital and Nursing Problems." *Hospitals* 15:25, 1941.

Castiglioni, A., *History of Medicine.* New York: Knopf, 1941.

Chadwick, H. D., and Pope, A. S., *Modern Attack on Tuberculosis.* New York: The Commonwealth Fund, 1946.

Chapman, F. E., *Hospital Organization and Operation.* New York: Macmillan Co., 1924.

Chayer, M. E., "Mary Eliza Mahoney." *American Journal of Nursing* 54:429, 1954.

Cheney, E. D., ed., *Louisa May Alcott: Her Life, Letters, and Journals.* Boston: Little, Brown & Co., 1889.

Chesney, J. P., "Woman as a Physician." *Richmond and Louisville Medical Journal* 11:1, 1871.

Chesnut, M. B., *A Diary from Dixie,* ed. by Williams, B. A. Boston: Houghton Mifflin Co., 1949.

Christy, T. E., *Cornerstone for Nursing Education: A History of Division of Nursing Education of Teachers College, Columbia University, 1899–1947.* New York: Teachers College Press, 1969.

_____, "Equal Rights for Women: Voices from the Past." *American Journal of Nursing* 71:288, 1971.

_____, "Portrait of a Leader: Annie Warburton Goodrich." *Nursing Outlook* 18:46, 1970.

_____, "Portrait of a Leader: Isabel Maitland Stewart." *Nursing Outlook* 17:44, 1969.

_____, "Portrait of a Leader: Isabel Hampton Robb." *Nursing Outlook* 17:26, 1969.

_____, "Portrait of a Leader: Lavinia Lloyd Dock. *Nursing Outlook* 17:72, 1969.

_____, "Portrait of a Leader: Lillian D. Wald." *Nursing Outlook* 18:50, 1970.

_____, "Portrait of a Leader: M. Adelaide Nutting." *Nursing Outlook* 17:20, 1969.

Circular and Announcement by the Trustees of the Massachusetts General Hospital, of a Two Years' Course of Training in General Nursing. Boston: The Hospital, 1889.

Clappison, G. B., *Vassar's Rainbow Division.* Lake Mills, Iowa: Graphic Publishing Co., 1964.

Clarke, A., "Draft Nurses . . . a New War and Old Theme." *R.N.* 14:24, 1951.

Cleveland (Ohio) Hospital Council, *Cleveland Hospital and Health Survey.* Cleveland: The Council, 1922.

"College of Surgeons Surveys the Nursing Situation." *Modern Hospital* 69:59, 1947.

Collins, S. D., "Frequency and Volume of Nursing Service in Relation to All Illnesses Among 9,000 Families: Based on Nation-wide Periodic Canvasses 1928–31." *Milbank Memorial Fund Quarterly* 21:5, 1943.

Colp, R., and Keller, M. W., *Textbook of Surgical Nursing.* New York: Macmillan Co., 1921.

Colton, O. A., "District Nurse of Yesterday and of Today." *Survey* 32:414, 1914.

Colvin, D., "Reminiscences of a Country Doctor During the Past Fifty Years, Including the Crude Condition of American Medical Literature at the Beginning of the Period." *Transactions of the New York Medical Association* 11:403, 1894.

Commission on Financing of Hospital Care, *Financing Hospital Care in the United States.* New York: Blakiston Co., 1954.

_____, *Financing Hospital Care in the United States. Volume 2: Prepayment and the Community.* New York: McGraw-Hill Book Co., 1955.

Commission on Hospital Care, *Hospital Care in the United States.* New York: The Commonwealth Fund, 1947.

Committee on the Costs of Medical Care, *Medical Care for the American People: The Final Report of the Committee on the Costs of Medical Care.* Chicago: The University of Chicago Press, 1932.

Committee on the Function of Nursing, *Program for the Nursing Profession.* New York: Macmillan Co., 1948.

Committee on the Grading of Nursing Schools, *Nurses: Production, Education, Distribution, and Pay.* New York: The Committee, 1930.

_____, *Nursing Schools—Today and Tomorrow.* New York: National League of Nursing Education, 1934.

_____, *Results of the First Grading Study of Nursing Schools,* 3 vols. New York: National League of Nursing Education, 1931.

_____, *Second Grading of Nursing Schools, Based on Information Gathered from 1,383 Schools of Nursing in the United States During the Year 1932.* New York: National League of Nursing Education, 1932.

Commonwealth Fund, "Five Years in Fargo." *Report of the Commonwealth Fund Child Health Demonstration in Fargo, North Dakota, 1923-27.* New York: The Fund, 1929.

Commonwealth of Massachusetts, *Report of a General Plan for the Promotion of Public and Personal Health, Devised, Prepared, and Recommended by the Commissioners Appointed Under a Resolve of the Legislature of Massachusetts Relating to a Sanitary Survey of the State.* Boston: Dutton & Wentworth, 1850.

Comstock, S., "Your Daughter's Career If She Wants to Be a Nurse." *Good Housekeeping* 61:728, 1915.

Conference on Better Care for Mothers and Babies, Washington, D.C., January 17-18, 1938. Washington, D.C.: Government Printing Office, 1938.

Connecticut Training School for Nurses, *Handbook of Nursing for Family and General Use.* Philadelphia: J. B. Lippincott Co., 1878.

Connecticut Training Schools for Nurses Attached to the New Haven Hospital, *Annual Reports of the Executive Committee to the Public.* New Haven: The School, 1875-1901.

_____, *Circular to the Public, Announcing Its Organization and Soliciting Contributions.* New Haven: The School, 1873.

Cooke, J. B., *A Nurse's Handbook of Obstetrics.* Philadelphia: J. B. Lippincott Co., 1924.

Cooper, P., *Navy Nurse.* New York: McGraw-Hill Book Co., 1946.

Cordell, E. F., "A Doctor's Life in the Backwoods One Hundred Years Ago." *Maryland Medical Journal* 41:227, 1899.

Corwin, E. H. L., *The American Hospital.* New York: The Commonwealth Fund, 1946.

_____, "Rise of the Hospital Idea." *Bulletin of the New York Academy of Medicine* 9:111, 1933.

Courtney, W., "The Trained Nurse." *St. Paul Medical Journal* 7:259, 1905.

Cowan, M. C., *Bandages and Bandaging for Nurses.* Philadelphia: W. B. Saunders Co., 1920.

Craig, L. N., "Opportunities for Men Nurses." *American Journal of Nursing* 40:669, 1940.

Crandall, E. P., "Do I Want My Daughter to Be a Nurse?" *Ladies' Home Journal* 37:99, 1920.

_____, "The National Organization for Public Health Nursing." *Modern Hospital* 8:133, 1917.

"Crisis Now Near in Medical Care?" *U.S. News and World Report* 60:38, 1966.

Cumming, K., *Gleanings from the Southland.* Birmingham: Roberts & Son, 1895.

_____, *Journal of Hospital Life in the Confederate Army of Tennessee from the Battle of Shiloh to the End of the War; with Sketches of Life and Character, and Brief Notices of Current Events During That Period.* Louisville: John P. Morton, 1866.

Cunningham, E. V., *Today's Diploma Schools of Nursing.* New York: National League for Nursing, 1963.

Cunningham, H. H., *Doctors in Gray—the Confederate Medical Service.* Baton Rouge: Louisiana State University Press, 1958.

Cunningham, R. M., "Can Political Means Gain Professional Ends?" *Modern Hospital* 77:51, 1951.

Cust, R. N., "Scutari Hospital." *Notes and Queries* 9:337, 1908.

Cyril, S., "How 20 Nurses May Save a Hospital Minimum of $4,234 in Year: Outline of Daily Routine of a Nurse Suggests Many Opportunities for Economy That Also Mean Better Service and Greater Satisfaction for the Patient." *Hospital Management* 36:21, 1933.

Daniel, H., "Better Hospitals for Everybody: The Work of the American College of Surgeons." *World's Work* 40:202, 1920.

Dante (Alighieri), *The Divine Comedy*. New York: Holt, Rinehart, & Winston, 1954.

D'Arby, L. B., "The Hospital X-ray Nurse." *American Journal of Nursing* 17:488–490, 1917.

Daughters of the American Revolution, *Second Report of the National Society of the Daughters of the American Revolution, October 11, 1897–October 11, 1898*. Washington, D.C.: Government Printing Office, 1900. Senate Document No. 425.

David, L. M., "Economic Status of Nurses." *Monthly Labor Review* 65:20, 1947.

Davidson, R., "Women and Nursing." *Nursing Science* 3:327, 1965.

Davies, M. O., "Trends in Nursing Education and Public Health Nursing Education." *American Journal of Public Health* 43:1289, 1953.

Davis, F. G., "Blue Cross Progress and Problems." *Modern Hospital* 83:51, 1954.

———, *The Nursing Profession: Five Sociological Essays*. New York: John Wiley & Sons, 1966.

Davis, G. G., *Principles and Practice of Bandaging*. Philadelphia: P. Blakiston's Sons & Co., 1911.

Davis, G. L., "Shortage of Nursing Personnel." *Journal of the American Medical Association* 135:519, 1947.

Davis, M. B., "*The Woman Who Battles for the Boys in Blue—Mother Bickerdyke*." San Francisco: Pacific Press Publishing House, 1886.

Davis, M. M., *Clinics, Hospitals, and Health Centers*. New York: Harper & Brothers, 1927.

———, "The Committee on Costs of Medical Care Makes Its Report." *Modern Hospital* 39:41, 1932.

———, "The Cost of Medical Care." *Hospital Social Service* 25:105, 1932.

———, *Immigrant Health and the Community*. New York: Harper & Brothers, 1921.

———, *Paying Your Sickness Bill*. Chicago: The University of Chicago Press, 1931.

———, *Public Medical Services*. Chicago: The University of Chicago Press, 1937.

Davis, M. M., and Haasis, B. A., "The Visiting Nurse and the Immigrant." *Public Health Nurse* 12:823, 1920.

Davis, M. M., and Warner, A. R., *Dispensaries: Their Management and Development*. New York: Macmillan Co., 1918.

Davis, N. S., "Internal Medicine in the Nineteenth Century." *Boston Medical and Surgical Journal* 144:571, 1901.

Dawson, W. W. "A Few Reflections upon the American Profession Today in Comparison to What It Was Twenty Years Ago; Contrast of the Teachings of the Present with That of the Past." *Transactions of the Ohio Medical Society* 26:45, 1872.

Dean, N. D., "The Roentgenological Field for Nurses." *American Journal of Nursing* 21:259, 1920.

Deans, A. G., and Austin, A. L., *The History of the Farrand Training School for Nurses*. Detroit: Alumnae Association of the Farrand Training School for Nurses, 1936.

"Deaths from Influenza and Pneumonia in Cities of the United States, 1918–1919." *Public Health Reports* 39:225, 1919.

DeKruif, P. H., *Fight for Life*. New York: Harcourt, 1940.

Delano, J. A., "How American Nurses Helped Win the War." *Modern Hospital* 12:7, 1919.

———, "Nursing as It Relates to the War." *American Journal of Nursing* 18:1064, 1918.

Delauney, P., "L'ancien Hotel-Dieu de Paris." *Janus* 6:405, 1901.

DeLee, J. B., *Obstetrics for Nurses*. Philadelphia: W. B. Saunders Co., 1917.

Deming, D., "Milestones of the Past 15 Years in Public Health Nursing." *American Journal of Public Health* 29:128, 1939.

———, "New Deals for Nurses." *Survey* 71:107, 1935.

———, "Nursing by Leg Power." *Survey* 63:205, 1929.

Dennie, F., "The Experience of an Army Nurse." *Trained Nurse and Hospital Review* 22:111, 1899.

Denny, F. P., "The Need of an Institution for the Education of Nurses Independent of the Hospitals." *Boston Medical and Surgical Journal* 148:657, 1903.

"Description of Appliances Exhibited at the Convention of the American Society of Superintendents of Training Schools for Nurses, Held in Pittsburgh, October, 1903." *American Journal of Nursing* 4:351, 1904.

Deutsch, A., *Mentally Ill in America: A History of Their Care and Treatment from Colonial Times*. New York: Doubleday, 1937.

———, "Trouble in Our Hospitals." *Woman's Home Companion* 78:44, 1951.

Deutscher, I. "Keep Nurses in Nursing." *Hospital Management* 86:44, 1958.

DeWitt, K., "Hospital Sketches." *American Journal of Nursing* 6:455–459, April, 1906.

———, *Private Duty Nursing*. Philadelphia: J. B. Lippincott Co., 1917.

Dickens, A. S., "University Training Is Good—But Is It Good for the Nurse as a Nurse?" *Modern Hospital* 74:79, 1950.

Dickens, C., *Martin Chuzzlewit*. New York: Macmillan Co., 1910.

Dickinson, Robert L., "The Corset: Questions of Pressure and Displacement." *New York Medical Journal* 46:507, 1887.

Diekmann, J. A., "Nursing Schools in Hospitals Under 100 Beds Should Close." *Hospital Management* 37:29, 1934.

Dietz, L. D., *Professional Problems for Nurses*, 2nd ed. Philadelphia: F. A. Davis Co., 1937.

Dix, D., *Memorial of D. L. Dix, Praying for a Grant of Land for the Relief and Support of the Indigent Curable and Incurable Insane in the United States*. Washington, D.C.: Tippin & Streeper, 1848.

Dix, G. "Hard Labour in the Hospitals." *Westminster Review* 140:627, 1893.

Dock. L. L., "The Development of Nursing in Hospitals." *Nosokomeion* 2:265, 1931.

————, "Experiment in Contagious Nursing." *Charities* 11:19, 1903.

————, "The History of Public Health Nursing." *Public Health Nurse* 14:522, 1922.

————, *Hygiene and Morality*. New York: Putnam, 1912.

————, "The Relation of the Nursing Profession to the Woman Movement." *Nurses Journal of the Pacific Coast* 5:197–201, 1909.

————, "Secretary's Report of the Meeting of the International Council of Nurses, Buffalo, New York, September 16, 1901." *American Journal of Nursing* 2:51, 1901.

————, *Text-book of Materia Medica for Nurses*. New York: Putnam, 1890.

Dock, L. L., et al., *History of American Red Cross Nursing*. New York: Macmillan Co., 1922.

"Dr. Flexner on German and American Hospitals." *Survey* 31:430, 1914.

"Doctors State Their Views on Nursing Education." *Modern Hospital* 75:72, 1950.

Donabedian, A., "Issues in National Health Insurance." *American Journal of Public Health* 66:345, 1976.

————, "Measuring and Evaluating Hospital and Medical Care." *Bulletin of the New York Academy of Medicine* 52:51, 1976.

Dorland, W. A. N., "The Progress of Medical Science During the World War." *Military Surgeons* 52:244, 1923.

Draper, Warren F., "The National Health Program and the Nurse." *American Journal of Nursing* 39:471, 1939.

Dreiblatt, M., "Shall We Have Cheap Labor or Good Nurses?" *American Mercury* 22:465, 1931.

Dublin, Louis, *The Effect of Life Conservation on the Mortality of the Metropolitan Life Insurance Company*. New York: Metropolitan Life Insurance Company, 1917.

————, *The First One Thousand Midwifery Cases of the Frontier Nursing Service*. New York: Metropolitan Life Insurance Company, 1932.

Dublin, L. I., and Lotka, A. J., *Twenty-five Years of Health Progress*. New York: Metropolitan Life Insurance Company, 1937.

Duffus, R. L., *Lillian Wald, Neighbor and Crusader*. New York: Macmillan Co., 1938.

Dunbar, C., "Rural Public Health Nursing." *Ohio Medical Journal* 18:33, 1922.

Dunlop, Margaret A., "History of the Nursing Corps of Base Hospital No. 10 U.S.A.," in *The Pennsylvania Hospital; History of the Pennsylvania Hospital Unit in the Great War*. New York: Paul B. Hoeber, 1921.

Earp, J. R., "Correlation of Infant Salvage with Nursing Effort." *American Journal of Public Health* 17:557, 1927.

"Economic Status of the Nursing Profession." *American Journal of Nursing* 47:456, 1947.

Editorial, *American Medical Times* 3:25, 1861.

————, *Buffalo Medical Journal* 24:191, 1869.

Edmunds, J. S., *Leaves from a Nurse's Life's History*. Rochester, New York: Press of the Democrat & Chronicle, 1905.

Edson, K. P., "Student Nurses and the Eight-hour Law in California." *Survey* 31:499, 1914.

Ehrenfeld, R. M., "The Evolution of Public Health Nursing." *American Journal of Nursing* 20:14, 1920.

Ehrenreich, B., and English, D., *Witches, Midwives, and Nurses: A History of Women Healers*. New York: Feminist Press, 1973.

"The Eight-hour Day for Nurses." *Trained Nurse and Hospital Review* 53:37, 1914.

Eldredge, A., "How Many Girls of 15 Years Are Enrolled in Nurse Schools?" *Hospital Management* 25:49, 1928.

Embree, Edwin R., *Brown America: The Story of a New Race*. New York: Viking Press, 1931.

Emerson, H., and Luginbuhl, M., *Local Health Units for the Nation: A Report*. New York: The Commonwealth Fund, 1945.

Emmet, Thomas Addis, "Personal Reminiscenses Associated with the Progress of Gynecology." *Gynecological and Obstetrical Journal* 18:301, 1900.

Ernst, H. C., "The Progress of Medicine (1850–1900)." *Boston Medical and Surgical Journal* 143:130, 1900.

"Essential Considerations for Federal Aid for Nursing Education." *American Journal of Nursing* 51:136, 1951.

"Essentials of a Nursing Education." *National Hospital Record* 11:21, 1908.

Ewell, Charles M., "What Patients Really Think About Their Nursing Care." *Modern Hospital* 109:106, 1967.

Ewing, O. R., *The Nation's Health: A Report to the President*. Washington, D.C.: Government Printing Office, 1948.

Executive Office of the President, Office of Management and Budget, *The Budget of the United States Government, 1974*. Washington, D.C., Government Printing Office, 1973.

"Experiences in the Hospitals of Philadelphia with Typhoid Fevers Originating Among the Soldiers in the Late War." *Philadelpia Medical Journal* 3:408, 1899.

"Extracts from the Journal of a Pupil Nurse." *Trained Nurse and Hospital Review* 42:95, 1909.

_____, *Trained Nurse and Hospital Review* 40:314, 1908.

Faddis, M. O., *A School of Nursing Comes of Age*. Oberlin, Ohio: Oberlin Printing Co., 1973.

_____, *History of the Frances Payne Bolton School of Nursing*. Cleveland: Western Reserve University Press, 1948.

Falk, I. S., *Security Against Sickness: A Study of Health Insurance*. New York: Doubleday, 1936.

Falk, I. S., Rorem, C. R., and Ring, M. D., *Costs of Medical Care*. Chicago: The University of Chicago Press, 1933.

"Falling Hospital Salaries and Some Compensations." *American Journal of Nursing* 32:1319, 1932.

Falls, W. H., "A Glance at Some of the Contributions of America to the Science of Medicine, from 1776 to 1876." *Cincinnati Lancet and Observer* 20:217, 1877.

Farrand Training School for Nurses, *Annual Report of the Training School Committee to the Board of Trustees of Harper Hospital*. Detroit: Harper Hospital, 1887.

_____, *Rules for Nurses in Harper Hospital*. Detroit: Harper Hospital, 1884.

Faville, K., "New Deans for Nurses." *Survey* 71:137, 1935.

Faxon, N. W., Half-empty Hospitals. *Survey Graphic* 23:604, 1934.

_____, ed., *The Hospital in Contemporary Life*. Cambridge: Harvard University Press, 1949.

"Federal Legislation—and the World We Live in." *American Journal of Nursing* 40:176, 1940.

Fein, R., *The Doctor Shortage: An Economic Diagnosis*. Washington, D.C.: The Brookings Institution, 1967.

Feingold, E., *Medicare: Politics and Policy*. San Francisco: Chandler Publishing Co., 1966.

Fifield, J. C., ed., *American and Canadian Hospitals*. Chicago: Physicians' Record Company, 1937.

Finer, H., *Administration and the Nursing Services*. New York: Macmillan Co., 1952.

First Annual Nurse Register: A Book of Reference for Families and Physicians. New York: J. H. Vail & Co., 1891.

Fishbein, M., "The Committee on the Costs of Medical Care." *Journal of the American Medical Association* 99:1950, 1932.

Fiske, A., *Structure and Functions of the Body: A Handbook of Anatomy and Physiology for Nurses and Others Desiring a Practical Knowledge of the Subject*. Philadelphia: W. B. Saunders Co., 1911.

Fitch, S. S., *Dr. S. S. Fitch's Health Almanac for 1854*. New York: S. S. Fitch & Co., 1854.

Fitzpatrick, L., *A History of the National Organization for Public Health Nursing*. New York: National League for Nursing, 1975.

Flanagan, L., *One Strong Voice*. Kansas City: American Nurses' Association, 1976.

Flexner, A., *Medical Education in the United States and Canada*. New York: The Carnegie Foundation for the Advancement of Teaching, 1910.

Flexner, S., and Flexner, J. T., *William Henry Welch and the Heroic Age of American Medicine*. New York: Viking Press, 1941.

"Flight Angel: Charlotte Cooley." *Cosmopolitan* 134:112, 1953.

Flikke, J. O., *Nurses in Action: The Story of the Army Nurse Corps*. Philadelphia: J. B. Lippincott Co., 1943.

Flint, A., "The Revolution in Medicine." *Forum* 10:527, 1891.

Florence, S. M., "Attributes Which Make for a Successful Surgical Nurse." *Modern Hospital* 24:62, 1925.

Foley, E. L., "Standing Orders." *American Journal of Nursing* 13:451, 1913.

_____, *Visiting Nurse Manual*. Chicago: Chicago Visiting Nurse Association, 1915.

Foote, J., *Essentials of Materia Medica and Therapeutics for Nurses*. Philadelphia: J. B. Lippincott Co., 1918.

_____, *The Essentials of Materia Medica for Nurses*. Philadelphia: J. B. Lippincott Co., 1910.

_____, "Hospitals, Their Origin and Evolution." *Popular Science Monthly* 82:478, 1913.

Forbes, M., "The Small General Hospital: Its Advantages and Difficulties as a Field for Training." *American Journal of Nursing* 3:341, 1902–1903.

Fox, E. G., "The Economics of Nursing." *American Journal of Nursing* 29:1037, 1929.

Francis, S. C., "The Private Duty Nurse in a New Era." *American Journal of Nursing* 36:773, 1936.

Freeman, J., *The Politics of Women's Liberation: A Case Study of an Emerging Social Movement and Its Relation to the Policy Process*. New York: McKay, 1975.

Fridenberg, P., *The Ophthalmic Patient: A Manual of Therapeutics and Nursing in Eye Disease*. New York: Macmillan Co., 1900.

Friedenwald, J., and Ruhrah, J., *Dietetics for Nurses*. Philadelphia: W. B. Saunders Co., 1905.

Frost, H., "The Training of Third-year Students in Public Health Nursing." *Modern Hospital* 12:71, 1919.

Frothingham, C., "The Administration of a Military Base Hospital: Comparison with a Civil Hospital." *Boston Medical and Surgical Journal* 179:223, 1918.

_____, "The Education of the Trained Nurse." *Boston Medical and Surgical Journal* 187:930, 1922.

Fullerton, A. M., *Nursing in Abdominal Surgery and Diseases of Women*. Philadelphia: P. Blakiston's Son & Co., 1891.

_____, *Surgical Nursing: A Compilation of the Lectures upon Abdominal Surgery, Gynecology, and General Surgical Conditions and Procedures, Delivered to the Classes in the Training School for Nurses Connected with the Woman's Hospital of Philadelphia*. Philadelphia: P. Blakiston's Son & Co., 1899.

Fulmer, H., "Does Public Health Nursing Belong in the Curriculum of the School of Nursing?" *Trained Nurse and Hospital Review* 95:539, 1935.

_____, "The Pioneer in Public Health Nursing." *Public Health Nurse* 7:19, 1915.

_____, "Visiting Nurse in a Great City: A Short History of the Visiting Nurse Association of Chicago." *Charities* 16:22, 1906.

"Funds for Nursing Cut to Bone in Federal Budget." *American Journal of Nursing* 73:414, 1973.

Furman, B., *A Profile of the United States Public Health Service, 1798–1948*. Washington, D.C.: Government Printing Office, 1973.

Furstner, J. M., "The Value of Public Health Nurses." *Wisconsin Medical Journal* 15:391, 1916–1917.

Gage, N. D., and Haupt, A. C., "Some Observations on Negro Nursing in the South." *Public Health Nursing* 24:674, 1932.

Gallison, J. C., "Nurses and Nurses." *Vermont Medical Monthly* 5:1, 1899.

Gamble, L. A., "Should Public Health Nurses Give Much Bedside Care?" *Nation's Health* 9:11, 1927.

Gardner, M. S., "The National Organization for Public Health Nursing." *Visiting Nurse Quarterly* 4:13, 1912.

_____, *Public Health Nursing*. New York: Macmillan Co., 1915.

Garrison, F. H., *An Introduction to the History of Medicine*, 4th ed. Philadelphia: W. B. Saunders Co., 1929.

Geister, J. M., "Economic Security Is More Than Money: Nurses Must Regain Their Identity." *Modern Hospital* 99:64, 1962.

_____, "Hearsay and Facts in Private Duty." *American Journal of Nursing* 26:515, 1926.

_____, "The Hospital and the Nurse." *Modern Hospital* 71:59, 1948.

_____, "More About General Duty." *Trained Nurse and Hospital Review* 107:346, 1941.

_____, "Nurses Out of Work." *Survey* 65:320, 1930.

_____, "The Trouble Is Not Lack of Nurses, It's Lack of Sense in Using Them." *Modern Hospital* 89:63, 1957.

Gelinas, A., *Nursing and Nursing Education*. New York: The Commonwealth Fund, 1946.

Gifford, H., "The Predominance of German Influence in Modern Medicine and Surgery." *Eye, Ear, Nose and Throat Monthly* 2:261, 1923–1924.

Gilbert, R., *Public Health Nurse and Her Patient*. New York: The Commonwealth Fund, 1940.

Giles, D., *A Candle in Her Hand: Bellevue Hospital School of Nursing*. New York: Putnam, 1949.

Ginzberg, E., *A Pattern of Hospital Care*. New York: Columbia University Press, 1949.
Goldmark, J. C., *Fatigue and Efficiency: A Study in Industry*. New York: Russell Sage Foundation, 1912.
_____, *Nursing and Nursing Education in the United States. Report of the Committee for the Study of Nursing Education and Report of a Survey by Josephine Goldmark*. New York: Macmillan Co., 1923.
Goldsmith, M., *Florence Nightingale: The Woman and the Legend*. London: Hodder & Stoughton, 1937.
Goldstein, S. E., "Social Function of the Hospital." *Charities* 18:160, 1907.
Goldwater, S. S., "The Nursing Crisis: Efforts to Satisfy the Nursing Requirements of the War; a Way Out of the Difficulty." *American Journal of Nursing* 18:1030, 1917–1918.
_____, *On Hospitals*. New York: Macmillan Co., 1947.
Gooch, M., "Ten Years of Progress in Reducing Maternal and Infant Mortality." *Children* 10:77, 1945.
"The Good Old Days." *Bright Corridors* 8:1, 1963.
Goodnow, M., *First-year Nursing; a Text-book for Pupils During Their First Year of Hospital Work*. Philadelphia: W. B. Saunders Co., 1912.
_____, *Outlines of Nursing History*. Philadelphia: W. B. Saunders Co., 1916.
Goodrich, A. W., "Case of the Vanishing Nurse." *Medical Economics* 24:121, 1946.
_____, "The Contribution of the Army School of Nursing." *Proceedings of the National League of Nursing Education* 25:146, 1919.
_____, "How Shall the Superintendents of Small Hospitals Be Trained?" *Transactions of the American Hospital Association* 18:359, 1916.
_____, "New Horizons in Professional Training." *Survey* 60:228, 1928.
_____, "The Past, Present, and Future of Nursing." *American Journal of Nursing* 31:1385, 1931.
_____, "The Plan for the Army School of Nursing." *Proceedings of the National League of Nursing Education* 24:171, 1918.
_____, "Report of the Survey of the Nursing Resources of the Country." *American Journal of Nursing* 18:959, 1918.
Goold, L. L., "Home Life of the Pupil Nurse: Ideal and Existent Conditions." *American Journal of Nursing* 8:752, 1908.
Goostray, S., *Fifty Years: A History of the School of Nursing, the Children's Hospital, Boston*. Boston: The Alumnae Association of the Children's Hospital School of Nursing, 1940.
_____, "Isabel Maitland Stewart: The Story of a National and International Leader in Nursing Education." *American Journal of Nursing* 54:302, 1954.
_____, *Memoirs: Half a Century in Nursing*. Boston Nursing Archives, Boston University Mugar Memorial Library, 1969.
_____, "Pediatric Nursing at the Turn of the Century." *American Journal of Nursing* 50:624, 1950.
Gordner, L. E., *Measuring Nursing Resources*. Washington, D.C.: Government Printing Office, 1949.
Gordon, H. P., "Nursing: Changing Profession." *School and Society* 69:266, 1949.
Gordon, P., "Nursing Costs: A Study Made at the Charles T. Miller Hospital, St. Paul, Minnesota." *American Journal of Nursing* 30:1495, 1930.
Gould, G. M., "The Duties and the Dangers of Organization in the Nursing Profession." *Johns Hopkins Hospital Bulletin* 10:103, 1899.
Grafton, S., "Too Busy for Back Rubs: Today's Nurse Is an Executive." *McCalls* 86:52, 1959.
"Graham Davis Attacks Brown Report on 'Nursing for the Future.' " *Modern Hospital* 71:138, 1948.
Grant, A., *Nursing: A Community Health Service*. Philadelphia: W. B. Saunders Co., 1942.
Gray, C. E., "What Are the Aims of Nursing Education?" *American Journal of Nursing* 21:308, 1920–1921.
Greenberg, D., "Influenza Statistics of the Visiting Nurse Association of New Haven." *Public Health Nurse* 12:209, 1920.
Greener, E. A., "The Hospital Is No Stronger Than Its Nursing Service." *Modern Hospital* 41:55, 1933.
_____, "Organization and Administration of the Nursing Department." *Modern Hospital* 2:163, 1914.
_____, "Report of the Committee on Education." *Proceedings of the Convention of the National League of Nursing Education* 13:76, 1913.

_____, "A Study of Hospital Nursing Service." *Modern Hospital* 16:28, 1921.

Gregory, S., *Licentiousness, Its Causes and Effects.* Boston: G. Gregory, 1857.

Grob, G. N., *The State and the Mentally Ill: A History of the Worcester State Hospital in Massa-chusetts, 1830–1920.* Chapel Hill: University of North Carolina Press, 1966.

Gross, L., "Introducing—the Supernurse: Nurse-practitioners as Physicians' Assistants." *McCalls* 98:75, 1971.

Grossman, J. E., "An Observation on the Yellow Fever Epidemic, Memphis and Shelby County, Tennessee, in 1878." *Chicago Medical School Quarterly* 26:227, 1967.

"Group Hospitalization Strongly Stressed at Protestant Hospital Convention." *Trained Nurse and Hospital Review* 91:345, 1933.

"Growing Hospital Crisis: Big Changes Coming, the Reasons." *U.S. News and World Report* 62:66, 1967.

Grunau, D. L., "Are Nurses Over-educated?" *Trained Nurse and Hospital Review* 122:210, 1949.

Guarini, E., "Electricity in Hospitals." *Scientific American* 94:44, 1906.

Guinther, L., "A Nurse Among the Heroes of the Yellow Fever Conquest." *American Journal of Nursing* 32:173, 1932.

Hahnemann Hospital Training School for Nurses, *Course of Instruction, Rules for Pupil-nurses and Questions to be Answered by Candidate.* Chicago: The Hospital, 1898.

Hale, S. J., "Lady Nurses." *Godey's Lady's Book* 92:188, March, 1871.

Hale, T., "The Five Sides of the Nursing Problem." *Modern Hospital* 89:71, 1957.

_____, "Nursing Education Heads for Catastrophe." *Modern Hospital* 84:93, 1955.

_____, "Problems of Supply and Demand in the Education of Nurses." *New England Journal of Medicine* 275:1044, 1966.

_____, "Too Much Education for Too Few Nurses?" *Modern Hospital* 86:75, 1956.

_____, "What's Wrong with American Hospitals? A Doctor's Opinion." *Saturday Review* 50:62, 1967.

_____, "Why the Nursing Shortage Persists." *New England Journal of Medicine* 270:1092, 1964.

_____, "Why the Nursing Supply Is Failing to Meet the Demand." *Modern Hospital* 95:100, 1960.

Hales, T., and Bell, E. A., "How Schools of Nursing Can Break Even." *Modern Hospital* 94:103, 1960.

Haller, J. S., "Neurasthenia: The Medical Profession and the 'New Woman' of Late Nineteenth Century." *New York State Journal of Medicine* 71:473, 1971.

Halsey, O. S., "Health Insurance and Public Health Nursing." *Public Health Nurse* 8:59, 1916.

Hamilton, A., and Stanmore, G., *Sidney Herbert of Lea: A Memoir.* New York: E. P. Dutton & Co., 1906.

Hamilton, T. S., "Three Ways to Close the Gap in Nursing." *Modern Hospital* 96:75, 1961.

Hampton, I. A., "The Aims of the Johns Hopkins Hospital Training School for Nurses." *Johns Hopkins Hospital Bulletin* 1:6, 1889.

_____, "Educational Standards for Nurses." *Trained Nurse and Hospital Review* 10:135, 1893.

_____, *Nursing: Its Principles and Practice for Hospital and Private Use.* Philadelphia: W. B. Saunders Co., 1893.

_____, "Three Years Course of Training in Connection with the Eight-hour System." *Transactions of the American Society of Superintendents of Training Schools for Nurses* 2:33, 1895.

Hardin, C. A., "Twenty Studies of Nursing Functions." *American Journal of Nursing* 54:1378, 1954.

Harding, G., *The Higher Aspects of Nursing.* Philadelphia: W. B. Saunders Co., 1919.

Harmer, B., *Textbook of Methods and Principles of Teaching the Principles and Practice of Nurs-ing.* New York: Macmillan Co., 1926.

Harris, L., *Harris College of Nursing: Five Decades of Struggle for a Cause.* Fort Worth: Texas Christian University Press, 1973.

Harris, S. E., *The Economics of American Medicine.* New York: Macmillan Co., 1964.

Harriss, E. D., "Yellow Fever—History and Nursing. *American Journal of Nursing* 16:859, June, 1916.

Hart, D. E., "An Address on Pasteur and Lister." *British Medical Journal* 23:1838, 1902.

Hartley, H. L., "The City Nurse as an Agent for the Prevention of Infant Mortality." *Transactions of the American Association for the Study and Prevention of Infant Mortality* 9:122, 1918.

Harvey, E. L., "Financing Diploma Schools of Nursing." *Hospital Management* 92:26, 1961.

Harwell, Richard B., ed., *Kate: The Journal of a Confederate Nurse.* Baton Rouge: Louisiana State University Press, 1959.

Hastings, C. J., "The Value of the Public Health Nurse in Public Health and Welfare Administration." *American Journal of Public Health* 11:712, 1921.

Haupt, A. C., "A Pioneer in Negro Nursing." *American Journal of Nursing* 35:857, 1935.

———, "Some New Emphases in Public Health Nursing." *American Journal of Public Health* 25:1346, 1935.

———, "Thirty Years of Pioneering in Public Health Nursing." *American Journal of Nursing* 39:619, 1939.

Haworth, E. P., "Nursing in the Movies." *Modern Hospital* 16:156, February, 1921.

Hayhow, E. C., "Military and Industrial Expansion Affect Hospital Personnel." *Hospitals* 16:42, 1942.

"Health Care in America: Progress and Problems." *U.S. News and World Report* 78:50, 1975.

Health Insurance Institute, *Source Book of Health Insurance Data, 1975–1976.* New York: The Institute, 1976.

Health Resources Advisory Committee, "Critical Shortage of Hospital Personnel." *Hospitals* 27:106, 1953.

Heffernon, G. A., "More Nurses Where They Are Most Needed." *Hospitals* 28:101, 1954.

Hempstead, G. S. B., "Reminiscences of the Physicians of the First Quarter of the Present Century, with a Review of Some Features of Their Practice." *Cincinnati Lancet and Clinic* 1:33, 1878.

Henry, J. N., *A Nurse's Hand-book of Medicine.* Philadelphia: J. B. Lippincott Co., 1913.

Henry Street Settlement, *Annual Report of the Henry Street Settlement for 1905.* New York: The Settlement, 1905.

Herringshaw, H., "Nursing in Prepayment Medical Care Plans." *American Journal of Nursing* 46:596, 1946.

Hertzberg, R., "The Graduate Nurse: Her Relation to Patient, Physician, and the Profession of Nursing." *New York Medical Journal* 99:584, 1914.

Hess, H. E., "That Changing Hospital Dollar." *Hospitals* 13:63, 1939.

Hickey, M., "Nurses: A Major National Need." *Ladies' Home Journal* 72:29, 1955.

Hilbert, H., "Public-health Nursing in Maternal and Child-health Services." *Children* 3:123, 1938.

Hildreth, J. L., "The Nurse's Work from the Point of View of a General Practitioner." *Trained Nurse and Hospital Review* 15:333, 1895.

Hill, S. C., *A Cook Book for Nurses.* Boston: Whitcomb & Barrows, 1906.

"Historical Sketch of the New York Hospital." *New York Journal of Medicine* 2:65, 1857.

Hodges' New York City Nurses' Directory: A Classified Directory of Graduate Nurses in Manhattan, Bronx, and Brooklyn. New York: Hodge & Co., 1916.

Hodson, J., ed., *How to Become a Trained Nurse: A Manual of Information in Detail; with a complete List of the Various Training Schools for Nurses in the United States and Canada.* New York: Abbott, 1898.

Hoffman, F. L., "Practical Statistics of Public Health Nursing and Community Sickness Experience." *Public Health Nursing* 6:24, 1914.

Hoffman, K., "St. Luke's, N.Y.: Model Hospital." *Munsey's Magazine* 22:487, 1900.

Holmes, O. W., *Currents and Counter-currents in Medical Science.* Boston: Ticknor & Fields, 1860.

Holt, L. E., *Care and Feeding of Children: A Catechism for the Use of Mothers and Children's Nurses.* New York: Appleton, 1903.

Horner, H. H., *Nursing Education and Practice in New York State, with Suggested Remedial Measures.* Albany: University of the State of New York Press, 1934.

Hornsby, J. A., and Schmidt, R. E., *The Modern Hospital: Its Inspiration, Its Architecture, Its Equipment, Its Operation.* Philadelphia: W. B. Saunders Co., 1914.

"Hospital Costs Up." *Time* 67:77, 1956.

"Hospital Work Up, Funds Down." *Survey* 69:323, 1933.

"Hospital Workers—a Militant New Force in Organized Labor." *U.S. News and World Report* 77:61, 1975.

"Hospitals in the Red." *Saturday Evening Post* 208:22, 1936.

Hôtel-Dieu, Paris, *Administration Generale de l'assistance Publique à Paris.* Paris: Hôtel-Dieu, 1882.

———, *Collection de Documents Pour Servir à l'Histoire des Hopitaux de Paris.* Paris: Hôtel-Dieu, 1881–1884.

Howard, J., *An Account of the Principal Lazarettos in Europe; with Various Papers Relative to the Plague; Together with Further Observations on Some Foreign Prisons and Hospitals; and Additional Remarks on the Present State of Those in Great Britain and Ireland.* Warrington:

T. Cadell, 1789.

Howard, S., *The New Profession of Nursing*. Montreal: Privately printed, 1875.

Howard, W. T., "During the Last Half of the Last Century Was More Done for the Advancement and Growth of Medicine Than Was Done in the Twenty-two Hundred and Fifty Years Which Preceded It?" *Transactions of the Medical and Chirurgical Faculty of Maryland* 49:25, 1902–1903.

Hoxie, G. H., *Manual of Medicine for Nurses and Housemothers*. Philadelphia: W. B. Saunders Co., 1908.

Hudson, D., "Where Are We Going in Nursing Education?" *Southern Hospitals* 26:29, 1958.

Hughes, E. C., Hughes, H. M., and Deutscher, I., *Twenty Thousand Nurses Tell Their Story*. Philadelphia: J. B. Lippincott Co., 1958.

Hughes, J., "Hospital Uses Ward Secretaries to Conserve Time of Nurses." *Hospital Management* 53:30, 1942.

Hume, R. F., *Great Women of Medicine*. New York: Random House, 1964.

Hummell, S. K., "Hospital Economics and the Future of Nursing Education." *Hospital Management* 74:91, 1952.

Hunter, F. E., "Army Nurses Did Superb Work." *Trained Nurse and Hospital Review* 116:264, 1946.

Huntington, E., *Cost of Medical Care*. Berkeley: University of California Press, 1951.

Hurd, Henry M., "Another Source of Friction in Hospital Administration." *Modern Hospital* 6:112, 1916.

———, "Disreputable Hospitals." *Modern Hospital* 2:296, 1914.

———, *The Institutional Care of the Insane in the United States and Canada*. Baltimore: Johns Hopkins Press, 1916.

———, "Is Nursing a Profession?" *Albany Medical Annals* 25:625, 1904.

———, President's Address. *Transactions of the American Hospital Association* 14:88, 1912.

———, "The Relation of the Training School for Nurses to the Johns Hopkins Hospital." *Johns Hopkins Hospital Bulletin* 1:7, 1899.

Huxley, E., *Florence Nightingale*. New York: Putnam, 1975.

Ill, E. J., "The Trained Nurse and the Doctor: Their Mutual Relations and Responsibilities." *Journal of the Medical Society of New Jersey* 2:36, 1905.

Illinois Training School for Nurses, Attached to Cook County and Presbyterian Hospitals, Chicago, *Annual Reports of the Officers to the Board of Directors*. Chicago: The School, 1881–1898.

"Industrial Nurse." *Industrial Magazine and Surgery* 22:448, 1953.

Inglis, D., "Social Forces of To-day and the Future of the Medical Profession." *Journal of the American Medical Association* 32:153, 1899.

Inke, L. V., and Mitchell, A. W., *Outlook for Women in Professional Nursing Occupations*. Washington, D.C.: Government Printing Office, 1953.

"Interim Classification of Schools of Nursing Offering Basic Programs (1949)." *American Journal of Nursing* 49:34, 1949.

Iverson, M., "Our Nursing Laws." *Trained Nurse and Hospital Review* 9:78, 1918.

Jacobs, J. B., "Elizabeth Fry, Pastor Fliedner, and Florence Nightingale." *Annals of Medical History* 3:17, 1921.

Jameson, H. F., "Uncle Sam's Bluebirds: Student Army Nurse Corps." *Ladies' Home Journal* 36:35, 1919.

Jamme, A. C., "Administrative and Legislative Problems in Meeting Modern Demands on the Graduate Nurse." *American Journal of Nursing* 17:912, 1917.

———, "The Army School of Nursing." *Public Health of Michigan* 7:97, 1919.

———, "The California Eight-hour Law for Women." *American Journal of Nursing* 19:525, 1918–1919.

———, "The Training of a Student Nurse." *Pacific Coast Journal of Nursing* 16:548, 1920.

Johns, E., "The University in Relation to Nursing Education." *Modern Hospital* 15:105, 1920.

Johns, E., and Pfefferkron, B., *The Johns Hopkins Hospital School of Nursing, 1889–1949*. Baltimore: Johns Hopkins Press, 1954.

Johns Hopkins Hospital, *Reports and Papers Relating to Construction and Organization. No. 13. Summary of Work for the Year 1884*. Baltimore: The Hospital, 1885.

———, *Rules for the Nurses' Home*. Baltimore: The Hospital, 1889.

Johnson, C., "Life, Death, and Miracles: Student Nurse in Her First Year." *Seventeen* 22:80, 1963.

Johnson, C. B., *Muskets and Medicine*. Philadelphia: F. A. Davis Co., 1917.

Johnson, R. W., *Friendly Cautions to the Heads of Families and Others, Very Necessary to Be Observed in Order to Preserve Health and Long Life; with Ample Directions to Nurses Who Attend the Sick Women in Childbed, Etc.* Philadelphia: J. Humphreys, 1804.

Joint Committee on Auxiliary Nursing Service, "Annual Report to the NLNE." *Proceedings of the 50th Annual Convention of the National League of Nursing Education* 50:239, 1946.

Joint Committee on Nursing in National Security, "Mobilization of Nurses for National Security." *American Journal of Nursing* 51:78, 1951.

Jones, E. K., "On Books and Reading: Outline of a Course of Lectures for Nurses in Hospitals." *American Journal of Insanity* 72:297, 1915-1916.

Jones, I. W., "What Ails Nursing?" *Scribner's Magazine* 97:183, 1935.

Jordan, H. J., *Cornell University—New York Hospital School of Nursing, 1877-1952.* New York: Society of the New York Hospital, 1952.

"The Journal of a Pupil Nurse." *Trained Nurse and Hospital Review* 40:314, 1908.

Judge, D., "The New Nurse: A Sense of Duty and Destiny." *Modern Healthcare* 2:21, 1974.

Judson, H., *Edith Cavel.* New York: Macmillan Co., 1941.

Kalisch, B. J., "Of Half-gods and Mortals: Aesculapian Authority." *Nursing Outlook* 23:22, 1975.

Kalisch, B. J., and Kalisch, P. A., "A Discourse on the Politics of Nursing." *Journal of Nursing Administration* 6:29, 1976.

_____, "The Girl with a Future: The Publicity and Advertising Campaign of the U.S. Cadet Nurse Corps." *Nursing Outlook* 21:444, 1973.

_____, "Slaves, Servants, or Saints? An Administrative Analysis of the System of Nurse Training in the United States, 1873-1948." *Nursing Forum* 14:222, 1975.

_____, "The U.S. Cadet Corps in World War II." *American Journal of Nursing* 76:240, 1976.

Kalisch, P. A., "Heroines of '98: Female Army Nurses in the Spanish-American War." *Nursing Research* 24:411, 1975.

_____, "How Army Nurses Became Officers: One Bar on a Shoulder Strap is Worth Two Regulations in a Book." *Nursing Research* 25:164, 1976.

Kalisch, P. A., and Kalisch, B. J., "Congress Copes with the Nurse Shortage 1941-1971: Dynamics of Congressional Nurse Education Policy Formulation." *Proceedings of Ninth Annual American Nurses' Association Research Conference.* Kansas City, Missouri: American Nurses' Association, 1974.

_____, *From Training to Education: The Impact of Federal Aid on Schools of Nursing in the United States During the 1940s.* (Final Report of NIH Grant NU 00443, in manuscript), 1974.

_____, "Nurses Under Fire: An Analysis of the World War II Experience of Military Nurses on Bataan and Corregidor." *Nursing Research* 25:400, 1976.

_____, *Nursing and War: The Role of American Nurses in Nine Wars.* (Manuscript), 1975.

_____, "Untrained But Undaunted: The Women Nurses of the Blue and the Grey." *Nursing Forum* 15:4, 1976.

_____, "The Women's Draft: An Analysis of the Controversy over the Nurses' Selective Service Bill of 1945." *Nursing Research* 22:402, 1973.

Kandel, P. M., "Graduate Nurses to Supplement Student Service." *Transactions of the American Hospital Association* 32:727, 1931.

_____, *Hospital Economics for Nurses.* New York: Harper, 1930.

Kaplan, R. H., "Adequate Nursing Service." *Hospitals* 12:45, 1938.

Keiser, P. H., "Nursing Education Costs Are Getting Too Big for Their Budgets." *Modern Hospital* 78:51, 1952.

Kelley, F., *Medical Problems of Immigration.* Easton, Pennsylvania: American Academy of Medicine Press, 1913.

Kellogg, F. S., *Mother Bickerdyke as I Knew Her.* Chicago: Unity Publishing, 1907.

Kellogg, J. H., "The Influence of Dress in Producing the Physical Decadence of American Women." *Transactions of the Michigan Medical Society* 15:41, 1891.

Kelly, C. W., "Today's Practical Nurse: How She Is Filling the Nursing Gap." *Hospitals* 33:47, 1959.

Kelly, H. A., *Walter Reed and Yellow Fever.* New York: Putnam, 1923.

Kelly, H. W., and Bradshaw, M. C., *Handbook for School Nurses.* New York: Macmillan Co., 1918.

_____, "Women in Medicine." *Bulletin of the Johns Hopkins Hospital* 7:50, 1896.

Kelly, I. V., *Textbook of Nursing Technique.* Philadelphia: W. B. Saunders Co., 1926.

Kelly, L. E., "Graduate Nursing in Rural Hospitals." *American Journal of Nursing* 32:960, 1932.

Kempf, E. J., *The Revival of Medical Learning: Including a Description of the History of the Dis-*

covery of the Circulation of the Blood; an Account of the Beginning of Modern Medical Juris-
prudence; a Sketch of the Advent of the Medical Journal; a Comment on the Commencement of
Modern Clinical Teaching; and a Synopsis of the Various Systems of Medicine Preceding the
Day of Scientific Medicine. Chicago: Medical Standard, 1905.

Kenney, J. A., "Some Facts Concerning Negro Nurse Training Schools and Their Graduates."
Journal of the National Medical Association 11:53, 1919.

Kenny, E., And They Shall Walk. New York: Dodd, 1943.

Kernodle, P. B., Red Cross Nurse in Action—1882-1948. New York: Harper, 1949.

Kimber, D. C., and Gray, C. E., Anatomy and Physiology for Nurses. New York: Macmillan Co.,
1893.

King, J. D., "The Industrial Nurse in Relation to Public Health." Public Health Nurse 11:100, 1919.

Kinney, D. H., "Nursing in the United States Army and the Legislation Effected in Connection
Therewith." British Journal of Nursing 33:127, 1904.

_____, "Some Questionable Nursing Schools and What They Are Doing." American Journal of
Nursing 5:224, 1905.

Kirkbride, F. B., "Utilization of the Dispensary and District Nursing as a Means of Reducing Hospital Deficits." Charities 14:1086, 1905.

Kirstein, G., "Why Hospitals Exploit Labor." Nation 189:3, 1959.

Klarman, H. E., The Economics of Health. New York: Columbia University Press, 1965.

Klaw, S., The Great American Medicine Show: The Unhealthy State of U.S. Medical Care and
What Can Be Done About It. New York: Viking Press, 1975.

Kleinert, M. N., "Linda Richards and the New England Hospital." Journal of the American Medical
Woman's Association 23:828, 1968.

Klem, M. C., "Is Prepaid Nursing Care Possible?" American Journal of Nursing 44:1154, 1944.

_____, "Medical Care Insurance and the Nurse." American Journal of Nursing 46:387, 1946.

Kossoris, M. D., "San Francisco Bay Area 1966 Nurses' Negotiations." Monthly Labor Review
90:8, 1967.

Kruger, D. H., "Bargaining and the Nursing Profession." Monthly Labor Review 84:699, 1961.

Kuehn, R. P., "Nurse Power in Mobilization." American Journal of Nursing 51:395, 1951.

Lamb, A. R., The Presbyterian Hospital and the Columbia-Presbyterian Medical Center, 1868-
1943: A History of a Great Medical Adventure. New York: Columbia University Press, 1956.

Lambertsen, E. C., Education for Nursing Leadership. Philadelphia: J. B., Lippincott Co., 1958.

_____, Nursing Team Organization and Functioning. New York: Teachers College, Columbia
University, 1953.

La Motte, E. N., "An American Nurse in Paris." Survey 34:333, 1915.

_____, "The Hotel-Dieu of Paris: An Historical Sketch." Medical Library and History Journal
4:225, 1906.

_____, The Tuberculosis Nurse: Her Function and Her Qualifications. New York: G. P. Putnam's
Sons, 1915.

_____, Tuberculosis Nursing. New York: G. P. Putnam's Sons, 1915.

La Perle, E. S., "Studies of Nursing Education." American Journal of Nursing 51:504, 1951.

Larrabee, E., The Benevolent and Necessary Institution: The New York Hospital, 1771-1971.
Garden City, N.Y.: Doubleday, 1971.

Lazaro, A. R., "The Role of the Flight Nurse in Air Evacuation." Military Surgeon 105:60, 1949.

Lee, E., History of the School of Nursing of the Presbyterian Hospital, 1892-1942. New York:
Putnam, 1942.

Le Hardy, J. C., "The Yellow-fever Panic." Atlanta Medical and Surgical Journal 5:605, 1888-1889.

Leland, R. G., "Seventeen Defects or Objections to Group Hospitalization." Hospital Management
35:25, 1933.

Lent, M. E., "True Function of the Nurse." Charities 21:250, 1908.

"Less Expensive Nursing Care Needed, ACS Report Concludes." Hospital Management 61:41,
1947.

Levine, E., "Some Answers to the 'Nurse Shortage.'" Nursing Outlook 12:30, 1964.

Levine, M. "Florence Nightingale—the Legend That Lives." Nursing Forum 2:24, 1963.

Lewis, C. E., and Cheyovich, T. K., "Who Is a Nurse Practitioner? Processes of Care and Patients'
and Physicians' Perceptions." Medical Care 14:365, 1976.

Lewis, F. P., "The Graduate Nurse Yesterday, Today, and Tomorrow." Buffalo Medical Journal
44:781, 1904-1905.

Lindsley, M. A., "Housekeeper Dietitian in the Hospital Field." Journal of Home Economics 4:425,
1912.

Link, E. P., "Elizabeth Blackwell, Citizen and Humanitarian." *Woman Physician* 26:451, 1971.

Livermore, M. A., *My Story of the War: A Woman's Narrative of Four Years Personal Experience as Nurse in the Union Army and in Relief Work at Home, in Hospitals, Camps, and at the Front During the War of the Rebellion. With Anecdotes, Pathetic Incidents, and Thrilling Reminiscences Portraying the Lights and Shadows of Hospital Life and the Sanitary Service of the War.* Hartford: A. D. Worthington, 1889.

———, "Nurses in the Civil War," in *Proceedings of the Sixth Annual Convention of the Nurses' Associated Alumnae of the United States, June 10, 11, and 12, 1903.* Philadelphia: J. B. Lippincott Co., 1903.

Lodge, H. C., *Selections from the Correspondence of Theodore Roosevelt and Henry Cabot Lodge, 1884–1918.* New York: Scribner's Sons, 1925.

Loftus, M. D., *A History of St. Vincent's Hospital School of Nursing, Indianapolis, Indiana, 1896–1970.* Indianapolis: Litho Press, 1972.

Logan, L. R., "Nursing in Cincinnati, 1820–1920." *University of Cincinnati Medical Bulletin* 1:68, 1920.

———, "A Program for the Grading of Schools of Nursing." *Hospital Progress* 6:549, 1925.

———, "Readjustments Which Training Schools and Nursing Departments are Facing from the Standpoint of the University." *Hospital Social Service Quarterly* 1:286, 1919.

———, "A Review of the Progress of Nursing and Nursing Education in 1924." *Modern Hospital* 24:18, 1925.

"The Long View." *Nursing Outlook* 2:403, 1954.

Longeway, M. L., *The Trained Nurses' Directory, Composed of Names Carefully Selected by Prominent Physicians and Surgeons of New York and Vicinity from Their Private Lists.* New York: Privately printed, 1897.

Longfellow, H. W., "Santa Filomena." *Atlantic Monthly* 1:22, 1857.

Longmore, T., *The Sanitary Contrasts of the British and French Armies During the Crimean War.* London: C. Griffin & Co., 1883.

Lounsbery, H. C., "Some Reminiscences of Sternberg Hospital." *American Journal of Nursing* 3:81, 1902–1903.

Loveridge, E. L., "Reminiscences of Forty Years in Hospital Work." *Bulletin of the American Hospital Association* 4:48, 1930.

Lowe, C., "Does the Nursing Profession Need Nursing?" *Ladies' Home Journal* 37:28, 1920.

Lowman, I. W., "The Relation of a School of Nursing to a Hospital." *Modern Hospital* 28:157, 1922.

Ludlam, G. P., "The Organization and Control of Training Schools." *New York Medical Journal* 83:850, 1906.

Lueth, H. C., "The New Demands for Nursing Services." *Modern Hospital* 71:56, 1948.

Lynd, R. S., and Lynd, H., *Middletown: A Study in Contemporary American Culture.* New York: Harcourt, 1929.

Lyon, E. P., "Taking the Profit Out of Nursing Education." *Modern Hospital* 37:122, 1931.

McBride, J. H., "The Good Nurse." *Chicago Medical Recorder* 19:176, 1900.

McCombs, R. S., *Diseases of Children for Nurses,* 6th ed. Philadelphia: W. B. Saunders Co., 1929.

McCormick, V., "Are There Too Many Nurses?" *Survey* 64:349, 1930.

McCrae, A., *Procedures in Nursing.* Boston: Barrows, 1925.

McDill, J. R., "Hospitals: Their Construction, Organization, and Management." *Journal of the American Medical Association* 22:99, 1899.

McDonald, A. L., *Essentials of Surgery: A Textbook of Surgery for Students and Graduate Nurses.* Philadelphia: J. B. Lippincott Co., 1919.

MacDougall, E. F., "Effect of Relief Programs on Public Health Nursing in the State: Preparation of Nurses." *American Journal of Public Health* 26:672, 1936.

MacEachern, M. T., *Hospital Organization and Management.* Chicago: Physicians' Record Co., 1947.

———, "How Hospital Standardization Can Improve the Professional Work and the Service to the Patient in the Hospital." *Surgery, Gynecology and Obstetrics* 34:149, 1922.

———, "Which Shall We Choose—Graduate or Student Service?" *Modern Hospital* 38:97, 1932.

MacFarlane, C., *A Reference Hand-book of Gynecology for Nurses,* 5th ed. Philadelphia: W. B. Saunders Co., 1927.

McGee, A. N., "The American Woman in the Army." *Collier's* 2:14, 1900.

———, "The Army Nurse Corps in 1899." *Trained Nurse and Hospital Review* 24:119, 1900.

———, "The Growth of the Nursing Profession in the United States." *Trained Nurse and Hospital*

Review 24:441, 1900.

_____, "The Nurse Corps of the Army." *Journal of the Association of Military Surgeons of the United States* 11:267, 1902.

_____, "Women Nurses in the American Army." *Proceedings of the Association of Military Surgeons of the United States* 8:242, 1899.

McGee, F., "Industrial Welfare Nursing." *American Journal of Nursing* 19:920, 1918–1919.

McGrath, B., "Fifty Years of Industrial Nursing in the United States." *Public Health Nursing* 37:119, 1945.

_____, *Nursing in Commerce and Industry.* New York: The Commonwealth Fund, 1946.

McHugh, M. B., "Relationship of Housekeeping and Nursing Service at University of Minnesota Hospitals." *Hospital Management* 52:64, 1941.

McIsaac, I., *Bacteriology for Nurses.* New York: Macmillan Co., 1909.

_____, *Hygiene for Nurses.* New York: Macmillan Co., 1908.

_____, "Illinois School for Nurses, Chicago, U.S.A." *Nursing Mirror* 27:261, 1900.

_____, *Primary Nursing Technique.* New York: Macmillan Co., 1907.

McIver, P., "Analysis of the Present Qualifications of Public Health Nurses in the United States." *American Journal of Public Health* 31:151, 1941.

_____, "Federal Aid for Nursing Education and Student War Nursing Reserve." *Hospitals* 17:21, 1943.

_____, "Public Health Nursing Under the Social Security Act: Developments Under the U.S. Public Health Service." *Public Health Nursing* 28:585, 1936.

_____, "Some Findings of the N. O. P. H. N. Survey of Public Health Nursing of Significance to State Health Administrators." *Public Health Report* 49:1081, 1934.

_____, "Trends in Public Health Nursing." *American Journal of Public Health* 25:551, 1935.

McKechnie, M. W., "What Has Been Accomplished in the Direction of a Uniform Curriculum?" *Trained Nurse and Hospital Review* 18:297, 1897.

MacLean, B. C., "Nurses—What Next?" *Modern Hospital* 47:51, 1936.

McMahon, K. H., "A War Nurse in the Fighting Fields of Europe." *American Journal of Nursing* 18:603, 1918.

MacMaster, J., "Half a League Onward in Public Health Nursing." *Trained Nurse and Hospital Review* 100:418, 1938.

McMillan, M. H., "A Practical 8-hour Nursing Schedule." *Hospital Management* 12:47, 1921.

McMurdy, R., "Negro Women as Trained Nurses in Chicago." *Survey* 31:159, 1913.

Magaw, A., "Observations on 1092 Cases of Anesthesia from Jan. 1, 1899 to Jan. 1, 1900." *Trained Nurse and Hospital Review* 31:150, 1903.

Maisel, A. Q., "Why Hospitals Are Chronically Broke." *Reader's Digest* 75:190, 1959.

Major, R. H., *Fatal Partners: War and Disease.* Garden City, N.Y.: Doubleday, 1941.

Mallory, J. B., "Account of the Yellow Fever Epidemic in Memphis in 1873." *American Journal of Medical Science* 67:343, 1874.

Manley, M. E., "The Subsidiary Worker, Attendant, in the Nursing Care of the Sick." *Transactions of the American Hospital Association* 41:523, 1939.

Mannino, A. J., "Men in Nursing." *American Journal of Nursing* 51:198, 1951.

Mansfield, E. O., "Economics Affecting the Growth of Hospital Schools of Nursing." *Hospital Management* 84:43, 1957.

Maroney, K. A., "How a Small Hospital Can Nurse Its Patients Without a School." *American Journal of Nursing* 32:640, 1932.

Marsh, A. W., "Changes That Have Occurred in the Past 25 Years Having an Effect on the Progress of Medicine." *Boston Medical and Surgical Journal* 187:821, 1922.

Marshall, E. D., and Moses, E. B., *RNs 1966: An Inventory of Registered Nurses.* New York: American Nurses' Association, 1969.

Marshall, H. E., *Dorothea Dix: Forgotten Samaritan.* Chapel Hill: University of North Carolina Press, 1937.

_____, *Mary Adelaide Nutting: Pioneer of Modern Nursing.* Baltimore: Johns Hopkins University Press, 1972.

"Mass Recruitment of Nurses Unsatisfactory." *Modern Hospital* 70:176, 1948.

Massachusetts General Hospital, Boston, *McLean Asylum Training School for Nurses. Circular and Announcement by the Trustees of the Massachusetts General Hospital of a Two Years' Course of Training in General Nursing.* Boston: The Hospital, 1889.

_____, *Nurses' Rules.* Boston: The Hospital, 1889.

Masson, D., ed., *The Poetical Works of John Milton.* New York: Macmillan Co., 1903.

"Matrimony Is Not the Goal of the Trained Nurse." *Literary Digest* 55:84, 1917.

Maxwell, A. C., "The Field Hospital at Chickamauga Park." *Trained Nurse and Hospital Review* 23:3, 1899.

————, "Struggles of the Pioneers." *American Journal of Nursing* 21:321, 1920–1921.

Maxwell, A. C., and Keith, M. L., "The Private Nurse and Twenty-four Hour Hospital Duty." *American Journal of Nursing* 17:191, 1916.

Maxwell, A. C., and Pope, A. E., *Practical Nursing: A Text-book for Nurses,* 4th ed. New York: Putnam, 1923.

Mayo, W. J., "The Medical Profession and the Public." *Journal of the American Medical Association* 76:921, 1921.

Mead, K. C., *History of Women in Medicine.* New York: Haddam Press, 1938.

Mechanic, D., *The Growth of Bureaucratic Medicine: An Inquiry into the Dynamics of Patient Behavior and the Organization of Medical Care.* New York: John Wiley & Sons, 1976.

Menninger, K., "The Future of Psychiatric Care in Hospitals." *Modern Hospital* 64:43, 1945.

Menninger, W. C., *Psychiatry in a Troubled World: Yesterday's War and Today's Challenge.* New York: Macmillan Co., 1948.

Methodist Episcopal Hospital, *Admission of Patients.* Philadelphia: The Hospital, 1892.

————, *Collection of Blank Forms Used in the Hospital, Including Admission Cards; Application for Copies of Hospital Report; Bed Card; Contract to Pay Hospital Charges; Dispensary Ticket; History of Case; Order for Stimulants; Patient's Clothing List; Physician's Certificate for Admission; Requisition; Subscription Blanks, Weekly Reports.* Philadelphia: The Hospital, 1890–1892.

Millard, S., *I Saw Them Die: Diary and Recollections of Shirley Millard.* New York: Harcourt, Brace, & Co., 1936.

Miller, M. C., *Through the Years with the Nurses at the Shadyside Hospital.* Pittsburgh: Miriam C. Miller, 1946.

————, "What's Got into the Nurses?" *Medical Economics* 29:135, 1951.

Mills, C. K., "The Hospital and the Nurse." *Philadelphia Monthly Medical Journal* 1:643, 1899.

————, *Nursing and Care of the Nervous and the Insane.* Philadelphia: J. B. Lippincott Co., 1887.

Minderman, E., "One Thousand Eight Hundred and Twenty-six Public Hospitals Aided by WPA During the Last Five Years." *Hospital Management* 50:22, 1940.

Minot, F., "The Progress of Medicine During the Last Fifty Years." *Boston Medical and Surgical Journal* 121:269, 1889.

Montag, M. L., *Community College Education for Nursing: An Experiment in Technical Education for Nursing.* New York: McGraw-Hill Book Co., 1959.

————, "Technical Education in Nursing." *American Journal of Nursing* 63:100, 1963.

Moody, S., "Isabel Hampton Robb—Her Contribution to Nursing Education." *American Journal of Nursing* 38:1131, 1938.

Moore, H. H., *Public Health in the United States.* New York: Harper, 1923.

"More Nurses Needed." *New York State Journal of Medicine* 48:155, 1948.

Morgan, J. D., "Are the Trained Nurses Over-educated?" *American Journal of Nursing* 6:858, 1906.

Morrill, W. P., "School of Nurses with University Affiliation." *Proceedings of the National League of Nursing Education, 1920* 26:303, 1921.

Morten, H., *Nurse's Dictionary of Medical Terms and Nursing Treatment.* Philadelphia: W. B. Saunders Co., 1894.

Mortimer, M., *A Green Tent in Flanders.* New York: Doubleday, 1918.

Morton, T. G., *The History of the Pennsylvania Hospital, 1751–1895.* Philadelphia: Times Printing House, 1897.

Mountin, J. W., "Nursing—a Critical Analysis." *American Journal of Nursing* 43:29, 1943.

"Mrs. America Takes Up Home Nursing." *Saturday Evening Post* 215:84, 1943.

Mumey, N., *Hygiene for Nurses.* St. Louis: C. V. Mosby Co., 1918.

Munson, H. W., and Stevens, K., *Story of the National League of Nursing Education.* Philadelphia: W. B. Saunders Co., 1934.

Mustard, H. S., *Government in Public Health.* New York: The Commonwealth Fund, 1945.

————, *Introduction to Public Health,* 2nd ed. New York: Macmillan Co., 1944.

————, *Rural Health Practice.* New York: The Commonwealth Fund, 1936.

Myrdal, G., et al., *An American Dilemma: The Negro Problem and Modern Democracy.* New York: Harper & Brothers, 1944.

Naffziger, H. C., "Comments on Report on Activities of the American College of Surgeons to Promote Training and Use of Vocational Nurses in Hospitals." *Bulletin of the American College of Surgeons* 33:26, 1948.

Nahm, H., "Temporary Accreditation." *American Journal of Nursing* 52:997, 1952.

Napheys, G. H., *Handbook of Popular Medicine, Embracing the Anatomy and Physiology of the Human Body; Illustrations of Home Gymnastics; Instructions for Nursing the Sick; the Domestic Treatment of the Ordinary Diseases and Accidents of Children and Adults; Plan for a Family Health Record, Etc. With Over 300 Choice Dietetic and Remedial Recipes, and More Than 100 Engravings on Wood. Especially Adapted for General and Family Instruction and Reference.* Philadelphia: H. C. Watts, 1882.

National Commission for the Study of Nursing and Nursing Education, *An Abstract for Action.* New York: McGraw-Hill Book Co., 1970.

National Committee on Maternal Health, *Biennial Report, 1927–28.* New York: The Committee, 1928.

National League for Nursing, *Report on Hospital Schools of Nursing, 1957.* New York: National League for Nursing, 1959.

———, *Roles and Relationships in Nursing Education. Viewpoints Expressed at the 1959 Regional Conference of Representatives of Nursing Service and Nursing Education.* New York: National League for Nursing, 1959.

———, *Study on Cost of Nursing Education. Part I. Cost of Basic Diploma Programs.* New York: The League, 1964.

———, *Study on Cost of Nursing Education. Part II. Cost of Basic Baccalaureate and Associate Degree Programs.* New York: The League, 1965.

———, Department of Diploma and Associate Degree Programs, in *Report on Hospital Schools of Nursing, 1957.* New York: National League for Nursing, 1959.

———, in *Today's Diploma Schools of Nursing: Report of the 1962 Survey of 728 Diploma Schools of Nursing. Prepared by Elizabeth V. Cunningham.* New York: The League, 1963.

National League of Nursing Education, *List of Schools of Nursing Meeting Minimum Requirements Set by Law in the Various States.* New York: The League, 1935.

———, *The Pupil Nurse in the Out-patient Department: A Study of the Nurse and Nursing Services in the Out-patient Department.* New York: The League, 1925.

———, *Study of Nursing Service in One Children's and Twenty-one General Hospitals.* New York: The League, 1948.

———, Committee on Curriculum, *A Curriculum Guide for Schools of Nursing.* New York: The League, 1927.

———, *A Curriculum Guide for Schools of Nursing.* New York: The League, 1937.

———, Committee on Education, *Nursing School Faculty: Duties, Qualifications, and Preparation.* New York: The League, 1933.

———, *Standard Curriculum for Schools of Nursing, Prepared by the Committee on Education of the National League of Nursing Education.* New York: The League, 1917.

———, Committee on Standards, *Essentials of a Good School of Nursing.* New York: The League, 1936.

———, Committee on Studies, *Study of the Nursing Service in Fifty Selected Hospitals.* New York: The League, 1937.

———, Committee to Study Administration in Schools of Nursing, *Fundamentals of Administration for Schools of Nursing.* New York: The League, 1940.

———, Department of Studies, *State-accredited Schools of Nursing,* rev. ed. New York: The League, 1946.

———, *Study on the Use of the Graduate Nurse for Bedside Nursing in the Hospital.* New York: The League, 1933.

National Organization for Public Health Nursing, *Principles and Practice of Public Health Nursing Including Cost Analysis.* New York: Macmillan Co., 1932.

———, *Report of the Committee to Study Visiting Nursing.* New York: The Organization, 1924.

———, *Survey of Public Health Nursing: Administration and Practice.* New York: The Commonwealth Fund, 1934.

Neff, R. E., "The Cost of Nursing Education to the Hospital." *American Journal of Nursing* 29:1119, 1929.

———, "A Hospital Administrator Explores the Field of Nursing." *Modern Hospital* 41:55, 1933.

Neergaard, C. F., "Some Glaring Faults in Hospital Construction." *Modern Hospital* 6:408, 1916.

Nelson, S. C., "Mary Sewall Gardner." *Nursing Outlook* 1:668, 1953.

New England Hospital for Women and Children, *Annual Reports of the Officers to the Society and Friends, 1862–3 to 1892–3.* Boston: The Hospital, 1863–1894.

_____, *History and Description of the New England Hospital for Women and Children.* Boston: The Hospital, 1876.

"New Group Will Combat Legislation Unfavorable to Unclassified Nursing Schools." *Modern Hospital* 74:128, 1950.

New Haven, Connecticut, State Hospital, Training School for Nurses, *Hand-book of Nursing for Family and General Use. Published Under the Direction of the Connecticut Training School for Nurses, State Hospital, New Haven, Connecticut.* Philadelphia: J. B. Lippincott Co., 1878.

"New Structure of Nursing Organizations." *Public Health Reports* 67:1258, 1952.

New York Academy of Medicine, Public Health Committee, "Problems of Disease." *Modern Medicine* 2:1, 1920.

New York Association for Improving the Condition of the Poor, *Annual Report for 1884.* New York: The Association, 1884.

New York City, Department of Public Charities, *The Charity Hospital Training School for Male Nurses, Blackwell's Island.* New York: The Department, n.d.

_____, *The Training School for Nurses, Charity Hospital, Blackwell's Island.* New York: The Department, 1882.

New York Hospital Training School for Nurses, Attached to Bellevue Hospital, *Manual of Nursing Prepared for the Training School for Nurses, Attached to Bellevue Hospital.* New York: The Hospital, 1878.

New York Nurse Register, Containing Names and Addresses of Professional Female and Male Nurses and Masseurs of New York, Brooklyn, and Jersey City. New York: George W. Rachel, 1888.

New York State Charities Aid Association, *A Century of Nursing, with Hints Towards the Organization of a Training School.* New York: The Association, 1876.

_____, *Hand-book for Hospitals.* New York: The Association, 1883.

_____, *Report of the Committee on Hospitals, Dec. 23, 1872, on the Training School for Nurses to Be Attached to Bellevue Hospital.* New York: The Association, 1873.

_____, *Sickness in Dutchess County, New York: Its Extent, Care and Prevention.* New York: The Association, 1915.

New York Tenement House Commission, *Report of the Tenement House Commission for 1900.* New York: The Commission, 1900.

"Night Duty." *Trained Nurse and Hospital Review* 41:239, 1908.

Nightingale, F., *A Contribution to the Sanitary History of the British Army During the Late War with Russia.* London: Harrison, 1859.

_____, "Hospital Statistics and Hospital Plans." *Transactions of the National Association for the Promotion of Social Science* 4:554, 1861.

_____, *Introductory Notes on Lying-in Institutions; Together with a Proposal for Organizing an Institution for Training Midwives and Midwifery Nurses.* London: Longmans, Green & Co., 1871.

_____, *Notes on Hospitals.* London: Parker, 1859.

_____, *Notes on Matters Affecting the Health, Efficiency, and Hospital Administration of the British Army.* London: Harrison & Sons, 1858.

_____, *Observations on the Evidence Contained in the Stational Reports Submitted to the Royal Commission on the Sanitary State of the Army in India.* London: Stanford, 1863.

_____, *Talks to Pupils: A Selection of Addresses to Probationers and Nurses.* New York: Macmillan Co., 1914.

Nixdorff, N. W., "Training of a Professional Nurse." *Ladies' Home Journal* 30:30, 1913.

Notable American Women, 1607–1950. Cambridge: Harvard University Press, 1971.

Noyes, C. D. "How Some Nursing Leaders Visualize the Ideal Student Nurse." *Hospital Management* 23:53, 1927.

_____, "Postgraduate Study for Nurses." *Proceedings of the Annual Meeting of American Society of Superintendents of Training Schools for Nurses* 11:121, 1905.

"The Nurse." *America* 41:407, 1944.

"Nurse and Immigrant." *Survey* 35:234, 1915.

"Nurse Training Provisions Pass Over Presidential Veto." *American Journal of Nursing* 75:1413, 1975.

"Nurse Training Schools, 1917–18." *U.S. Bureau of Education Bulletin* 73:1, 1919.

Nurse's Manual and Mother's Medical Adviser; a Guide to the Inexperienced. Philadelphia: Lindsay & Blakiston, 1845.

"Nurses and Labor Laws." *Trained Nurse and Hospital Review* 52:37, 1914.

"Nurses and Nursing." *British and Foreign Medico-Chirurgical Review* 57:283, 1876.

"Nurses Prove Their Way: Work-relief Project in Nursing." *Survey* 70:164, 1934.

"Nurses' Schools and Illegal Practice of Medicine." *The Journal of the American Medical Association* 47:1835, 1906.

Nursing Techniques Used in the Strong Memorial Hospital and the Rochester Municipal Hospital Which Are Associated with the University of Rochester School of Nursing. Rochester: The School, 1945.

Nutting, M. A., Address, *Proceedings of the Annual Convention of the American Society of Superintendents of Training Schools for Nurses* 17:18, 1911.

_____, "Apprenticeship to Duty." *American Journal of Nursing* 19:159, 1918–1919.

_____, *The Education and Professional Position of Nurses.* Washington, D.C.: Government Printing Office, 1907.

_____, "Educational Status of Nursing." *U.S. Bureau of Education Bulletin* 7:1, 1912.

_____, "How the Nursing Profession Is Trying to Meet the Problems Arising out of the War." *Proceedings of the National League of Nursing Education* 24:125, 1918.

_____, "Notes of a Typhoid Fever Case." *Trained Nurse* 6:121, 1891.

_____, "Nursing and Public Health." *Boston Medical and Surgical Journal* 166:401, 1912.

_____, "Nursing as It Relates to the War." *Proceedings of the National League of Nursing Education* 24:246, 1918.

_____, President's Address, in *Transactions of the American Hospital Association* 14:88, 1912.

_____, "The Relation of the Nursing Profession to the Community at Large." *Trained Nurse and Hospital Review* 19:1, 1897.

_____, "The Relation of the War Program to Nursing in Civil Hospitals." *Modern Hospital* 11:339, 1918.

_____, "The Report of the Committee on Education." *Proceedings of the Convention of the National League of Nursing Education* 19:76, 1913.

_____, *Sound Economic Basis for Schools of Nursing and Other Addresses.* New York: Putnam, 1926.

_____, "Thirty Years of Progress in Nursing." *American Journal of Nursing* 23:1027, 1923.

_____, "Visiting Nurses for Tuberculosis." *Charities* 16:51, 1906.

Nutting, M. A., and Dock. L. L., *A History of Nursing: The Evolution of Nursing Systems from Earliest Times to the Foundations of the First English and American Training Schools for Nurses,* 4 vols. New York: G. P. Putnam's Sons, 1907 and 1912.

O'Brien, H. J., ed., *Medical and Surgical Nursing: A Treatise on Modern Nursing from the Physician's and Surgeon's Standpoint, for the Guidance of Graduate and Student Nurses, Together with Practical Instruction in the Art of Cooking for the Sick.* New York: G. P. Putnam's Sons, 1900.

Ochsner, A. J., and Sturm, M. J., *The Organization, Construction, and Management of Hospitals.* Chicago: Cleveland Press, 1907.

O'Gorman, J. J., "Early American Hospitals." *Catholic World* 131:290, 1930.

"Old Hospitals." *Southern Hospitals* 5:4, 1937.

Olmsted, K. M., "Rural Nursing." *Transactions of the American Association for the Study and Prevention of Infant Mortality* 7:242, 1916.

Olson, A. P., and Tibbitts, H. G., "Study of Head Nurse Activities in a General Hospital." Washington, D. C.: Government Printing Office, 1951.

"On the Shortage of Practical Nurses." *Hospitals* 25:28, 1951.

"Opening of the Nurses' Home and Inauguration of the Training School for Nurses." *Johns Hopkins Hospital Bulletin* 1:6, 1889.

"Organized Public Nursing and Variation of Field Programs in 94 Selected Counties." *Public Health Reports* 54:815, 1939.

Osborn, S. G., *Scutari and Its Hospitals.* London: Dickinson Brothers, 1855.

Osler, W., *Doctor and Nurse: Remarks to the First Class of Graduates from the Training School for Nurses at the Johns Hopkins Hospital.* Baltimore: The Hospital, 1891.

_____, *Evolution of Modern Medicine.* New Haven: Yale University Press, 1921.

Ott, F. M., "Nursing in the Early Days." *Trained Nurse and Hospital Review* 107:103, 1941.

Ottenberg, R., *Chemistry for Nurses.* New York: Macmillan Co., 1914.

"Our Health and Our Hospitals." *Collier's* 117:90, 1946.

Owen, M. A., "Lest We Forget: Memories of Front-line Nursing." *Trained Nurse and Hospital Review* 95:415, 1935.

Packard, F. R., *Some Account of the Pennsylvania Hospital: From Its First Rise to the Beginning of the Year 1938*. Philadelphia: The Hospital, 1938.

Pahl, H. W., "The Eight-hour Law for Pupil Nurses in California, After One and One-half Years Practical Demonstration in a General Hospital of 100 Beds." *Proceedings of the National League of Nursing Education* 21:178, 1915.

Palmer, G., "Hospital That Walks Upstairs: Day in New York Slums with a Visiting Nurse." *Reader's Digest* 31:26, 1937.

Palmer, S. F., "The Effect of State Registration upon Training Schools." *American Journal of Nursing* 5:656, 1904–1905.

———, "The Essential Features of a Bill for the State Registration of Nurses and How to Pass It." *American Journal of Nursing* 7:428, 1907.

Parker, E. M., and Breckinridge, S. D., *Surgical and Gynecological Nursing*, 3rd ed. Philadelphia: J. B. Lippincott Co., 1925.

Parker, W. W., "Woman's Place in the Christian World: Superior Morally, Inferior Mentally to Man; Not Qualified for Medicine or Law; the Contrariety and Harmony of the Sexes." *Transactions of the Medical Society of Virginia* 23:86, 1892.

Parran, T., "Public Health in the Reconversion Period." *American Journal of Public Health* 35:987, 1945.

———, "Public Health Nursing Marches On." *Public Health Nursing* 29:617, 1937.

———, *Shadow on the Land*. New York: Reynal & Hitchcock, 1937.

Parsons, F. G., *The History of St. Thomas' Hospital*, 3 vols. London: Methuen, 1932.

Parsons, S. E., *History of the Massachusetts General Hospital Training School for Nurses*. Boston: Barrows, 1922.

———, "Impressions and Conclusions Based on Experience Abroad by Overseas Nurses." *American Journal of Nursing* 19:829, 1918–1919.

———, *Nursing Problems and Obligations*. Boston: Barrows, 1916.

Paterson, R. G., "The Development of State Public Health Nursing." *Public Health Nurse Quarterly* 8:69, 1916.

———, *Nursing in the Acute Infectious Diseases*, 3rd ed. Philadelphia: W. B. Saunders Co., 1915.

———, "Twenty Years of County Public Health Nursing in Ohio." *Public Health Nursing* 25:329, 1933.

Paul, G. P., *A Text-book of Materia Medica for Nurses*, 4th ed. Philadelphia: W. B. Saunders Co., 1924.

Pearch, F. S., "Practical Application of Electricity." *Trained Nurse and Hospital Review* 24:338, 1900.

Peck, C. H., "The Hospitals of the American Expeditionary Forces." *Annals of Surgery* 68:463, 1918.

Peebles, A., and McDermott, V. D., *Nursing Services and Insurance for Medical Care in Brattleboro, Vermont*. Chicago: The University of Chicago Press, 1932.

Pennock, M., ed., *Makers of Nursing History*. New York: Lakeside, 1940.

"Pennsylvania Hospital: The Pioneer Hospital of the United States." *National Hospital Record* 5:3, 1901–1902.

Pennsylvania Hospital for the Insane, *Annual Report of the Physician-in-Chief and Superintendent to the Board of Managers for 1842*. Philadelphia: The Hospital, 1843.

Perrott, G., St. J., and Holland, D. F., "Health as Element in Social Security." *Annals of the American Academy of Political and Social Science* 202:116, 1939.

Perry, C. M., "Pupil Nursing Outside the Hospital." *The International Hospital Record* 14:23, 1910.

"Personnel Shortage Closes Thousands of Hospital Beds." *Southern Hospitals* 15:44, 1947.

Petry, L., "Increasing and Using Nursing Auxiliaries." *Hospitals* 17:37, 1943.

———, "Nursing Service in Hospitals," in *Chicago-Cook County Health Survey*. New York: Columbia University Press, 1949.

———, "Training of Practical Nurses for Hospital Staffs Urged." *Hospital Management* 62:74, 1946.

Petry, L., Arnstein, M., and Gillan, R., "Surveys Measure Nursing Resources." *American Journal of Nursing* 49:770, 1949.

Petry, L., Arnstein, M., and McIver, P., "Research for Improved Nursing Practices." *Public Health Reports* 67:183, 1952.

Petry, L., and Vreeland, E. M., "Nursing Education." *Higher Education* 8:181, 1952.

Pfefferkorn, B., "Cost Study of Nursing Service and Nursing Education." *Transactions of the*

American Hospital Association 40:657, 1938.

―――, "Improvement of the Nurse in Service—an Historical Review." *American Journal of Nursing* 28:700, 1928.

Phelps, C., "Address: The Medical Profession at the Close of the Nineteenth Century." *Transactions of the New York Medical Association* 13:36, 1896.

"The Philadelphia Biennial: Nursing in a Democracy." *American Journal of Nursing* 40:673, 1940.

Philadelphia Department of Charities and Correction, Philadelphia Hospital Training School for Nurses, *Course of Study for Probationers, Junior and Senior Classes*. Philadelphia: The Department, 1889.

Philadelphia General Hospital, *Annual Report of the Philadelphia General Hospital for 1866*. Philadelphia: The Hospital, 1866.

Philadelphia General Hospital, *Annual Report of the Philadelphia General Hospital for 1883*. Philadelphia: The Hospital, 1883.

―――, *Manual of Nursing Procedures*. Philadelphia: The Hospital, 1924.

Philadelphia Lying-in and Nurse Charity, *Appeal for the Supply of a Greater Number of Intelligent Women to Become Trained as Nurses for the Sick*. Philadelphia: The Charity, 1855.

Pickhardt, L., "Recent Legislation Governing Hours of Duty of Pupil Nurses in Hospitals." *Proceedings of the 20th Convention of the National League of Nursing Education*. 20:106, 1914.

Pilcher, J. E., "The Red Cross." *Military Surgeon* 20:230, 1907.

Pines, M., "Hospital: Enter at Your Own Risk." *McCalls* 95:79, 1968.

Pipe, A. E., *Manual of Nursing Procedures*. New York: Putnam, 1919.

―――, *Textbook of Anatomy and Physiology for Nurses*. New York: Putnam, 1913.

Pipe, A. E., and Carpenter, M. L., *Essentials of Dietetics*, 2nd ed. New York: G. P. Putnam's Sons, 1917.

"Platform of the American Nurses' Association." *American Journal of Nursing* 52:953, 1952.

Pogrebin, L. C., "Why Do Women in White See Red?" *Ladies' Home Journal* 89:40, 1972.

Pointer, D. D., and Graham, H., "Recognition, Negotiation, and Work Stoppages in Hospitals." *Monthly Labor Review* 94:54, 1971.

Pollard, E. F., *Florence Nightingale*. London: S. W. Partridge Co., 1902.

Poole, A. R., "Public Health Nurse: Friend of the People." *Survey* 52:537, 1924.

Poole, E., *Nurses on Horseback*. New York: Macmillan Co., 1935.

Potter, T., "The Nursing Problem." *New York Medical Journal* 91:995, 1910.

Powers, E. J., *Hospital Pencilings*. Boston: Edward L. Mitchell, 1866.

"Practice of Medicine by Nurses." *Boston Medical and Surgical Journal* 185:728, 1921.

Preston, A., *Nursing the Sick and the Training of Nurses*. Philadelphia: King & Baird, 1863.

Price, J., "The Professional Nurse and Her Training." *Transactions of the American Association of Obstetricians and Gynecologists* 11:130, 1899.

"Prock's Letters from Camp, Battlefield, and Hospital." *Indiana Magazine of History* 34:96, 1938.

"A Prophet Honored." *American Journal of Nursing* 71:58, 1971.

"Pupil Nurses on Outside Cases." *The International Hospital Record* 17:10, 1914.

Putnam, H. C., "Attendants and Nursemaids: Less Expensive and Less Expert Service Needed; Classes by Philanthropic Organizations; Medical Institutions for the Sick the Proper Ones to Give Such Instruction; This Grade of Helpers Would Raise the Standing of Graduate Nurses." *Journal of the American Medical Association* 38:1364, 1902.

Pyle, E., *Here Is Your War: The Story of G. I. Joe*. Cleveland: World Publishing Co., 1944.

Quain, R., *A Dictionary of Medicine*. New York: D. Appleton & Co., 1883.

Quandt, E., "Active Service on the Western Front." *American Journal of Nursing* 18:388, 1917–1918.

Quintard, L. W., "Limitations of Pupil Nurses in Caring for Male Patients." *Proceedings of the American Society of Superintendents of Training Schools for Nurses* 3:70, 1896.

Radey, H. M., "Study of Nursing Care—How Much, When, and by Whom?" *Hospitals* 27:72, 1953.

Randall, M. G., "Home Nursing Service in the Health Insurance Plan of Greater New York." *American Journal of Public Health* 39:167, 1949.

―――, "The Public Health Nurse in a Rural Health Department: An Introductory Report on the Study in Progress in Cattaraugus County." *American Journal of Public Health* 21:737, 1931.

―――, "Public Health Nursing Service for Rural Children." *Quarterly Bulletin of the Milbank Memorial Fund* 10:276, 1932.

Ransome, J. E., "The Beginnings of Hospitals in the United States." *Bulletin of the History of Medicine* 13:514, 1943.

Rathbone, W., *History and Progress of District Nursing*. New York: Macmillan Co., 1890.

Ravenel, M. R., ed., *Half Century of Public Health*. New York: American Public Health Association, 1921.

Rawlings, B. B., "Nurses in Hospitals." *The Nineteenth Century* 10:824, 1908.

Rayfield, S., "A Study of Negro Public Health Nursing." *Public Health Nursing* 22:525, 1930.

Redmond, J., *I Served on Bataan*. Philadelphia: J. B. Lippincott Co., 1943.

Reed, C. A. L., "The Relations of the Nursing Profession to That of Medicine and to Society." *Cincinnati Lancet-Clinic* 53:82, 1904.

Register, W. R., *Practical Fever Nursing*. Philadelphia: W. B. Saunders Co., 1907.

"Registration of Trained Nurses." *Outlook* 73:503, 1903.

"Regulations Governing Bellevue and Allied Hospitals in the City of New York." *Charities* 6:317, 1901.

Reid, E. P., et al., *A Manual of Nursing Procedures*. Philadelphia: W. B. Saunders Co., 1923.

Reid, L. D., "The Trouble with Nursing? No Nurses." *Modern Hospital* 88:58, 1957.

Reid, M. E., *Bacteriology in a Nutshell*, 8th ed. New York: Paul B. Hoeber, 1915.

———, "Some Reasons for the Training School in Small Hospitals." *National Hospital Record* 9:26, 1906.

Reisman, L., and Rohrer, J. H., *Change and Dilemma in the Nursing Profession*. New York Putnam, 1957.

Rennie, T. A. C., and Woodward, L. E., *Mental Health in Mental Society*. New York: The Commonwealth Fund, 1948.

"Report of Committee on Nursing Education." *Nation's Health* 4:408, 1922.

"Report of the Committee on the Training of Nurses." *Transactions of the American Medical Association* 20:161, 1869.

Rhoades, W., "Can Hospitals Be Humane?" *Survey* 54:303, 1925.

Rhode Island Hospital Training School for Nurses, *Rules in Relation to the Admission of Pupils and the Government and Conduct of the School for the Training of Women Desirous of Becoming Professional Nurses*. Providence: Rhode Island Hospital, 1885.

Rice, A. G., *Medical Inspection of Schools*. Providence: Snow & Farnham Co., 1912.

Richard, J. F., *The Florence Nightingale of the Southern Army: Experiences of Mrs. Ella K. Newsom*. New York: Broadway, 1914.

Richards, L., "Early Days in the First American Training School for Nurses." *American Journal of Nursing* 26:174, 1915.

———, *Reminiscences of Linda Richards, America's First Trained Nurse*. Boston: Barrows, 1911.

———, "Thirty Years of Progress." *American Journal of Nursing* 4:263, 1904.

Richardson, A. H., "Do You Want to Be a Trained Nurse?" *Woman's Home Companion* 33:42, 1906.

Richardson, L. G., "A Nurse's Protest Against Girls as Nurses." *Nurses Journal of the Pacific Coast* 4:74, 1908.

Richet, C., "The Work of Pasteur and the Modern Conception of Medicine." *Journal of the American Medical Association* 29:611, 1897.

Riddle, M., *Boston City Hospital Training School for Nurses: Historical Sketch*. Boston: City Hospital Nurses Alumnae Association, 1928.

Riese, M., "Despite the Release of Nurses in the Armed Forces, Hospitals Still Face Shortage." *Hospitals* 19:57, 1945.

Ringer, P. H., *Clinical Medicine for Nurses*, 3rd ed. Philadelphia: F. A. Davis, 1929.

Ristine, H., "Then and Now: A Review of Practice of Fifty Years Ago." *Transactions of the Iowa Medical Society* 7:141, 1886–1889.

Robb, I. H., "The Affiliation of Training Schools for Nurses for Educational Purposes." *American Journal of Nursing* 5:670, 1905.

———, *Educational Standards for Nurses, with Other Addresses on Nursing Subjects*. Cleveland: Koeckert, 1907.

———, "Nursing as a Profession." *Albany Medical Annals* 21:491, 1900.

———, *Nursing Ethics: For Hospital and Private Use*. Cleveland: Koeckert, 1900.

———, "Some of the Lessons of the Late War and Their Bearing upon Trained Nursing." *Cleveland Medical Gazette* 14:463, 1898–1899.

Roberts, J. G., *Manual of Bacteriology and Pathology for Nurses*, 5th ed. Philadelphia: W. B. Saunders Co., 1928.

Roberts, J. T., and Thetis, M. G., "The Women's Movement and Nursing." *Nursing Forum* 12:303, 1973.

Roberts, M. M., *American Nursing: History and Interpretation*. New York: Macmillan Co., 1954.
———, "Lavinia Lloyd Dock—Nurse, Feminist, Internationalist." *American Journal of Nursing* 56:176, 1956.
———, "S. Lillian Clayton, 1876–1930." *American Journal of Nursing* 54:1360, 1954.
———, "Stella Goostray—Distinguished Administrator, Professional Leader, and Good Neighbor." *American Journal of Nursing* 58:352, 1958.
———, "We Pay Tribute to Charles-Edward Amory Winslow." *Nursing Outlook* 5:155, 1957.
Robertson, J. D., "Home and Public Health Nurses and Their Training." *Journal of the American Medical Association* 74:481, 1920.
———, "What Shall Nurse the Sick?" *Survey* 46:411, 1921.
Robinson, V., *White Caps: The Story of Nursing*. Philadelphia: J. B. Lippincott Co., 1946.
Rockefeller Foundation, Division of Medical Education, *Nursing Education and Schools of Nursing*. New York: The Foundation, 1932.
"Rockefeller Foundation and Nursing Education." *American Journal of Nursing* 20:525, 1920.
Rodabaugh, J. H., and Rodabaugh, M. J., *Nursing in Ohio: A History*. Columbus: The Ohio State Nurses Association, 1951.
Roddis, L. H., "The U. S. Hospital Ship *Red Rover* (1862–1865)." *Military Surgeon* 77:92, 1935.
Roe, J. H., *Principles of Chemistry: An Introductory Textbook of Inorganic, Organic, and Physiological Chemistry for Nurses and Students of Home Economics and Applied Chemistry, with Laboratory Experiments*, 2nd ed. St. Louis: C. V. Mosby Co., 1929.
Rogers, W. A., "Camp Wikoff." *Harper's Weekly* 42:890, 1898.
Root, E. H., "The Evolution of Nursing: Woman's Role in the Care of the Sick and Wounded in Times Ancient and Modern." *Nursing World* 3:133, 1896.
Rose, J., "Men Nurses in Military Service." *American Journal of Nursing* 47:146, 1947.
Ross, J. W., "Lessons Drawn from Practical Professional Experience with Trained Women Nurses in Military Service." *Journal of the Association of Military Surgeons of the United States* 11:274, 1902.
Ross, M., *All Manner of Men*. New York: Reynal & Hitchcock, 1948.
———, "Crisis in the Hospitals." *Survey* 22:364, 1933.
———, "Private Life or Private Duty for the R. N." *Survey* 55:549, 1926.
Roswell, C. G., "Hospital Costs . . . Yesterday, Today, and Tomorrow." *Hospitals* 35:42, 1961.
Rottman, E., "Why Should a Hospital Close Its Nursing School?" *Modern Hospital* 39:77, 1932.
Rovetta, C. A., "Cost Concepts of Hospital and Nursing Administration." *Hospitals* 12:56, 1938.
Rowe, G. H. M., "The Training of Nurses." *Boston Medical and Surgical Journal* 108:1, 1883.
Rowe, H. R., and Flitter, K. H., *Study on Cost of Nursing Education. Part I: Cost of Basic Diploma Programs*. New York: National League for Nursing, 1964.
"Rural Community Hospitals Established by the Commonwealth Fund." *American Journal of Public Health* 16:315, 1926.
Rush, B., *An Account of the Yellow Fever as It Appeared in Philadelphia in 1797*. Philadelphia: Thomas Dobson, 1798.
Rusk, H. A., "About Shortages: Shortages of Doctors, Nurses, Will Grow Worse in Coming Years." *Hospital Progress* 32:234, 1951.
Russell, J. E., et al., "M. Adelaide Nutting as Known by Friends, Students, and Co-workers." *American Journal of Nursing* 25:445, 1925.
Russell, W. H., *The British Expedition to the Crimea*. London: Routledge, 1858.
Safran, C., "Their Patients Call Them Supernurses: Nurse Practitioners." *Today's Health* 53:20, 1975.
Sanders, G. J., *Modern Methods in Nursing*. Philadelphia: W. B. Saunders Co., 1922.
Sandwith, F. M., "The Nursing and Care of the Sick Prior to 1850." *Hospitals* 56:273, 1914–1915.
Sanger, M., *Margaret Sanger: An Autobiography*. New York: W. W. Norton Co., 1938.
———, *Motherhood in Bondage*. New York: Brentano's, 1928.
Sargent, E. G., "The Nursing Profession Works for Recovery." *American Journal of Nursing* 33:1165, 1933.
Sayles, M. B., "Visiting Nurse and the Nurses' Settlement." *Outlook* 81:419, 1905.
"Scandalous Hospitals." *Newsweek* 52:58, 1958.
"Schedule of Lectures at the Johns Hopkins Hospital Training School for Nurses, 1889–90." *Johns Hopkins Hospital Bulletin* 1:39, 1889–1890.
Schryver, G. F., *History of the Illinois Training School for Nurses*. Chicago: Board of Directors of School, 1930.
Scoit, A. H., "Status of Graduate Nurse Service as Indicated by Recent Studies Conducted Through

the American Nurses' Association Headquarters." *Transactions of the American Hospital Association* 40:410, 1938.

Scott, W. C., and Smith, D. W., "Social Security and the Nurse." *American Journal of Nursing* 48:32, 1948.

_____, "Taft-Hartley Act and the Nurse." *American Journal of Nursing* 56:1556, 1956.

Scovil, E. R., *In the Sickroom: The Art of Nursing.* New York: Montgomery, 1888.

_____, "The Private Hospital as Owned and Managed by Nurses." *American Journal of Nursing* 3:892, 1903.

Seaman, V., *The Midwives Monitor, and Mothers Mirror, Being Three Concluding Lectures of a Course of Instruction on Midwifery; Containing Directions for Pregnant Women; Rules for the Management of Natural Births, and for Early Discovering When the Aid of a Physician Is Necessary; and Cautions for Nurses, Respecting Both the Mother and Child. To Which Is Prefixed, a Syllabus of Lectures on That Subject.* New York: I. Collins, 1800.

Sedgwick, M. K. R., "Instructive District Nursing." *Forum* 22:297, 1896.

Sellew, G., *Pediatric Nursing Including the Care of the Well Infant and Child.* Philadelphia: W. B. Saunders Co., 1926.

Sellew, G., and Furfey, P. H., *Sociology and Social Problems in Nursing Service,* 2nd ed. Philadelphia: W. B. Saunders Co., 1946.

Senn, N., *A Nurse's Guide for the Operating Room.* Chicago: Keener, 1902.

_____, "Nursing and Nurses in War." *Journal of the American Medical Association* 32:155, 1899.

Shilling, J. W., "Standing Orders for Nurses in Industry." *Industrial Medicine and Surgery* 18:467, 1949.

Shinn, G. W., "Founding of Small Hospitals." *New England Magazine* 22:255, 1900.

Shober's Directory of Trained Nurses. Being a Selected List of Names and Addresses of Competent Graduated Trained Nurses Practicing in the Cities of Greater New York, Boston, Philadelphia, Baltimore, and Washington. New York: Shober-Cornell, 1902.

Shoemaker, M. T., *History of Nurse-midwifery in the United States.* Washington, D.C.: Catholic University of America Press, 1947.

"Shortage of Nurses: No Solution in Sight." *U.S. News and World Report* 69:37, 1970.

Shryock, R. H., *The History of Nursing: An Interpretation of the Social and Medical Factors Involved.* Philadelphia: W. B. Saunders Co., 1959.

_____, "Nursing Emerges as a Profession: The American Experience." *Clio Medica* 3:131, 1968.

Shultz, G. D., ed., "Cruelty in Maternity Wards: Letters." *Ladies' Home Journal* 75:44, 1958.

Sim, F. L., "Medicine Forty Years Ago and Now." *Memphis Medical Monthly* 13:398, 1893.

Sinclair, C. G., *Microbiology for Nurses.* Philadelphia: F. A. Davis Co., 1931.

Sleeper, F. H., "Present Trends in Psychiatric Nursing." *American Journal of Psychiatry* 109:203, 1952.

Sleeper, R., "Nursing Care Throughout Fifty Years." *American Journal of Nursing* 50:586, 1950.

_____, "Nursing Education in Evolution." *New England Journal of Medicine* 271:27, 1964.

_____, "Stretching the Nurse." *Hospitals* 28:80, 1954.

Sleeper, R., and Lyons, V., "Is Nursing School Accreditation Worth the Work and Worry? Nurses Answer 'Yes!'" *Hospitals* 27:73, 1953.

Sloan, R. P., *This Hospital Business of Ours.* New York: Putnam, 1952.

Smillie, W. G., *Public Health Administration in the United States.* New York: Macmillan Co., 1935.

Smilie, W. G., and Kilbourne, E. D., *Preventive Medicine and Public Health,* 3rd ed. New York: Macmillan Co., 1963.

Smith, A. A., *Operating Room: A Primer for Public Nurses.* Philadelphia: W. B. Saunders Co., 1924.

_____, "Rehabilitation of the Nursing Profession." *Trained Nurse and Hospital Review* 57:113, 1921.

Smith, J. M., "The Civil Hospital and Its Duties in Wartime." *Trained Nurse and Hospital Review* 60:13, 1918.

_____, "A Comparative View of the State of Medicine in the Years 1733 and 1833: An Introductory Lecture." *New York Journal of Medicine and Surgery* 1:245, 1839.

Smith, S., "In Memory of Dr. Elizabeth Blackwell and Dr. Emily Blackwell." *Bulletin of the New York Academy of Medicine* 25:3, 1911.

_____, "Old Bellevue Hospital as a Maker of Medical History." *New York Evening Sun,* March 11, 1911.

_____, "Random Recollections of a Long Medical Life." *Medical Record* 90:356, 1911.

Smith, W. H., "The Educational Function of the Hospital." *Modern Hospital* 6:1, 1916.
_____, "How Nurses Are Meeting the Present Needs." *American Journal of Nursing* 18:979, 1918-1919.
_____, "Reorganization of the Civilian Hospital on a War Basis." *Transactions of the American Hospital Association* 19:111, 1917.
Smith-Rosenberg, C., and Rosenberg, C., "The Female Animal: Medical and Biological Views of Woman and Her Role in Nineteenth Century America." *Journal of American History* 60:332, 1973.
Snively, M. A., "A Nurse's Day in a Hospital." *Trained Nurse* 13:8, 1894.
"So Proudly We Hail: Realistic Story of Nurses in the Philippines." *Life* 15:69, 1943.
"Social Security Official Estimates National Nurse Shortage at 40,000." *Modern Hospital* 72:146, 1949.
Society of the New York Training School for Nurses, Attached to Bellevue Hospital, *Annual Reports of the Secretary, 1873 to 1900.* New York: The Society, 1900.
_____, *Rules for the Hospital: Head Nurses and Assistant Nurses.* New York: The Society, 1885.
_____, *Rules for the Hospital: Night Nurses.* New York: The Society, 1885.
"Some Hospital Statistics." *National Hospital Record* 5:13, 1902.
"Some Problems in Grading Our Schools of Nursing." *Trained Nurse and Hospital Review* 77:507, 1926.
Souchon, E., "Original Contributions of America to Medical Sciences." *Transactions of the American Surgical Association* 35:65, 1917.
Soyer, A., *Soyer's Culinary Campaign.* London: G. Routledge & Co., 1857.
Spalding, H. S., *Talks to Nurses: The Ethics of Nursing.* New York: Benziger, 1920.
"Spread of Visiting Nursing." *Charities* 16:1, 1906.
Stanton, M., "Political Action and Nursing." *Nursing Clinics of North America* 9:579, 1974.
"The State Board Test Pool Examination." *American Journal of Nursing* 52:613, 1952.
"Statement of AHA Concerning Collective Bargaining in Hospitals." *Hospitals* 33:98, 1959.
"Statistics of Hospitals in the United States, 1872-73. Derived from Replies to Inquiries by the U.S. Bureau of Education." *Transactions of the American Medical Association* 14:314, 1873.
"Statistics of Nurse Training Schools, 1926-1927." *U.S. Bureau of Education Bulletin* 2:1, 1928.
Staupers, M. K., *No Time for Prejudice: A Story of the Integration of Negroes in Nursing in the United States.* New York: Macmillan Co., 1961.
Stephenson, L. G., *Nobel Prize Winners in Medicine and Physiology.* New York: Henry Schuman, 1953.
Stephenson, M. V., *The First Fifty Years of the Training School for Nurses of the Hospital of the University of Pennsylvania.* Philadelphia: J. B. Lippincott Co., 1940.
Sterling, E. B., *American Medical Practice in the Perspectives of a Century.* New York: The Commonwealth Fund, 1945.
_____, "Probationary Experiences at Johns Hopkins." *Trained Nurse and Hospital Review* 16:514, 1896.
Stern, B. J., *Medical Services by Government: Local, State, and Federal.* New York: The Commonwealth Fund, 1946.
_____, *Medicine in Industry.* New York: The Commonwealth Fund, 1946.
_____, *Society and Medical Progress.* Princeton: Princeton University Press, 1941.
Stevens, E. F., *American Hospital of the Twentieth Century: A Treatise on the Development of Medical Institutions, both in Europe and in America, Since the Beginning of the Present Century,* 2nd ed. New York: Architectural Record Co., 1928.
Stevens, R., *American Medicine and the Public Interest.* New Haven: Yale University Press, 1971.
Stewart, H. R., "The Value of the Public Health Nurse to the Community." *Modern Medicine* 1:429, 1919.
Stewart, I. M., "Developments in Nursing Education Since 1918." *U.S. Bureau of Education Bulletin* 20:1, 1921.
_____, *The Education of Nurses.* New York: Macmillan Co., 1944.
_____, "Isabelle M. Stewart Recalls the Early Years (1900-1920)." *American Journal of Nursing* 60:1426, 1960.
_____, "The Nursing Profession and National Defense." *Hospitals* 15:33, 1941.
_____, "Problems of Nursing Education." *Teachers College Record* 11:7, 1910.
_____, "Readjustments in the Training School Curriculum to Meet the New Demands in Public Health Nursing." *American Journal of Nursing* 20:102, 1919-1920.
_____, "Trends in Nursing Education." *American Journal of Nursing* 31:601, 1931.

_____, "Which Way Are We Going in Nursing?" *Survey* 46:411, 1921.

Stewart, M. S., *Social Security.* New York: W. W. Norton Co., 1939.

Stiles, S. V., and Johnson, K. A., "National Health Planning and Resources Development Act of 1974: Regulatory and Review Functions of Agencies Created by the Act." *Public Health Reports* 91:24, 1976.

Stimson, J. C., *History and Manual of the Army Nurse Corps.* Carlisle, Pa.: Army Medical School, 1937.

Stokes, W. R., "Four Great Anglo-American Medical Discoveries (Jenner, Lister, Reed, Morton)." *Maryland Medical Journal* 48:7, 1905.

Stone, F., "Is There Need for Another Class of Sick Attendants Besides Nurses?" *American Journal of Nursing* 17:991, 1917.

Stone, T. C., "A Glimpse at the Western Battle Front and Some of the Horrors of Modern Warfare, as Seen from the Second Division, A. E. F." *International Journal of Surgery* 33:24, 1920.

Stoney, E., *Bacteriology and Surgical Technic for Nurses,* 4th ed. Philadelphia: W. B. Saunders Co., 1916.

_____, *Practical Points in Nursing for Nurses in Private Practice,* 2nd ed. Philadelphia: W. B. Saunders Co., 1897.

Storer, H., *Nurses and Nursing.* Boston: Lee & Shepard, 1868.

"Story of Ward L." *Charities* 17:287, 1917.

Stout, P. S., "A Plea for Male Nurses." *New York Medical Journal* 103:1225, 1916.

Stout, S. H., "Reminiscences of Medical Officers of the Confederate Army and Department of Tennessee." *St. Louis Medical and Surgical Journal* 64:228, 1893.

Struthers, L., *School Nurse.* New York: G. P. Putnam's Sons, 1917.

Stuart, N. G., and Aynes, E. A., "Coming Scandal in Nursing." *McCalls* 91:100, 1964.

"The Supply of Nurses." *National Hospital Record* 21:2, 1908.

"Survival of Hospital Nursing Schools Called Matter of Utmost Urgency." *Hospital Management* 69:30, 1950.

Swanson, R., "Nursing Education—What It Costs the Hospital." *Hospitals* 27:68, 1953.

Sydenstricker, E., "Extent of Medical and Hospital Service in a Typical Small City." *Public Health Reports* 42:121, 1928.

Taft, W. H., "A Distinct Call to Women." *Ladies' Home Journal* 34:22, 1918.

_____, "Wanted: 30,000 Nurses." *Ladies' Home Journal* 35:22, 1918.

"Taking a Stand." *American Journal of Nursing* 59:1245, 1959.

Talley, C., *Ethics: A Textbook for Nurses.* New York: G. P. Putnam's Sons, 1925.

Tappert, T. G., and Lehmann, H. T., ed. and trans., *Luther's Works.* Philadelphia: Fortress Press, 1967. Vol. 54.

Tattershall, L. M., and Altenderfer, M. E., "Private Duty Nursing in General Hospitals." *American Journal of Nursing* 44:651, 1944.

Tattershall, L. M., and West, M. D., "Wartime Nursing Care in 604 General Hospitals." *American Journal of Nursing* 44:211, 1944.

Taylor, E. J., "The School of Nursing at the Yale University." *American Journal of Nursing* 25:9, 1925.

Taylor, K. O., "Methods of Measuring the Quality of Nursing Care." *Modern Hospital* 66:52, 1946.

Taylor, M. E., "Telling the Public About the Public Health Nurse." *Public Health Nursing* 12:218, 1920.

Thatcher, V. S., *History of Anesthesia with Emphasis on the Nurse Specialist.* Philadelphia: J. B. Lippincott Co., 1953.

Thomas, T. G., "Fifty Years of Medicine: A Retrospect of Progress During the Past Half Century." *New York Medical Journal* 74:1009, 1901.

Thompson, D. E., "How the Army Nursing Service Met the Demands of the War." *Proceedings of the National League for Nursing Education* 25:116, 1919.

_____, "Nursing as It Relates to the War." *Proceedings of the National League of Nursing Education* 24:226, 1918.

Thompson, J., *The ANA in Washington.* Kansas City, Mo.: American Nurses' Association, 1972.

Thompson, W. G., "Efficiency in Nursing." *Journal of the American Medical Association* 61:2146, 1913.

_____, "The Overtrained Nurse." *New York Medical Journal* 83:845, 1906.

_____, *Training Schools for Nurses with Notes on Twenty-two Schools.* New York: Putnam, 1883.

Thoms, A. B., ed., *Pathfinders: A History of the Progress of Colored Graduate Nurses with Biographies of Many Prominent Nurses.* New York: McKay, 1929.

Thoms, A. B., and Bullock, C. E., "Development of Facilities for Colored Nurse Education." *Trained Nurse and Hospital Review* 80:722, 1928.

Thornton, G. B., "The Yellow Fever Epidemic in Memphis." *Boston Medical and Surgical Journal* 101:787, 1879.

"Three Hundred and Seventy-seven Hospitals Meet Minimum Standard: American College of Surgeons Makes Public List of Approved General Institutions of 100 Beds or More." *Hospital Management* 9:40, 1920.

"335,000 Nurses Aren't Nearly Enough." *Medical Economics* 31:264, 1954.

Thwing, M. D., "Factory Nursing." *Public Health Nursing* 5:28, 1913.

Tibbitts, H. G., "Distribution of Hospital Nursing Services." *Public Health Reports* 68:933, 1953.

Tibbitts, H. G., and Levine, E., *Health Manpower Source Book. Section 2. Nursing Personnel.* Washington, D.C.: Government Printing Office, 1953.

Tiffany, F., *Life of Dorothea Lynde Dix.* Boston: Houghton, 1937.

Titus, H., "Return of the Practical Nurse." *Saturday Evening Post* 221:38, 1949.

Titus, S. C., "Economic Facts of Life for Nurses." *American Journal of Nursing* 52:1109, 1952.

_____, "Economic Security Is Not Too Much to Ask." *Modern Hospital* 61:71, 1943.

_____, "The Present Position of Nursing in Hospitals in the United States." *Nosokomeion* 2:288, 1931.

"To the Graduate of '39." *American Journal of Nursing* 39:529, 1939.

Todd, A. J., "Nursing as a Learned Profession—a Sociologist's View." *Public Health Nursing* 11:13, 1919.

"Too Many Nurses in These Localities." *American Journal of Nursing* 30:344, 1930.

Toombs, A., "Flight Nurse." *Woman's Home Companion* 70:36, 1943.

Torrop, H. M., "Are Practical Nurses the Answer?" *Hospitals* 26:56, 1952.

_____, "How Much Nursing Service Should an Orderly Give?" *American Journal of Nursing* 37:15, 1937.

Townsend, J. G., "The Public Health Nurse." *Public Health Reports* 41:651, 1926.

_____, "Public Health Nursing." *Public Health Reports* 40:2471, 1925.

"Training Camps for Nurses." *Outlook* 119:94, 1918.

"Training Program Announced for 100,000 Nurses' Aides." *Hospital Management* 52:44, 1941.

Training School for Nurses, Attached to the Massachusetts General Hospital, Boston, *Circular of the Committee to Physicians, Calling Their Attention to the Establishment of the School.* Boston: The School, 1873.

"Training Schools." *Charities* 17:267, 1906.

"Training Schools." *Transactions of the American Hospital Association* 13:397, 1911.

Tucker, F., "Hospital Situation in New York." *Charities* 12:27, 1904.

_____, "Public Conscience and the Hospitals." *Charities* 13:285, 1904.

Tuley, H. E., *Obstetrical Nursing for Nurses and Students,* 2nd ed. Louisville: Morton, 1910.

Turner, V. A., "American Nurses' Association Settles Important Issues." *Trained Nurse and Hospital Review* 124:260, 1950.

Turner, W. K., "Financing Nursing Education—an Unfair Burden for 1100 Hospitals." *Hospitals* 33:40, 1959.

Tuttle, G. T., "The Male Nurse." *American Journal of Insanity* 63:192, 1906.

"Twenty Years of It in the Henry Street Nurses' Settlement." *Survey* 31:606, 1914.

"Twenty-five Years of Rural Public Health Nursing." *Red Cross Courier* 17:17, 1937.

"Two Bills Introduced in Congress to Aid Nursing Schools." *Hospitals* 27:131, 1953.

Tyrrell, H., *Pictorial History of the War with Russia 1854–1856.* London: W. & R. Chambers, 1856.

Underhill, E., "History of the Movement for the State Registration of Nurses." *Journal of the Medical Society of New Jersey* 8:72, 1911.

U.S. Commissioner of Education, *Annual Report of the U.S. Commissioner of Education for 1873.* Washington, D.C.: Government Printing Office, 1874.

_____, "Final Examination Questions of the Evansville Sanitarium Training School for Nurses." *Annual Report of the U.S. Commissioner of Education for 1903.* Washington, D.C.: Government Printing Office, 1904.

_____, *Annual Report of the U.S. Commissioner of Education for 1906.* Washington, D.C.: Government Printing Office, 1907.

_____, *Report of the U.S. Commissioner of Education for 1902.* Washington, D.C.: Government

Printing Office, 1903.

U.S. Congress, House, *Message from the President of the United States Transmitting a Message on the State of the Union.* Washington, D.C.: Government Printing Office, 1945.

U.S. Congress, House, Committee on Appropriations, *Departments of Labor and Health, Education, and Welfare Appropriations for 1974.* Hearings before the Committee. Washington, D.C.: Government Printing Office, 1973.

U.S. Congress, House, Committee on Interstate and Foreign Commerce. *National Health Plan.* Washington, D.C.: Government Printing Office, 1949.

U.S. Congress, House, Committee on Interstate and Foreign Commerce, Subcommittee on Public Health and Welfare, *Health Manpower Act of 1968.* Hearings before the Subcommittee. Washington, D.C.: Government Printing Office, 1968.

U.S. Congress, House, Committee on Interstate and Foreign Commerce, Subcommittee on Public Health and Safety, *Nurse Training Act of 1964.* Hearings before the Subcommittee. Washington, D.C.: Government Printing Office, 1964.

U.S. Congress, House, Committee on Interstate and Foreign Commerce, Subcommittee on Public Health and Safety, *Nurse Training Act of 1964.* Report to Accompany H.R. 11241. Washington, D.C.: Government Printing Office, 1964.

U.S. Congress, House, Committee on Labor, *Hygiene of Maternity and Infancy.* Hearings before the Committee. Washington, D.C.: Government Printing Office, 1919.

U.S. Congress, House, Committee on Labor, *Labor Disputes Act, Hearings Held March 13–April 4, 1935.* Washington, D.C.: Government Printing Office, 1935.

U.S. Congress, House, Committee on Military Affairs, *Army Nurse Corps.* Hearings before the Committee. Washington, D.C.: Government Printing Office, 1944.

U.S. Congress, House, Committee on Military Affairs, *Report Amending H.R. 11770 for Employment of Women Nurses in Military Hospitals of the Army.* Washington, D.C.: Government Printing Office, 1899.

U.S. Congress, House, Committee on Rules, *The Strike at Lawrence, Massachusetts.* Hearings before the Committee. Washington, D.C.: Government Printing Office, 1912.

U.S. Congress, House, Committee on Ways and Means, *Economic Security Act.* Hearings before the Committee. Washington, D.C.: Government Printing Office, 1935.

U.S. Congress, Senate, *Economic Security Act.* Hearings on S. 1130. Washington, D.C.: Government Printing Office, 1935.

U.S. Congress, Senate, *National Health Planning and Development and Health Facilities Assistance Act of 1974.* Report on S. 2994. Washington, D.C.: Government Printing Office, 1974.

U.S. Congress, Senate, Committee on Education and Labor, *National Health Program.* Hearings before the Committee. Washington, D.C.: Government Printing Office, 1946.

U.S. Congress, Senate, Committee on Education and Labor, *Protection of Maternity.* Hearings before the Committee. Washington, D.C.: Government Printing Office, 1921.

U.S. Congress, Senate, Committee on Finance, *Medicare and Medicaid, Issues and Alternatives.* Washington, D.C.: Government Printing Office, 1970.

U.S. Congress, Senate, Committee on Labor and Public Welfare, *Health Insurance Plans in the United States.* Washington, D.C.: Government Printing Office, 1951.

U.S. Congress, Senate, Committee on Labor and Public Welfare, *Nurse Training Act of 1964.* Report to Accompany H.R. 11241. Washington, D.C.: Government Printing Office, 1964.

U.S. Congress, Senate, Special Committee on Aging, *Nursing Home Care in the United States: Failure in Public Policy; Supporting Paper No. 4—Nurses in Nursing Homes: The Heavy Burden.* Washington, D.C.: Government Printing Office, 1975.

U.S. Council of National Defense, *First Annual Report of the Council of National Defense, Fiscal Year 1917.* Washington, D.C.: Government Printing Office, 1917.

U.S. Department of Commerce, Bureau of the Census, *Fourteenth Census of the United States, 1920.* Washington, D.C.: Government Printing Office, 1923.

————, Bureau of the Census, *Mortality Statistics, 1914.* Washington, D.C.: Government Printing Office, 1916.

————, *United States Life Tables, 1901–02, 1909–10, 1919–20.* Washington, D.C.: Government Printing Office, 1923.

U.S. Department of Commerce and Labor, *Report on the Condition of Woman and Child Wage-earners in the United States.* Washington, D.C.: Government Printing Office, 1911.

————, Bureau of the Census, *Mortality Statistics, 1910: General Death Rates; Specific and Standardized Death Rates; Infant and Child Mortality; Causes of Death.* Washington, D.C.: Government Printing Office, 1913.

————, *Statistics of Women at Work.* Washington, D.C.: Government Printing Office, 1907.

U.S. Department of Health, Education, and Welfare, Secretary's Committee to Study Extended Roles for Nurses, *Extending the Scope of Nursing Practice: A Report of the Secretary's Committee.* Washington, D.C.: Government Printing Office, 1972.

U.S. Department of the Interior, Bureau of Education, *The Inception, Organization, and Management of Training Schools for Nurses.* Washington, D.C.: Government Printing Office, 1882.

————, *Training Schools for Nurses.* Washington, D.C.: Government Printing Office, 1879.

U.S. Department of Labor, Bureau of Labor Statistics, *The Economic Status of Registered Professional Nurses, 1946–47.* Washington, D.C.: Government Printing Office, 1948.

————, *Industry Wage Survey—Hospitals: March, 1969.* Washington, D.C.: Government Printing Office, 1971.

————, Children's Bureau, *Annual Report of Administration of the Maternity and Infancy Act.* Washington, D.C.: Government Printing Office, 1923.

————, *The Children's Bureau: Yesterday, Today, and Tomorrow.* Washington, D.C.: Government Printing Office, 1937.

————, *Maternal and Child-health Services Under the Social Security Act, Title V. Part 1: Development of Program.* Washington, D.C.: Government Printing Office, 1941.

U.S. President, Interdepartmental Committee to Coordinate Health and Welfare Activities, *Proceedings of the National Health Conference, July 18, 19, 20, 1938, Washington, D.C.* Washington, D.C.: Government Printing Office, 1939.

————, National Advisory Commission on Health Manpower, *Report of the National Advisory Commission on Health Manpower.* Washington, D.C.: Government Printing Office, 1967.

U.S. Public Health Service, *Toward Quality in Nursing: Needs and Goals. Report of the Surgeon General's Consultant Group on Nursing.* Washington, D.C.: Government Printing Office, 1963.

————, Health Resources Administration, Bureau of Health Planning and Resources Development, *The Consumer and Health Planning.* Washington, D.C.: Government Printing Office, 1976.

U.S. Public Works Administration, *P.W.A. Provides Modern Hospitals.* Washington, D.C.: Government Printing Office, 1937.

U.S. Sanitary Commission, *Account of the Field Relief Corps of the U.S. Sanitary Commission in the Army of the Potomac.* New York: The Commission, 1863.

————, *Qualifications of Candidates for Service in the Women's Department for Nursing in the Military Hospitals of the United States.* Washington, D.C.: The Commission, 1862.

————, *Report Concerning the Woman's Central Association of Relief at New York to the United States Sanitary Commission at Washington, October 12, 1861.* New York: The Commission, 1861.

U.S. War Department, Typhoid Commission, *Report on Origin and Spread of Typhoid Fever in the U.S. Military Camps During the Spanish War of 1898: By Walter Reed, Victor C. Vaughan, and Edward O. Shakespeare.* Washington, D.C.: Government Printing Office, 1904.

Valléry-Radot, D., *Life of Pasteur.* Garden City, N.Y.: Doubleday, 1923.

Van Blarcon, C. C., *Obstetrical Nursing: A Textbook on the Nursing Care of the Expectant Mother, the Woman in Labor, the Young Mother and Her Baby.* New York: Macmillan Co., 1922.

Van DeVrede, J., "The Value of the Nurse in Public Health Work in the South." *Southern Medical Journal* 14:463, 1921.

Van Doren, M., *Walt Whitman.* New York: Viking Press, 1945.

Vannier, M. L., and Thompson, B. A., *Nursing Procedures.* Minneapolis: University of Minnesota Press, 1929.

Vaughan, V. C., *A Doctor's Memories.* Indianapolis: Bobbs-Merrill, 1926.

Vaughan, V. C., Vaughan, H. F., and Palmer, G. T., *Epidemiology and Public Health.* St. Louis: C. V. Mosby Co., 1922.

Vietor, A. C., *A Woman's Quest: The Life of Marie E. Zakrsewska, M.D.* New York: Appleton & Co., 1924.

Villet, B., "More Than Compassion: Head Nurse Judy Strickland." *Life* 72:63, 1972.

Virchow, R., "Recent Advances in Science and Their Bearing on Medicine and Surgery." *Popular Science Monthly* 61:558, 1902.

Voswinkel, B. M., "The Journal of a Red Cross Nurse." *Trained Nurse and Hospital Review* 21:309, 1898.

Vreeland, E. M., "Some Qualitative and Quantitative Factors in Nurse Education." *Public Health Reports* 63:1667, 1948.

Waagen, L. O., "The Hospital Survey and Construction Act." *American Journal of Nursing* 48:361, 1948.

Wakefield, D., "Victims of Charity: Employees of Voluntary Hospitals." *Nation* 188:226, 1959.

Wakeford, C., *The Wounded Soldiers' Friends: The Story of Florence Nightingale, Clara Barton, and Others*. London: Headley Brothers, 1917.

Wald, L. D., "Development of Public Health Nursing in the United States." *Trained Nurse and Hospital Review* 80:689, 1928.

———, "Henry Street Settlement." *Charities* 16:35, 1906.

———, *House on Henry Street*. New York: Holt, 1915.

———, "Nurse and the Community." *Survey* 30:516, 1913.

———, "Nursing." *Survey* 31:355, 1913.

———, "What Keeps the Nurses Going?" *Survey* 68:590, 1932.

———, *Windows on Henry Street*. Boston: Little, Brown and Company, 1934.

Wales, M., *Public Health Nurse in Action*. New York: Macmillan Co., 1941.

Waller, C. E., "The Social Security Act in Its Relation to Public Health." *American Journal of Public Health* 25:1186, 1935.

Walter, W., "The Hospital Laboratory as a Community Asset." *Chicago Medical Recorder* 40:466, 1918.

War Investigating Commission, *Report of the Commission Appointed by the President to Investigate the Conduct of the War with Spain*. Washington, D.C.: Government Printing Office, 1899.

"War Nurse's Diary." *Trained Nurse and Hospital Review* 60:90, 1918.

Ward, A. G., "Some of the Newer Problems in the Training of the Nurse." *Trained Nurse and Hospital Review* 64:311, 1920.

Warrington, J., *The Nurses' Guide. Containing a Series of Instructions to Females Who Wish to Engage in the Important Business of Nursing Mother and Child in the Lying-in Chamber*. Philadelphia: T. Cowperthwait & Co., 1839.

Warwick, M., "The Nurse as a Laboratory Technician." *American Journal of Nursing* 27:95, 1927.

Washburn, F. A., "The Broadened Concept of Hospital Functions Since the Year 1896." *Hospitals* 14:13, 1940.

Washington, B. T., "Training Colored Nurses at Tuskegee." *American Journal of Nursing* 10:167, 1910–1911.

Waterman, T. L., *Nursing for Community Health*. Philadelphia: F. A. Davis Co., 1944.

Waters, Y., "The Rise, Progress, and Extent of Visiting Nurses in the United States." *Charities* 16:16, 1906.

———, *Visiting Nursing in the United States*. New York: Russell Sage Foundation, 1912.

Watson, D.C., *Lectures on Medicine: A Handbook for Nurses*. New York: Wood, 1918.

Watson, F. S., "On Some of the Good Qualities Necessary for Being a Good Nurse." *Boston Medical and Surgical Journal* 138:217, 1898.

Watson, J. K., *A Handbook for Nurses*. Philadelphia: J. B. Lippincott Co., 1900.

Wayland, M. M., *Hospital Head Nurse*, 2nd ed. New York: Macmillan Co., 1944.

Weber, J. J., *First Steps in Organizing a Hospital*. New York: Macmillan Co., 1924.

Webster, W., *Anesthesia for Nurses*. St. Louis: C. V. Mosby Co., 1924.

Weeks-Shaw, C. S., *A Textbook of Nursing for the Use of Training Schools, Families, and Private Students*. New York: Appleton, 1885.

Weisbrod, B. A., "Research in Health Economics: A Survey." *International Journal of Health Services* 5:643, 1975.

Weiss, M. O., "The Skills of Psychiatric Nursing." *American Journal of Nursing* 47:174, 1947.

Welch, W. H., *Public Health in Theory and Practice*. New Haven: Yale University Press, 1925.

———, "Some of the Conditions Which Have Influenced the Development of American Medicine, Especially During the Last Century." *Johns Hopkins Hospital Bulletin* 19:33, 1908.

Wershub, L. P., *One Hundred Years of Medical Progress: A History of the New York Medical College, Flower and Fifth Avenue Hospitals*. Springfield, Ill.: Charles C Thomas, 1967.

West, M., and Hawkins, C., *Nursing Schools at the Mid-century*. New York: National Committee for the Improvement of Nursing Services, 1950.

West, R. M., *History of Nursing in Pennsylvania*. Harrisburg: Pennsylvania State Nurses' Association, 1926.

Wetzel, S. M., "What's Wrong with the Nursing in Our Hospitals?" *Trained Nurse and Hospital Review* 97:244, 1936.

"What Is a Public Health Nurse?" *Survey* 51:698, 1924.

"What's All This About the Deplorable State of Nursing Schools?" *Hospital Management* 67:31,

1949.

"What's Wrong with American Hospitals?" *Saturday Review* 50:59, 1967.

"What's Your Opinion—Should Training of Registered Nurses Be Underwritten by the Comparatively Small Number of Hospitals That Have Schools of Nursing?" *Southern Hospitals* 28:28, 1960.

Wheeler, C. A., "The Faculty of a School of Nursing." *Modern Hospital* 16:537, 1921.

Wheeler, M. C., *Nursing Technique.* Philadelphia: J. B. Lippincott Co., 1918.

_____, "Summary of Nursing Events in 1918." *Modern Hospital* 12:29, 1919.

Wheeler, R., and Wheeler, H., *Talks to Nurses on Dietetics and Dietotherapy.* Philadelphia: W. B. Saunders Co., 1926.

"When Doctor's on the Floor." *Trained Nurse and Hospital Review* 16:90, 1896.

"When Does the Home Front Have Priority?" *Public Health Nursing* 35:77, 1943.

White, W. A., *Forty Years of Psychiatry.* New York: Nervous and Mental Disease Publishing Company, 1937.

White House Conference on the Care of Dependent Children, *Proceedings of the Conference held at Washington, D.C., January 25, 26, 1909.* Washington, D.C.: Government Printing Office, 1909.

White House Conference on Child Health and Protection, *Obstetric Education: Report of the Subcommittee on Obstetric Teaching and Education.* New York: The Century Company, 1932.

"The White Parade." *Trained Nurse and Hospital Review* 93:563, 1934.

Whitehall, A. V., and Foster, M. J., "Nine Strikes Against Federal Aid for Nursing Education." *Hospitals* 26:55, 1952.

Whitman, H., and Ingalls, D. J., "Don't Curse the Nurse." *Collier's* 119:26, 1947.

Whitman, W., *The Works of Walt Whitman.* New York: Funk and Wagnall's, 1968.

_____, *The Wound-dresser, a Series of Letters Written from the Hospitals in Washington During the War of the Rebellion.* Boston: Small, Maynard, 1898.

Whitney, J. S., and Stofer, H. J., *Tuberculosis Among Nurses.* New York: National Tuberculosis Association, 1941.

"Who Has Heard the Nightingale?" *Ladies' Home Journal* 65:11, 1948.

"Why Crisis in Medical Care Keeps Growing." *U.S. News and World Report* 62:60, 1967.

"Why Not Be Fair?" *Bulletin of the American Hospital Association* 6:6, 1932.

"Why Not Homelike Hospitals?" *Literary Digest* 60:19, 1919.

Whyte, A. M., "Public Health Nursing: Its Place in the Public Health Movement." *Public Health Nursing* 5:69, 1913.

Wilcox, R. W., *A Manual of Fever Nursing,* 2nd ed. Philadelphia: P. Blakiston's Son & Co., 1904.

Wile, I. S., "The Relation of the Public Health Nurse to the Practicing Physician: The Viewpoint of the Physician." *American Journal of Public Health* 14:106, 1924.

Williams, J., ed., *The Autobiography of Elizabeth Davis, a Balaclava Nurse.* London: Hurst & Blackett, 1857.

Williams, S. W., "A Brief Historical Notice of the Progress of Medical Science in Massachusetts, from the Landing of the Pilgrims at Plymouth to the Present Time." *New York Journal of Medicine* 4:145, 1950.

_____, "A Medical History of the County of Franklin, in the Commonwealth of Massachusetts." *Medical Communications of the Massachusetts Medical Society* 7:1, 1842–1848.

_____, "Notice of Some of the Medical Improvements and Discoveries of the Last Half Century and More Particularly in the United States of America." *New York Journal of Medicine* 8:153, 1852.

Williamson, A. A., "California and the Eight-hour Law." *Trained Nurse and Hospital Review* 53:257, 1914.

_____, *50 Years to Starch.* Culver City, Ca.: Murray & Gee, 1948.

Wilson, D. C., *Lone Woman: The Story of Elizabeth Blackwell, the First Woman Doctor.* Boston: Little, Brown and Company, 1970.

Wilson, H. W. A., "Moral Influence of the Trained Nurse." *Westminster Review* 148:328, 1897.

Wilson, J. C., *Fever Nursing.* Philadelphia: J. B. Lippincott, Co., 1915.

_____, *Practical Lessons in Nursing. Fever-nursing; Designed for the Use of Professional and Other Nurses, and Especially as a Textbook for Nurses in Training.* Philadelphia: J. B. Lippincott Co., 1888.

Wilson, W. R., *A Reference Handbook of Obstetric Nursing,* 3rd ed. Philadelphia: W. B. Saunders Co., 1916.

Winslow, A., *Frontier Nursing Service.* Washington, D.C.: The Committee on the Costs of Medical Care, 1932.

Winslow, C. E. A., *City Set on a Hill: The Significance of the Health Demonstration at Syracuse, New York*. Garden City, N.Y.: Doubleday, 1934.

_____, *Conquest of Epidemic Disease: A Chapter in the History of Ideas*. Princeton: Princeton University Press, 1943.

_____, "National Health Challenges: How the Public Health Nurse Is Meeting Them." *Public Health Nursing* 27:120, 1935.

_____, "Nursing Education: Its Past and Its Future." *Modern Hospital* 25:237, 1925.

_____, "Public Health at the Crossroads." *American Journal of Public Health* 16:1075, 1926.

Winslow, W., "We Can Save the Mentally Sick." *Saturday Evening Post* 220:20, 1947.

Wise, P. M., "The Construction of Hospitals." *Albany Medical Annals* 19:64, 1898.

_____, *A Textbook for Training Schools for Nurses, Including Physiology and Hygiene and the Principles and Practice of Nursing; with an Introduction by Edward Cowles*. New York: G. P. Putnam, 1896.

Witte, F. W., "Opportunities in Graduate Education for Men Nurses." *American Journal of Nursing* 34:133, 1934.

Wolf, A. D., "How Can General Duty Be Made More Attractive to Graduate Nurses?" *American Journal of Nursing* 28:903, 1928.

Wolf, L. K., "Development of Floor Nursing and Supervision." *Hospitals* 15:53, 1941.

"Woman's Hospital in Philadelphia." *Annual Reports of the Board of Managers and Resident Physician to the Contributors, 1861–92*. Philadelphia: The Hospital, 1862–1893.

_____, Nurses' Training School, *History of the Nurses' Training School of the Woman's Hospital of Philadelphia, 1861–1925*. Philadelphia: The Hospital, 1925.

"Women as Physicians." *Medical and Surgical Reporter* 44:354, 1881.

"Women in White." *Coronet* 30:71, 1951.

Wood, B. M., and Weeks, A. L., *Fundamentals of Dietetics: A Textbook for Nurses and Dietitians*. Philadelphia: W. B. Saunders Co., 1926.

Wood, C. A., "A Few Civil War Hospitals." *Military Surgeon* 13:539, 1918.

Wood, F. C., "The Hospital Laboratory." *Bulletin of the American College of Surgeons* 3:20, 1917.

Woodbury, C., "Student Nurse: Could You Take It?" *Woman's Home Companion* 76:36, 1949.

Woodham-Smith, C., *Florence Nightingale, 1820–1910*. New York: McGraw-Hill Book Co., 1951.

Woodward, E. S., "The WPA and Nursing." *American Journal of Nursing* 37:994, 1937.

Woolsey, J. S., *Hospital Days*. New York: D. Van Nostrand, 1870.

Worcester, A., "An Address at the Celebration of the Fiftieth Anniversary of the Establishment of the Training School for Nurses at the New England Hospital for Women and Children, October 31, 1922." *Boston Medical and Surgical Journal* 187:943, 1922.

_____, "Is Nursing Really a Profession?" *American Journal of Nursing* 2:908, 1901–1902.

_____, *Nurses for Our Neighbors*. Boston: Houghton Mifflin Co., 1914.

"Working and Recreation Hours for Pupil Nurses." *National Hospital Record* 11:3, 1908.

Wrench, E. M., "The Development and Present Scope of Industrial Nursing in the United States." *International Journal of Public Health* 2:43, 1921.

_____, "The Lessons of the Crimean War." *British Medical Journal* 2:205, 1899.

Wright, F. S., *Industrial Nursing*. New York: Macmillan Co., 1919.

Wright, M. J., *Improvement of Patient Care: Study at Harper Hospital, Detroit, Michigan*. New York: Putnam, 1954.

_____, "Meeting the Need for Nursing Personnel." *Hospitals* 26:49, 1952.

Wylie, W. G., *Hospitals: Their History, Organization, and Construction*. New York: Appleton, 1877.

Yett, D. E., *An Economic Analysis of the Nurse Shortage*. Lexington: D. C. Heath, 1975.

Young, A. H., "Industrial Welfare Nursing." *Public Health Nurse* 6:81, 1914.

Zabriskie, L., *Nurses Handbook of Obstetrics*. Philadelphia: J. B. Lippincott Co., 1929.

Index